Hormones in Blood

Hormones in Blood

THIRD EDITION

Volume 1

Edited by

C. H. GRAY
*Division of Clinical Chemistry,
Clinical Research Centre, Harrow,
Middlesex, UK*

V. H. T. JAMES
*Department of Chemical Pathology,
St. Mary's Hospital Medical School,
London, UK*

1979

ACADEMIC PRESS
LONDON · NEW YORK · SAN FRANCISCO
A Subsidiary of Harcourt Brace Jovanovich, Publishers

ACADEMIC PRESS INC. (LONDON) LTD.
24/28 Oval Road
London NW1

United States Edition published by
ACADEMIC PRESS INC.
111 Fifth Avenue
New York, New York 10003

British Library Cataloguing in Publication Data
Hormones in blood. – 3rd ed.
  Vol. 1
  1. Hormones   2. Blood
  I. Gray, Charles Horace   II. James, Vivian
  Hector Thomas
  612'.405   QP571   78–73882

  ISBN 0-12-296201-X

Printed in Great Britain by
Page Bros (Norwich) Ltd,
Mile Cross Lane, Norwich.

Contributors to Volume 1

A. ARIMURA, *Veterans Administration Hospital, 1601 Perdido Street, New Orleans, Louisiana 70146, USA.*

K. D. BAGSHAWE, *Department of Medical Oncology, Charing Cross Hospital, Fulham Palace Road, London W6 8RF, UK.*

D. R. BANGHAM, *National Institute for Biological Standards and Control, Holly Hill, Hampstead, London NW3 6RB, UK.*

W. R. BUTT, *Department of Clinical Endocrinology, Birmingham and Midland Hospital for Women, Sparkhill, Birmingham, UK.*

T. CHARD, *The Medical College, St. Bartholomews Hospital, West Smithfield, London EC1A 7BE, UK.*

P. G. CONDLIFFE, *National Institute of Arthritis, Metabolism and Digestive Diseases, Department of Health, Education and Welfare, National Institutes of Health, Bethesda, Maryland 20014, USA.*

P. MARY COATES, *Division of Clinical Chemistry, Clinical Research Centre, Harrow, Middlesex HA1 3UJ, UK.*

S. FRANKS, *Cobbald Labororatories, Thorn Institute of Clinical Science, Middlesex Hospital Medical School, London W1N 8AA, UK.*

LINDA FRYKLUND, *Department of Endocrinology and Metabolism, Karolinska Sjukhuset, S-104 01 Stockholm 60, Sweden.*

D. F. GUÈRET WARDLE, *Division of Surgical Sciences (Oncology Section), Clinical Research Centre, Harrow, Middlesex HA1 3UJ, UK.*

KERSTIN HALL, *Department of Endocrinology and Metabolism, Karolinska Sjukhuset, S-104 01 Stockholm 60, Sweden.*

P. J. LEFEBVRE, *Division of Diabetes, Institute of Medicine, University Hospital of Bavière, University of Liege, B-4020 Liege, Belgium.*

A. S. LUYCKX, *Division of Diabetes, Institute of Medicine, University Hospital of Bavière, University of Liege, B-4020 Liege, Belgium.*

Ü. A. PARMAN, *Division of Clinical Chemistry, Clinical Research Centre, Harrow, Middlesex HA1 3UJ, UK.*

J. E. RALL, *National Institute of Arthritis, Metabolism and Digestive Diseases, Department of Health, Education and Welfare, National Institutes of Health, Bethesda, Maryland 20014, USA.*

J. ROBBINS, *National Institute of Arthritis, Metabolism and Digestive Diseases, Department of Health, Education and Welfare, National Institutes of Health, Bethesda, Maryland 20014, USA.*

A. V. SCHALLY, *Veterans Administration Hospital, 1601 Perdido Street, New Orleans, Louisiana 70146, USA.*

F. SEARLE, *Department of Medical Oncology, Charing Cross Hospital, Fulham Palace Road, London W6 8RF, UK.*

P. H. SÖNKSEN, *Department of Medicine, St. Thomas' Hospital Medical School, Lambeth Palace Road, London SE1, UK.*

M. WASS, *Department of Medical Oncology, Charing Cross Hospital, Fulham Palace Road, London W6 8RF, UK.*

B. D. WEINTRAUB, *National Institute of Arthritis, Metabolism and Digestive Diseases, Department of Health, Education and Welfare, National Institutes of Health, Bethesda, Maryland 20014, USA.*

T. E. T. WEST, *Department of Medicine, St. Thomas' Hospital Medical School, Lambeth Palace Road, London SE1, UK.*

Preface

When the second edition of "Hormones in Blood" was published in 1967, endocrinology had reached a stage when new methodology had opened up our knowledge of the normal levels in blood of those hormones and metabolites known at that time. During the 11 years which have elapsed since then not only have methods of hormone analysis advanced mainly towards greater precision and accuracy but well established hormones have been shown to be heterogeneous, prohormones and new hormones have been identified, and much has been learned of control mechanisms, interaction and synergism between hormones, metabolic pathways as well as of the details of the molecular basis of action. During this period the rate of the development of the subject of endocrinology has accelerated so much that at no time did it seem opportune to attempt to bring out a new and up-dated edition, even allowing for the publisher's agreement to publish if possible within six months of receipt of manuscripts.

At present, endocrinology has reached a stage for taking stock of its position. The value and limitations of radioimmunoassay (RIA) have been recognised, competitive protein binding and receptor assays have been developed, the latter especially has combined the sensitivity of RIA with a specificity which approximates with rather less discrepancy to biological activity; there is ever increasing development of sensitive biological assays using isolated or culture cells and even intracellular membranes. These new methods have been so rigidly characterised for the hormones being analysed, there is no special chapter devoted to them as there was in 1967 for gas-liquid chromatography (GLC) gel filtration, thin-layer chromatography, immunoassay, and spectrophotometry. However, three general techniques, high pressure liquid chromatography, non-isotopic immunoassay and gas-liquid chromatography-mass spectrometry have warranted separate chapters, the first because despite its great resolving power it has not yet been widely used with hormones, even with the polypeptides for which it is specially suited; with the development of more sensitive detectors it will inevitably be found to have many applications. The second will ultimately replace RIA by a method less demanding of expensive equipment, although the disagreement between international bodies concerned with standardisation in enzyme assays suggest that the widespread application of enzyme-immunoassay may have to be delayed. The combination of GLC with mass spectrometry has mostly been of value in the detailed analyses of urinary steriods, but Dr Smythe in his new

vii

chapter on serotonin has no doubt that it is only the expense of the equipment which prevents its wide use.

The third edition of "Hormones in Blood" has other new chapters, two on gastro-intestinal peptides; one on vitamin D because it is the precursor of the true hormone 1,25-dihydroxycholecalciferol, which, with parathyroid hormone play so important a role in calcium metabolism, a chapter on somatomedin and one on erythropoietin. Dr Schally and his colleague have reviewed the enormous changes brought about by the identification, synthesis, mode of action and practical application of what in 1967 were only known as hypothalamic releasing and inhibiting factors.

We have given much thought as to whether the prostaglandins should be regarded as hormones and have decided that they are, because they function as chemical messengers and are carried in the blood to remote target organs as well as targets within the cells or structures in which they are synthesised. The field has expanded enormously since their discovery, and the recognition of the various prostaglandins and their precursors and metabolites has been more than usually dependent on the development of more sensitive and specific forms of analysis, especially with the now widely appreciated heterogeneity of the peptide hormones. The editors hope that there will be some cross-fertilisation of ideas and that some of the experimental techniques may prove to be of value in endocrinology.

The acceptance of SI units by some countries and not others has presented a problem. Where possible we have provided all concentrations in SI units along with traditional units. To avoid enlarging tables undesirably we have provided conversion factors. When early work is described in which methods had not been properly established (e.g. with the steroids and smaller poly-peptides) traditional units alone have been given; more recent results obtained when methods and standard preparations were available have been presented in both systems of units.

The symbols and abbreviations which have been used are those which are generally accepted in current scientific publications. We have in addition used u for international units and, unless otherwise stated, $\pm$ refers to the s.e.m. All temperatures are in °C (Celcius).

We are grateful to those authors who complied so splendidly with the request for prompt delivery of their manuscripts, as well as to those who relieved our anxiety by producing their manuscripts better late than never. As some contributors were unable to meet our deadline and did not conform to our stated requirements, rather than delay publication we decided not to return these chapters for revision, which accounts for a few of the chapters being less comprehensive than we would have liked. Our thanks are also due to Miss Nancy Blamey for all the help she gave us during preparation of this publication, and to Miss Helen Wortham of Academic Press who has been so patient with us, especially in respect of some late changes we required.

C. H. GRAY and V. H. T. JAMES   *June, 1979*

Standards for Hormones

D. R. BANGHAM

Almost all assays to estimate the concentration of a hormone are comparative assays, in which the test sample is compared with a measured quantity of a reference preparation of the hormone. For hormones such as steroids and peptides of a few residues, any preparation of the pure chemical may be suitable for this purpose providing it complies with precise specifications of identity and purity. But for hormones of more complex structure (such as glycoproteins or peptides of more than say 20 residues) that cannot be completely characterised by chemical and physical means alone, it is necessary to use suitably prepared reference materials. Moreover, in order to be able to correlate results obtained using them, it is necessary to relate such reference materials ultimately in terms of a single preparation, which has recognised international status. It is for this purpose that a service of international biological standards and reference materials has been provided since 1925. This service is administered under the aegis of the Expert Committee on Biological Standardisation of the World Health Organization; and the following list includes those International Standards and International Reference Preparations of hormones as well as other reference preparations currently distributed from the National Institute for Biological Standards and Control.

Certain hormones, such as thyrotrophin (TSH), follicle stimulating hormone (FSH), luteinising hormone (LH) and human chorionic gonadotrophin (hCG), are particularly complex, e.g. they appear to consist of heterogeneous mixtures of slightly dissimilar glycoproteins. In these instances, and until there is general and sustained agreement on its exact chemical structure, a hormone is identified by the biological response that it elicits; since it is the standard that is used as the yardstick with which to measure that activity, it is thus the material used in the standard that helps to "define" that hormone. It is essential that such a standard is thoroughly characterised by chemical, physical and biological procedures to obtain information on its identity, purity, activity, stability and suitability to serve as a standard for use with various assay methods. Such evidence is a prerequisite for the establishment of each WHO International Reference Material and is summarised in the report on each standard, which is usually published (see list of standards). Guidance on how to prepare, ampoule and characterise international, national and laboratory standards has been published (Annex 4, 29th Report of WHO ECBS, 1978).

The introduction of radioimmunoassays, hormone receptor assays and other protein binding assays highlighted many fundamental problems of standardisation in hormone assays. While a hormone is identified as that (form of a) molecule that directly elicits the characteristic biological response that defines it, many problems arise from the lack of—or inappropriate—specificity of many protein-binding assay systems for a single "form" of a hormone. Thus a sample of biological fluid or a tissue extract may contain precursor forms and metabolised fragments of the hormone, or artefactually altered forms caused by *in vitro* handling. Other hormones such as TSH, LH, FSH and HCG are naturally heterogeneous, that is they exist as populations of slightly dissimilar molecules.

The problems for standards arising from such diversity of molecular forms has been discussed in detail (Bangham and Cotes, 1974; 26th Report of WHO ECBS, 1975). The subject is currently under active consideration by special committees of WHO, the International Federation of Clinical Chemistry, the International Society of Endocrinology and the International Atomic Energy Agency.

Meanwhile new international preparations consisting where possible of the most highly purified preparations of hormones are established each year and are listed in successive reports of the ECBS of WHO.

BIOLOGICAL STANDARDS AND REFERENCE MATERIALS

The following reference materials are available to scientists in limited quantities for use as standards to define units of biological activity or as reference materials for binding assays. Some of these preparations have been provided and characterised as a result of international collaboration; some of them have been designated British or International Standards or Reference Preparations. They are not for administration to man.

Ampoules of these preparations, together with relevant information, are issued in response to written application from the scientist concerned, stating the purpose for which the material is required, addressed to:

> National Institute for Biological Standards and Control,
> Holly Hill, Hampstead, London NW3 6RB, UK.

REFERENCES

Bangham, D. R. and Cotes, P. M. (1974). Standardization and standards. *Br. med. Bull.* **30**, 12.

26th Report of WHO Expert Committee on Biological Standardization (1975). WHO Tech. Rep. Ser. No. 565.

29th Report of WHO Expert Committee on Biological Standardization (1978). WHO Tech. Rep. Ser. No. 626.

30th Report of WHO Expert Committee on Biological Standardization (1979). WHO Tech. Rep. Ser. (in press).

Standard	Ampoule code No.	Defined activity	Approximate composition of ampoule contents	Other information
1st IS for glucagon, porcine, for bioassay	69/194	1·49 u/amp	1·5 mg glucagon, 5 mg lactose, 0·24 mg sodium chloride	*Acta endocr., Copenh.* **77**, 705, 1974; *J. biol. Stand.* **3**, 263, 1975
1st IRP of glucagon, porcine, for immunoassay	69/194	1·49 u/amp	1·5 mg glucagon, 5 mg lactose, 0·24 mg sodium chloride	*J. biol. Stand.* **3**, 263, 1975; *Acta endocr., Copenh.* **77**, 705, 1974.
4th IS for insulin, bovine and porcine, for bioassay	58/6	24·0 u/mg	100 mg crystals, 42% porcine insulin, 58% bovine insulin	*Bull. Wld Hlth Org* **20**, 1209, 1959; *Diabetologia* **11**, 581, 1975
1st IRP of insulin, human, for immunoassay	66/304	3·0 u/amp	130 µg insulin, 5 mg sucrose	WHO/BS/74.1084
Insulin C-peptide for immunoassay	76/561	2·5 nm/amp	10 µg synthetic human insulin C-peptide analogue, 50 µg human albumin	synthetic (64-formyllysine) human proinsulin 31-65 WHO/BS/78. 1223
2nd IS for chorionic gonadotrophin, human, for biossay	61/6	5,300 u/amp	2 mg chorionic gonadotrophin, 5 mg lactose	*Bull. Wld Hlth Org.* **31**, 111, 1964
1st IRP of chorionic gonadotrophin, human, for immunoassay	75/537	650 u/amp	70 µg chorionic gonadotrophin, 5 mg human albumin	*Bull. Wld Hlth Org.* **54**, 463, 1976
1st IRP of α-subunit of chorionic gonadotrophin, human, for immunoassay	75/569	70 u/amp	70 µg chorionic gonadotrophin α-subunit, 5 mg human albumin	*Bull. Wld Hlth Org.* **54**, 463, 1976
1st IRP of β-subunit of chorionic gonadotrophin, human, for immunoassay	75/551	70 u/amp	70 µg chorionic gonadotrophin β-subunit, 5 mg human albumin	*Bull. Wld Hlth Org.* **54**, 463, 1976

Standard	Ampoule code No.	Defined activity	Approximate composition of ampoule contents	Other information
1st IRP for FSH/LH, human, pituitary, for bioassay	69/104	FSH 10 u/amp LH 25 u/amp	0·5 mg FSH/LH, lactose 1·25 mg	*J. clin. Endocr. Metab.* **36**, 647, 1973
1st IRP of LH, human pituitary, for immunoassay	68/40	77 u/amp	11·6 µg LH, 5 mg lactose, 1 mg human albumin, 1 mg sodium chloride	*Acta endocr., Copenh.* **88**, 250, 1978
IS FSH/LH, human, urinary, for bioassay	70/45	FSH-54 u/amp LH-46 u/amp	1 mg human post-menopausal urine extract, 5 mg lactose	*Acta endocr., Copenh.* **83**, 700, 1976
Gonadorelin	77/596	38 nm/amp	36 nmoles synthetic gonadorelin, 2·5 mg lactose, 0·5 mg human albumin	ovine sequence WHO/BS/78. 1219
Angiotensin I (Asp Isoleu[5])	71/328	9 µg/amp nominal	9 µg synthetic angiotensin I, 2 mg mannitol	*Clin. Sci. mol. Med.* **48**, 135.S. 1978
Angiotensin II (Asp Ileu[5])	70/302	24 µg/amp nominal	24 µg synthetic angiotensin II, 2 mg mannitol	*Clin. Sci. mol. Med.* **48**, 135.S. 1978
1st IRP of renin, human, for bioassay	68/356	0·1 u/amp	0·27 mg renal extract, 5 mg lactose, phosphate buffer	*Clin. Sci. mol. Med.* **48**, 135.S. 1978
IRP calcitonin, human, for bioassay	70/234	1·0 u/amp	10 µg synthetic calcitonin of sequence found in tumours, 5 mg mannitol	WHO/BS/78. 1229
1st IRP of calcitonin, porcine, for bioassay	70/306	1·0 u/amp	10 µg purified extract, 5 mg mannitol	WHO/BS/74. 1077
1st IRP of calcitonin, salmon, for bioassay	72/158	80 u/amp	20 µg synthetic salmon calcitonin I, 2 mg mannitol	WHO/BS/74. 1077

Description	Code number	Unitage	Composition	Reference
1st IRP of parathyroid hormone, bovine, for bioassay	67/342	200 u/amp	0·6 mg gland extract, 5 mg lactose	WHO/BS/74. 1078
1st IRP of parathyroid hormone, bovine, for immunoassay	71/324	2·0 u/amp	1 μg purified extract, 200 μg human albumin, 1 mg lactose	WHO/BS/74. 1078
Parathyroid hormone, human, for immunoassay	75/549	0·25 u/amp	250 ng extract of human adenomata, 250 μg human albumin, 1·25 mg lactose	
3rd IS for corticotrophin (ACTH), porcine, for bioassay. International Working Standard	59/16, various	5·0 u/amp, 5·0 u/amp	50 μg pituitary extract, 5 mg lactose	*Bull. Wld Hlth Org.* **27**, 395, 1962
Corticotrophin human	74/555		11·6 μg corticotrophin, 5 mg human albumin, 2·5 mg mannitol	WHO/BS/78. 1233
2nd IRP of erythropoietin, human, urinary, for bioassay	67/343	10 u/amp	2 mg urinary extract containing erythropoietin, 3 mg sodium chloride	*Bull. Wld Hlth Org.* **47**, 99, 1972
Gastrin I, human (G-17)	68/439	12 u/amp	12·6 μg synthetic gastrin as hexamonium salt, 5 mg lactose, phosphate buffer	
Gastrin II, porcine (G-17)	66/138	10 u/amp	10 μg gastrin II, 5 mg sucrose, phosphate buffer	
2nd IS for serum gonadotrophin, equine, for bioassay	62/1	1600 u/amp	0·8 mg extract, 5 mg lactose	*Bull. Wld Hlth Org.* **35**, 761, 1966
2nd IS for prolactin, ovine, for bioassay	57/8	22 u/mg	10 mg extract	*Bull. Wld Hlth Org.* **29**, 721, 1963

Standard	Ampoule code No.	Defined activity	Approximate composition of ampoule contents	Other information
IRP prolactin, human, for immunoassay	75/504	0.650 u/amp	20 µg extract, 1 mg human albumin, 5 mg lactose	*J. Endocr.* **80**, 157, 1979
IRP of placental lactogen, human, for immunoassay	73/545	0·850 mu/amp	850 µg placental lactogen, 5 mg mannitol	*Br. J. Obstet. Gynaec.* **85**, 451, 1978
1st IS for growth hormone, bovine, for bioassay	55/1	1·0 u/mg	30 mg purified growth hormone	WHO/BS/77.1156
1st IRP of growth hormone, human, for immunoassay	66/217	0·35 u/amp	175 µg growth hormone, 5 mg sucrose, phosphate buffer	
1st IS for thyrotrophin, bovine, for bioassay	53/11	13·5 u/mg	1 part pituitary extract, 19 parts lactose	*Bull. Wld Hlth Org.* **13**, 917, 1955
1st IRP of TSH, human, for immunoassay	68/38	147 u/amp	46·2 µg TSH extract, 5 mg lactose, 1 mg human albumin	
4th IS oxytocin for bioassay	76/575	12·5 u/amp	24 µg synthetic oxytocin acetate, 5 mg human albumin, citric acid	WHO/BS/78. 1227
1st IS arginine vasopressin for bioassay	77/501	8·2 u/amp	20 µg synthetic arginine vasopressin, 5 mg human citric acid	WHO/BS/78. 1231
1st IS lysine vasopressin	77/512	7·7 u/amp	30 µg synthectic lysine vasopressin acetate, 5 mg human albumin, citric acid	WHO/BS/78. 1230

Contents of Volume 1

I. Hypothalamic Releasing and Inhibiting Hormones and Factors
A. ARIMURA and A. V. SCHALLY

II. Insulin
Ü. A. PARMAN

III. Glucagon
P. J. LEFEBVRE and A. S. LUYCKX

IV. Growth Hormone
P. H. SÖNKSEN and T. E. T. WEST

V. Somatomedins
KERSTIN HALL and LINDA FRYKLUND

VI. Prolactin
S. FRANKS

VII. Human Placental Lactogen
T. CHARD

VIII. Human Chorionic Gonadotrophin
K. D. BAGSHAWE, F. SEARLE and M. WASS

IX. Gonadotrophins
W. R. BUTT

X. Erythropoietin
P. MARY COTES and D. E. GUÈRET WARDLE

XI. Pituitary Thyroid-stimulating Hormone and Other Thyroid-stimulating Substances
P. G. CONDLIFFE and B. D. WEINTRAUB

XII. The Iodine-containing Hormones
J. ROBBINS and J. E. RALL

Contents of Volume 2

Contents of Volume 3

I. Hypothalamic Releasing and Inhibiting Hormones and Factors

A. ARIMURA and A. V. SCHALLY

INTRODUCTION

Harris (1955) clearly forecast the existence of agents, formed in the hypo-thalamus and secreted into the hypophysial portal blood, which act as important regulators of anterior pituitary function. This forecast proved to be correct and the past nine years have seen the isolation, identification and synthesis of at least three hormones. Other hypothalamic hormones will probably be identified and synthesised during the next few years. The information gathered from animal experiments and studies in human beings has shed much new light on physiological and clinical phenomena, the origins of which were not completely understood. However, investiga-tions with hypothalamic hormones, while extensive, are still in an early stage, and the interpretation of some studies is uncertain because our understanding of various physiological processes and the pathophysiology of many endo-crine syndromes is very sketchy. It is likely that further studies with hypo-physiotrophic hormones, especially the development or improvement of the methods for their measurement in blood, will help us unravel many of the remaining mysteries of various physiological events and of endocrine disease. In our previous contribution to these series (Schally, Kastin, Locke and Bowers, 1967), we collected significant data concerning the hypothalamic agents available through mid-1967. In the following paragraphs we have attempted to gather, and fit into the editorial framework of this book, the most recent information on not only the three hypothalamic hormones whose structures have been established and which have been synthesised, but also on those hormones which may be identified in the near future.

A. CORTICOTROPHIN RELEASING FACTOR (CRF)

1. Chemical Constitution and Main Physico-chemical Properties

CRF was the first hypothalamic hormone to be discovered (Saffran and Schally, 1955) and its characteristics are those of a small peptide, but, it has not yet been obtained in pure form. The problems involved in the isolation of CRF, have been reviewed previously (Schally, Arimura and Kastin, 1973).

Recently, work on the purification of CRF has been resumed in several laboratories. Cooper, Synetos, Christie and Schulster (1976) described the purification of 0·1 M HCl extract of porcine hypothalami by ultrafiltration and chromatography on Sephadex G-50. Two materials with CRF activity with mws of 30,000 and 1500 and the characteristics of peptides were obtained. Jones, Gillham and Hillhouse (1977) also found two forms of CRF after purifications by gel filtration, chromatography on carboxymethycellulose (CMC), and high voltage electrophoresis.

Our laboratory is in the process of isolating, sequencing and synthesising several peptides with CRF activity. In our most recent studies (Schally, Coy and Meyers, 1978a, c), hypothalamic extracts from nearly half a million pig hypothalami were first separated into 14 fractions by preparative gel filtration of Sephadex G-25. Significant CRF activity was found in high mw fraction with $R_f = 0.77$, in fraction ($R_f = 0.4$) with mw about 1000, and even in the retarded or low mw fractions ($R_f = 0.3$) which also contained catecholamines. High mw CRF-active fractions from Sephadex were purified by column chromatography on CMC, countercurrent distribution (CCD) in a system of 0·1 % acetic acid: 1-butanol:pyridine = 11:5:3 (by volume), chromatography and rechromatography on SE-Sephadex, gel filtration on Sephadex G-50 and partition chromatography. CRF activity was completely lost after 16 hr digestion with trypsin and partially destroyed by thermolysin. The results indicate that CRF activity in this fraction is due to a basic polypeptide and this CRF has been tentatively named large mw CRF.

Fraction with R_f of 0·4 from Sephadex containing intermediate mw CRF was also repurified by chromatography on CMC (Schally, Redding, Chihara, Huang, Chang, Carter, Coy and Saffran, 1978d). CRF activity was found in well-separated acidic fractions, neutral fractions and basic fractions. The basic fractions had the highest CRF activity, increasing ACTH release *in vitro* 10–100 fold. These fractions were further purified by CCD and SE-Sephadex. The highly purified material is devoid of ACTH-like activity, is active *in vitro* in doses of 3 ng/ml and shows an excellent dose-response relationship. Attempts are being made to identify structurally the active material in basic fractions, which is most likely to represent the physiological CRF.

Small mw or retarded CRF fractions from Sephadex with $R_f = 0.3$, were repurified by countercurrent distribution, gel filtration on Sephadex G-15 and partition chromatography or ion-exchange chromatography on SE-Sephadex, and more than 15 mg of a tetradecapeptide with CRF activity were obtained. Its amino acid sequence was determined as Phe–Leu–Gly–Phe–Pro–Thr–Thr–Lys–Thr–Tyr–Phe–Pro–His–Phe (Schally et al., 1978c). This tetradecapeptide was then synthesised, but subsequently this amino acid sequence was found to be identical with the residues No. 33–46 of α-chain of porcine hemoglobin and hence this tetradecapeptide is unlikely to have an origin different from porcine hemoglobin and most probably is an artifact of extraction and isolation. Nevertheless, the natural and synthetic tetradecapeptide stimulated the release of ACTH in monolayer cultures of mouse and rat pituitary cells and from rat pituitary quarters in doses of 0.5–3.0 μg but dose-response curves were not obtained. Moreover, it was inactive in vivo even in doses of 100 μg. It is difficult at present to interpret the finding of multiple CRF activities, but it is possible that high mw fractions represent pro-CRF (a precursor of CRF) and the intermediate mw the physiological CRF (CRH). A part of the CRF activity of low mw fractions is due to catecholamines and part to α-hemoglobin fragment. Further work should lead to the isolation of these CRF's and in the determination of their physiological role.

2. Localisation, Biosynthesis and Release

(a) Organs and cells at origin

CRF has been found in the highest concentration in the median eminence and neurohypophysial tissue in various animals including man (Schally et al., 1978a, c). Krieger, Liotta and Brownstein (1977) studied the distribution of CRF in various regions of the rat brain as tested by a bioassay using acutely dispersed rat pituitary cells in vitro (see later). Highest concentrations were found in the median eminence, with decreased concentrations noted proceeding dorsally and cephalad from the median eminence. The CRF potencies in terms of NIAMDD-HE-RP-1/1 μg extract: median eminence—2.2; arcuate N—0.88; dorsomedial N—0.41; ventromedial N—0.35; periventricular N—0.24; hypothalamus—0.05; thalamus—0.01; cortex—0.005; measurable, but lesser amounts than in the above cited nuclei, were present in supraoptic and paraventricular nuclei where vasopressin and oxytocin are synthesised. Complete hypothalamic deafferentation resulted in an increase in CRF in the median eminence and the medial basal hypothalamus, suggesting that CRF is mainly synthesised in these areas. The presence of CRF in the brain cortex was also reported by Portanova and Sayers (1973) but not confirmed by others (Hiroshige, Fujieda, Kaneko and Honma, 1977; Vernikos-Danellis and Marks, 1969; Arimura, Saito and Schally, 1967; Lymangrover and Brodish, 1973; Rivier, Vale and Guillemin, 1973). The discrepancy appears to be due to different assay methods for CRF used. Yasuda and Greer (1976) reported that "specific CRF" is concentrated primarily in the basal hypothalamus and the neurohypophysial tissue and is not identical with widely distributed extrahypothalamic extraneurohypophysial CRF. Nearly normal amounts of CRF were also present in the hypothalamus of homozygous Battleboro rats which do not synthesise vasopressin (Arimura, Saito, Bowers and Schally; Krieger, Liotta and Brownstein, 1977), refuting the concept that vasopressin is the CRF.

(b) Tissue CRF

Failure in abolishing stress response in dogs after most of the central nervous system (CNS) was removed (Egdahl, 1960) and in the rats with median eminence lesion (Brodish, 1964) led to the speculation that extra CNS–CRF exists. Brodish and Long (1962) speculated that dual controls for ACTH secretion might exist, one via afferent neural pathways to the hypothalamus and another via a systematic humoral route to the pituitary. Lymangrover and Brodish (1973) demonstrated CRF activity in the peripheral blood of rats bearing extensive hypothalamic lesion which were hypophysectomised and subjected to laparotomy stress. CRF activity was not found in similar rats that were not subjected to stress. Hypothalamic CRF elicits an immediate but transient secretion of ACTH, whereas the extrahypothalamic CRF produces a prolonged stimulation of the pituitary. Based upon its extreme potency and prolonged time-course of action, the term tissue-CRF was proposed to distinguish it from CRF of hypothalamic origin (Lymangrover and Brodish, 1973; Brodish, 1977). But the site of origin of tissue CRF and its chemical characteristics remain unknown.

(c) CRF in ectopic ACTH-secreting tumours

Substances with CRF activity were found in the extracts of ectopic ACTH-producing tumours (Upton and Amaturda, 1971; Yamamoto, Hirara, Matsukura, Imura, Nakamura and Tanaka, 1976; Suda, Demura, Demura, Wakabayashi, Nomura, Odagiri and Shizume, 1977). Yamamoto et al. (1976) reported that extracts of 7 of 12 ACTH-producing tumours showed CRF-like activity. No correlation was found between ACTH and CRF activities in these tumour extracts. The dose-response curve of one tumour extract was nearly parallel to that of crude CRF and was clearly different from those of lysine-vasopressin and arginine vasopressin, both of which showed CRF-like activities. Trypsin digestion considerably reduced the CRF-like activity of the tumour extract. In addition to CRF-like substances some of the ACTH-secreting ectopic tumour extracts contained β-lipotrophin, β-MSH, α-MSH and serotonin (Hirata, Matsukura, Imura, Nakamura and Tanaka, 1971). Upton and Amatadura (1971) chromatographed extracts of ectopic ACTH-producing tumours on a Sephadex column. Two CRF peaks were demonstrated, one being similar to ACTH in molecular size and another smaller in size than vasopressin.

(d) Biosynthesis

Although the exact mode of biosynthesis remains unknown, CRF activity in the hypothalamus fluctuates under various experimental conditions. CRF activity increases immediately after stress (Hiroshige et al., 1969; Hiroshige and Sato, 1970; Zarrow, Campbell and Penenberg, 1972; Sato, Sato, Shinsako and Dallman, 1975), shows diurnal variation (Hiroshige and Sato, 1970; Seiden and Brodish, 1972; Ixart Szafarczyk, Belugou and Assenmacher, 1977), increases after hypophysectomy and administration of dexamethasone (Krieger et al., 1977), and decreases after bilateral adrenalectomy (Hillhouse and Jones, 1976). Since ACTH secretion increases immediately after stress, the prompt increase in hypothalamic CRF following noxious stimuli may indicate a rapid synthesis of CRF or conversion to an active CRF from its inactive or less active precursor. Electrical stimulation or addition of acetylcholine in the incubation medium increase CRF release from the rat hypothalamus in vitro (Bradbury, Burden, Hillhouse and Jones, 1974). Hypothalami from adrenalectomised rats released several fold more CRF into the medium during electrical stimulation than the initial content of the tissue, showing that the tissue can synthesise CRF in vitro (Bradbury et al., 1974). Gillham, Jones, Hillhouse and Burden (1975) and Jones, Gillham and Hillhouse (1977) subjected CRF released from the rat hypothalamus into the incubation medium to gel filtration on Sephadex G-25 column and demonstrated two CRF peaks, one being of approximately 2500 daltons and another 1300 daltons in size.

(e) Secretion of CRF

Acetylcholine (Ach) appears to be a most potent stimulator of CRF release from the hypothalamus. As small a dose as 1 pg/ml caused release of CRF from the rat hypothalamus in vitro. 5HT also stimulates CRF release (Jones and Gillham, 1976). Ach or serotonin-induced CRF release in vitro was prevented by noradrenalin (10 ng/ml), γ-aminobutyric acid, GABA or melatonin (Burden, Hillhouse and Jones, 1974). Synaptosomes from sheep and rat hypothalami contained CRF and electrical stimulation or high concentration of K^+ causes release of the CRF in vitro (Bennett et al., 1975).

Modulation of ACTH secretion by glucocorticoids is well documented and the steroid has been proposed to act both at the hypothalamus and the pituitary. Change in CRF levels in the hypothalamus by bilateral adrenalectomy, its prevention by exogenous glucocorticoids and enhanced release of CRF from the hypothalamic tissue from adrenalectomised rats (Yates and Mayan, 1974; Smelik, 1977) indicate that glucocorticoids act on the hypothalamus and modulate the turnover of hypothalamic CRF. On the other hand, glucocorticoids inhibit the release of ACTH by incubated hemipituitary glands by vasopressin (Fleisher and Vale, 1968), hypothalamic extracts (Arimura, Bowers, Schally, Saito and Miller, 1969) and other substances (Kracer and Morris, 1976; Vale and Rivier, 1977) showing that these steroids also act on the pituitary gland.

3. Methods of Determination

At present CRF activity can be detected and measured only by biological assay. Both *in vivo* and *in vitro* methods have been used. All depend on estimates of ACTH activity in the medium for *in vitro* assays, or ACTH or glucocorticoids in the peripheral circulation for *in vivo* methods. The criteria set for determination of CRF activity of a substance were set forth by Guillemin and Schally (1959), Schally and Guillemin (1960), and Leeman, Glenister and Yates (1962).

(a) In vitro *bioassays*

(*1*) *The original method.* This was designed by Saffran and Schally (1955) for the detection of substances affecting the release of ACTH employs anterior pituitary tissue incubated in Krebs–Ringer bicarbonate (KRB) medium. It is useful not only for detecting CRF but also for other hypothalamic factors. The method has been modified so that rat pituitary quarters are incubated in 1 ml KRB containing glucose and bovine serum albumin (BSA). After 3 hr preincubation, the incubation media are replaced with fresh media and incubated for 1 hr. The media are then replaced by fresh KRB in the control beakers or KRB containing test substances, and the tissues are incubated for another 1 hr. Amounts of ACTH released by the pituitary tissue into the media for the second 1 hr incubation period are expressed as a percentage of the amount of ACTH released during the first hr (Uehara, Arimura and Schally, 1973/74; Arimura, Takahara, Davis, Nishi and Schally, 1975). ACTH is assayed by RIA. This method reduces variation in response parameters in the same treatment group and is suitable for assaying several test samples simultaneously. The method is being successfully used for screening CRF activities in the purification work for CRF.

(2) *Cultures of enzymatically dispersed pituitary cells.* This method (Vale, Grant, Amoss, Blackwell and Guillemin, 1972) is widely used for assaying hypothalamic hypophysiotrophic hormones. Rat pituitary cells are enzymatically dispersed and cultured in plastic tissue culture dishes for four days. At the beginning of the experiment, the dishes are removed from the incubator, the cells are washed with the medium and then the medium containing test substances is added. The incubation period is usually 2·5–4 hr. At the end of the incubation, the media are removed, centrifuged, diluted and assayed for ACTH.

(3) *Acutely dispersed pituitary cells.* Pituitary cells are dispersed by trypsin and their ACTH response to test materials are measured *in vitro* (Portanova and Sayer, 1973). Both cultured and acutely dispersed pituitary cells are sensitive to CRF, but their ACTH responses occasionally appear to be non-specific.

(4) *Superfusion system.* Rat pituitary halves or cells embedded on swollen Sephadex G-15 are perifused *in vitro* by KRB containing glucose and bovine serum albumin (BSA). Exposure of the superfused glands to repeated stimuli with hypothalamic extract results in a series of equal peaks of ACTH secretion. The response was proportional to a log dose òver the range of 0·25–2·0 rat hypothalamic equivalents/ml (Edwardson and Gilbert, 1976; Mulder and Smelik, 1977; Lowry, 1974).

(5) *A semi-automated* in vitro *assay for CRF.* This method consists of an *in vitro* assay for CRF using the adrenal superfusion system (Pearlmutter, Rapino and Saffran, 1975) with rat pituitary fragments and the assay for ACTH released.

(b) In vivo *assay*

(1) *Pharmacologically-blocked rats.* Rats pretreated with Nembutal and morphine respond to CRF but not to non-specific stress. Other combinations of CNS depressants such as chlorpromazine, morphine and Nembutal (Arimura *et al.*, 1967) and dexamethasone and Nembutal (Arimura *et al.*, 1967) are used to block the effects of non-specific stress. CRF preparations are injected i.v. into these animal preparations and the rise of plasma corticosterone levels 15–20 min after injection are used as the response parameter for CRF activity. Hiroshige, Kunita, Yoshimura and Itoh (1968) used intrapituitary microinjections of CRF samples in the dexamethasone-blocked rats. Dexamethasone is a very potent suppressor for various stress effects including that of vasopressin, but it also suppresses pituitary ACTH response to CRF.

(2) *Rats with hypothalamic lesion.* Rats rendered refractory to stress by placing a lesion on the basal medial hypothalamus are also employed as

assay animals for CRF (Brodish, 1963; Witorsch and Brodish, 1972). They are injected with CRF samples under anaesthesia and the rise of plasma corticosterone or ACTH levels (Rivier *et al.*, 1973) are used as the response parameters.

(3) *Rats with a pituitary tumour graft under the kidney capsule.* (Grindeland, Wherry, Anderson, 1962). This method of preparation causes secretion of ACTH in response to vasopressin and can be used for determination of CRF activity in the blood (Anderson, 1966), but its specificity has not been conclusively demonstrated.

4. Plasma Levels

(a) Normal

The peripheral blood from normal unstressed rats did now show CRF activity as tested by the cross-circulation techniques (Brodish and Long, 1962) and in rats with a pituitary tumour graft (Anderson, 1966). However, Yasuda and Greer (1977) reported that normal rat and human plasma stimulated the release of ACTH from rat pituitary cells maintained on a monolayer culture. As little as 0.1% (v/v) plasma in the assay system was effective. CRF activity was also found in normal rat plasma as tested in an *in vitro* assay system using acutely dispersed pituitary cells (Kendall, Gray and Gaudett, 1976). CRF activity in plasma was associated with materials of a molecular weight larger than 15,000. Hagen, Carthwaite and Martinson (1977) also found CRF activity in methanol extracts of normal human plasma as tested *in vitro* using rat pituitary quarters. They have confirmed that the CRF activity was associated with molecules of 10,000 daltons. The dose-response curve for plasma CRF was parallel to that for hypothalamic extracts.

(b) Effect of stress, hypophysectomy, adrenalectomy and adrenal steroids

CRF activity was demonstrated in the peripheral blood from hypophysectomised rats using a cross-circulation technique (Brodish and Long, 1962). Although adrenals were not essential, the plasma CRF activity was undetectable in the presence of a high steroid level. Blood CRF activity was not demonstrated in hypophysectomised rats with a hypothalamic lesion, suggesting that the CRF activity originated in the hypothalamus. More recently, Lymangrover and Brodish (1973) demonstrated CRF activity in the blood from stressed, hypophysectomised rats with median eminence lesions.

CRF activity in the plasma was assessed in rats with hypothalamic lesions (Brodish, 1963). The time course of plasma corticosterone response to extracts of hypothalamic tissue in these rats was characterised by a quick rise of the plasma steroid levels after injection, reaching its peak at 20 min. Administration of plasma from stressed hypophysectomised rats showed a similar response to those for hypothalamic CRF. However, rats with lesions still showed a slow steroid response to severe stress or after administration of plasma from severely stressed, hypophysectomised, lesioned rats. The latter CRF activity was thus considered different from hypothalamic CRF and designated as tissue CRF (Brodish, 1977).

Plasma from hypophysial portal vessels of hypophysectomised dogs showed CRF activity which after alcohol fractionation was present in the Cohn fraction IV (Porter and Jones. 1956; Porter and Rumsfeld, 1956, 1959).

B. THYROTROPHIN RELEASING HORMONE (TRH)

1. Chemical Constitution and Main Physico-chemical and Biological Properties

TRH was isolated from porcine hypothalami (Schally, Bowers, Redding and Barrett, 1966; Schally, Redding, Bowers and Barrett, 1969) and from ovine hypothalami (Burgus, Dunn, Desiderio and Guillemin, 1969; Burgus, Dunn, Desiderio, Ward, Vale and Guillemin, 1970). TRH from both of these species was structurally identified as pyro-Glu–His–Pro–NH_2 and synthesised by the same two groups (Folkers, Enzmann, Bøler, Bowers and Schally, 1969; Bøler, Enzmann, Folkers, Bowers and Schally, 1969; Nair, Barrett, Bowers and Schally, 1970; Burgus et al., 1969, 1970). Natural and synthetic TRH had identical physico-chemical and biological properties (Schally and Bowers, 1970; Bowers, Schally, Enzmann, Bøler and Folkers, 1970). TRH was also later synthesised by Gillesen, Felix, Lergier and Studer (1970) and by Baugh, Krumdieck, Hershman and Pittman (1970). Physico-chemical and immunological studies indicate that the bovine and human TRH may have the same structure as porcine and ovine hormone (Schally et al., 1973). The structure of this tripeptide (optical rotation = $[\alpha]_D^{25} = -44\cdot3°$; mol wt (as acetate) = 422·43) contains several features which may contribute to its powerful biological activity. TRH lacks both the amino-terminal (glutamic acid being cyclised to (pyro)glutamic or pyrrolidone carboxylic acid) and a free carboxy-terminal group. All three amino acids contain five membered heterocyclic rings which could allow an intimate contact with corresponding sites on the receptor molecule. The only proton-exchanging group is the imidazol moiety of the histidine residue. TRH is resistant to the action of most proteolytic enzymes (Schally et al., 1969, 1973), but it is inactivated by incubation with plasma (Redding and Schally, 1969; Nair, Redding and Schally, 1971b). Synthetic pyro-Glu–His–Pro–NH$_2$ has been shown to stimulate thyrotrophin (TSH) release in all mammals studied, including mice, rats, nutria (myocaster coypus), sheep, goats, cows, humans, and birds (Schally *et al.*, 1973; Schally, Coy, Meyers and Kastin, 1978b). However, it was inactive in the tadpole and the lungfish (Gorbman and Hyder, 1973).

TRH may not only cause release, but may also stimulate the synthesis of TSH. Among the physiological stimuli which appear to release TRH is exposure to mild cold. TRH can be administered intravenously, subcutaneously, intraperitoneally and even orally; however, doses 50–100 times larger than for parenteral route are needed in the case of oral administration to humans and most clinical tests employ a single i.v. dose of 200 μg. TRH will also release prolactin in rats, sheep and humans (Jacobs, Snyder, Wilber, Utiger and Daughaday, 1971; Tashjian, Barowsky and Jensen, 1971; Bowers, Friesen, Hwang, Guyda and Folker, 1971; Debeljuk, Arimura, Redding and Schally, 1973), but it remains to be established whether this effect is physiological or pharmacological. In addition, TRH will stimulate GH secretion in animals under certain conditions, and in patients with acromegaly or renal failure (Schalch, Gonzales-Barcena, Kastin, Schally and Lee, 1972).

Various neuropharmacological studies also suggest that TRH may act on the brain and on the spinal cord (Kastin, Miller, Sandman, Schally and Plotnikoff, 1977; Martin, Renaud and Brazeau, 1975). This possible role of TRH as a neurotransmitter in the central nervous system is supported by the presence of significant concentrations of immunoreactive TRH in the extra-hypothalamic brain areas of various vertebrates examined, including rat, chicken, snake, frog, tadpole, salmon and lamprey (Jackson and Reichlin, 1974a, b).

2. Localisation, Biosynthesis, Release and Metabolism

(a) Localisation

Large scale synthesis of TRH made it possible to develop radioimmunoassay (RIA) for TRH and to establish methods for studying the localisation, biosynthesis and secretion of TRH. TRH is distributed throughout the brain tissue in the rat. The greatest concentration of TRH was found in the hypothalamus, followed in turn by the posterior pituitary gland, thalamus, brain stem, cerebrum, anterior pituitary gland, and the cerebellum (Oliver, Eskay, Ben-Jonathan and Porter, 1974). TRH content in the whole rat hypothalamus measured by RIA ranged from 3·6–15·7 ng (Bassiri and Utiger, 1974; Jackson and Reichlin, 1974a, b; Oliver *et al.*, 1974). The hypothalamic localisation of TRH was more precisely examined using a technique for isolating discrete nuclei by microdissection (Palkovits, 1973). The highest concentration was found in the median eminence (38·4 ng/mg protein) and certain individual nuclei including the ventromedial (9·02 ng/mg) and the periventricular (4·25 ng/mg). Significant amounts were found in the preoptic area, in the nuclei of the septum, and the outside of the hypothalamus. About one-third (33·6%) of the total TRH in the rat brain was present in the thalamus, 26·7% in the cerebrum, 18·8% in the hypothalamus, 18·6% in the brain, 1·6% in the cerebellum, 0·42% in the posterior pituitary gland, and 0·09% in the anterior pituitary gland (Oliver *et al.*, 1974b). The highest concentration of TRH in cells is found in an enriched synaptosomal fraction of the hypothalamus (Barnea, Ben-Jonathan and Porter, 1975).

Immunoreactive TRH was found in hypothalamic extracts from man, pig, rat, hamster, chicken, frog, snake, salmon, and the whole brain of the larval form of the primitive cyclostome lamprey, and in the head region of the protochordate amphioxus. The TRH levels in the frog hypothalamus were 1520–3260 pg/mg tissue. These findings indicate that TRH is distributed throughout the vertebrate kingdom (Jackson and Reichlin, 1974a, b). Concentrations of TRH in the brain outside the hypothalamus and the pituitary complex are greater in the lower than in the higher species (Jackson and Reichlin, 1974a). TRH is present in the skin of the frog (*Rana pipiens*) in a concentration twice that found in the hypothalamus of this amphibian. A skin extract shows biological activity appropriate to its immunoreactive content. TRH was found in the blood and retina in significant concentrations. This observation implies that frog skin is a huge endocrine organ that synthesises and secretes TRH (Jackson and Reichlin, 1977).

TRH is also present in the rat spinal cord (Utiger, 1976), in ovine, bovine, porcine and frog pineal glands (White, Hedlund, Weber, Rippel, Johnson and Willus, 1974; Jackson, Saperstein and Reichlin, 1977). Only trace amounts of TRH are present in the rat pineal gland, and these are unaffected by environmental lighting (Jackson, Saperstein and Reichlin, 1974). High concentrations of TRH are found in the neurohypophysis of many species (Jackson and Reichlin, 1974a).

Using indirect immunofluorescence techniques in rats, TRH-containing nerve terminals were found in the medial part of the external layer of the median eminence, dorsomedial nucleus, and perifornical area, in extra-hypothalamic nuclei, such as nucleus accumbens, lateral septal nucleus and in several motor nuclei of the brain stem and spinal cord. (Hökfelt, Fuxe, Johansson, Jeffcoate and White, 1975).

TRH is also found in the gastro-intestinal tissue of the frog (Jackson and Reichlin, 1977).

(b) Biosynthesis of TRH

Fragments of rat hypothalamic tissue were shown to incorporate ^{14}C-labelled glutamic acid, histidine and proline into peptides which had the mobility of TRH in a chromatographic purification system (Mitnick and Reichlin, 1971; Reichlin and Mitnick, 1973). TRH synthetic activity was found in the stalk median eminence, ventral hypothalamus and dorsal hypothalamus, and in the soluble, particulate-free extracts of either rat or porcine hypothalamic tissue (Reichlin and Mitnick, 1973). However, Bauer and Lipman (1976), who used more vigorous purification techniques for TRH, failed to confirm the findings of Mitnick and Reichlin (1971). Neuronal integrity appears to be necessary for synthesis of TRH (McKelvy, Sheridan, Joseph, Phelps and Perrie, 1975). TRH biosynthesis is RNA-dependent in the newt (McKelvy, Grimm-Jorgensen, 1976; Grimm-Jorgensen and McKelvy, 1976).

Various conditions and drugs modify the content of hypothalamic TRH. Hypothalamic TRH content was not altered by thyroidectomy, or by treatment with tri-iodothyronine and thyroxine (Montoya, Seibel and Wilber, 1975) but decreased after hypophysectomy (Bassiri and Utiger, 1974) and insulin injection (Leung, Guansing, Ajlouni, Hagen, Rosenfeld and Barboriak, 1975; Kardon, Marcus, Winokur and Utiger, 1977). Exposure of rats to cold increased serum TSH without changing hypothalamic TRH (Bassiri and Utiger, 1974). Administration of α-methylparatyrosine, p-chlorophenylalanine, or reserpine, which alter brain content of noradrenaline or serotonin, did not modify hypothalamic TRH (Kardon, Marcus, Winokur and Utiger, 1977). Rats treated with large doses of T_4 during the neonatal period showed an increased concentration of hypothalamic TRH with decreased TRH levels in the circulation (Bakke, Lawrence, Bennett and Robinson, 1975).

(c) Release of TRH

TRH is released from the nerve terminals in the median eminence into the portal vessels as a hypophysiotrophic hormone, and also at synapses in a discrete region of the brain and spinal cord as a neurotransmitter (Hökfelt, Fuxe, Johansson, Jeffcoate and White, 1975). TRH was released from a synaptosome-rich hypothalamic fraction by depolarising concentration (60 mM) of K^+ in a Ca^{++} dependent manner (Warberg, Eskay, Barnea, Reynolds and Porter, 1977). Release of TRH from the neurons appears to be controlled by adrenergic (stimulatory) and serotonergic (inhibitory) influence (Mitsuma, Hirooka and Nihei, 1976).

(d) Metabolism

After administration of tritiated ^{125}I or ^{14}C-labelled TRH to rats and mice, the radioactivity accumulates in the pituitary (Redding and Schally, 1971,

1972; Virkkunen *et al.*, 1972). Since some radioactivity also becomes concentrated in kidney and liver, these organs may play a role in the inactivation and excretion of TRH (Redding and Schally, 1971). TRH is rapidly inactivated by rat and human plasma, its half life in the blood of the rat being about 4 min (Redding and Schally, 1971). Among the products of digestion of TRH with plasma or hypothalamic fragments are (pyro)Glu–His–Pro, proline and proline amide (Schally *et al.*, 973; Bauer and Lipmann, 1976; Nair *et al.*, 1971b). This rapid inactivation of TRH complicates the measurement of TRH in body fluids and the interpretation of the results. The capacity of rat blood to inactivate is increased by administration of T_3, is decreased after thyroidectomy and appears to be greater in female animals than in males (Bauer, 1976). A similar finding was reported in human blood (White, Jeffcoate, Griffiths and Hooper, 1976). TRH is also inactivated in the hypothalamus (Bauer and Lipmann, 1976). It is possible that the inactivation process in the hypothalamic tissue affects the secretion rate of TRH.

3. Method of Determination

(a) In vitro *assays*

(*1*) *Release of TSH from rat anterior pituitary glands.* This method, originally developed by Saffran and Schally (1955) for CRF, can also be used for TRH (Bowers, Redding and Schally, 1965; Guillemin, Yamazaki, Gard, Jutisz and Sakiz, 1963; Schreiber, 1961; Sinha and Meites, 1965/68; Solomon and McKenzie, 1966); the TSH released is assayed now by RIA, but it was assayed formerly by bioassays. This assay system can detect 0·01 ng of TRH (Schally, Bowers, Redding and Barrett, 1966a) and the results correlate perfectly with *in vivo* data. TRH can re-establish TSH production in tissue cultures of rat anterior pituitaries (Schally, Redding and Bowers, 1966).

(*2*) *Release of TSH from cultured pituitary cells.* Monolayer cultures of rat pituitary cells (Vale *et al.*, 1972; Vale, Rivier, Brown, Chan, Ling and Rivier, 1976) can also be used for TRH assay. TSH release into the medium is determined by RIA.

(*3*) *Receptor assay for TRH.* Plasma membranes isolated from bovine anterior pituitaries (Labrie, Barden, Poirier and DeLean, 1972), or prolactin-growth hormone (PRL/GH) secreting tumour cells (Hinkle and Tashjian, 1975; Hinkle, Woroch, and Tashjian, 1974), a TSH-secreting tumour (Grant, Vale and Guillemin, 1973), and anterior pituitary homogenates prepared from rat (DeLean, Beaulieu and Labrie, 1974) all bind TRH with almost identical binding constants. In competition experiments, various analogues were found to displace labelled TRH with equal potency using receptors from PRL/GH secreting GH3 cells (Hinkle *et al.*, 1974) and from a TSH-secreting tumour (Grant *et al.*, 1973). The abilities of most analogues to compete with ^{3}H-TRH for binding to pituitary cells can be related to their relative potencies to stimulate TSH or PRL secretion (Hinkle *et al.*, 1974), indicating that changes in receptor affinities determine the difference in potency.

(*b*) In vivo *assays*

(*1*) *Release of* ^{131}I *in iodine-deficient mice, treated with* ^{131}I, *codeine and 1 µg thyroxine.* Provided the extract being tested is free of TSH, the rise in the radioactivity of the blood 2 hr after injection of the extract is proportional to the TSH released by TRF (Redding, Bowers and Schally, 1966).

(*2*) *Release of* ^{131}I *in immature rats.* This assay is based on measurement of radioactivity in blood of rats treated with ^{131}I and 5 µg thyroxine (Yamazaki, Sakiz and Guillemin, 1963). This assay is apparently less sensitive than *in vitro* assays or the assay of Redding *et al.* (1966).

(*3*) *Increase in plasma levels of TSH.* Thyroidectomised rats treated with 1 µg thyroxine (Bowers, Redding and Schally, 1965) or normal animals (Ducommun, Sakiz and Guillemin, 1965) can be used. Serum TSH can be determined by RIA for rat TSH. This method may be the most desirable way to test for TRH.

(*c*) *Radioimmunoassay*

Synthetic TRH was conjugated to bovine serum albumin (BSA) by means of bis-diazotized-benzidine (BDB) and used as the immunogen preparation. In rabbits, this immunogen generated a specific TRH-antibody which was successfully used for RIA for TRH (Bassiri and Utiger, 1972). The tracer was prepared by iodinating TRH by ^{125}I using chloramine T (Hunter and Greenwood, 1962) and purified on a Sephadex G-10 column. Bound hormones were separated by precipitation with the second antibody. The sensitivity of the assay was 10 pg TRH (Bassiri and Utiger, 1972). TRH RIA methods, most of which are similar to the aforementioned method, were reported by others (Oliver, Charvet, Codaccioni and Vague, 1974; Koch, Baram and Fridkin, 1976).

4. TRH in Biological Fluids

(*a*) *Plasma TRH*

TRH was demonstrated to be in the hypophysial portal blood of the rat by bioassay (Wilber and Porter, 1970) and RIA (Bassiri and Utiger, 1972). Its concentration was increased by electrical stimulation of the hypothalamus

(Wilber and Porter, 1970). Presence of immunoreactive TRH in the peripheral blood of rats (Jackson and Reichlin, 1974b; Montoya, Seibel and Wilber, 1975) and humans (Mitsuma, Hirooka and Nihei, 1976b; Oliver *et al.*, 1974) were also reported. However, there are considerable discrepancies between the values reported. According to Oliver, Eskay, Mical and Porter (1973) plasma TRH levels were around 60–70 pg/ml in normal rats, undetectable in hypothyroid rats and elevated in T_4-treated animals. Other studies reported that plasma TRH levels were 60–80 pg/ml in normal rats, unaffected by thyroid status, and rose after cold exposure (Montoya, Seibel and Wilber, 1973). Jackson and Reichlin (1974b) reported that plasma TRH levels in normal rats were around 13 pg/ml. In the frog, TRH is found in the blood in significant concentration of about 45 ng/ml (Jackson and Reichlin, 1977).

Plasma TRH levels in humans were reported to range from 5–60 pg/ml, undetectable in hyperthyroidism, elevated in primary and secondary hypothyroidism, and undetectable in tertiary hypothyroidism (Mitsuma *et al.*, 1967b). In another report, plasma TRH levels in humans were said to be around 20 pg/ml (Oliver *et al.*, 1974). Biological half life of TRH was estimated to be 4–5 min (Bassiri and Utiger, 1973; Redding and Schally, 1972), its distribution volume being 18·5 % of body weight. Assuming plasma levels being 25 pg/ml, the total amount of TRH secreted into circulation would be 70 μg/day (Nihei, 1977). It is difficult to accept that this amount of TRH originates only from the hypothalamus.

(b) Urine TRH

TRH is secreted in the urine after injection of exogenous hormone in man (Bassiri and Utiger, 1973; Jackson, Gagel, Papapetrou and Reichlin, 1974), approximately 15 % of the injected dose being identified immunologically. Endogenous TRH was also demonstrated in urine in humans (Jackson *et al.*, Oliver *et al.*, 1974), and rats (Jackson and Reichlin, 1974b; Montoya, Seibel and Wilber, 1973). The daily urinary excretion of TRH appeared to be greater in men (195 ng) than in women (149 ng). Unlike rat (Jackson *et al.*, 1974b), and human plasma TRH (Mitsuma *et al.*, 1976), urinary levels of TRH in humans were said not to be affected by altered thyroid status (Jackson, Papapetrou and Reichlin, 1974), but were increased by cold exposure (Gale, Hayward, Green, Wu, Schiller and Jackson, 1975). However, the validity of the assay for urinary TRH was questioned (Vagenakis, Roti, Mannix and Brauerman, 1975). Recently Leppäluoto, Ling and Vale (1976) reported an ion-exchange method for purifying TRH from urine and found urine concentrations of 2–20 pg/ml.

(c) Cerebrospinal fluid (CSF) TRH

TRH has been found in rat and human CSF. TRH content in human CSF was reported to range between 65 and 290 pg/ml (Oliver *et al.*, 1974). The origin of CSF TRH remains unknown.

C. PROLACTIN RELEASING FACTOR (PRF)

1. Chemical Constitution and Main Physico-chemical and Biological Properties

Both a prolactin-releasing factor (PRF) and a prolactin-release inhibiting factor (PIF) appear to be present in the hypothalami of mammals and birds, but PIF may predominate in the former and PRF in the latter (Meites and Clemens, 1972). A part of the PRF activity in the extracts of hypothalami of domestic animals is clearly due to TRH which, under specific conditions, can stimulate prolactin secretion (see section on TRH). It has also been reported recently that administration of antisera to TRH will greatly lower prolactin levels in rats (Koch, Goldhaber, Fireman, Zor, Shani and Tal, 1977). This finding, if confirmed, might support the concept of a physiological role of TRH in the control of prolactin secretion.

However, prolactin- and TSH-release can be dissociated under various physiological and clinical conditions. Moreover, the work of several groups suggests that partially purified hypothalamic fractions, apparently different from TRH, can still stimulate the release of prolactin from rat pituitaries *in vivo* and *in vitro*. TRH is less resistant to inactivation by incubation with fresh serum than PRF and can be separated from PRF by adsorption on charcoal (Szabo and Frohman, 1976; Boyd, Spencer, Jackson and Reichlin, 1976).

We have also established that several other fractions with different physico-chemical properties from TRH, as shown by different partition coefficients on CCD, basicity on CMC and SE-Sephadex, and behaviour on molecular sieving on Sephadex, can also stimulate the release of prolactin from rat pituitary fragments from monolayer cell cultures (Schally, Arimura and Redding, unpublished). Further purification and identification of these materials is in progress.

Various drugs, among them inhibitors of catecholamines and a variety of natural substances of CNS and extra-CNS origin such as vasopressin, oestrogens, β-endorphin and Met-enkephalin, can augment prolactin release (Schally *et al.*, 1978a), but they do not represent the physiological PRF, the chemistry of which remains to be elucidated.

2. Localisation, Biosynthesis and Release

PRF activity was demonstrated in the hypothalamus in mammals and birds (Meites and Nicoll, 1966; Boyd, Spencer, Jackson and Reichlin, 1976; Dular, LaBella, Vivian and Eddie, 1974; Frohman and Szabo, 1975; Hagen, Kokubu, Sawano, Shiraki, Yanasaki and Ishizaka, 1975; Milmore and Reece, 1975; Rivier and Vale, 1974; Szabo and Frohman, 1976; Takahashi, Saito, Wokai, Hoshiai, Wada, Sakurada and Suzuki, 1976; Meites and Clemens, 1972). PRF activity was also found in the bovine, rat and human pineal gland (Blask, Vaughan, Reiter, Johnson and Vaughan, 1976). Since PRF, different from TRH, has not been isolated, the precise mode of biosynthesis and release remains unknown.

Although PIF may be a major regulator of pituitary prolactin-secreting cells in mammals, there appears to be a stimulatory serotoninergic component. Administration of tryptophan and 5-hydroxy-tryptophan (5-HTP), both precursors of serotonin, release prolactin in rats (Kamberi, Mical and Porter, 1971; Lu and Meites, 1973) and men (MacIndoe and Turkington, 1973; Kato, Nakai, Imura, Chihara and Ohgo, 1974). Administration of 5-HTP does not affect plasma TSH levels and stimulates prolactin release in normal subjects and in patients with isolated TRH deficiency (Kato et al., 1974). p-Chlorophenylalanine, which blocks 5-HTP synthesis, inhibits suckling-induced prolactin-release in rats (Kordon, Blake, Terkel and Sawyer, 1973). On the other hand, reserpine raises serum prolactin but does not prevent stress-induced prolactin release (Valverde, Chieffo and Reichlin, 1973). PIF secretion appears to be regulated by a catecholaminergic mechanism and PRF secretion by a serotoninergic pathway. PRF activity in the hypothalamus has been reported to increase during late pregnancy in rats (Takahashi, Saito, Wakai, Hoshiai, Wada, Sakurada and Suzuki, 1976).

3. Methods of Determination

(a) In vitro methods

The in vitro methods using rat pituitary halves or quarters can be used to assay both PRF and PIF activities as well as other releasing and inhibiting hormone activities (Arimura and Schally, 1975). In our laboratories, young adult male rats are used as pituitary donors. Pituitary fragments are incubated as described in Section A.3. At the end of the incubation period, the medium is collected and its prolactin content is determined by RIA. The results are expressed as a percent ratio of the medium prolactin in the second hour to medium prolactin in the first hour. We abandoned the use of microgram of prolactin per milligram of pituitary tissue, because histological examination of the pituitary halves revealed considerable necrosis of the central part of the pituitary after the preliminary 3 hr incubation period.

Monolayer cultures of rat pituitaries are also used for PRF and PIF activity (Vale *et al.*, 1972). Prolactin released into the medium is assayed by RIA.

Superfusion of rat pituitary fragments or pituitary cells (Lowry, 1974; Sawano and Kokubu, 1977) appears to be sensitive, especially to PRF activity. Prolactin-release rates can be measured from time to time, and transient stimulation of prolactin release can be detected in this system.

(b) In vivo *assay*

Both male and female rats are used. They are intact or treated with oestrogen–progesterone, or ovariectomised and treated with these steroids. Under anaesthesia samples are injected and elevation of serum prolactin levels are determined by RIA (Frohman and Szabo, 1975; Rivier and Vale, 1974; Szabo and Frohman, 1976).

D. PROLACTIN RELEASE-INHIBITING FACTOR (PIF)

1. Chemical Constitution and Main Physico-chemical and Biological Properties

Although the presence of PIF activity in hypothalamic extracts was demonstrated many years ago (for reviews, see Schally *et al.*, 1973; Meites and Clemens, 1972), the nature of PIF is still unclear. Many substances are present in the brain or hypothalamic extracts which can inhibit prolactin secretion *in vitro* and *in vivo*. It has been demonstrated that the catecholamines influence the release of prolactin (MacLeod, 1969). Our recent work also showed that hypothalamic catecholamines inhibit prolactin release by a direct action on the pituitary. PIF activity present in acetic acid extracts of pig hypothalami was purified by various methods. Some of the highly purified fractions which strongly inhibited the release of prolactin *in vitro* and *in vivo* were found to contain much noradrenaline and dopamine (Schally, Dupont, Arimura, Takahara, Redding, Clemens and Shaar, 1976c). Synthetic noradrenaline and dopamine, in doses of 10–100 ng also strongly inhibited the release of prolactin *in vitro*.

Another hypothalamic substance with PIF activity is gamma-aminobutyric acid (GABA) (Schally, Redding, Arimura, Dupont and Linthicum, 1977). Natural GABA and synthetic GABA inhibited prolactin release *in vitro* from isolated rat pituitary halves in doses as low as 0·1 µg/ml. GABA also had PIF activity *in vivo*, although larger doses were needed for an effect. The results indicate that GABA can inhibit prolactin release by a direct action on the pituitary gland, but again it is not known whether this effect is physiological or pharmacological.

Other compounds with PIF activity different from catecholamines and GABA, but still unidentified are present in pig hypothalamic extracts. One of them appears to be a polyamine and the other a polypeptide (Schally, Arimura and Redding, unpublished). Further work is needed to identify the physiological PIF. Drugs like L-dopa and 2 bromo-α-ergocriptine (CB-154), an ergot alkaloid, are now used in order to inhibit the release of prolactin and to suppress undesired lactation.

2. Localisation, Biosynthesis and Release

The presence of PIF in the hypothalamus has been demonstrated by several workers (for reviews, see Meites and Clemens, 1972). PIF activity has been also demonstrated in the extra-hypothalamic brain (Vale, Rivier, Palkovits, Saavedra and Brownstein, 1974) and the pineal gland of mammals (Blask, Vaughan, Reiter, Johnson and Vaughan. 1976).

Fractions of pig hypothalamic extracts with the greatest PIF activity have been found to be rich in catecholamines (Schally *et al.*, 1976c). Dopamine appears to play an important role in the inhibition of prolactin secretion since specific agonists or antagonists of dopanine have been shown to alter the secretion of prolactin *in vivo* (Meites, 1970; Lu, Amenomeri, Chen and Meites, 1970, Birge, Jacobs, Hammer and Daughaday, 1970; Dickerman, Kledzik, Gelato, Chen and Meites, 1974) and *in vitro* (MacLeod, 1969; MacLeod, 1976; Shaar and Clemens, 1974). Dopamine has been found in the hypophysial portal blood in sufficient concentration for suppressing prolactin release (Gibbs and Neill, 1978; Ben-Jonathan, Oliver, Weiner, Mical and Porter, 1977).

Dopamine levels are particularly high in the median eminence and arcuate nucleus, and moderately high in the suprachiasmatic nucleus, paraventricular nucleus, the medial part of the ventromedial nucleus, the dorsomedial nucleus, and the posterior part of the medial forebrain bundle (Palkovits, Brownstein, Saavedra and Axelrod, 1974). Part of the dopamine in the hypothalamus is present in cell bodies in the arcuate and periventricular nuclei (Dahlstrom and Fuxe, 1964; Fuxe, 1964; Fuxe and Hökfelt, 1966). Complete deafferentation of the rat mediobasal hypothalamus did not decrease dopamine content in the hypothalamic island appreciably and in these animals, serum prolactin levels remain in the normal range (Weiner, 1975). Inhibition of dopamine synthesis results in a marked elevation of serum prolactin (Weiner, 1975). PIF in subcellular fractions of the rat mediobasal hypothalamus has been reported to be distributed evenly in the 17,000 g supernatant (S_2) and in the crude mitochondrial fraction (P_2) which contains synaptosomes. Elimination of dopamine by alumina adsorption results in complete loss of PIF in S_2, but not in P_2. In contrast, strial PIF was detected in only P_2, and disappeared completely upon alumina adsorption. Addition of dopamine antagonists reduced PIF activity of crude mediobasal hypothalamic extracts by about half, but no longer affected it after alumina adsorption (Enjalbert, Moos, Carbonell, Priam and Kordon, 1977).

3. Methods of Determination

(a) In vitro *methods*

The *in vitro* methods using rat pituitary halves or quarters (Saffran and Schally, 1955; Arimura *et al.*, 1975a) or pituitary cell cultures (Vale *et al.*, 1973) as described in C-3 are successfully used for determining PIF activity.

(b) In vivo *assay methods*

Both male and female rats are used. Under anaesthesia they are injected with drugs which stimulate prolactin release. The drugs used include the following: chlorpromazine, 1 mg/100 g bw, i.p.; perphenazine, 1 mg/100 g bw i.p.; haloperidol, 10 μg/100 g bw i.v.; monoiodotyrosine, 10–20 mg/100 g bw, i.p.; and Sulpiride, 1 mg/100 g bw i.p. Rats with hypothalamic lesion and hypophysectomised rats with pituitary grafts can also be used. Test materials are injected into the jugular vein as a bolus, or by infusion. Their suppressive activity on elevated serum prolactin levels induced by the drugs or by placing the hypothalamic lesion is measured by determining serum prolactin by RIA.

Primiparous lactating female Wister rats 6–8 days post-partum are also used. They are separated from their pups for 8 hr and then a mammary nerve is dissected and stimulated for 10 min electrically under urethane anaesthesia. Test material is injected 10 min before stimulation. PIF activity of the material is evaluated by its suppressive effect on the rise of plasma prolactin levels due to stimulation of the mammary nerve (Enjalbert *et al.*, 1977).

The following points should be kept in mind, when *in vivo* assay for PIF is performed:

(i) The hypothalamic extracts contain both PIF and PRF, and the ratio of these factors may vary. Therefore, administration of crude extracts may not suppress serum prolactin levels.

(ii) When dopamine represents the major protion of PIF activities in the test materials, their administration may not suppress serum prolactin in rats treated with dopamine antagonists such as perphenazine. Dopamine antagonists prevent PIF activity of dopamine at the pituitary level as observed *in vitro* (Arimura *et al.*, 1975a).

(iii) Some material may stimulate release of endogenous PIF, resulting in a decrease of prolactin release as a secondary sequence.

E. MELANOCYTE STIMULATING HORMONE (MSH)-RELEASING FACTOR (MRF) AND RELEASING INHIBITING FACTOR (MIF)

1. Chemical Constitution and Physico-chemical Properties

The release of MSH from the pars intermedia of the pituitary gland is controlled by hypothalamic stimulating factor (MRF) and inhibitory factor (MIF), the latter having a predominant role (Kastin *et al.*, 1977). However, considerable confusion still exists as to the identity of MIF and MRF. The first prospective MIF was isolated from bovine hypothalami and identified as $H–Pro–Leu–Gly–NH_2$ in this laboratory (Schally and Kastin, 1966; Nair, Kastin and Schally, 1971a). Celis, Taleisnik and Walter (1971a) originally observed that $H–Pro–Leu–Gly–NH_2$ could be formed by incubating oxytocin with an enzyme present in hypothalamic tissue and that it inhibits MSH release in the rat. In addition to MIF action, this tripeptide also has important CNS activities (Kastin *et al.*, 1977). Not all authors agree that $H–Pro–Leu–Gly–NH_2$ is in fact MIF. Other substances such as tocinoic acid, the cyclic pentapeptide ring of oxytocin, and catecholamines have been proposed as MIF.

There is also evidence for an MRF. Celis, Taleisnik and Walter, 1971a) proposed that the opened *N*-terminal ring portion of oxytocin H–Cys–Tyr–Ile–Gln–Asn–Cys–OH constitutes MRF. However, open end or unopened cyclic pentapeptide fragments of oxytocin have not been identified in the hypothalamus. In conclusion, the identity of the physiological MIF and MRF is still unknown.

2. Localisation and Methods of Determination

There are materials found in hypothalamic tissue which inhibit MSH release in certain assay systems, but at the moment physiological MIF has not yet been described. An MIF peptide, $H\text{-}Pro–Leu–Gly–NH_2$, has been reported to be present in the hypothalamic tissue (Nair, Kastin and Schally, 1971). This was ascertained by a single assay system (Kastin, Schally and Viosca, 1971) which does not seem to be sensitive to every batch of Pro–Leu–Gly–NH$_2$ (Kastin, Plotnikoff, Nair, Redding and Anderson, 1972). MIF activity of Pro–Leu–Gly–NH$_2$ has also been demonstrated by Celis, Macagno and Taleisnik (1973) but not confirmed by others (Grant, Clark and Rosanoff, 1973). MRF activity has been demonstrated in extracts of the median eminence (Taleisnik and Orias, 1965). This effect has been reported to be lost after incubation, which results in the production of MIF activity (Celis and Taleisnik, 1971).

(a) In vitro *assay*

Rats and hamsters' pituitaries are incubated with test materials *in vitro* and the amount of MSH released into the incubation medium is determined by photoreflectance methods described originally for the frog skin bioassay for MSH. In this system, tocinamide and tocinoic acid, both of which have the ring structure of oxytocin, have been reported to be potent inhibitors of MSH release (Hruby *et al.*, 1972). However, the same investigators later reported that they failed to reconfirm the results.

(b) In vivo *assay for MIF*

The *in vivo* assay using rats based on the restoration by MIF of depleted pituitary MSH content following pretreatment with Nembutal and morphine has been described by Kastin, Miller and Schally (1968). The same authors described another *in vivo* assay for MIF by the direct application of MIF preparations to the exposed pituitary of a frog with the hypothalamic lesion (Kastin, Schally and Viosca, 1971). It has been reported that the hypothalamus of rabbit and rat contain membrane-bound exopeptidase which degrades radioactively-labelled oxytocin to give labelled H-Pro–Leu–Gly–NH$_2$ (Walter, Griffiths and Hooper, 1973).

F. LUTEINISING HORMONE RELEASING HORMONE (LH-RH) AND FOLLICLE STIMULATING HORMONE RELEASING HORMONE (FSH-RH)

1. Chemical Constitution and Main Physico-chemical and Biological Properties

LH-RH was first isolated from porcine hypothalami by two different methods (Schally, Arimura, Baba, Nair, Matsuo, Redding, Debeljuk and White, 1971a; Schally, Nair, Redding and Arimura, 1971c). The structure of porcine

LH-RH was determined as (pyro)Glu–His–Trp–Ser–Tyr–Gly–Leu–Arg–Pro–Gly–NH$_2$ (Matsuo, Baba, Arimura, Nair and Schally, 1971b; Baba, Matsuo and Schally, 1971). LH-RH corresponding to this structure was first synthesised by us (Matsuo et al., 1971a, b; Schally, Arimura, Kastin, Matsuo, Baba, Redding, Nair, Debeljuk and White, 1971b) and then by others (Geiger, König, Wismann, Geisen and Enzmann, 1971).

Several months after our report of the isolation and structure of porcine LH-RH, the isolation of ovine LH-RH was announced (Amoss, Burgus, Blackwell, Vale, Fellows and Guillemin, 1971). Its structure proved to be the same as that of porcine hormone (Burgus, Butcher, Amoss, Ling, Monahan, Rivier, Fellows, Blackwell, Vale and Guillemin, 1972) and subsequent biochemical and immunological studies indicated that bovine, human and rat LH-RH probably have the same structure (Schally et al., 1973, 1978a, b).

LH-RH is a basic decapeptide with the N-terminus blocked by pyroglutamic acid. Its carboxyl terminus is also blocked with an amide group. The specific rotation of LH-RH $[\alpha]_D^{25} = -50 \cdot 5°$ (1% solution in 1% acetic acid) and its calculated mol wt is 1182, although after synthesis it is obtained as a diacetate tetrahydrate (mw 1374) or a trihydrate (mw 1356). The His–Trp sequence seems to constitute its active centre while the other amino acids are involved in binding to the receptors and preserving the conformation.

Our original observations that natural porcine LH-RH and the synthetic decapeptide release both LH and FSH (Schally et al., 1971a, b) have been confirmed in and extended to a variety of animals, including rats, mice, rabbits, golden hamsters, mink, spotted skunk, impala, rock hyrax, sheep, cattle, pigs, horses, monkeys and humans (Schally et al., 1973, 1978a, b). The fact that ovulation has been induced in most of these species with LH-RH demonstrates that this decapeptide can release enough FSH to induce follicular maturation. Increases in sex steroid levels in blood have also been reported after administration of LH-RH. LH-RH is also active in birds such as domestic fowl and pigeons, and in some species of fish such as brown trout and carp. Our concept (Schally et al., 1971b) that LH-RH is also the physiological FSH-RH has not been seriously challenged, although claims have been made that other natural materials with FSH-RH activity exist (Bowers, Currie, Johansson and Folkers, 1973). Recent biochemical results indicate that the LH-RH decapeptide represents the bulk of the FSH-RH activity in the pig hypothalamus (Schally, Arimura, Redding, Debeljuk, Carter, Dupont and Vilchez-M., 1976a).

Investigations of the routes of administration in rats and humans revealed that LH-RH is effective not only after intravenous, subcutaneous, intramuscular and intracarotid injection, but also after intravaginal, intrarectal, intranasal, cutaneous (on the skin in dimethyl sulphoxide), and even oral administration. However, the doses required for effect by extravascular routes are 100–10,000 times larger than the parenteral. In addition to being the regulator of the release of LH and FSH, LH-RH might act as a neurotransmitter with effects on sex drive (Moss, 1977).

2. Localisation, Biosynthesis, Release and Degradation

(a) Localisation

The presence of LH-RH in the hypothalamus was first demonstrated by bioassays (McCann, Taleisnik and Friedman, 1960). Based on anatomical and physiological experiments, Barraclough (1967) proposed dual hypothalamic control of LH-RH secretion and suggested that basal secretion of LH is controlled by the arcuate and ventromedial nucleus (VMN), and that the cyclic release of LH is stimulated by the preoptic suprachiasmatic nuclei. Availability of antibody to LH-RH and the radioimmunoassay for LH-RH has made it possible to study the localisation of LH-RH in tissue more precisely. By dissecting discrete regions of the brain, the highest concentration of LH-RH has been shown to be present in the median eminence, with lesser amounts in the arcuate nucleus (Palkovits, Arimura, Brownstein, Schally and Saavedra, 1974). Small amounts are detectable in the anterior region as well, corresponding to earlier reports of LH-RH in the preoptic area (King, Arimura and Williams, 1975). Immunocytological studies revealed that the median eminence of the rat, mouse, hamster and guinea-pig is particularly rich in LH-RH (Barry, Dubois and Carette, 1974; Naik, 1974). LH-RH-containing neurones were demonstrated in the preoptic area with their processes extending toward the median eminence (Naik, 1974; Sétáló, Vigh, Schally, Arimura and Flerkó, 1975). Alpert, Brawer, Jackson and Patel (1975) demonstrated that there is a high concentration of LH-RH in the pre-mammillary areas. There is a lack of agreement as to the cells of origin of LH-RH. Barry et al. (1974) reported that colchicine permits the staining of cell bodies in the preoptic and septal region after castration in guinea pigs, but others failed to confirm this finding in rats (Sétáló et al., 1975). However, Nembutal injection on the day of proestrus and frontal deafferentation in female rats has permitted the staining of LH-RH cell bodies which are scattered in the suprachiasmatic area between the anterior commissure and the optic chiasm, and in the medial prechiasmatic area near the organum vasculosum of the lamina terminalis (Sétáló, Vigh, Schally, Arimura and Flerkó, 1976).

LH-RH has been demonstrated in the processes corresponding to the tuberohypophysial tract (Sétáló et al., 1975). LH-RH positive secretory granules are localised to nerve endings (Pelletier, Labrie, Puviani, Arimura and Schally, 1974). Particulate fractions corresponding to "synaptosomes" prepared from mammalian hypothalamic tissue contain approximately half of the immunoreactive LH-RH and a heavier particulate fraction contains the rest (Barnea, Ben-Jonathan and Porter, 1975).

There are differences among species in the localisation of LH-RH cell bodies. Preoptic-anterior hypothalamic localisation of the LH-RH cells is characteristic for the rat (Sétáló *et al.*, 1976), guinea-pig and cat (Barry and Dubois, 1975). In the dog, 40% of the LH-RH cells are found in the tubero-mammillary regions, whereas in primates, the majority of cells are found in these regions (Barry and Carrette, 1975; Barry and Dubois, 1975). LH-RH appears to be synthesised in the cell bodies of the tubero-mammillary regions and the preoptic suprachiasmatic regions, and transported to the neuronal terminals in the median eminance by axoplasmic flow. LH-RH has been detected in methanolic extracts of hypothalamic tissue from human foetuses as early as 4–5 weeks after conception (Winter, Eskay and Porter, 1974). By immunological techniques, LH-RH positive cells have been demonstrated in the region rostral to the anterior commissure, the paraolfactory area and the organum vasculosum of the lamina terminalis (OVLT) (Sétáló *et al.*, 1976).

The LH-RH neurones appear to be distinct from catecholaminergic neurones (Kizer, Arimura, Schally and Brownstein, 1975). Simultaneous identification of LH-RH and dopamine in the median eminence of the rat revealed that the inner band of dopamine terminals in the lateral median eminence overlaps the LH-RH terminals, and an outer band appears juxtaposed with portal capillaries (McNeill and Sladek, 1978). The presence of LH-RH in tanycytes (Naik, 1974; Naik, 1976; Zimmerman, Hsu, Feris and Kozlowshi, 1974) may be caused by absorption from cerebrospinal fluid or by uptake from adjacent neural elements.

White, Hedlund, Weber, Rippel, Johnson and Willus (1974) reported that ovine, bovine and porcine pineal glands contained high levels of LH-RH as determined by RIA and bioassay. However, we failed to confirm their findings in the rat and others have found no LH-RH in the pineal of the rat, sheep or monkey. White recently reported that the earlier findings may be artifactual.

(b) Biosynthesis of LH-RH

Incubation of rat hypothalamic tissue with ^{3}H-tyrosine *in vitro* has been reported to lead to incorporation of the radioisotope into the LH-RH fraction which has been purified on a Sephadex G-25 column (Moguilevisky, Enero and Szwarcfarb, 1974). The hypothalamic fraction which contains mitochondria has been reported to incorporate ^{14}C-glutamine into gonado-trophin-releasing hormone (Johansson, Currie, Folkers and Bowers, 1973).

A similar type of finding was recently made by Reichlin who isolated a radioactive peptide by anti-LH-RH affinity chromatography, following ^{3}H-proline labelling, which migrated with synthetic LH-RH upon chromatography and electrophoresis (Reichlin, 1976). Kordon, Epelbaum, Enjalbert and McKelvy (1976) briefly perfused the cerebral ventricular system of rats with ^{3}H-L-tyrosine and then extracted the hypothalamus just before and also after an *in vitro* incubation. They found that *in vitro* incubation resulted in an increased yield of biosynthetically labelled LH-RH compared with non-incubated hypothalamus and that this increase was greater in the tissue from castrated rats.

(c) Release of LH-RH

LH-RH in the neuronal terminals adjacent to the capillaries in the median eminence is considered to be released into the hypophysial portal vessel. The LH-RH content in the rat mid-hypothalamus has been reported to be highest in the morning of pro-oestrus and to decline in the mid to late afternoon, and then increase gradually (Asai and Wakabayashi, 1975; Araki, Ferin, Zimmerman and Vande Wiele, 1975). Since the LH surge occurs during the afternoon of pro-oestrus, the decline of LH-RH content in the mid-hypothalamus suggests the release of LH-RH at this time. An increase in LH-RH concentration in the hypophysial portal blood has been detected during the afternoon of pre-oestrus in rats anesthetised with Althesin which does not block ovulation in rats (Sarkar, Chiappa, Fink and Sherwood, 1976). Noradrenaline appears to stimulate the release of LH-RH; alpha-adrenergic receptor blocking drugs inhibit LH-release. Similarly, drugs that interfere with catecholamine synthesis such as α-methyl tyrosine, block LH release. This blockade can be reversed by drugs such as dihydroxyphenyl-serine, which reinitiates the synthesis of noradrenaline, but not of dopamine (McCann, 1977). Electrical stimulation of the preoptic area or median eminence, which stimulates LH release, increases LH-RH concentration in the hypophysial portal blood (Porter, Eskay, Oliver, Ben-Jonathan, Warberg, Parker and Barnea, 1977; Sherwood, Chiappa and Fink, 1976). Lateral ventricle infusion of prostaglandin E_2 causes 2–3 fold increase in the concentration of LH-RH in the hypophysial portal plasma (Eskay, Warberg, Mical and Porter, 1975). Release of LH-RH from synaptosomes from the median eminence *in vitro* is stimulated by dopamine (Bennett, Edwardson, Holland, Jeffcoate and White, 1975). High K^+ concentrations stimulate release of LH-RH from the medio-basal hypothalamus of rat *in vitro*, and K^+ stimulated release is Ca^{++} dependent (Rotsztejn, Charli, Pattou, Epelbaum and Kordon, 1976). Prostaglandin E_2, melatonin and high K^+ have been found to stimulate LH-RH release from superfused rat hypothalamic tissue but noradrenaline, dopamine, acetylcholine or serotonin did not (Gallardo and Ramirez, 1977; Kao and Weisz, 1977).

(d) Degradation and metabolism of LH-RH

LH-RH is rapidly degraded in blood by enzymatic cleavage of the (pyro)Glu–His group from the amino terminus and is excreted by the kidneys (Redding, Kastin, Gonzales-Barcena, Coy, Coy, Schalch and Schally, 1973). The half life of LH-RH in the human is 4 min (Redding et al., 1973) and in the rat 7 min (Redding and Schally, 1973). It has also been demonstrated that homogenates of rat and pig hypothalami degrade LH-RH (Griffith, Hooper, Jeffcoate and Holland, 1974). Koch, Baram, Chobsieng and Fridkin (1974) identified the products formed by incubation of LH-RH with hypothalamic slices to be pyro-Glu–His–Trp–Ser–Tyr–Gly–OH and probably Leu–Arg–Pro–Gly–NH$_2$. This indicates that the cleavage occurred between amino acids residues 6 and 7.

3. Methods of Determination

(a) In vitro assay

(1) Release of LH and FSH from rat pituitary quarters in vitro. Quartered rat pituitaries are incubated in 1 ml Krebs bicarbonate buffer containing glucose and BSA according to the in vitro method for CRF by Saffran and Schally (1955), with some modification as described previously (Arimura and Schally, 1976).

(2) Release of LH and FSH from monolayer cultures of rat pituitary cells. LH-RH stimulates the release of LH and FSH from cultured pituitary cells in a dose related manner (Vale et al., 1972, 1976).

(b) In vivo assay

(1) LH release in ovariectomised, oestrogen and progesterone-treated rats. This animal preparation is highly sensitive to LH-RH. Elevation of serum LH after injection of test materials is used as the response parameter. Serum LH is assayed by RIA. In our hands, the minimum detectable dose of LH-RH is 0·2 ng/rat. This preparation is, however, insensitive to FSH-RH activity (Ramirez and McCann, 1963).

(2) LH and FSH release in immature male rats. Prolonged infusion of LH-RH into immature rats increased serum LH and FSH in a dose related manner (Arimura, Debeljuk and Schally, 1972). Serum LH and FSH are determined by RIA.

(c) Radioimmunoassay of LH-RH

A considerable number of reports on radioimmunoassay for LH-RH have appeared (Arimura, Sato, Kumasaka, Worobec, Debeljuk, Dunn and Schally, 1973; Nett, Akbar, Niswender, Hedlund and White, 1973; Koch, Wilchek, Fridkin, Chobsieng, Zor and Lindner, 1973; Jonas, Burger, Cumming, Findlay and deKretser, 1975). Specific antisera against synthetic LH-RH conjugated with a carrier protein or adsorbed on a large molecular substance such as polyvinylpyrolidone or charcoal have been generated in rabbits, guinea pigs and sheep. Using these antisera, radioimmunoassay methods have been established. Synthetic LH-RH is labelled by ^{125}I by chloramine T or lactoperoxidase methods (Miyachi, Charamback, Mecklenberg and Lipsett, 1973) and purified by gel filtration on a Sephadex G-25 column (Nett *et al.*, 1973) or ion-exchange chromatography (Arimura *et al.*, 1973). Bound and free hormones are separated either by double-antibody method (Nett *et al.*, 1973) or by dextran-coated charcoal (Arimura *et al.*, 1973). The methods of RIA for LH-RH are very sensitive so that an amount smaller than 1 pg LH-RH per tube can be detected. Details of the methods are described elsewhere (Arimura *et al.*, 1973; Nett *et al.*, 1973; Arimura and Schally, 1975).

Although the RIA methods are specific and not interfered with by other known hypothalamic hormones and pituitary hormones, they detect various LH-RH analogues to different degrees depending on the antibody used. The recognition sites vary from one antibody to another. Some antibodies generated against PVP adsorbed LH-RH (Arimura *et al.*, 1973) or LH-RH conjugated with a carrier protein by using bis-diazotized-benzidine (Nett *et al.*, 1973) appear to recognise only the complete molecule of LH-RH, whereas other antibodies recognise certain parts of the LH-RH molecule (Arimura, Sato, Coy, Worobec, Schally, Yanaihara and Sukura, 1975a). Therefore, LH-RH contents of the tissue determined by RIA using different antibodies occasionally vary. For instance, one antibody (Arimura No. 422) recognises only the complete molecule of LH-RH, whereas another (Arimura No. 743) can detect peptides containing an amino acid sequence corresponding to positions 3–9. LH-RH activity of the extract from the preoptic-suprachiasmatic region of the rat brain as determined by RIA using anti-serum No. 422 was reported to be smaller than those values estimated by antiserum No. 743 (King, Elkind, Gerall and Miller, 1978). This finding would indicate that this preoptic-suprachiasmatic region contains LH-RH plus LH-RH-like peptides which cross-react with antiserum No. 743. On the other hand, estimates of LH-RH activity in the median eminence and in the organum vasculosum of the lamina terminalis, both of which consist of fibrous tissue, was the same for antisera No. 422 and No. 743. This may indicate that these areas contain mainly complete molecules of LH-RH (King *et al.*, 1978). Therefore, RIA for LH-RH is not only useful for determining LH-RH concentrations in tissues, but also for studying the interrelationship between LH-RH decapeptides and LH-RH-like peptides which include prohormone, intermediates and breakdown products.

4. Plasma LH–RH

Plasma LH-RH levels in animals and humans as measured by bioassay and RIA have been reported. Nallar and McCann (1965) demonstrated LH-RH activity in plasma of long-term hypophysectomised rats as determined by ovarian ascorbic acid depletion in gonadotrophin-pretreated immature rats after injection of plasma. However, this finding was not confirmed by using a more sensitive LH-RH assay, which consists of the elevation of immunoreactive LH levels in plasma of oestrogen–progesterone treated ovariectomised rats (Arimura, unpublished). FSH-releasing activity as measured *in vitro* (Negro-Vilar, Dickerman and Meites. 1968a, b) and *in vivo* (Saito, Sawano, Arimura and Schally, 1967) has been reported, and the validity of these assay methods has been questioned.

The presence of LH-RH in the hypophysial portal plasma has been demonstrated by bioassay (Fink, 1967; Fink, Nallar and Worthington, 1967; Ben-Jonathan, Mical and Porter, 1973) and by RIA (Sarker, Chiappa, Fink and Sherwood, 1976; Fink and Jamieson, 1973; Neill, Patton, Dailey, Tsau and Tindall, 1977; Eskay, Mical and Porter, 1977). Immunoreactive LH-RH levels in the hypophysial portal plasma of rhesus monkeys has been reported to be within a detectable range (10 pg/ml), significantly elevated during the preovulatory-like LH surge (101 $\pm$ 34 pg/ml) as compared with the follicular phase (23 $\pm$ 5 pg/ml). LH-RH concentrations in the ovariectomised animals ranged from 19–226 pg/ml (Neill *et al.*, 1977).

Many reports on immunoreactive LH-RH levels in the peripheral plasma have appeared but reported values varied considerably between investigators, ranging from non-detectable to as high as several ng/ml (Arimura and Schally, 1975). The difference may be caused by different antisera which have different antigenic determinants and different affinities. The variability of the results also appears to be due to interference by non-specific macromolecules in plasma, especially when unextracted plasma was assayed for LH-RH (Arimura and Schally, 1975; de la Cruz and Arimura, 1975). For a valid assay, it is necessary to remove these interfering substances by ethanol (Arimura and Schally, 1975), acetone (Neill *et al.*, 1977) or Florisil extraction (Groot, Arimura and Bettendorf, 1976). Mean LH-RH activity in the ethanol extract of peripheral plasma from normal women was highest during the midcycle and lowest during the follicular phase (Arimura, Kastin,

Schally, Saito, Kumasaka, Yaoi, Nishi and Ohkura, 1974). However, even during the midcycle, LH-RH was undetectably low in some of the plasma samples, suggesting that increased LH-RH secretion is of short duration, probably pulsatile. This possibility has been supported by demonstration of a pulsatile peak of LH-RH in plasma samples obtained at shorter intervals throughout a 24 hr period. In this experiment, plasma LH-RH levels ranged from non-detectable to 2 pg/ml during the follicular phase, from non-detectable to 18 pg/ml at midcycle and from non-detectable to 5 pg/ml during the luteal phase (Groot et al., 1976).

G. GROWTH HORMONE RELEASING FACTOR (GH-RF)

1. Chemical Constitution and Main Physico-chemical and Biological Properties

The secretion of growth hormone (GH) from the anterior pituitary is regulated by a dual system of hypothalamic control, one inhibitory and one stimulatory (Schally et al., 1973, 1978a, b). The stimulatory effect on GH release of some hypothalamic fractions appears to be due to a GH-RF (Schally, Arimura, Bowers, Kastin, Sawano and Redding, 1968; Schally et al., 1973; Takahara, Arimura and Schally, 1975), which, under some conditions, might predominate over the inhibitory action of somatostatin because of the short half life of the latter. However, despite the intense effort by several groups, the nature of the physiological GH-RF is still unknown.

Several substances found in the hypothalamus and/or higher brain centres such as catecholamines, TRH, endorphins and enkephalins (Cusan, Dupont, Kledzik, Labrie, Coy and Schally, 1977), and other substances such as insulin, arginine, L-dopa, can, under certain conditions, stimulate the release of GH in vivo and in vitro. However, the effect of these substances may be explained by an action via higher brain centres, or a non-specific one.

Attempts to purify GH-RF have been hampered by the presence of large amounts of somatostatin and pro-somatostatin in hypothalamic extracts. However, using antisera to somatostatin or columns of Sepharose linked to antisomatostatin-gamma-globulin to eliminate somatostatin, we have detected several fractions with GH-RF activity, and purified them by gel filtration on Sephadex, CCD, chromatography on CMC and partition. These fractions stimulate the release of growth hormone from pituitary quarters or from monolayer cultures of rat anterior pituitaries at a dose of 1 μg/ml and increase plasma GH in mice (Schally et al., 1978a, b). GH-RF activity appears to be due to materials with properties of polypeptides, but further work is needed to identify them.

2. Localisation, Biosynthesis and Release

Since GH-RF has not been isolated or characterised, and the assay methods are far from satisfactory, only limited information on localisation, biosynthesis and secretion is available. The activity appears to be restricted to the region of the ventromedial nucleus (VMN) of the hypothalamus (Krulich, Illner, Fawcett, Quijada and McCann, 1972; Krulich, Quijada and Illner, 1971). VMN and the basal medial hypothalamus are the only regions directly excitable to augment GH release in electrical stimulation experiments.

3. Methods of Determination

(a) In vitro *methods*

(1) *Stimulation of release of GH in tissue cultures.* (Deuben and Meites, 1964, 1965.) Anterior pituitaries of rats are cultured in a synthetic medium at 35°C in an atmosphere of 95% O_2 and 5% CO_2 as described by Nicoll and Meites (1963). Addition of crude rat hypothalamic extracts to the culture medium will increase the release of GH in tissue cultures of rat anterior pituitaries or reinitiate the GH release after it has declined to insignificant levels. Since 4–6 times more GH was released than originally present in pituitary tissue, an effect of GRF on synthesis of GH is suggested.

(2) *Stimulation of release of GH on short-term incubation of rat anterior pituitary tissue.* The Saffran and Schally (1955) method devised for determination of CRF was adapted by Schally, Steelman and Bowers (1960) for determination of GRF and modification by others (Dickerman, Negro-Vilar and Meites, 1969; Wilber, Nagel and White, 1971; Uehara, Arimura and Schally, 1973/74; Stachura, Dhariwal and Frohman, 1972; Bowers, Chang and Fong, 1977).

(3) *Stimulation of release of GH from cultured pituitary cells.* The method originally described by Vale *et al.* (1972, 1976) is used for assessing GH-RH activity (Machlin, Jacobs, Cirulis, Kimes and Miller, 1974). Rats, cattle or sheep are used as the pituitary donors. GH released into the incubation medium, GH in the culture cells or both, can be determined by RIA.

(4) *Stimulation of GH released from superfused rat pituitaries.* The rat pituitary is superfused in the superfusion chamber and the release of GH into the efflux is determined by RIA. This method is suitable for following moment to moment changes in the secretion rate of GH (Beck, Larkins, Martin and Burger, 1973; Sawano and Kokubu, 1977).

All these *in vitro* methods are convenient, but their specificity is questionable.

(*b*) In vivo *assay*

(*1*) *Elevation of plasma GH in monkey.* The materials are given intravenously into unanaesthetised restrained monkeys (Knobil, 1966), Nembutal
anaesthetised monkeys (Garcia and Geschwind, 1966) or monkeys pretreated
with morphine (Knobil and Meyer, 1967). Plasma GH is then measured by a
radioimmunoassay method. A variety of stimuli will also result in elevation
of plasma GH levels in monkeys (Meyer and Knobil, 1966). Marked responses
to 0·1–0·3 u vasopressin/kg were observed (Meyer and Knobil, 1966) and
similar results were obtained in human subjects (Greenwood and Landon,
1966).

(*2*) *Elevation of plasma immunoreactive GH in the rat.* Rats anaesthetised
with urethane, with or without various pretreatments, are injected i.v. with
test samples and the elevation of plasma immunoreactive GH is used as the
response parameter of GH-RH activity (Kato, Dupre and Beck, 1973;
Malacara, Valverde, Reichlin and Bollinger, 1972; Szabo and Frohman,
1975).

4. GRF Activities in Biological Fluids

In vitro GH release from the pituitary was reported to be induced by a
dialysable factor in acromegalic plasma (Hagen, Lawrence and Kirsteins,
1972). It was also claimed that bioassayable GH-RH activity can be detected
in rat hypophysial portal blood after VMN stimulation, and in the peripheral
blood in freely moving rats. The rise in GH-RH activity in the peripheral
blood preceded pulsatile GH secretory episodes (Willoughby, Matin,
Brazeau and Renaud, 1975). GH biosynthesis *in vitro* was said to be stimulated by CSF from acromegalic patients (Barbato, Lawrence and Kirsteins,
1974).

H. GROWTH HORMONE RELEASE INHIBITING HORMONE (GH-RIH; SOMATOSTATIN)

1. Chemical Constitution and Main Physico-chemical and Biological Properties

Somatostatin (growth hormone release-inhibiting hormone; GH-RIH) was
isolated from ovine (Brazeau, Vale, Burgus, Ling, Butcher, Rivier and
Guillemin, 1973) and subsequently porcine (Schally, Dupont, Arimura,
Redding and Linthicum, 1975; Schally, Dupont, Arimura, Redding, Nishi,
Linthicum and Schlesinger, 1967b) hypothalami by its ability to inhibit

tetradecapeptide is identical in both species (Brazeau *et al.*, 1973; Schally *et al.*, 1976b):

H–Ala–Gly–Cys–Lys–Asn–Phe–Phe–Trp–Lys–Thr–Phe–Thr–Ser–Cys–OH.

Somatostatin was synthesised by several groups (Rivier, Brazeau, Vale, Ling, Burgus, Gilon, Yardley and Guillemin, 1973; Coy, Coy, Arimura and Schally, 1973; Yamashiro and Li, 1973). Both the reduced dihydro linear form and oxidised cyclic form are active.

The calculated mw of this tetradecapeptide is 1639, but the synthetic product as the hepta-acetate and $5H_2O$ has a mw of 2147. The specific rotation $[\alpha]^{25}$ has been reported to be from $-33\cdot3°$ (Rivier *et al.*, 1973) to $-39\cdot5°$ (1% solution on 0·1% acetic acid) (Coy *et al.*, 1973).

Synthetic somatostatin was found to produce a variety of actions, not only on the pituitary, but also on diverse hormones and other substances from many tissues, including the pancreas, stomach, gut and brain. These effects appear to be of physiological significance since somatostatin is present in high concentrations within those tissues affected by the hormone (Arimura, Sato, Dupont, Nishi and Schally, 1975c; see also sections which follow).

Thus somatostatin inhibits both basal and stimulated secretion of GH from the pituitary *in vitro* and *in vivo* in several species, including humans (Schally and Arimura, 1977; Vale, Rivier and Brown, 1977; Hall, Besser, Schally, Coy, Evered, Goldie, Kastin, McNeilly, Mortimer, Phenekos, Tunbridge and Weightman, 1973; Siler, Vandenberg, Yen, Brazeau, Vale and Guillemin, 1973). Somatostatin also suppresses the TRH-induced secretion of TSH, *in vitro* and *in vivo*, and it could play a physiological role in the regulation of TSH secretion (Carr, Gomez-Pan, Weightman, Roy, Hall, Besser, Thorner, McNeilly, Schally, Kastin and Coy, 1975). The release of prolactin *in vitro* is also decreased by somatostatin.

Somatostatin inhibits both basal and stimulated secretion of insulin and glucagon by a direct action on the β and α pancreatic islet cells respectively (Hall and Gomez-Pan, 1976; Schally and Arimura, 1977; Alberti, Christensen, Christensen, Prange-Hansen, Iversen, Lundbaek, Seyer-Hansen and Orskow, 1973). Somatostatin affects the exocrine pancreas as well, inhibiting pancreatic bicarbonate and protein secretion (Boden, Sivitz, Owen, Essa-Koumar and Landor, 1975; Konturek, Tasler, Obtulowicz, Coy and Schally, 1976b). Somatostatin also decreases the circulating levels of gastrin in man (Bloom, Mortimer, Thorner, Besser, Hall, Gomez-Pan, Roy, Russell, Coy, Kastin and Schally, 1974) and in dogs (Konturek, Tasler, Cieszkowska, Coy and Schally, 1976a). From the inhibition of pentagastrin-induced gastric acid and pepsin secretion in cats and dogs, we concluded that, in addition to inhibiting gastrin release, somatostatin also exerts a direct antisecretory effect on both parietal and peptic cells (Gomez-Pan, Reed, Albinus, Shaw, Hall, Besser, Coy, Kastin and Schally, 1975; Konturek et al., 1976a). Thus, this hormone can exert exocrine, as well as endocrine, effects (Gomez-Pan et al., 1975). Somatostatin also suppresses the release of secretin and cholecystokinin/pancreozymin from the duodenal mucosa (Boden et al., 1975; Konturek et al., 1976b), the release of gastric inhibitory polypeptide, vasoactive intestinal polypeptide, motilin and renin (Besser and Mortimer, 1976; Hall and Gomez-Pan, 1976).

2. Localisation, Biosynthesis, Release and Metabolism

(a) Localisation and cells of origin

Somatostatin or somatostatin-like activity (SLA) as tested by both biological (Krulich, Illner, Fawcett, Quijada and McCann, 1972; Vale, Rivier, Palkovits, Saavedra and Brownstein, 1974) and immunological techniques (Alpert, Brawer, Jackson and Patel, 1975; Arimura and Schally, 1975; Brownstein, Arimura, Sato, Schally and Kizer, 1975; Dube, Leclerc, Pelletier, Arimura and Schally, 1975) has been shown to be concentrated in the median eminence. Electronmicroscopic immunocytochemistry has demonstrated that somatostatin is present in granules in numerous nerve endings adjacent to the primary capillary plexus of the hypophysial portal system (Pelletier, Labrie, Arimura and Schally, 1974) suggesting a neurosecretory mechanism for the delivery of somatostatin to the adenohypophysis. Somatostatin is also found in relatively high concentrations in hypothalamic areas other than the median eminence. Those include the arcuate nucleus, VMN, premammillary nucleus and periventricular nucleus (Brownstein et al., 1975).

Somatostatin activity was also found in the extrahypothalamic brain as revealed by bioassay (Vale et al., 1974) and immunological techniques (Brownstein et al., 1975; Vale, Ling, Rivier, Rivier, Villarreal and Brown, 1976; Hökfelt, Efendic, Hellerstrom, Johansson, Luft and Arimura, 1974). More than 90% of the total somatostatin-like substance in the brain is found in the extrahypothalamic area, and distributed throughout the brain with high concentrations in the preoptic and septal region, amygdala and circumventricular organs (Alpert, Brawer, Patel and Reichlin, 1976; Brownstein et al., 1975; Dube et al., 1975; Kizer, Palkovits and Brownstein, 1976). SLA was demonstrated in the substantia gelatinosa of the dorsal horn of the spinal cord and in the adjacent parts of the lateral funiculus, in a few spinal ganglion cells (Hökfelt et al., 1974), in neurones in the myenteric plexus and neuronal cell bodies in the mucosa and submucosa of intestines (Costa, Patel, Furness and Arimura, 1977).

In addition, SLA was identified in the pancreas, stomach and intestines by immunocytochemistry (Dubois, 1975; Dubois, Paulin, Assan and Dubois,

1975; Hökfelt et al., 1975; Luft, Efendic, Hökfelt, Johansson and Arimura, 1974), by radioimmunoassays (Arimura, Sato, Dupont, Nishi and Schally, 1975c; Patel, Weir and Reichlin, 1975; Vale et al., 1976; Patel and Weir, 1976) and by bioassays (Vale et al., 1976). SLA was demonstrated in pancreatic D-cells, the products of which had remained unknown until recently (Goldsmith, Rose, Arimura and Ganong, 1975; Hökfelt et al., 1975; Polak, Pearse, Grimelius, Bloom and Arimura, 1975; Orci, Baetens, Dubois and Rufener, 1975). The close proximity of D-cells to A- and B-cells in the pancreatic islets and suppression of insulin and glucagon secretion by exogenous somatostatin has led to a view that D-cells have a functional role in regulating A- and B-cell activities (Dubois, 1975; Luft, et al., 1974). Pancreatic somatostatin-like activity has been reported to increase in streptozotocin diabetic rats and juvenile-type diabetes in humans (Orci, Baetens, Rufener, Amherat, Ravvazzolo, Studer, Malaise-Lagae and Unger, 1976), and to decrease in spontaneously diabetic mice (Patel, Cameron, Stefan, Malaisse-Lagae and Orci, 1977).

In the gastrointestinal tract, SLA was found in the highest concentrations in the fundus and antrum of the stomach (Arimura et al., 1975b). Somatostatin-like activity has been found in various vertebrate species, including birds, amphibians, fish and teleost (Dupont, Barry and Leonardelli, 1974; Vale et al., 1976). In mammals, the highest concentration of somatostatin-like activity (2·5 ng/mg) occurs in the hypothalamus, but the greatest amount is found in the gastrointestinal tract. On the other hand, in lower species, the highest concentration has been found in the pancreas, particularly in the pigeon (50 ng/mg) and catfish (45 ng/mg) (Vale et al., 1976).

(b) Biosynthesis

Incubation of pancreatic islets of anglerfish with ^{14}C-Ile, ^{3}H-Trp and ^{35}S-Cys for longer than 1 hr has been reported to result in the incorporation of ^{3}H-Trp and ^{35}S-Cys, but not ^{14}C-Ile, into a peptide which is indistinguishable from somatostatin, immunologically, electrophoretically and chromatographically. During pulse-chase incubation, no incorporation into somatostatin has been observed immediately after 30 min of pulse, but incorporation of Trp and Cys into somatostatin has increased with the length of the chase in isotope-free medium (Noe, Weir and Bauer, 1977). The incorporation is blocked by cyclohexamide. These findings suggest that somatostatin is synthesised in the islets by de novo synthesis, probably through a larger precursor. An immunoreactive somatostatin of higher mol wt was found in the extracts of the hypothalamus (Schally, Dupont, Arimura, Redding, Nishi, Linthicum and Schlesinger, 1976b; Vale et al., 1976), pancreas and stomach (Arimura et al., 1975c). The extension of the N-terminus in a larger somatostatin-like molecule has been suggested (Vale *et al.*, 1976; Arimura, Lundqvist, Rothman, Chang, Elde, Coy, Meyers and Schally, 1977). Recently, using a synthetic gene for somatostatin, transformation of *E. coli* with the chimeric plasmid DNA led to the synthesis of a polypeptide including the sequence of amino acids corresponding to somatostatin (Itakura, Hirose, Crea, Riggs, Heyneker, Boliver and Boyer, 1977).

(c) *Release of somatostatin*

Presence of somatostatin-like activity in the neuronal process adjacent to the plexus of capillaries in the median eminence suggests that somatostatin is released into the hypophysial blood to be delivered to the adenohypophysis. The concentration of somatostatin-like activity in the hypophysial portal blood has been reported to be 5–11 times greater than that in the systemic blood (Chihara, Arimura and Schally, 1978).

Immunoreactive somatostatin is released from hypothalamic synaptosomes by high concentration of K^+ and dopamine *in vitro* and the release by K^+ was Ca^{++} dependent (Wakabayashi, Miyazawa, Kanda, Miki, Demura, Demura and Shizume, 1977).

The release of pancreatic somatostatin is stimulated by glucose, arginine, leucine, glucagon, secretin, gastrin, cholecystokinin-pancreozymin and tolbutamide (Ipp, Dobbs, Arimura, Vale, Harris and Unger, 1977; Patton, Ipp, Dobbs, Orci, Vale and Unger, 1976; Patton, Ipp, Dobbs, Orci, Vale and Unger, 1977; Chihara, Arimura, Chihara and Schally, 1978). Somatostatin secretion by the pancreatic islets appeared to be cAMP dependent (Barden, Alvarado-Urbina, Cote and Dupont, 1976).

(d) *Degradation and metabolism*

Somatostatin has a short biological half life (less than 4 min) (Hall *et al.*, 1973; Redding and Coy, 1974). This may be due to cleavage by endopeptidases of amino acid sequences within the ring portion of somatostatin (Benuck and Marks, 1976).

3. Methods of Determination

(a) In vitro *assay*

(*1*) *Inhibition of GH release from rat or sheep pituitaries* in vitro. The *in vitro* assay for CRF of Saffran and Schally (1955) as described in Section A.3 can be used with some modification (Uehara, Arimura and Schally, 1973/74). Monolayer cultures of rat pituitary cells are very sensitive to GH-RIH activity and show an excellent dose response curve for somatostatin (Vale, Grant, Amoss, Blackwell and Guillemin, 1972).

(2) *Inhibition of insulin and glucagon release from isolated pancreatic islets* in vitro. Pancreatic islets from rats are prepared by the method as described by Lacy and Kostianovsky (1972). Acutely dispersed cells are insensitive to somatostatin, but the sensitivity is restored after culturing the cells for 1–2 days (Durcot-Lemay, Lemay and Lacy, 1975). These pancreatic cells are incubated with test samples for insulin and glucagon-suppressing activity.

(3) *Inhibition of insulin and glucagon release from superfused pancreatic islets.* Enzymatically digested and cultured rat pancreatic islets are imbedded in Sephadex G-10 in a superfusion-chamber and exposed to the pulse of test samples (Chihara, Arimura, Chihara and Schally, 1978). Decreases in concentrations of insulin and glucagon in the efflux as compared to those before the pulse are used as the response parameters.

(4) *Inhibition of insulin and glucagon release from rat pancreatic slices* in vitro. Suppression of insulin and glucagon release by test samples during incubation for 30 min is used as the response parameter (Basabe, Cresto and Aparicio, 1977).

(5) *Inhibition of insulin and glucagon release from monolayer cultures of rat pancreatic islet.* Islet cells are prepared from neonatal rat pancreas by enzymatic digestion and cultured as described by Lambert, Blondel, Kanazawa, Orci and Renold (1972). Release of insulin and glucagon from the monolayer cultures of the islet cells are inhibited by somatostatin in a dose-related manner (Wollheim, Blondel, Renold and Sharp, 1977; Fujimoto, Ensinck and Williams, 1974).

(b) In vivo *method*

(1) *Suppression of Nembutal or morphine-induced elevation of plasma GH levels in rats.* Both anesthetised and conscious rats are used. Test samples and Nembutal or morphine are injected (s.c.) simultaneously or at various intervals. Blood is collected 10–30 min after injection. Suppression of Nembutal or morphine-elicited GH rise by test samples as compared to serum GH levels after Nembutal or morphine alone is used as the response parameter (Brazeau, Rivier, Vale and Guillemin, 1974; Brazeau and Martin, 1975).

(2) *Suppression of plasma GH levels in gentled rats.* Handling rats for several days to accustom the animals to manipulation results in an elevation of basal plasma GH levels. Administration of substances with GH-RIH activity causes a decrease of plasma GH levels which can be used as the response parameter for GH-RIH (Brazeau *et al.*, 1974).

(3) *Suppression of arginine-induced elevation of plasma insulin and glucagon levels in rats.* Arginine is infused i.v. in anaesthetised rats alone or with substances to be tested, and plasma is analysed for insulin and glucagon by

RIA. Suppression of plasma insulin and glucagon by test materials is estimated by comparing those after arginine infusion alone. A dose-related suppression has been demonstrated and the method is used as a semiquantitative assay for insulin and glucagon suppression (Gordin, Meyers, Arimura, Coy and Schally, 1977).

(4) *Suppression of insulin and glucagon levels in hepatic portal plasma in rats.* Basal levels of insulin and glucagon in the hepatic plasma are higher than those in the peripheral plasma. Suppression of basal hormone levels in the hepatic portal plasma by administration of somatostatin or related substances is dose-related and can be used as a response parameter for somatostatin-like activity (Brown, Vale and Rivier, 1977).

(5) *Inhibition of glucagon and insulin secretion from the pancreas perfused in situ.* The pancreas of rat (Johnson, Ensinick, Koerker, Palmer and Goodner, 1975; Erich, Lovinger and Grodsky, 1975) or dog (Sakurai, Dobbs and Unger, 1974) is perfused by a buffer solution or a buffer containing somatostatin or test substances, and the decrease of the release of insulin and glucagon by somatostatin or test substances is used as the response parameter.

(c) *Radioimmunoassays for somatostatin*

Specific antisera against synthetic somatostatin conjugated with carrier protein by means of glutaraldehyde (Arimura, Sato, Coy and Schally, 1975b) or carbodiimide (Kronheim, Berelowitz and Pimstone, 1976; Patel et al., 1975) have been generated. Radioimmunoassay methods for somatostatin have been established using ^{125}I-labelled Tyr^1-somatostatin or N-Tyr-somatostatin as the tracer (Arimura et al., 1975a; Kronheim et al., 1976; Patel et al., 1975). These antisera have been reported to recognise the amino acid sequence corresponding to position 5 through 11 or 13 of somatostatin including the ring portion (Arimura, 1978; Arimura et al., 1977; Vale et al., 1976). Another antiserum, the recognition site of which is directed toward the N-terminus, has also been generated by using human serum albumin-conjugated Tyr^{11}-somatostatin in rabbits (Vale et al., 1976). The radioimmunoassays for somatostatin are highly sensitive and specific (Arimura et al., 1977; Kronheim et al., 1976). Radioimmunoassays are successfully used for determining somatostatin-like substances in tissue extracts and the estimated values reported by different investigators show quite good agreement, even though different antisera were used.

4. Somatostatin in Biological Fluids

(a) Plasma

Plasma somatostatin levels reported by different laboratories vary considerably, probably due to the presence of substances which interfere with the tracer-antibody binding in a non-specific manner. The extent of such non-specific interference appears to vary among plasma of different species and also differs depending on the affinity constant of the antiserum used (Arimura, unpublished).

The concentrations of somatostatin-like activity (SLA) in unextracted dog plasma as determined by RIA were around 130 pg/ml in systemic plasma, and 275 pg/ml in the hepatic portal plasma. During glucose infusion, an increase of SLA was demonstrated only in the plasma from the pancreatic duodenal vein. SLA levels in the peripheral plasma in alloxan diabetic and insulin-deprived dogs have been higher than those in normal dogs and in diabetic and insulin treated dogs (Schusdziarra, Dobbs, Harris and Unger, 1977). On the other hand, SLA in the acetone-extract of systemic plasma of the dog was usually lower than 10 pg/ml. The highest concentration (35–69 pg/ml) was found in the plasma from vena gastrica brevis, which collect blood from the body of the stomach, followed by plasma from vena pancreatico-duodenalis and vena gastroepiploica dextra (Arimura, Itoh, Aizawa and Rothman, 1978). Since the recovery of somatostatin added to plasma after extraction with acetone is about 80%, the difference in plasma SLA levels between unextracted and acetone-extracted plasma appears to be due to acetone-precipitable macromolecules which show immuno-reactivity in unextracted plasma. Although we believe that extraction is necessary for a valid assay of plasma somatostatin, this problem has not been settled.

(b) Cerebrospinal fluid (CSF)

SLA has been demonstrated in CSF in humans, the mean concentration being 35 pg/ml in normal subjects. SLA in CSF was said to be elevated in patients with nerve root compression, intrinsic spinal cord disease and cerebral disease (Patel, Roa and Reichlin, 1977). These results suggest that under normal circumstances, SLA in CSF comes from the hypothalamus. However, some of the CSF specimens do not show parallel inhibition curves to the standard curve, suggesting that some SLA in the CSF is attributable to some substances other than true somatostatin (Arimura, 1978).

In collaboration with Dr. R. Randall, we estimated the mean SLA concentration in CSF from patients with a variety of diseases as being 46 pg/ml. SLA in CSF from a patient with active acromegaly was undetectable

(Arimura, 1978). Patel *et al.* (1977) reported that CSF SLA levels were normal or low in acromegaly and low or undetectable in patients with pituitary tumours involving the hypothalamus.

CONCLUSIONS

Three hypothalamic hypophysiotrophic hormones, TRH, LH-RH and somatostatin have been isolated, characterised, synthesised and validated for their physiological roles. The work of isolating other hypothalamic hormones is in progress. Antisera against these three synthetic hormones have been generated to develop radioimmunoassay (RIA) and immunocytological methods. The results of studies using these methods prompted research on these hypothalamic hormones at the molecular level and provided new information on biosynthesis, secretion, receptors and mechanism of action. In addition, demonstration of hypothalamic hormones in extrahypothalamic tissues, including brain cortex, spinal cord, as well as gastrointestinal organs, pancreas and others has led to a new concept on the relationship between neurones and endocrine cells. This new concept, taken together with the concept of APUD cell group proposed by Pearse (1976), appears to lift the barrier between endocrine cells and neurones. Since one hypothalamic hormone may show multiple actions on various target tissues and organs, therefore, this hormone must be assayed for its multiple activities. Wide distribution of those hormones in various organs may obscure the origin of the hormonal activity in plasma and other biological fluids. In addition, a rapid inactivation of these peptide hormones in circulation and non-specific interference with RIA by plasma components require extreme caution in performing valid assays for the relatively minute amounts of these peptide hormones in plasma. Nevertheless, reported fluctuations in the levels of those hypothalamic releasing or inhibiting activities in the hypophysial portal plasma, in the systemic plasma or in the venous plasma from the hormone-rich organs under various physiological and pathological conditions suggest that plasma hormone levels reflect the secretory status of these hormones, and provide new understanding of the physiology, and perhaps pathophysiology of those systems.

REFERENCES

Alberti, K. G. M. M., Christensen, N. J., Christensen, S. E., Prange-Hansen, A., Iversen, J., Lundbaek, K., Seyer-Hansen, K. and Ørskov, H. (1973). *Lancet*, **ii**, 1299.

Alpert, L. C., Brawer, J. R., Jackson, I. M. D. and Patel, Y. (1975). *Endocrinology*, **95**, 239A.

Alpert, L. C., Brawer, J. R., Patel, Y. C. and Reichlin, S. (1976). *Endocrinology*, **98**, 255.

Amoss, M., Burgus, R., Blackwell, R., Vale, W., Fellows, R. and Guillemin, R. (1971). *Biochem. biophys. Res. Commun.* **44**, 205.

Anderson, E. (1966). *Science*, **152**, 379.

Araki, S., Ferin, M., Zimmerman, E. A. and Vande Wiele, R. L. (1975). *Endocrinology*, **96**, 644.

Arimura, A. (1978). Proc. Int. Symp. Applic. Radioassay Syst. Clin. Endocr., Los Angeles.

Arimura, A., Bowers, C. Y., Schally, A. V., Saito, M. and Miller, M. C. (1969). *Endocrinology*, **85**, 300.

Arimura, A., Debeljuk, L. and Schally, A. V. (1972). *Endocrinology*, **91**, 529.

Arimura, A., Itoh, Z., Aizawa, I. and Rothman, J. (1978). Prog. 60th Ann. Meet. Endocr. Soc.

Arimura, A., Kastin, A. J., Schally, A. V., Saito, M., Kumasaka, T., Yaoi, Y., Nishi, N. and Ohkura, K. (1974). *J. clin. Endocr. Metab.* **38**, 510.

Arimura, A., Lundqvist, G., Rothman, J., Chang, R., Elde, R., Coy, D. H., Meyers, C. and Schally, A. V. (1977). Proc. Int. Symp. Somatostatin, Freiburg.

Arimura, A., Saito, T., Bowers, C. Y. and Schally, A. V. (1967a). *Acta endocr., Copnh.* **54**, 155.

Arimura, A., Saito, T. and Schally, A. V. (1967b). *Endocrinology*, **81**, 235.

Arimura, A., Sato, H., Coy, D. H., Worobec, R. B., Schally, A. V., Yanaihara, N., Hashimoto, T., Yanaihara, C. and Sukura, N. (1975a). *Acta endocr., Copnh.* **78**, 222.

Arimura, A., Sato, H., Coy, D. H. and Schally, A. V. (1975b). *Proc. Soc. exp. Biol. Med.* **148**, 784.

Arimura, A., Sato, H., Dupont, A., Nishi, N. and Schally, A. V. (1975c). *Science*, **189**, 1007.

Arimura, A., Sato, H., Kumasaka, T., Worobec, R. B., Debeljuk, L., Dunn, J. and Schally, A. V. (1973). *Endocrinology*, **93**, 1092.

Arimura, A. and Schally, A. V. (1975). "Hypothalamic Hormones", p. 27. Academic Press, London and New York.

Arimura, A. and Schally, A. V. (1976). "Basic Applications and Clinical Uses of Hypothalamic Hormones" (A. L. Charro-S, R. Fernandez-D. and J. G. Lopez-d-C, eds), p. 130. Exerpta Med. Int. Cong. Ser. No. 374, Amsterdam.

Arimura, A., Takahara, J., Davis, S., Nishi, N. and Schally, A. V. (1976). "Basic Applications and Clinical Uses of Hypothalamic Hormones" (A. L. Charro-S, R. Fernandez-D. and J. G. Lopez-d-C, eds), p. 200. Exerpta Med, Int. Cong. Ser. No. 374, Amsterdam.

Asai, T. and Wakabayashi, K. (1975). *Endocr. jap.* **22**, 319.

Bakke, J. L., Lawrence, N. L., Bennett, J. and Robinson, S. (1975). *Endocrinology*, **97**, 659.

Barbato, T., Lawrence, A. M. and Kirsteins, L. (1974). *Lancet.* **i**, 599.

Barden, N., Alvarado-Urbino, G., Cote, J. P. and Dupont, A. (1976). *Biochem. biophys. Res. Commun.* **71**, 840.

Barnea, A., Ben-Jonathan, N., Colston, C., Johnston, J. M. and Porter, J. C. (1975a). *Proc. natn. Acad. Sci., USA*, **72**, 3153.

Barnea, A., Ben-Jonathan, N. and Porter, J. C. (1975b). *Feb. Proc.* **34**, 239.

Barraclough, C. A. (1967). "Neuroendocrinology", Vol. II, p. 61. Academic Press, New York and London.

Barry, J. and Carette, B. (1975). *Cell Tiss. Res.* **164**, 163.

Barry, J. and Dubois, M. P. (1975). *Neuroendocrinology*, **18**, 290.

Barry, J., Dubois, M. P. and Carette, B. (1974). *Endocrinology*, **95**, 1416.

Basabe, J. C., Cresto, J. C. and Aparicio, N. (1977). *Endocrinology*, **101**, 1436.

Bassiri, R. M. and Utiger, R. D. (1972). *Endocrinology*, **90**, 722.

Bassiri, R. M. and Utiger, R. D. (1973). *J. clin. Invest.* **52**, 1616.

Bassiri, R. M. and Utiger, R. D. (1974). *Endocrinology*, **94**, 188.

Bauer, K. (1976). *Nature, Lond.* **259**, 591.

Bauer, K. and Lipmann, F. (1976). *Endocrinology*, **99**, 230.

Baugh, C. M., Krumdieck, C. L., Hershman, J. M. and Pittman, Jr., J. A. (1970). *Endocrinology*, **87**, 1015.

Beck, C., Larkins, R. G., Martin, T. J. and Burger, H. G. (1973). *J. endocr.* **59**, 325.

Ben-Jonathan, N., Mical, R. S. and Porter, J. C. (1970). *Endocrinology*, **93**, 497.

Ben-Jonathan, N., Oliver, C., Weiner, H. J., Mical, R. S. and Porter, J. C. (1977). *Endocrinology*, **100**, 458.

Bennett, G. W. and Edwardson, J. A. (1975). *J. endocr.* **65**, 33.

Bennett, G. W., Edwardson, J. A., Holand, D. T., Jeffcoate, S. L. and White, N. (1975). *Nature, Lond.* **257**, 323.

Benuck, M. and Marks, N. (1976). *Life Sci.* **19**, 1271.

Besser, G. M. and Mortimer, C. H. (1976). "Frontiers in Neuroendocrinology", p. 227. Raven Press, New York.

Birge, C. A., Jacobs, L. S., Hammer, C. T. and Daughaday, W. H. (1970). *Endocrinology*, **86**, 120.

Blash, D. E., Vaughn, M. K., Reiter, R. J., Johnson, L. Y. and Vaughn, G. (1976). *Endocrinology*, **99**, 152.

Bloom, S. R., Mortimer, C. H., Thorner, M. O., Besser, G. M., Hall, R., Gomez-Pan, A., Roy, V. M., Russell, R. C. G., Coy, D. H., Kastin, A. J. and Schally, A. V. (1974). *Lancet*, **ii**, 1109.

Boden, G., Sivitz, M. C., Owen, O. E., Essa-Koumar, N. and Landor, J. H. (1975). *Science*, **190**, 163.

Bøler, J., Enzmann, F., Folkers, K., Bowers, C. Y. and Schally, A. V. (1969). *Biochem. biophys. Res. Commun.* **37**, 705.

Bowers, C. Y., Chang, I. K. and Fong, T. T. W. (1977). Prog. 59th Ann. Meet. Endocr. Soc. Abstr. No. 351.

Bowers, C. Y., Currie, B. L., Johansson, K. N. G. and Folkers, K. (1973). *Biochem. biophys. Res. Commun.* **50**, 20.

Bowers, C. Y., Friesen, H., Hwang, P., Guyda, H. and Folkers, K. (1971). *Biochem. biophys. Res. Commun.* **45**, 1033.

Bowers, C. Y., Redding, T. W. and Schally, A. V. (1965). *Endocrinology*, **77**, 609.

Bowers, C. Y., Schally, A. V., Enzmann, F., Bøler, J. and Folkers, K., (1970). *Endocrinology*, **86**, 1143.

Boyd, A. E., Spencer, E., Jackson, I. M. D. and Reichlin, S. (1976). *Endocrinology*, **99**, 861.

Bradbury, M. W., Burden, J., Hillhouse, E. W. and Jones, M. T. (1974). *J. Physiol., Lond.* **239**, 269.

Brazeau, P. and Martin, J. B. (1975). "Hypothalamus and Endocrine Functions", p. 379. Plenum Press, New York.

Brazeau, P., Rivier, J., Vale, W. and Guillemin, R. (1974). *Endocrinology*, **94**, 184.

Brazeau, P., Vale, W., Burgus, R., Ling, N., Butcher, M., Rivier, J. and Guillemin, R. (1973). *Science*, **179**, 77.

Brodish, A. (1963). *Endocrinology*, **73**, 727.

Brodish, A. (1964). *Endocrinology*, **74**, 28.

Brodish, A. (1977). *Ann. N.Y. Acad. Sci.* **297**, 420.

Brodish, A. and Long, C. N. H. (1962), *Endocrinology*, **71**, 298.

Brown, M., Vale, W. and Rivier, J. (1977). Proc. Int. Symp. Somatostatin, Freiburg.

Brownstein, M., Arimura, A., Sato, H., Schally, A. V. and Kizer, J. S. (1975). *Endocrinology*, **96**, 1456.

Burden, J., Hillhouse, F. W. and Jones, M. T. (1974). *J. Physiol. Lond.* **239**, 116P.

Burgus, R., Butcher, M., Amoss, M., Ling, N., Monahan, M., Rivier, J., Fellows, R., Blackwell, R., Vale, W. and Guillemin, R. (1972). *Proc. natn. Acad. Sci. USA*, **69**, 278.

Burgus, R., Dunn, T. F., Desiderio, D. and Guillemin, R. (1969). *C.r. hebd. Seanc. Acad. Sci. Paris*, **269**, 1870.

Burgus, R., Dunn, T. F., Desiderio, D., Ward, D. N., Vale, W. and Guillemin, R. (1970). *Nature, Lond.* **226**, 321.

Carr, D., Gomez-Pan, A., Weightman, D. R., Roy, V. C. M., Hall, R., Besser, G. M., Thorner, M. O., McNeilly, A. S., Schally, A. V., Kastin, A. J. and Coy, D. H. (1975). *Br. med. J.* **3**, 67.

Celis, M. E., Macagno, R. and Taleisnik, S. (1973). *Endocrinology*, **93**, 1229.

Celis, M. E. and Taleisnik, S. (1971). *Int. J. Neurosci.* **1**, 223.

Celis, M. E., Taleisnik, S., Walter, R. (1971a). *Biochem. biophys. Res. Commun.* **45**, 564.

Celis, M. E., Taleisnik, S., Walter, R. (1971b). *Proc. natn Acad. Sci.* USA, **68**, 1428.

Chihara, M., Arimura, A., Chihara, K. and Schally, A. V. (1978a). *Fed. Proc.* **37**, 338.

Chihara, K., Arimura, A. and Schally, A. V. (1978b). *Fed. Proc.* **37**, 638.

Cooper, D. M. F., Synetos, D., Christie, R. B., Schulster, D. (1976). *J. Endocr.* **71**, 171.

Costa, M., Patel, Y., Furness, J. B. and Arimura, A. (1977). *Neurosci. Lett.* **6**, 215.

Coy, D. H., Coy, E. J., Arimura, A. and Schally, A. V. (1973). *Biochem. biophys. Res. Commun.* **54**, 1267.

Cusan, L., Dupont, A., Kledzik, G. S., Labrie, F., Coy, D. H. and Schally, A. V. (1977). *Nature, Lond*, **268**, 544.

Dahlstrom, A. and Fuxe, K. (1964). *Acta physiol. scand.* **323S**, 1.

Debeljuk, L., Redding, T. W., Arimura, A. and Schally, A. V. (1973). *Proc. Soc. exp. Biol. Med.* **142**, 421.

De la Cruz, K. and Arimura, A. (1975). Prog. 57th Ann. Meet. Endocr. Soc. Abstr. No. 106.

DeLeon, A., Beaulieu, D. and Labrie, F. (1974). *Clin. Res.* **22**, 730A.

Deuben, R. R. and Meites, J. (1964). *Endocrinology*, **74**, 408.

Deuben. R. R. and Meites, J. (1965). *Proc. Soc. exp. Biol. Med.* **118**, 409.

Dickerman, S., Kledzik, G., Gelato, M., Chen, H. J. and Meites, J., (1974). *Neuroendocrinology*, **15**, 10.

Dickerman, E., Negro-Villar, A. and Meites, J. (1969). *Neuroendocrinology*, **4**, 75.

Dube, D., Leclerc, R., Pelletier, G., Arimura, A. and Schally, A. V. (1975). *Cell Tiss. Res.* **161**, 385.

Dubois, M. P. (1975). *Proc. natn Acad. Sci. USA*, **72**, 1340.

Ducommun, P., Sakiz, E. and Guillemin, R. (1965). *Endocrinology*, **77**, 792.

Dular, R., Labella, F., Vivian, S. and Eddie, L. (1974). *Endocrinology*, **94**, 563.

Durcot-Lemay, L., Lemay, A. and Lacy, P. E. (1975). *Biophys. biochem. Res. Commun.* **63**, 1130.

Edwardson, J. A. and Gilbert, D. (1976). *J. endocr.* **68**, 197.

Egdahl, R. H. (1960). *Endocrinology,* **66**, 200.

Enjalbert, A., Moos, F., Carbonell, M., Priam, M. and Kordon, C. (1977). *Neuroendocrinology,* **24**, 147.

Eskay, R. L., Mical, R. S. and Porter, J. C. (1977). *Endocrinology,* **100**, 263.

Eskay, R. L., Warberg, J., Mical, R. S. and Porter, J. C. (1975). *Endocrinology,* **97**, 816.

Fink, G. (1967). *J. physiol.* **191**, 125.

Fink, G. and Jamieson, M. G. (1976). *J. Endocr.* **68**, 71.

Fink, G., Nallar, R. and Worthington Jr., W. C. (1967). *J. Physiol.* **191**, 407.

Fleischer, N. and Vale, W. (1968). *Endocrinology,* **83**, 1232.

Folkers, K., Enzmann, F., Bøler, J., Bowers, C. Y. and Schally, A. V. (1969). *Biochem. biophys. Res. Commun.* **37**, 123.

Frohman, L. A. and Szabo, M. (1975). *Endocrinology,* **96**, A86.

Fujimoto, W. Y., Ensinck, J. W. and Williams, R. H. (1974). *Life Sci.* **15**, 1999.

Fuxe, K. (1964). *Z. Zellforsch.* **61**, 710.

Fuxe, K. and Hokfelt, T. (1966). *Acta physiol. scand.* **66**, 245.

Gale, C. C., Hayward, J. S., Green, W. L., Wu, S. Y., Schiller, H. and Jackson, I. (1975). *Fed. Proc.* **34**, 301.

Gallardo, E. and Ramirez, V. D. (1977). *Proc. Soc. exp. Biol. Med.* **155**, 79.

Garcia, J. F. and Geschwind, I. I. (1966). *Nature, Lond.* **211**. 372.

Geiger, R., Konig, W., Wissman, H., Geisen, K. and Enzmann, F. (1971). *Biochem. biophys. Res. Commun.* **45**, 767.

Gibbs, D. M. and Neill, J. D. (1978). *Fed. Proc.* **37**, 555.

Gillessen, D., Felix, A. M., Lergier, W. and Studer, R. O. (1970). *Helv. Chim. Acta.* **53**, 63.

Gillham, B., Jones, M. T., Hillhouse, E. W. and Burden, J. (1975). *J. Endocr.* **65**, 12P.

Goldsmith, P. C., Rose, J. C., Arimura, A. and Ganong, W. F. (1975). *Endocrinology,* **97**, 1901.

Gomez-Pan, A., Reed, J. D., Albinus, M., Shaw, B., Hall, R., Besser, G. M., Coy, D. H., Kastin, A. J. and Schally, A. V. (1975). *Lancet,* **i**, 888.

Gorbman, A. and Hyder, M. (1973). *Gen. comp. Endocr.* **20**, 588.

Gordin, A., Meyers, C., Arimura, A., Coy, D. H. and Schally, A. V. (1977). *Acta endocr., Copenh.* **86**, 833.

Grant, N. H., Clark, D. E. and Rosanoff, E. I. (1973). *Biochem. biophys. Res. Commun.* **51**, 100.

Grant, G., Vale, W. and Guillemin, R. (1973). *Endocrinology,* **92**, 1629.

Greenwood, F. C. and Landon, J. (1966). *Nature, Lond.* **210**, 540.

Griffiths, E. C., Hooper, K. C., Jeffcoate, S. L. and Holland, D. T. (1974). *Acta endocr., Copenh.* **77**, 435.

Grimm-Jorgensen, Y. and McKelvy, J. F. (1976). *Brain Res. Bull.* **1**, 171.

Grindeland, R. E., Wherry, F. E. and Anderson, E. (1962). *Proc. Soc. exp. Biol. Med.* **110**, 377.

Groot-de la Cruz, K., Arimura, Z. and Bettendorf, G. (1976). *Prog. 5th Int. Cong. Endocr. Abst.* No. 312, p. 128.

Guillemin, R. and Schally, A. V. (1959). *Endocrinology,* **65**, 555.

Guillemin, R., Yamazaki, E., Gard, D., Jutisz, M. and Sakiz, E. (1963). *Endocrinology,* **73**, 564.

Hagen, T. C., Garthwaite, T. L. and Martinson, D. R. (1977). *Proc. Soc. exp. Biol. Med.* **156**, 518.

Hagen, T. C., Guansing, A. R. and Sill, A. J. (1976). *Neuroendocrinology*, **21**, 256.

Hagen, T. C., Lawrence, A. M. and Kirsteins, L. (1972). *J. clin. Endocr. Metab.* **33**, 448.

Hall, R., Besser, G. M., Schally, A. V., Coy, D. H., Evered, D., Goldie, D. J., Kastin, A. J., McNeilly, A. S., Mortimer, C. H., Phenekos, C., Tunbridge, W. M. G. and Weightman, D. (1973). *Lancet*, **ii**, 581.

Hall, R. and Gomez-Pan, A. (1976). "Advances in Clinical Chemistry", p. 173. Academic Press, New York and London.

Hall, R. W. and Steinberger, E. (1976). *Neuroendocrinology*, **21**, 111.

Harris, G. W. (1955). "Neural Control of the Pituitary Gland." Arnold Press, London.

Hillhouse, E. W. and Jones, M. T. (1976). *J. Endocr.* **71**, 21.

Hinkle, P. M. and Tashjian Jr., A. (1975). *Biochemistry*, **14**, 3845.

Hinkle, P., Woroch, E. and Tashjian Jr., A. (1974). *J. biol. Chem.* **249**, 3085.

Hirata, Y., Matsujura, S., Imura, H., Nakamura, M. and Tanaka, A. (1976). *J. clin. Endocr. Metab.* **42**, 33.

Hiroshige, T., Fujieda, K., Kaneko, M. and Honma, K. (1977). *Ann. N.Y. Acad. Sci.* **257**, 436.

Hiroshige, T., Kunita, H., Yoshimura, K. and Itoh, S. (1968). *Jap. J. Physiol.* **18**, 179.

Hiroshige, T. and Sato, T. (1970). *Endocrinology*, **86**, 1174.

Hiroshige, T., Sato, T., Ohta, R. and Itoh, S. (1969). *Jap. J. Physiol.* **19**, 866.

Hökfelt, T., Efendic, S., Hellerstrom. C., Johansson, O., Luft, R. and Arimura, A. (1975a). *Acta endocr., Copenh.* Suppl. 200.

Hökfelt, T., Efendic, S., Johansson, O., Luft, R. and Arimura, A. (1974). *Brain Res.* **80**, 165.

Hökfelt, T., Fuxe, K., Johansson, O., Jeffcoate, S. and White, N. (1975b). *Eur. J. Pharmacol.* **34**, 389.

Hruby, V. J., Smith, C. W., Bowers, S. A. and Hadley, M. E. (1972). *Science*, **176**, 1331.

Hunter, W. M. and Greenwood, F. C. (1962). *Nature, Lond*, **194**, 495.

Ipp, E., Dobbs, R. E., Arimura, A., Vale, W., Harris, V. and Unger, R. (1977). *J. clin. Invest.* **60**, 760.

Itakura, K., Hirose, T., Crea, R., Riggs, A. D., Heyneker, H. L., Bolivar, F. and Boyer, H. W. (1977). *Science*, **198**, 1056.

Ixart, G., Szafarczyk, A., Belugou, J. L. and Assenmacher, I. (1977). *J. Endocr.* **72**, 113.

Jackson, I. M. D., Gagel, R., Papapetrou, P. and Reichlin, S. (1974a) *Clin. Res.* **23**, 342A.

Jackson, I. M. D., Papapetrou, P. D. and Reichlin, S. (1974b). Proc. 50th Am. Thyroid Assoc. (abstract).

Jackson, I. M. D. and Reichlin, S. (1974a). *Endocrinology*, **95**, 854.

Jackson, I. M. D. and Reichlin, S. (1974b). *Life Sci.* **14**, 2259.

Jackson, I. M. D. and Reichlin, S. (1977). *Science*, **198**, 414.

Jackson, I. M. D., Saperstein, R. and Reichlin, S. (1974c). Proc. Endocr. Soc. 56th Meet. Abst. No. 23, 67.

Jackson, I. M. D., Saperstein, R. and Reichlin, S. (1977). *Endocrinology*, **100**, 97.

Jacobs, L., Snyder, P., Wilbur, J., Utiger, R. and Daughaday, W. (1971). *J. clin. Endocr. Metab.* **33**, 996.

Johansson, K. N. G., Currie, B. L., Folkers, K. and Bowers, C. Y. (1973). *Biochem. biophys. Res. Commun.* **50**, 8.

Johnson, D. G., Ensinck, J. W., Koerker, D., Palmer, J. and Goodner, C. J. (1975). *Endocrinology*, **96**, 370.

Jonas, H. A., Burger, H. G., Cumming, I. A., Findlay, J. K. and de Krestser, D. M. (1975). *Endocrinology*, **96**, 384.

Jones, M. T., Gillham, B. and Hillhouse, E. W. (1977). *Fed. Proc.* **36**, 2104.

Jones, M. T., Hillhouse, E. W. and Burden, J. (1976). *J. Endocr.* **69**, 1.

Kamberi, I. A., Mical, R. S. and Porter, J. C. (1971). *Endocrinology*, **88**, 1288.

Kao, L. W. and Weisz, J. (1977). *Endocrinology*, **100**, 1723.

Kardon, F., Marcus, R. J., Winokur, A. and Utiger, R. D. (1977). *Endocrinology*, **100**, 1604.

Kastin, A. J., Miller, L. H., Sandman, C. A., Schally, A. V. and Plotnikoff, N. P. (1977). "Essays in Neurochemistry and Neuropharmacology", Vol. 1, p. 139. John Wiley, London.

Kastin, A. J., Miller, M. C. and A. V. Schally (1968). *Endocrinology*, **83**, 137.

Kastin, A. J., Plotinikoff, N. P., Nair, R. M. G., Redding, T. W. and Anderson, M. S. (1972). "MIF: Its Pituitary and Extra-pituitary Effect", p. 159. Excerpta Medica Int. Cong. Ser. No. 263, Amsterdam.

Kastin, A. J., Schally, A. V. and Viosca, S. (1971). *Proc. Soc. exp. Biol. Med.* **13T**, 1437.

Kato, Y., Dupre, J. and Beck, J. C. (1973). *Endocrinology*, **93**, 135.

Kato, Y., Nakai, Y., Imura, H., Chihara, K. and Ohgo, S. (1974). *J. clin. Endocr. Metab.* **38**, 695.

Kendal, J. W., Gray, D. K. and Gaudette, N. D. (1976). *Proc. Soc. exp. Biol. Med.* **152**, 691.

King, J. A., Arimura, A. and Williams, T. H. (1975). *J. Anat.* **120**, 275.

King, J. C., Elkind, K. E., Gerall, A. A. and Millar, R. P. (1978). "Brain-Endocrine Interaction, III, Neurohormones and Reproduction", p. 97. Kager, Basel.

Kizer, J. S., Arimura, A., Schally, A. V. and Brownstein, M. J. (1975). *Endocrinology*, **96**, 523.

Kizer, J. S., Palkovits, M. and Brownstein, M. (1976). *Endocrinology*, **98**, 311.

Knobil, E. (1966). *Physiologist*, **9**, 25.

Knobil, E. and Meyer, V. (1967). *Ann. N.Y. Acad. Sci.* **148**, 459.

Koch, Y., Baram, T., Chobsieng, P. and Fridkin, M. (1974). *Biochem. biophys. Res. Commun.* **61**, 95.

Koch, Y., Baram, T. and Fridkin, M. (1976). *FEBS Lett.* **63**, 295.

Koch, Y., Goldhaber, G., Fireman, I., Zor, U., Shani, J. and Tal, E. (1977). *Endocrinology*, **100**, 1476.

Koch, Y., Wilchek, M., Fridkin, M., Chobsieng, P., Zor, U. and Lindner, H. R. (1973). *Biochem. biophys. Res. Commun.* **55**, 616.

Kokubu, T., Sawano, S., Shiraki, M., Yamasaki, M. and Ishizuku, Y. (1975). *Endocr. jap.* **22**, 213.

Konturek, S. J., Tasler, J., Cieszkowski, M., Coy, D. H. and Schally, A. V. (1976a). *Gastroenterology*, **70**, 737.

Konturek, S. J., Tasler, J., Obtulowicz, W., Coy, D. H. and Schally, A. V. (1976b). *J. clin. Invest.* **58**, 1.

Kordon, C., Blake, C. A., Terkel, J. and Sawyer, C. H. (1973). *Neuroendocrinology*, **13**, 213.

Kordon, C., Epelbaum, J., Enjalbert, A. and McKelvy, J. (1976). "Subcellular Mechanism in Reproductive Neuroendocrinology", p. 167. Elsevier, Amsterdam.

Kraicer, J. and Morris, A. R. (1976). *Neuroendocrinology*, **20**, 79.

Krieger, D. T., Liotta, A. and Brownstein, M. J. (1977). *Endocrinology*, **100**, 227.

Kronheim, S., Berelowitz, M. and Pimstone, B. L. (1976). *Clin. Endocr.* **5**, 619.

Krulich, L., Illner, P., Fawcett, C. P., Quijada, M. and McCann, S. M. (1972). "Growth and Growth Hormone", p. 306. Excerpta Medica, Amsterdam.

Krulich, L., Quijada, M. and Illner, P. (1971). Prog. 53rd Ann. Meet. Endocr. Soc. Abst. No. 83.

Labrie, F., Barden, N., Poirier, G. and De Leon, A. (1972). *Proc. natn. Acad. Sci. USA*, **69**, 283.

Lacy, P. E. and Kostianovsky, M. (1967). *Diabetes*, **16**, 35.

Lambert, A. E., Blondel, B., Kanazawa, Y., Orci, L. and Renold, A. E. (1972). *Endocrinology*, **90**, 239.

Leeman, S. E., Glenister, D. W. and Yates, F. E. (1962). *Endocrinology*, **70**, 249.

Leppäluoto, J., Ling, N. and Vale, W. (1976). Prog. 5th Int. Cong. Endocr. p. 333 (abstract).

Leung, Y., Guansing, A. R., Ajlouni, K., Hagon, T. C., Rosenfeld, P. S. and Barboriak, J. J. (1975). *Endocrinology*, **97**, 380.

Lowry, P. J. (1974). *J. Endocr.* **62**, 163.

Lu, K. H., Amenomori, Y., Chem, C. L. and Meites, J. (1970). *Endocrinology*, **87**, 667.

Lu, K. H. and Meites, J. (1973). *Endocrinology*, **93**, 152.

Luft, R., Effendic, S., Hökfelt, T., Johansson, O. and Arimura, A. (1974). *Med. Biol.* **52**, 428.

Lymangrover, J. R. and Brodish, A. (1973). *Neuroendocrinology*, **12**, 225.

Machlin, L. J., Jacobs, L. S., Cirulis, N., Kimes, R. and Miller, R. (1974). *Endocrinology*, **95**, 1350.

MacIndoe, J. H. and Turkington, R. W. (1973). *J. clin. Invest.* **52**, 1972.

MacLeod, R. M. (1969). *Endocrinology*, **85**, 916.

MacLeod, R. M. (1976). "Frontiers in Neuroendocrinology", p. 169. Raven Press, New York.

Malacara, N. M., Valverde, R. C., Reichlin, S. and Bollinger, J. (1972). *Endocrinology*, **91**, 1189.

Martin, J. B., Renaud, L. P. and Brazeau, P. (1975). *Lancet*, **11**, 393.

Matsuo, H., Arimura, A., Nair, R. M. G. and Schally, A. V. (1971a). *Biochem. biophys. Res. Commun.* **45**, 822.

Matsuo, H., Nair, R. M. G., Arimura, A. and Schally, A. V. (1971b). *Biochem. biophys. Res. Commun.* **43**, 1334.

McCann, S. M. (1977). *New Engl. J. Med.* **296**, 797.

McCann, S. M., Taleisnik, S. and Friedman, H. M. (1960). *Proc. Soc. exp. Biol. Med.* **104**, 432.

McKelvy, J. F. and Grimm-Jorgensen, Y. (1976). "Hypothalamic Hormone Chemistry Physiology, Pharmacology and Clinical Uses", p. 13. Academic Press, New York and London.

McKelvy, J. F., Sheridan, M., Joseph, S., Phelps, C. H. and Perrie, S. (1975). *Endocrinology*, **97**, 908.

McNeill, T. H. and Sladek, J. R. (1978). *Science*, **200**, 72.

Meites, J. (1970). "Hypophysiotropic Hormones of the Hypthalamus, Assay and Chemistry", p. 261. William and Wilkins, Baltimore.

Meites, J. and Clemens, J. A. (1972). *Vit. Horm.* **30**, 165.

Meites, J. and Nicoll, C. S. (1966). *Ann. Rev. Physiol.* **28**, 57.

Meyer, V. and Knobil, E. (1966). *Endocrinology*, **79**, 1016.

Milmore, J. E. and Reese, R. P. (1975). *Endocrinology*, **96**, 732.

Mitnik, M. and Reichlin, S. (1971). *Science*, **172**, 1241.

Mitsuma, T., Hirooka, Y. and Nihei, N. (1976a). *Folia endocr. Jap.* **52**, 806.
Mitsuma, T., Hirooka, Y. and Nihei, N. (1967b). *Acta endocr., Copnh.* **83**, 225.
Miyachi, Y., Charambach, A., Mecklenberg, R. and Lipsett, M. B. (1973). *Endocrinology*, **92**, 1725.
Moguilevsky, J. A., Enero, M. A. and Szwarcfarb, B. (1974). *Proc. Soc. exp. Biol. Med.* **147**, 434.
Montoya, E., Seibel, M. J. and Wilber, J. (1973). Prog. 55th Ann. Meet. Endocr. Soc. p. A-138.
Montoya, E., Seibel, M. J. and Wilber, J. F. (1975). *Endocrinology*, **96**, 1413.
Moss, R. L. (1977). *Fed. Proc.* **36**, 1978.
Mulder, G. H. and Smelik, P. G. (1977). *Endocrinology*, **100**, 1142.
Naik, D. V. (1974). *Anat. Rec.* **178**, 424.
Naik, D. V. (1976). *Cell Tissue Res.* **173**, 143.
Nair, R. M. G., Barrett, J. F., Bowers, C. Y. and Schally, A. V. (1979). *Biochemistry*, **9**, 1103.
Nair, R. M. G., Kastin, A. J. and Schally, A. V. (1971a). *Biochem. biophys. Res. Commun.* **43**, 1376.
Nair, R. M. G., Redding, T. W. and Schally, A. V. (1971b). *Biochemistry*, **10**, 3621.
Nallar, R. and McCann, S. M. (1965). *Endocrinology*, **76**, 272.
Negro-Vilar, A., Dickerman, E. and Meites, J. (1968a). *Endocrinology*, **83**, 1349.
Negro-Uilar, A., Dickerman, E. and Meites, J. (1968b). *Proc. Soc. exp. Biol. Med.* **127**, 751.
Neil, J. D., Patton, J. M., Dailey, R. A., Tsau, R. L. and Tindall, G. T. (1977). *Endocrinology*, **101**, 430.
Nett, T. M., Akbar, A. M., Niswender, G. D., Hedlund, M. T. and White, W. F. (1973). *J. clin. Endocr. Metab.* **36**, 880.
Nicoll, C. S. and Meites, J. (1963). *Endocrinology*, **72**, 544.
Nihei, N. (1977). *Gendai-Igaku*, **25**, 189.
Noe, B. D., Weir, G. C. and Bauer, G. E. (1977). Prog. Int. Symp. Somatostastin, Freiburg (abstract).
Oliver, C., Charvet, J. P., Codaccioni, J. L. and Vague, J. (1974a). *J. clin. Endocr. Metab.* **39**, 406.
Oliver, C., Eskay, R. L., Ben-Jonathan, N. and Porter, J. C. (1974b). *Endocrinology*, **95**, 540.
Oliver, C., Eskay, R. L., Mical, R. S. and Porter, J. C. (1973). Prog. 49th Meet. Am. Thyroid Assoc. p. T4 (abstract).
Orci, L., Baetens, D., Dubois, M. P. and Rufener, C. (1975). *Horm. Met. Res.* **7**, 400.
Orci, L., Baetens, D., Rufener, C., Amherdt, M., Ravvazzola, M., Studer, P., Malaisse-Lagae, F. and Unger, R. (1976). *Proc. natn Acad. Sci. USA*, **73**, 1338.
Palkovits, M. (1973). *Brain Res.* **59**, 449.
Palkovits, M., Arimura, A., Brownstein, M., Schally, A. V. and Savedra, J. M. (1974a). *Endocrinology*, **95**, 554.
Palkovits, M., Brownstein, M., Saavedra, J. M. and Axelrod, J. (1974b). *Brain Res.* **77**, 137.
Patel, Y. C. and Weir, G. C. (1971). *Clin. Endocr.* **5**, 191.
Patel, Y. C., Weir, G. C. and Reichlin, S. (1975). Prog. 57th Ann. Meet. Endocr. Abst. No. 154, p. 127.
Patel, Y. C., Rao, K. and Reichlin, S. (1977). *New Engl. J. Med.* **296**, 529.
Patton, G. S., Dobbs, R., Orci, L., Vale, W. and Unger, R. H. (1976a). *Metabolism*, **25** (Suppl. 1), 1499.

Patton, G. S., Ipp, E., Dobbs, R. E., Orci, L., Vale, W. and Unger, R. H. (1976b). *Life Sci.* **19**, 1957.

Patton, G. S., Ipp, E., Dobbs, R. E., Orci, L., Vale, W. and Unger, R. H. (1977). *Proc. natn. Acad. Sci. USA*, **74**, 2140.

Pearlmutter, A. F., Rapino, E. and Saffran, M. (1975). *Endocrinology*, **97**, 1336.

Pearse, A. G. E. (1976). "Peptide Hormones", p. 33. Macmillan Press, London.

Pelletier, G., Labrie, F., Arimura, A. and Schally, A. V. (1974a). *Am. J. Anat.* **140**, 445.

Pelletier, G., Labrie, F., Puvani, R., Arimura, A. and Schally, A. V. (1974b). *Endocrinology*, **95**, 314.

Polak, J. M., Pearse, A. G. E., Grimelius, L., Bloom, S. R. and Arimura, A. (1975). *Lancet*, **i**, 1220.

Portanova, R. and Sayers, G. (1973). *Neuroendocrinology*, **12**, 236.

Porter, J. C., Eskay, R. L., Oliver, C., Ben-Jonathan, N., Warberg, J., Parker, R. and Barnea, A. (1977). "Hypothalamic Peptide Hormones and Pituitary Regulation", p. 181. Plenum Press, New York.

Porter, J. C. and Jones, J. C. (1956). *Endocrinology*, **58**, 62.

Porter, J. C. and Rumsfeld Jr., H. W. (1956). *Endocrinology*, **58**, 359.

Porter, J. C. and Rumsfeld Jr., H. W. (1959). *Endocrinology*, **64**, 948.

Ramirez, V. D. and McCann, S. M. (1963). *Endocrinology*, **73**, 193.

Redding, T. W., Bowers, C. Y. and Schally, A. V., (1966). *Endocrinology*, **79**, 229.

Redding, T. W. and Coy, E. J. (1974). *Endocrinology*, **94 (Suppl.)**, A154.

Redding, T. W., Kastin, A. J., Gonzalez-Barcena, D., Coy, D. H., Coy, E. J., Schalch, D. S. and Schally, A. V. (1973). *J. clin. Endocr. Metab.* **37**, 626.

Redding, T. W. and Schally, A. V. (1969). *Proc. Soc. exp. Biol. Med.* **131**, 415.

Redding, T. W. and Schally, A. V., (1971). *Endocrinology*, **89**, 1075.

Redding, T. W. and Schally, A. V. (1972). *Neuroendocrinology*, **9**, 250.

Redding, T. W. and Schally, A. V. (1973). *Life Sci.* **12**, 23.

Reichlin, S. (1976). "Subcellular Mechanisms in Reproductive Neuroendocrinology", p. 109. Elsevier, Amsterdam.

Reichlin, S. and Mitnick, M. (1973). "Hypothalamic Hypophysiotropic Hormones", p. 124. Excerpta Medica, Amsterdam.

Rivier, C., Brazeau, P., Vale, W., Ling, N., Burgus, R., Gilon, C., Yardley, J. and Guillemin, R. (1973a). *C.r. Acad. Sci. Paris*, **276**, 2737.

Rivier, C. and Vale, W. (1974). *Endocrinology*, **95**, 978.

Rivier, C., Vale, W. and Guillemin, R. (1973b). *Proc. Soc. exp. Biol. Med.* **142**, 842.

Rotsztejn, W. H., Charli, J. L., Pattou, E., Epelbaum, J. and Kordon, C. (1976). *Endocrinology*, **99**, 1663.

Saffran, M. and Schally, A. V. (1955). *Can. J. Biochem. Physiol.* **33**, 408.

Saito, T., Sawano, A., Arimura, A. and Schally, A. V. (1967). *Endocrinology*, **81**, 1226.

Sakurai, H., Dobbs, R. and Unger, R. H. (1974). *J. clin. Invest.* **54**, 1394.

Sarkar, D. K., Chiappa, S. A., Fink, C. and Sherwood, N. M. (1976). *Nature, Lond.* **264**, 461.

Sato, T., Sato, M., Shinsako, J. and Dallman, M. F. (1975). *Endocrinology*, **97**, 265.

Sawano, S. and Kokubu, T. (1977). *Proc. Soc. exp. Biol. Med.* **156**, 72.

Schalch, D. S., Gonzalez-Barcena, D., Kastin, A. J. Schally, A. V. and Lee, L. A. (1972). *J. clin. Endocr. Metab.* **35**, 609.

Schally, A. V. and Arimura, A. (1977). "Clinical Neuroendocrinology", p. 2. Academic Press, New York and London.

Schally, A. V., Arimura, A., Baba, Y., Nair, R. M. G., Matsuo, H., Redding, T. W. and Debeljuk, L. (1971a). *Biochem. biophys. Res. Commun.* **43**, 393.

Schally, A. V., Arimura, A., Bowers, C. Y., Kastin, A. J., Sawano, S. and Redding, T. W. (1968). "Recent Progress in Hormone Research", Vol 24, p. 497. Academic Press, New York and London.

Schally, A. V., Arimura, A. and Kastin, A. J. (1973). *Science*, **179**, 341.

Schally, A. V., Arimura, A., Kastin, A. J., Matsuo, H., Baba, Y., Redding, T. W., Nair, R. M. G., Debeljuk, L. and White, W. F. (1971b). *Science*, **173**, 1038.

Schally, A. V., Arimura, A., Redding, T. W., Debeljuk, L., Carter, W., Dupont, A. and Vilchez-Martinez, J. A. (1976a). *Endocrinology*, **98**, 380.

Schally, A. V., Bowers, C. Y., Redding, T. W. and Barrett, J. F. (1966a). *Biochem. biophys. Res. Commun.* **25**, 165.

Schally, A. V., Coy, D. H. and Meyers, C. A. (1978a). *Ann. Rev. Biochem.* **48**, 89.

Schally, A. V., Coy, D. H., Meyers, C. A. and Kastin, A. J. (1978b)". Hormonal Proteins and Peptides", (C. H. Li, ed.), Vol. 47, p. 89. Academic Press, New York and London.

Schally, A. V., Dupont, A., Arimura, A., Redding, T. W. and Linthicum, G. L. (1975). *Fed. Proc.* **34**, 584.

Schally, A. V., Dupont, A., Arimura, A., Redding, T. W., Nishi, N., Linthicum, G. L. and Schlesinger, D. H. (1976b). *Biochemistry*, **15**, 509.

Schally, A. V., Dupont, A., Arimura, A., Takahara, J., Redding, T. W., Clemens, J. and Shaar, C. (1976c). *Acta endocr., Copnh.* **82**, 1.

Schally, A. V. and Guillemin, R. (1960). *Tex. Rep. biol. Med.* **18**, 133.

Schally, A. V., Huang, W. Y., Redding, T. W., Arimura, A., Coy, D. H., Chihara, K., Chang, R. C. C., Raymond, V. and Labrie, F. (1978c). *Biochem. biophys. Res. Commun.* (in press).

Schally, A. V. and Kastin, A. J. (1966). *Endocrinology*, **79**, 768.

Schally, A. V., Kastin, A. J., Locke, W. and Bowers, C. Y. (1967). "Hormones in Blood", p. 491, 2nd edition. Academic Press, New York and London.

Schally, A. V., Nair, R. M. G., Redding, T. W. and Arimura, A. (1971c). *J. biol. Chem.* **246**, 7230.

Schally, A. V., Redding, T. W., Arimura, A., Dupont, A. and Linthicum, G. L. (1977). *Endocrinology*, **100**, 681.

Schally, A. V., Redding, T. W. and Bowers, C. Y. (1966b). *Gunma Symp. Endocr.* **3**, 15.

Schally, A. V., Redding, T. W., Bowers, C. Y. and Barrett, J. F. (1969). *J. biol. Chem.* **244**, 4077.

Schally, A. V., Redding, T. W., Chihara, K., Huang, W. Y., Chang, R. C. C., Carter, W. H., Coy, D. H. and Saffran, M. (1978d). *Endocrinology*, **102**, 102A.

Schally, A. V. Steelman, S. L. and Bowers, C. Y. (1965). *Proc. Soc. exp. Biol. Med.* **119**, 208.

Schreiber, V. (1961). *Acta Univ. Carol. Med. Prague*, **7**, 33.

Schusdziarra, V., Dobbs, R. E., Harris, V. and Unger, R. H. (1977). *FEBS Lett.* **81**, 69.

Seiden, G. and Brodish, A. (1972). *Endocrinology*, **90**, 1401.

Sétáló, G., Vigh, S., Schally, S. V., Arimura, A. and Flerkó, B. (1975). *Endocrinology*, **96**, 135.

Sétáló, G., Vigh, S., Schally, A. V., Arimura, A. and Flerkó, B. (1976a). *Acta biol. Acad. sci. hung.* **27**, 75.

Sétáló, G., Vigh, S., Schally, A. V., Arimura, A. and Flerkó, B. (1976b). *Brain Res.* **103**, 597.

Shaar, C. J. and Clemens, J. A. (1974). *Endocrinology*, **95**, 1202.

Sherwood, N. M., Chippa, S. A. and Fink, G. (1976). *J. Endocr.* **70**, 501.

Siler, T. M., Vandenberg, G., Yen, S. S. C. Brazeau, P., Vale, W. and Guillemin, R. (1973). *J. clin. Endocr. Metab.* **37**, 632.

Sinha, D. and Meites, J. (1965/66). *Neuroendocrinology*, **1**, 4.

Smelik, P. G. (1977). *Ann. N.Y. Acad. Sci.* **297**, 580.

Solomon, S. H. and McKenzie, J. M. (1966). *Endocrinology*, **78**, 699.

Stachura, M. E., Dhariwal, A. P. S. and Frohman, L. A. (1972). *Endocrinology*, **91**, 1071.

Suda, T., Demura, H., Demura, R., Wakabayashi, I, Nomura, K., Odagira, E. and Shizume, K. (1977). *J. clin. Endocr. Metab.* **44**, 440.

Szabo, M. and Frohman, L. A. (1975). *Endocrinology*, **96**, 955.

Szabo, M. and Frohman, L. A. (1976). *Endocrinology*, **98**, 1451.

Takahara, J., Arimura, A. and Schally, A. V. (1975). *Acta endocr., Copenh.* **78**, 428.

Takahashi, K., Saito, M., Wakai, T., Hoshiai, H., Wada, Y., Sakurada, N. and Suzuki, M. (1976). *Tohoku J. exp. Bed.* **120**, 231.

Taleisnik, S. and Orias, R. (1975). *Am. J. Physiol.* **208**, 213.

Tashuian, A., Barowski, N. and Jensen, D. (1971). *Biochem. biophys. Res. Commun.* **43**, 516.

Uehara, T., Arimura, A. and Schally, A. V. (1973/74). *Neuroendocrinology*, **13**, 278.

Upton, G. V. and Amatadura, J. J. (1971). *New Engl. J. Med.* **285**, 419.

Utiger, R. (1976) *Ann. Rev. Physiol.* **38**, 389.

Vagenakis, A. G., Roti, E., Mannix, J. and Brauerman, L. E. (1975). *J. clin. Endocr. Metab.* **41**, 801.

Vale, W., Grant, G., Amoss, M., Blackwell, R. and Guillemin, R. (1972). *Endocrinology*, **91**, 562.

Vale, W., Ling, N., Rivier, J., Villarreal, J., Rivier, C., Douglas, C. and Brown, M. (1976a). *Metabolism*, **25** (Suppl. 1), 1491.

Vale, W. and Rivier, C. (1977). Prog. 59th Ann. Meet. Endocr. Soc. Abst. No. 321.

Vale, W., Rivier, C. and Brown, M. (1977). *Ann. Rev. Physiol.* **39**, 473.

Vale, W., Rivier, C., Brown, M., Chan, L., Ling, N. and Rivier, J. (1976b). "Hypothalamus and Endocrine Functions", p. 397. Plenum Press, New York.

Vale, W., Rivier, C., Palkovits, M., Saavedra, J. M. and Brownstein, M. (1974). *Endocrinology*, **94**, A128.

Valverde, R. C., Chieffo, V. and Reichlin, S. (1972). *Endocrinology*, **91**, 982.

Valverde, R. C., Chieffo, V. and Reichlin, S. (1973). *Life Sci.* **12**, 327.

Vernikos-Danellis, J. and Marks, B. H. (1969). "Assay and Chemistry", p. 60. Williams and Wilkins, Baltimore.

Wakabayashi, I., Miyazawa, Y., Kanda, M., Niki, N., Demura, R., Demura, H. and Shizume, K. (1977). *Endocr. jap.* **24**, 601.

Walter, R., Griffiths, E. C. and Hooper, K. C. (1973). *Brain Res.* **60**, 449.

Warberg, J., Eskay, R. L., Barnea, A., Reynolds, R. C. and Porter, J. C. (1977). *Endocrinology*, **100**, 814.

Weiner, R. I. (1975). "Hypothalamic Hormones", p. 249. Academic Press, New York and London.

White, W. F., Hedlund, M. T., Weber, G. F., Rippel, R. H., Johnson, E. S. and Willus, J. F. (1974). *Endocrinology*, **94**, 1422.

White, N., Jeffcoate, S. L., Griffiths, E. C. and Hooper, K. C. (1976). *J. Endocr.* **71**, 13.

Wilber, J. F. and Porter, J. C. (1970). *Endocrinology*, **87**, 807.

Wilber, J. F., Nagel, T. and White, W. F. (1971). *Endocrinology*, **89**, 1419.

Willoughby, J. O., Martin, J. R., Brazeau, P. and Renaud, L. P. (1975). *Clin. Res.* **23**, 619A.

Winter, A. J., Eskay, R. L. and Porter, J. C. (1974). *J. clin. Endocr. Metab.* **39**, 960.
Witorsch, R. and Brodish, A. (1972). *Endocrinology*, **90**, 552.
Wollheim, C. B., Blondell, B., Renold, A. E. and Sharp, G. W. C. (1977). *Endocrinology*, **101**, 911.
Yamamoto, H., Hirata, Y., Matsukara, S., Imura, H., Nakamura, M. and Tanaka, A. (1976). *Acta endocr.* **82**, 183.
Yamashiro, D. and Li, C. H. (1973). *Biochem. biophys. Res. Commun.* **54**, 882.
Yamazaki, E., Sakiz, E. and Guillemin, R. (1963) *Experientia*, **19**, 480.
Yasuda, N. and Greer, M. (1976). *Endocrinology*, **99**, 994.
Yasuda, N. and Greer, M. A. (1977). *Acta endocr., Copenh.* **84**, 1.
Yates, F. E. and Maran, J. W. (1974). *Handle. Physiol.* **4**, 367.
Zarrow, M. X., Campbell, P. S. and Penenberg, V. H. (1972). *Proc. Soc. exp. Biol. Med.* **141**, 356.
Zimmerman, E. A., Hsu, K. C., Feris, M. and Kozlowski, G. P. (1974). *Endocrinology*, **95**, 1.

II. Insulin

U. A. PARMAN

INTRODUCTION

Insulin was isolated from dog pancreas and identified as the antidiabetic hormone by Frederick Banting and Charles Best in 1922. Description of the monomeric three dimensional structure of porcine insulin, sequencing of a significant number of vertebrate insulins and isolation and characterisation of a "universal" insulin receptor by the 1970s have allowed an insight into the evolution of this remarkable protein, and the beginnings of highly promising investigations of the relationship of its structure to receptor binding, modification of cell metabolism, uptake into cells, and its structural alterations. These studies may clarify the problems of tissue insulin sensitivity, which varies physiologically and pathologically, the relationship of dose and form to homeostatic and anabolic roles, and the significance of the insulin-like growth factors. Despite intensive research during the last ten years, our understanding of the control of insulin synthesis and release, especially in relation to diabetes mellitus in man, is unclear and highly speculative.

A. CHEMICAL CONSTITUTION AND PHYSICAL PROPERTIES

Ryle, Sanger, Smith and Kitai (1955) were the first to describe the primary structure of bovine insulin as two peptide chains, designated A and B, consisting of 21 and 30 amino acids respectively, and linked by two disulphide bonds (Fig. 1(a)). The amino acid sequence of 28 different insulins of vertebrate origin is established (see Blundell and Wood, 1975).

The high resolution X-ray crystallographic study of the secondary, tertiary and quaternary structure of insulin provides a model to explain its physicochemical properties in solution and in the crystalline state, the structural basis of its biological and immunological behaviour in the circulation, and the evolution of its primary structure in the vertebrate.

1. Structure of Insulin

Crystalline rhombohedral porcine insulin contains two atoms of Zn per hexamer and consists of three slightly asymmetric dimers (Blundell, Dodson, Hodgkin and Mercola, 1972). The secondary structure of the monomer (Fig. 1(b)) consists of three α-helical regions, A2–A8, A13–A19 and B9–B19, the relative conformations of which are stabilised by the A7–B7 and A20–B19 disulphide bonds, at the extremities of the B9–B19 helix, and by creation of non-polar interactions between the juxtaposed B24, B26, B15, B11, A2, A16,

```
                          S                              S
A    H-Gly. Ile.  Val. Glu. Gln. Cys. Cys. Thr. Ser. Ile.  Cys. Ser. Leu. Tyr. Gln.
                          S
                          S
B    H-Phe. Val. Asn. Gln. His. Leu. Cys. Gly. Ser. His. Leu. Val. Glu. Ala. Leu.
       1     2    3    4    5    6    7    8    9   10   11   12   13   14   15
A       Leu. Glu. Asn. Tyr.  Cys. Asn-CH
                              S
                              S
B    Tyr. Leu. Val. Cys. Gly. Glu. Arg. Gly. Phe. Phe. Tyr. Thr. Pro. Lys. Ala-OH
      16   17   18   19   20   21   22   23   24   25   26   27   28   29   30
(a)
```

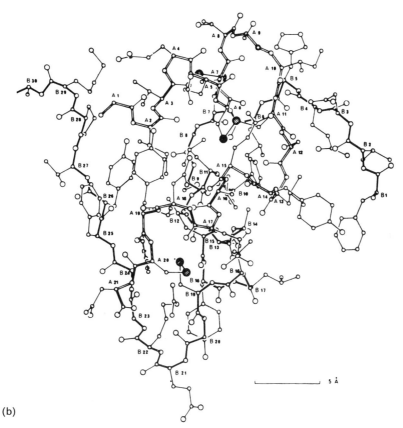

(b)

Fig. 1. Primary (a) and secondary (b) structure of porcine insulin. (From Blundell *et al.*, 1972.)

B18 and B6 residues, and less significantly, by the ionic bonding A4 to B29 and A21 to B22, and the hydrogen bonding of A19–B25, A7–B5 and A11–B4 residues. All polar residues are on the surface and non-polar residues, mainly of B chain origin, are involved in dimerisation, and dimer–dimer interactions. Dimerisation involves formation of an anti-parallel β-sheet with hydrogen bonding between B24 and B26 residues of the two monomers and the creation of a tight and continuous non-polar interface along one surface of the monomer by the participation of 20 residues, but mainly of the B12, B24, B26, B16 and B25. In the hexamer, the dimer–dimer associations are less crowded, more symmetrical, involving mainly the B14, B17, B18 of the 24 participants, which consequently facilitates ionic bonding at A17–B1 and hydrogen bonding between neighbouring A14s of the monomers. The hexamer has a central hydrophilic core formed by residues B9, B10 and B13, wherein the two zinc atoms are coordinated with B10 histidine imidazole. There is about 30% solvent in the crystal suggesting that most of the polar surface is in an aqueous environment. Hexamer packing also occurs by solvent exclusion between the few non-polar residues, e.g. A10, the different substitution of which alters the rhombohedral crystals, e.g. porcine versus bovine (Pullen, Lindsay, Wood, Tickle, Blundell, Wollman, Krail, Brandenburg, Zahn, Gliemann and Gammeltoft, 1976).

Interspecies differences in the primary structure are not random but occur at the variant sites grouped together at the surface of the tertiary structure. The invariant sites are involved mainly in aggregation and conformation stability and the few on the surface, e.g. A1, A5, A19, A21 are clustered closely and probably participate in receptor binding (Frank, Veros and Pekar, 1972; Pekar and Frank, 1972; Pullen et al., 1975). Evolutionary change has conserved a broadly comparable tertiary structure to the vertebrate insulin (Blundell and Wood, 1957; Pekar and Frank, 1972).

2. Physical Properties of Insulin

(a) Aggregation in solution and crystallisation

Aggregation in solution as estimated by sedimentation equilibrium velocities, circular dichroism and UV difference or NMR spectra, and crystallisation of the native and modified forms, are consistent with the tertiary structure outlined (Blundell et al., 1972; Bradbury and Brown, 1977). Insulin aggregation in solution depends on concentration, pH, ionic strength, presence of divalent cations (e.g. Zn^{++}, Cd^{++}, Co^{++}, Ni^{++} or Cu^{++}) and anions used at acid pH, the order of increasing effectiveness in aggregation being $H_2PO_4^-$, Cl^-, Br^-, NO_3^-, I^- and CNS^-. In very dilute solutions of about 0·33 mol zinc/mol insulin, or in the absence of zinc, with not less than 15 μmol/l insulin, and at low ionic strength (IS), a dimer–monomer equilibrium is detected at pH 7–8 (Blundell et al., 1972; Pullen et al., 1976; Jeffrey, 1974). The dimer predominates in 150–400 μmol/l insulin and low IS at pH 2·5 or below. Hexamers appear at 150 μmol/l insulin and pH 7 (Jeffrey, 1974). Hexamerisation is a linear function of the net charge/monomer, and is increasingly positive or negative at pH below and above, respectively, its isoelectric point ca 5·4 (Arquilla, Miles and Morris, 1972). The calculated intrinsic energy of association is independent of pH or IS, and exceeds the repulsive energies of association (Blundell et al., 1972). Since insulin crystallises by solvent exclusion, the high entropy factor must favour the same mode of aggregation in solution as in the crystal, and accounts for the stability in dilute acid and alkali, and during flash evaporation (Humbel, Bosshard and Zahn, 1972). Hence dissociation to monomers in organic solvents and by guanidine HCl or urea is due to lowered energy of association of the non-polar residues (Blundell et al., 1972; Federici, Duprè, Barboni, Fiori and Costa, 1973).

(b) Zinc binding

Zinc binds insulin above pH 4·5, and most avidly at pH 6–8, when zinc concentration becomes critical. If the zinc:insulin molar ratio of 0·33 is exceeded, larger than hexameric aggregates predominate up to pH 9, above which dissociation to hexamer accelerates. At neutral pH, dimer–dimer interactions are accelerated by zinc and occur at lower insulin concentrations (Blundell et al., 1972; Jeffrey, 1974; Goldman and Carpenter, 1974; Jeffrey, Milthorpe and Nichol, 1972). At pH 6–8, the zinc bound at 0·33 molar ratio is undialysable, and association constant is ca 10^5, i.e. higher than histidine–zinc association in solution (ca 10^3). In solution–crystal transition two constants of 10^8 and 10^{13} obtained are reconciled to the differences in position of the zinc binding sites of the hexamer, and the asymmetry of the dimer (Blundell et al., 1972). Zinc binding is prevented by EDTA. Hence zinc is a stabiliser in solution and in the crystalline form, and shifts the aggregation equilibria. At low pH the positive charge on B10 may prevent zinc coordination and at pH 10 clustering of negatively charged B13s may cause predominance of dimers and hexamers. Insulins lacking B10 histidine (e.g. guinea-pig, hagfish) do not bind zinc (Blundell et al., 1972; Wood, Blundell, Wollmer, Lazarus and Neville, 1975; Peterson, Steiner, Emdin and Falkmer, 1975; Peterson, Coulter and Steiner, 1974) and do not aggregate well (see Table 1). The uniquely larger and hydrophilic B14, B17, B20 residues and altered B4 and A1 clustering on the surface render the tertiary structure of guinea-pig insulin monomer stable in aqueous media. The hagfish insulin with altered B9, B1, B2 involved in hexamer formation in the porcine

Table 1

Properties of insulins in relation to structure.

Insulin (with increasing concentration)	Amino acid different from porcine insulin	Crystalline structure	Aggregation behaviour			Circular dichroism $-[\theta]_{274}^{\bar{w}}$
Porcine	—	rhombohedral-2Zn/hexamer	monomer,	dimer,	hexamer	↑
Bovine	A_8, A_{10}	rhombohedral-2Zn/hexamer	monomer,	dimer,	hexamer	↑
PRO (porcine bovine)	+ C-peptide	1:1 cocrystallisation	monomer,	dimer,	hexamer	↑
Guinea-pig	A_1, B_4, B_{10}, B_{14}, B_{17}, B_{20}, B_{22}	no crystallisation *in vitro*	monomer			—
Hagfish	B_1, B_2, B_9, B_{10}	tetragonal, no Zn	monomer,	dimer		
DOP (bovine)	"B_{23}–B_{30}" missing	no crystallisation	monomer,	↓↓dimer,	trimer	↑
DAA (bovine)	"A_{21}–B_{30}" missing	no crystallisation	monomer,	↓dimer,	↓ trimer	↑
DA (bovine)	B_{30} missing	rhombohedral-2Zn/hexamer	monomer,	↓dimer,	hexamer	↑
AA (bovine)	A_1-acetylated	rhombohedral-2Zn/hexamer	monomer,	↓dimer,	hexamer	∼↓

insulin, only forms perfect symmetrical dimers which pack in tetragonal, as against hexameric, symmetry (Peterson *et al.*, 1975). Hence, loss of zinc binding and hexamerising ability appear related adaptive alterations of the molecule.

(c) Insulin in storage

Proinsulin, the precursor of insulin, does not crystallise alone but bovine and porcine proinsulins have been cocrystallised as 1:1 complexes with their homologous insulins (Low, Fullerton and Rosen, 1974). Self-association and

$-[\theta]^{w}_{222}$	Percentage biological activity (relative to porcine)			Percentage immunoreactivity in insulin specific assays		References
	Mouse blood sugar (convulsion)	Fat pad	Isolated fat cells	Radio-immunoassay	Immune haemolysis	
↑	100	100	100	100	100	Pullen et al. (1976)
↑	100	100	100	100	100	Pullen et al. (1976)
↑	3, 17		5–10	26	0·06	Snell and Smyth (1975); Low et al. (1974); Blundell et al. (1972); Frank et al. (1972)
—	8·5	10				Blundell et al. (1972); Wood et al. (1975)
		7·0	6·0	0·1		Blundell et al. (1972); Peterson et al. (1974, 1975); Emdin et al. (1975)
↓	<0·1	0·7	0·8	2·0	0·08	Blundell et al. (1972); Goldman and Carpenter (1974); Rubenstein and Steiner (1971)
↓	4·0	5·5	3·0	3·5	0·17	Blundell et al. (1972); Goldman and Carpenter (1974); Rubenstein and Steiner (1971)
↑	100					Blundell et al. (1972)
~↓	100		40	47		Blundell et al. (1972); Goldman and Carpenter (1974)

hexamerisation with zinc of proinsulin indicate that insulin retains its conformation in this form (Blundell et al., 1972; Snell and Smyth, 1975; Frank et al., 1972). Unlike insulin, proinsulin can bind as much as 30 atoms of zinc per hexamer, retain solubility, and resist proteolysis, which are probably relevant to the easy intracellular transport and the formation of insulin granules. In the mature granule, i.e. after proinsulin to insulin conversion, the contents are usually condensed to a definite shape. The variation in the electron microscopic morphology of the stored insulins with different primary structures is reflected in their crystallisation in vitro (Blundell and Wood,

1975; Blundell *et al.*, 1972; Peterson *et al.*, 1975). It is therefore probable that the stored insulin is stabilised at very high concentration as a metal complex, possibly partly crystalline (Watari and Hotta, 1976).

(d) Insulin in serum

The sequence of possible structural changes the molecule may undergo after release into the extracellular fluid until joining the circulation is not known. In solution at neutral pH, $3\cdot8$ μmol/l bovine zinc-free insulin may be 55% monomeric (Pullen *et al.*, 1976), dimerisation starting at about $0\cdot1$ μmol/l. In plasma at physiological levels of about $2\cdot0$ nmol/l in the portal vein (see Schulz, Michaelis, Siegler, Teichmann, Nowak, Albrecht and Bibergeil, 1976; Heding, 1977) dimerisation may be low despite high zinc concentrations of 15–37 μmol/l but possibility of dimerisation has not been excluded (Blundell *et al.*, 1972).

Monomer may be the active form since insulins which do not dimerise *in vitro* are biologically active, e.g. guinea-pig, sulphated or tetranitrotyrosyl-insulins (Ginsberg, 1977b). The weakly dimerising bovine DAA insulin (Table 1) has biological activity in the guinea pig (Snell and Smyth, 1975). Changes in secondary or tertiary structure indicated by circular dichroism of modified insulins appear to be correlated with a decrease in biological activity (Blundell *et al.*, 1972). Receptor binding is a requisite of biological activity. Residues A1, A5, A19, A21 and the adjacent B12, B16, B22–B26 of the monomer appear to participate in binding which involves non-polar interactions and hydrogen bonding (Weitzel, Bauer and Eisela, 1976; Blundell *et al.*, 1972; Kobayashi and Meck, 1977; Pullen *et al.*, 1976; Ginsberg, 1977a).

(e) Adhesive properties of insulin in solution

These are relevant to precaution in quantitative work with insulin *in vitro*, since the molecule is adsorbed on most inert surfaces like glass (even after siliconisation), paper, polyethylene and polyvinyl chloride (Hirsch, Fratkin, Wood and Thomas, 1977).

B. LOCATION OF INSULIN AND ITS BIOSYNTHESIS

1. Phylogenesis of the B Cell

In man insulin is produced and stored in the B cells of the endocrine pancreas, or the islets of Langerhans (Falkmer and Östberg, 1976). In the chordates, from cyclostomes to the mammals, insulin-producing cells are cloned into these islets, which in the adult are separated from the gut and secrete insulin into the bloodstream. The APUD-cells may be the precursor of the mature B cell. In the prechordates, e.g. amphioxus, insulin producing cells are restricted to the midgut (Van Noorden and Pearse, 1976). In the invertebrate, knowledge of B cell homologues is scant, but cells with B cell histochemistry occur in the molluscs (Falkmer and Östberg, 1976). Insulin-like hormones have been observed in insects (Tager, Markese, Kramer, Speirs and Childs, 1976). The specialised endocrine/exocrine organ pancreas is seen in higher vertebrates only.

The adult human islets may contain three or four other cell types than the B cells which could produce and release glucagon, somatostatin, vasoactive inhibitory peptide (VIP) and pancreatic polypeptide (Pelletier, 1977; Bloom, Iversen, Polak, Hermanson and Adrian, 1977; Deconinck, Potvliege and Gepts, 1971). In the neonatal pancreas somatostatin cells are more numerous and pancreatic polypeptide is possibly absent (Deconinck, Van Assche, Potvliege and Gepts, 1972). Immunoreactive insulin-like activity has been reported in cell membranes of the rat pancreatic duct (Dorn et al., 1977) and extracted from the gastric mucosa of the totally pancreatectomised pig (Kühl, Jensen and Nielsen, 1976) but synthesis of proinsulin or granulation has not been shown. In human gut, insulin-like immunoactivity has not been detected (Kühl et al., 1976) but extra pancreatic tumours containing immuno-reactive insulin do occur (Kiang, Bauer and Kennedy, 1973).

Differentiation of B and A cells in human pancreas occurs by the end of the 9th week in utero and secretory granules are found at 9–10 weeks. Immuno-reactive insulin is detected in the 7th week and increases significantly from the 8th week onwards (Pronina and Sapronova, 1976).

2. Biosynthesis of Insulin and its Control

Most investigations of islet function have been made on animal preparations. The consistent issues of these data will be outlined in this review with emphasis on aspects relevant to insulin metabolism in man.

Insulin biosynthesis has been studied in foetal calf and in the rat, mouse and fish pancreatic islets, and the data have been reviewed (Lernmark, Chan, Choy, Nathans, Carroll, Tager, Rubenstein, Swift and Steiner, 1976; Steiner, Kemmler, Clark, Oyer and Rubenstein, 1972; Steiner, 1977). The gene(s), e.g. two in the rat, coding for insulin are transcribed in the nucleus to mRNA(s). Rat tumour and catfish mRNAs are characterised as 9·3 and 12·5 S molecules, respectively, the former consisting of approximately 600 nucleotides, about 55% of which is translated into "preproinsulin", the earliest precursor form. This precursor is extended into the cisternal space of the rough endoplasmic reticulum from its initial link to the ribosomes until chain extension is terminated. Preproinsulin has been isolated from catfish islets (Albert, Chyn, Goldford and Permutt, 1977; Permutt, Biesbroeck, Chyn, Buime, Szczesna and McWilliams, 1976) and from cell-free systems translating rat or hagfish islets mRNA (Lernmark et al., 1976; Steiner, 1977) as an 11,000–13,000 dalton peptide. Unidentified proteases cleave from the amino terminal of the B chain a peptide of approximately 23 amino acids, only partially sequenced, converting preproinsulin to proinsulin which is released into the cisternum (Chan, Keim and Steiner, 1976). The prohormone is transported in the budding-off terminals of the tubular endoplasmic cisternae (Steiner, 1977) to a special site of the Golgi region (Brinn, Owen and Schweisthal, 1976; Orci, 1974) where the insulin granule is formed and conversion to insulin starts. Trypsin-like endopeptidase and carboxypeptidase B-like exopeptidase activities have been detected in the granule fractions (Zühlke, Steiner, Lernmark and Lipsey, 1976; Steiner, 1977). These are believed to cleave sequentially the connecting peptide between the carboxyl- and amino-ends of B and A chains, respectively, liberating the double-chain insulin (Zühlke et al., 1976; Steiner et al., 1972)

Proinsulin transport is energy dependent and takes between 20 and 50 min in the rat and guinea-pig respectively (Steiner et al., 1972; Howell, Hellerström and Tyhurst, 1974), and its conversion to insulin takes one or 48 hr in the rat and hagfish respectively (Steiner, 1977).

Isolated insulin granules are unstable above pH 6·0, which is below the intracellular pH of 7·2 in the islets (Hellman, Sehlin and Täljedal, 1972b; Hellman, 1975). In vitro, calcium stabilises these granules (Hellman et al., 1972b; Hellman, 1975) which contain zinc, calcium (Schäfer and Klöppel, 1974), ATP (Leitner, Sussman, Vatter and Schneider, 1975) and can take up and store biogenic amines (Hellman, Lernmark, Sehlin and Täljedal, 1972a).

D-Glucose, more specifically the α-anomer, D-mannose, D-glyceraldehyde and several glucose derivatives stimulate insulin synthesis. Joint regulation of synthesis and release appear to depend on a common glucose receptor and partially common glucose dependent processes. In the rat islets, the effective glucose concentration range for synthesis is 1·4–8 mM, which is lower than that for the release (Truehart, Maldonato, Kaelin, Renold and Sharp, 1976). Maximal rates are attained in 10–15 min (Lernmark et al., 1976; Truehart et al., 1976) and are not dependent on extracellular calcium (Ashcroft, 1976). The early effect is on initiation of synthesis on existing mRNA, de novo mRNA synthesis starting after a lag of about 20 min in the rat, contributing significantly to the translatory rate after 60 min (Permutt and Kipnis, 1975). Intracellular cAMP levels when increased by methylxanthines significantly alter rates at lower glucose concentrations. Hence, in vivo, at basal glucose levels, insulin synthesis may be half-maximally stimulated and rapidly accelerate upon stimulation of insulin release (Truehart et al., 1976), and maintenance of islet cAMP levels by gut hormones postprandially or by glucagon may influence these rates (Niki and Niki, 1976). There may be other possible points of joint regulation of synthesis and release since at maximal rates of insulin release, glucose also accelerates proinsulin (PRO) conversion to insulin (Jain and Logothetopoulos, 1977; Sando, Borg and Steiner, 1972). The physiological significance of inhibition of insulin synthesis by D-glyceraldehyde (Niki and Niki, 1976) and arginine (Lin, 1977) at high concentrations is not clear. Insulin probably does not have a negative feedback control on its synthesis (Schatz and Pfeiffer, 1977; Duran-Garcia, Jarrousse and Rosselin, 1976).

Genetic factors influence insulin synthesis or its responsiveness to glucose (Truehart et al., 1976). In man, familial hyperproinsulinaemia, of autosomal dominant inheritance, is associated with an incomplete and possibly atypical PRO conversion product (Gabbay, de Luca, Fisher, Mako, Rubenstein and Steiner, 1976, 1977). Incompletely processed PRO (Creuzfeldt, Arnold, Creuzfeldt, Deuticke, Frerichs and Track 1973) and atypical storage forms of insulin (Permutt et al., 1976) exist in human insulinomas. In diabetes, incomplete conversion products are increased in the peripheral circulation and may be physiologically effective (see Section E.1). Decreased conversion of PRO to insulin and/or decreased synthesis and storage (see Sando et al., 1972) may cause increased preferential release of PRO by creating a discrepancy between frequency of demand and time of maturation of the insulin granule.

C. CONTROL OF INSULIN RELEASE

The mechanism of direct control of insulin release is not clearly understood. Greater research emphasis has been placed on the stimulation-response aspect of the problem, but the data cannot be satisfactorily pieced together. Information on the processes of mobilisation of the storage granules and extrusion of insulin is scant. The topics of stimulation by sugars (Ashcroft, 1976), cyclic nucleotide regulation (Montague and Howell, 1975) and kinetics (Grodsky, 1975) of insulin release have been reviewed. An attempt will be made here to correlate the advances in various aspects of the problem in man and in experimental animals.

1. Sugars and Ions

D-Glucose is the most potent physiological stimulus to insulin release (Ashcroft, 1976). Other sugars with relative potencies apparently correlating with their metabolism in the islets have been studied, and some of these can augment the glucose effect (Padron, Hunt and Lewis, 1972; Ashcroft, 1976;

Sener and Malaisse, 1977). Islet response to glucose is biphasic. The early phase has all or none characteristics with a critical glucose threshold and requiring a finite time of stimulation, gaining maximal rates within 2 min and decaying sharply. The second phase sets in slowly after a period of desensitisation, reaching maximal rates in 40–60 min. It is comparable to closely overlapping monophasic responses (Garcia-Hermida and Gomez-Acebo, 1974), sharply accelerating with an additional stimulus and rapidly decaying on its withdrawal. Of the monovalent and divalent cations tested, only potassium at concentrations above 4–8 mM stimulated a monophasic insulin response in the presence of low (e.g. 3 mM or 50 mg/dl) glucose concentrations (see Henquin and Lambert, 1974b).

A strong stimulation of islets by glucose for as short as 5 min (Henquin and Lambert, 1974b), interrupted by a short rest period, potentiates the response to a subsequent stimulation of equal strength by glucose (Grodsky, 1975) or potassium (Henquin and Lambert, 1974b). Hence a process with memory operates simultaneously with that of rapid decay after stimulus withdrawal. Previous exposure of the intact pancreas to glucose also regulates in a dose-dependent manner, the time taken for the start of the first phase (Lenzen, 1978a) and the rate of stimulation influences the rate of release, especially during the first phase (O'Connor, Landahl and Grodsky, 1977).

Stimulation causes membrane depolarisation superimposed with regular bursts of further depolarisations associated with action potentials. The dynamics of onset and acceleration of this activity closely resembles that of biphasic insulin release (Meissner and Attwater, 1976). More cells cooperate with increasing glucose concentration (Dean and Matthews, 1970a). The first phase is less synchronised than the second, suggesting stimulus propagation (Meissner, 1976). Depolarisation and action potentials are separate phenomena (Dean and Matthews, 1970a; Dean, Matthews and Sakomoto, 1975). The latter are consistent with transient cation-membrane associations, correlating in amplitude and frequency with external calcium levels (Pace and Price, 1972; Dean and Matthews, 1970b). Depolarisation in glucose solutions of normal ionic composition is more consistent with glucose uptake and phosphorylation (Dean et al., 1975; Dean and Matthews, 1970a).

Release of insulin occurs by extrusion of insulin granule contents after fusion of the granule with the cell membrane, or "emiocytosis" (Lacy, 1970; Berger, Dahl and Meissner, 1975; Orci, Amherdt, Malaisse-Lagae, Rouiller and Renold, 1973a). Endocytosis of surface membrane has also been demonstrated (Orci, Malaisse-Lagae, Ravazzola, Amherdt and Renold. 1973b). Electron microscopic evidence for alignment of granules (Orci, 1974), their fusion or "binesis" before discharge (Gabbay, Korff and Schneeberg, 1975), the periodicity of electric activity and the spiky nature of release (Garcia-Hermida and Gomez-Acebo, 1974) suggest that insulin release is not continuous but quantal and episodic. The coincidence of granular discharge and action potentials have not been proven but suggested (Berger et al., 1975).

The mechanisms linking changes in glucose concentration to the rates of insulin discharge is not known. Both phases of insulin release (Cerasi, 1975a), the increased number of cells with electrical activity (Dean and Matthews, 1970a), net islet calcium accumulation (Hellman, Sehlin and Täljedal, 1971), glucose oxidation to carbon dioxide (Ashcroft, 1976) bear the same sigmoidal dose-response relationship to glucose concentration, and are abolished by prevention of glucose phosphorylation (Ashcroft, 1976).

Islets possess adenyl and guanyl cyclase phosphodiesterase, protein phosphokinase and phosphoprotein phosphatase activities (Montague and Howell, 1975). Glucose mediated release is inhibited and potentiated by stimulators (Malaisse, Malaisse-Lagae and King, 1968) and inhibitors, respectively of phosphodiesterase activity (Montague and Howell, 1975). Glucagon, which binds to a specific receptor in the islets, coupled to adenyl cyclase (Goldfine et al., 1972), raises cAMP levels within 1 min, but insulin release occurs only in the presence of glucose and with a delay of more than 1 min (Schauder, McIntosh and Frerichs, 1977b). However islet cAMP may mediate the rapid insulin release, and its rapid potentiation, probably by regulating the liberation of intracellularly sequestered calcium into the cytosol and the insulin granule compartments (Herman, Sato and Hales, 1973; Ravazzola, Malaisse-Lagae, Amherdt, Perrolet, Malaisse and Orci, 1976; Hellman, Sehlin and Täljedal, 1976; Montague and Howell, 1975; Brisson and Malaisse, 1973). The potentiation of insulin release is also limited by the maximally stimulatory glucose concentration and not the absolute cAMP levels attained (Hellman, Idahl, Lernmark and Täljedal, 1974c).

Glucose increases islet cAMP content with the same dynamics of the onset of insulin release (Cerasi, 1975a; Zawalich, Karl, Ferrendelli and Matschinsky, 1975). Stimulation of release, initiation of action potentials and increase in cAMP levels are dependent on physiological extracellular calcium concentration (Ashcroft, 1976; Zawalich et al., 1975; Henquin and Lambert, 1975; Dormer, Kerbey, McPherson, Marley, Ashcroft, Schofield and Randle, 1973). However, glucose does not directly stimulate any of the cAMP associated enzymes (Montague and Howell, 1975) and calcium is inhibitory to cyclase action (Davis and Lazarus, 1972). At the outset, therefore, an effect of glucose is associated with calcium uptake and a sudden increase in cAMP levels.

There is evidence to suggest calcium enters the cells (Malaisse, Sener, Davis and Somers, 1976a; Somers, Devis, van Obberghen and Malaisse, 1976; Hellman, Sehlin and Taljedal, 1971; Naber, McDaniel and Lacy, 1976). It appears to be coupled, in a regulatory role, to a Na^+–Na^+ exchange pump and a Na^+/K^+-ATPase inhibited by ouabain, and stimulated by K^+ but not sensitive to glucose (Sehlin and Taljedal, 1974; Curry, Joy, Holley and Bennett, 1977; Lernmark, Parman and Täljedal, 1977; Lowe, Richardson, Donatsch and Buchelli, 1976). Indeed, sudden depletion of extracellular sodium causes transient action potentials of high amplitude (Dean and Matthews, 1970b) and monophasic insulin release (Lambert, Henquin and Malveaux, 1974a). But manipulating this pump by sodium or potassium depletion or by ouabain subsequently render islets refractory to glucose stimulation (Lambert *et al.*, 1974a, b; Henquin and Lambert, 1974a). Electric pulsations are lost (Dean and Matthews, 1970; Attwater and Meissner, 1975) and glucose metabolism is inhibited (Hellman, Idahl, Lernmark and Täljedal, 1974b; Ashcroft, Bassett and Randle, 1972; Matschinsky and Ellerman, 1973). However, the significant inhibition of calcium efflux after glucose stimulation (Malaisse, Brisson and Baird, 1973a) may account for the rapid intracellular accumulation through voltage-sensitive channels after depolarisation (Lowe *et al.*, 1976). A greater net calcium uptake is noted later during release (Hellman, *et al.*, 1976a; Sehlin and Täljedal, 1974; Malaisse-Lagae and Malaisse, 1971). These observations also emphasise the importance of ionic movements in the coordination of glucose metabolism and sustained insulin release.

It is possible to elicit a small but distinct monophasic release in the absence of glucose and presence of 10 nM extracellular calcium after mobilisation of intracellular calcium by the ionophore A23187 (Karl, Zawalich, Ferrendelli and Matschinsky, 1975) or by raising endogenous cAMP levels by theophylline (Charles, Lawecki, Picton and Grodsky, 1975; Hellman, Sehlin, Söderberg and Täljedal, 1975b) or by veratridine depolarisation (Malaisse, Sener, Koser, Ravazzola and Malaisse-Lagae, 1976b). However, the second phase with normal dynamics of release, requires the presence of glucose and extracellular calcium. At less than physiological levels of calcium, potentiating stimuli cause a delayed second phase (Charles *et al.*, 1975). Hence the ultimate effector of release is calcium, glucose mediating calcium coupling to release mechanisms.

The mode of glucose recognition is the subject of controversy. A membrane-associated hexose receptor (Price, 1973) with strong stereospecificity for the α-stereoisomer of D-glucose has been proposed (Niki and Niki, 1976). On the other hand, glucose metabolism may produce the entity, or entities, responsible for initiation of discharge (Montague and Taylor, 1969; Ashcroft, 1976; Malaisse *et al.*, 1976b; Sugden and Ashcroft, 1977) apart from supplying the energy for the discharge process and its potentiation (Hellman and Idahl, 1970; Ashcroft, Chatra, Weerasinghe and Randle, 1973; Leitner *et al.*, 1975; Georg, Sussman, Leitner and Kirsch, 1971; Basabe, Farina and Chieri, 1975; Frerichs, Schauder, McIntosh, Panten and Creutzfeldt, 1977). Hence the glucose metabolites glucose-6-phosphate, and phosphoenol pyruvate are stimulatory to the protein kinase activity (Davis and Lazarus, 1975), and these and 2-phosphoglycerate and alpha-glycerophosphate inhibit phospho-protein phosphatase (Sussman and Leitner, 1976). Consistent effects of these compounds were also noted in a reconstructed *in vitro* emiocytosis system (Davis and Lazarus, 1976). Islet protein kinase phosphorylates amongst others, insulin granule and membrane associated proteins not yet charac-terised (Montague and Howell, 1975).

The common point of glucose and external calcium ion effects on rapid cAMP generation may be at the level of the glycolytic trioses (Hellman, 1970) implicated in the control of cAMP dependent proteins, metabolism of which generates cytosolic ATP and NADH. It is at this level that islet glucose metabolism is consistently altered by depletion of extracellular calcium, sodium, or addition of ouabain, the sodium diuretic diazoxide, adrenalin (Hellman *et al.*, 1974b), anoxia (Hellman, Idahl, Sehlin and Täljedal, 1975a) and low levels of sulphydryl reagents (Hellman, Idahl, Lernmark, Sehlin and Täljedal, 1973). Also in the absence of external glucose, but with endo-genous glycogen, theophylline can bring about calcium uptake and insulin release (Malaisse *et al.*, 1976b). Potentiating input may also occur here (Ashcroft, 1976), as is observed after desensitisation to glucose during experi-mental hyperthyroidism (Lenzen, Joost and Haselblatt, 1976b). Calcium uptake may depend on the integrity of those stages of glucose metabolism which generate reduced nucleotides and maintain the membrane redox state (Malaisse, Sener, Kawazu and Boschero, 1977; Hellman, Idahl, Lern-mark, Sehlin and Täljedal, 1974a). Granule margination before emiocytosis is proposed to be mediated by a microtubular microfilamentous system (Ostlund, 1977). Microtubules are formed by reversible polymerisation of tubulin, possibly under the control of cAMP dependent protein kinases (Montague and Howell, 1975; Ostlund, 1977). These are reduced in concen-tration in starvation, or in the genetic diabetes of obese mice, and increase after glucose feeding (Selawry, 1973; Malaisse-Lagae, Ravazzola, Amherdt, Gutzeit, Stauffacher, Malaisse and Orci, 1975). Participation in granule extrusion of the microfilamentous contractile lining of the cell membrane has also been considered (Ostlund, 1977). The process of granule-membrane fusion is not known, but a facilitating role for calcium by charge neutralisa-tion has been speculated (Matthews, 1970).

2. Glucose and Human Foetal Pancreas

Immunoreactive insulin is detected in foetal pancreas in the 7th week of gestation, and granular storage between 9–10 weeks (Pronina and Sapronova, 1976). Insulin concentration increases by about 60 fold between the 7th and

15th weeks. As sensitivity to glucose appears by the 10–12th weeks, the relative potentiating effect of methylxanthines is reduced. Between the 15th and 22nd weeks, pancreatic insulin concentration is constant, while release into foetal blood starts (*ca* 5–10 μu/ml) and glucose sensitivity increases. From the 22nd–32nd weeks, insulin in the islets and circulation is further raised to 10 mu/g and 35 μu/ml respectively. This rise in insulin levels depends on an intact hypophysis (Turner and Cohen, 1974). Unlike the rat, arginine sensitivity was not detected in one study (Pronina and Sapronova, 1976) whereas others noted greater insulin response to arginine than to glucose, while pre-exposure to glucose retarded the response to arginine. Pancreatic insulin concentration increased between 1 5–20 weeks but levels in the foetal blood were not reported (Schäfer, Wilder and Williams, 1973). In the rat, serum insulin concentration increases before birth, but glucose sensitivity is established *post partum* (Foa, Blazquez, Sodoyez and Sodoyez-Goffeaux, 1976).

3. Glucose and Human Adult

Biphasic insulin release occurs when a priming pulse of glucose is followed by continuous infusion for up to 1 hr (Cerasi and Luft, 1967). Both phases display a sigmoidal dose-response relationship to glucose over the fasting threshold (Cerasi, 1975a; Cerasi, Fick and Rudemo, 1974). The alpha anomer of glucose is more insulinogenic than the beta form (Rossini and Soeldner, 1976). Intravenous galactose and xylitol cause low insulin release detectable in the portal but not the peripheral venous blood (Seino, 1976; Berger, Geissner, Moppert and Künzli, 1973).

The rate of infusion of i.v. glucose, i.e. the rate of stimulation of the B cell, influences the rate of first phase insulin discharge (Chen and Porte, 1976; Savage, Brannison, Flock and Bennett, 1977). The response to the i.v. glucose pulse is monophasic and the amount of insulin discharged between 3–5 min after the pulse is dose-dependent up to 20 g (Lerner and Porte, 1971). Insulin and C-peptide are released in equimolar amounts into the portal vein after i.v. insulin and the percentage of proinsulin-like immunoreactivity (PLC) (see Section E.1) of total insulin is within the range for extracted pancreas, confirming emiocytosis as the predominant mode of release (Horwitz, Starr, Mako, Blackard and Rubenstein, 1975). In isolated rat pancreas the percentage of PLC released increased with time within 1 hr of stimulation (Burr, Staufacher, Balant, Renold and Grodsky, 1969) whereas insulin release relative to PLC increases after 1 hr (Sando *et al.*, 1972). Hence, exposure to glucose may increase proinsulin conversion (Jain and Legothetopoulos, 1977). In diabetes, PLC conversion to insulin may be retarded since

1 hr after stimulation of release, peripheral PLC percentage is higher than normal (see Table 3). The early phase of release is diminished in diabetes (Simpson, Benedetti, Grodsky, Karam and Forsham, 1969) and the second phase is retarded (Chin, Hamashiro, Khan and Blankenhorn, 1974; Cerasi, 1975a). Fasting hyperglycaemia blunts early insulin response to i.v. or oral glucose (Brunzell, Robertson, Lerner, Hazzard, Ensinck, Bierman and Porte, 1976; Szabo, Oppermann, Victor and Camerini-Davalos, 1974).

4. Amino Acids

L-Isomers of amino acids stimulate insulin release but, except leucine, not all are effective in every species (Rocha, Faloona and Unger, 1972; Pfeiffer and Telib, 1968; Basabe, Lopez, Victora and Wolff, 1971). Leucine is metabolised in isolated islets (Nikkila and Tashkinen, 1975; Hellman et al., 1971). The metabolite α-oxoisocaproic acid also stimulates insulin release by increasing islet cAMP levels (Frerichs et al., 1977). Leucine does not directly influence the cAMP associated islet enzymes (Montague and Howell, 1975). Arginine is poorly metabolised in islets (Hellman et al., 1971), and potentiates glucose-stimulated insulin release (Basabe et al., 1971). An effect on the transmembrane cation equilibrium may mediate the effect of amino acids on insulin release (Aynsley-Green and Alberti, 1974; Hill, 1971). Also, arginine inhibits intracellular transport of leucine but does not change its insulinogenic effect (Lin, 1977; Panten and Christians, 1973; Gylfe, 1974). In man, arginine, then lysine, leucine and phenylalanine are most effective in stimulating insulin release (Fajans and Floyd, 1972). Arginine acts rapidly in man (Rabinowitz, Spitz, Gönen and Paran, 1973; Palmer, Walter and Ensinck, 1976b); and in the rat (Aynsley-Green and Alberti, 1974) and unlike leucine also stimulate glucagon release, causing hyperglycaemia (Rabinowitz et al., 1973; Palmer et al., 1976b). The magnitude of potentiation of the glucose effect by arginine is very variable between individuals and is not dose-dependent (Palmer et al., 1976b; Knopf, Conn, Floyd, Fajans, Rull, Guntsche and Thiffault, 1966). Arginine potentiates the response to subsequent tolbutamide stimulation (Widström and Cerasi, 1973c) and the potentially diabetic subject or the early maturity onset type of diabetic, show higher than normal sensitivity to arginine priming of glucose (Seino, Ikeda, Nakane, Nakahara, Seino and Imura, 1977; Efendic, Cerasi and Luft, 1974a; Palmer, Benzon, Walter and Ensinck, 1976a). Theophylline augments insulin response to arginine but not to tolbutamide (Widström and Cerasi, 1973c). The physiological effect of amino acids may be to increase the insulin:glucagon ratio to stimulate protein anabolism (Unger, 1974).

5. Fats

Short chain free fatty acids (FFA) and ketone bodies stimulate insulin release in the presence of glucose. Their effects *in vitro* or *in vivo* vary with different species (Hawkins, Alberti, Houghton, Williamson and Krebs, 1973; Goberna, Tamarit, Osorio, Fussganger, Tamarit and Pfeiffer, 1974; Crespin, Greenoghn and Steinberg, 1973; Madison, Mebaner, Unger and Lochrer, 1964; Horino, Machlin, Hertelendy and Kipnis, 1968). Infusion of FFA in man does not alter fasting insulin levels but augments the response to glucose, arginine or tolbutamide (Balasse and Ooms, 1973; Hicks, Taylor, Vij, Pek, Knopf, Floyd and Fajans, 1977). Ketone body effects *in vitro* are short-lived (Goberna *et al.*, 1974). The inconsistent results in man (Balasse and Ooms, 1968) may be due to poor reflection of the portal insulin levels in the periphery (Horwitz, *et al.*, 1975). Triglycerides do not directly stimulate insulin release (Eaton and Nye, 1973).

6. Hormonal Effects

(a) *Pancreatic hormones*

Exogenous proinsulin, and less strongly insulin, inhibit glucose-mediated insulin release in man, more effectively at lower glucose concentrations (Dunbar, McLaughlin, Walsh and Foa, 1975). *In vitro* islet glucose metabolism is also inhibited (Dunbar *et al.*, 1975; Akhtar, Verspohl, Hegner and Ammon, 1977). Islets are hyperpolarised and action potentials cease (Pace, Matschinsky, Lacy and Conant, 1977). The effect appears to be opposite to that of glucose and glucagon on rat islets (Akhtar *et al.*, 1977; Montague and Taylor, 1969) and may have physiological significance, since insulin also inhibits glucagon release (see Table 2).

Glucagon binds to a specific receptor and rapidly activates the adenyl cyclase system (Goldfine *et al.*, 1972) but insulin release occurs only in the presence of glucose when the magnitude and duration of cAMP elevation is greater and correlates with insulin release (Schauder *et al.*, 1977a; Schauder *et al.*, 1977b).

Exogenous somatostatin (STN) inhibits insulin and glucagon release (Table 2). Differential control of A and B cells by STN has been proposed (Taborsky and Smith, 1977; Schauder *et al.*, 1977b; Bhathena, Perrino, Voyles, Smith, Wilkins, Coy, Schally and Recant, 1976). In man and rat, arginine-stimulated insulin release is more sensitive to STN than glucagon release (Efendic *et al.*, 1976). Inhibition of cAMP production and insulin response to glucose is competitive with glucose (Claro, Grill, Efendic and Luft, 1977). Indeed glucagon-potentiated insulin release is more sensitive to

STN than release after glucose alone (Sieradzki, Schatz, Nierle and Pfeiffer, 1975). The minimally effective dose is more inhibitory to the second phase (Efendic, Luft and Grill, 1974b). *In vivo*, inhibition is rapidly reversed after cessation of STN infusion (Scurol, Le Cercio, Adam, Garrannini, Bianchi, Cominacini and Corgnati, 1976) and can be prevented by high extracellular calcium or potassium (Bhathena *et al.*, 1976) and is not mediated through α-adrenergic receptors (Wollheim, Kikuchi, Renold and Sharp, 1977; Efendic and Luft, 1975). Attempts to use STN have been made therapeutically for suppression of insulin response of islet cell tumours to glucose (Scurol *et al.*, 1976; Efendic, Lins, Sigurdsson, Ivemark, Granberg and Luft, 1971).

Exogenous vasoactive inhibitory peptide (VIP) and pancreatic poly-peptide (PP) are the least studied of this class of hormones. After injection *in vivo* (Schebalin, Said and Makhlouf, 1977) or perfusion of dog pancreas, VIP (Bloom and Iversen, 1976; Kaneto, 1977; Schebalin *et al.*, 1977) and hPP (Bloom and Iversen, 1976) in physiological or pharmacological doses have no effect on insulin release. The consistent release of glucagon after VIP is not reversible by atropine or β-blockade (Kaneto, 1977).

(b) *Gastro-intestinal hormones*

Oral glucose (McIntyre, Holdsworth, and Turner, 1964) or amino acids (Raptis, Dollinger, Schröder, Schleyer, Rothenberger and Pfeiffer, 1975) releases more insulin than an i.v. infusion which attains similar serum levels of glucose, and oral fat potentiates the insulin response to i.v. glucose (Rabino-witz *et al.*, 1973; Brown, Drysburgh, Ross and Dupre, 1975). Portal vein insulin rises within 2 min of administering oral glucose, 6 min before a change occurs in the portal vein glucose levels (Reyes-Leal, Castro, Bernal and Quandiola, 1973). Corresponding peripheral changes occur 1–2 min later (Karamanos, Butterfield, Asmal and Cox, 1971).

This early insulin response is attributed to a duodenal insulin-releasing activity (Zermatten, Heptner, Delahoye, Sechaud and Feiber, 1977). The later release is massive, peaks normally between 30–60 min (Szabo *et al.*, 1974), and gradually declines after 90 min. The peripheral and portal vein levels of insulin vary in parallel (Schulz, Michaelis, Siegler, Teichmann, Nowak, Albrecht and Bibergeil, 1976). The identity of "incretin" or gut factors which potentiate insulin release, is a subject of controversy (Brown, *et al.*, 1975). A combined action of all hormones in response to different types of nutrients has been proposed (Rehfeld, Stadil, Baden and Fischerman, 1975). The "incretin" probably makes up for inherent B cell insensitivity to a slowly rising stimulus to ensure efficient glucose clearance (Chin *et al.*, 1974).

Table 2

Pancreatic endocrine response to stimuli.

Species	Stimulus	Effect on release			References
		Insulin	Glucagon	Somatostatin	
Rat	↑Mg^{++}	↓			Bhathena et al. (1976)
Rat	↑K$^+$	↑	↑		Bhathena et al. (1976)
Rat	glyceraldehyde	↑	→		Schauder et al. (1977)
Rat	theophylline + glucose	↑			Schauder et al. (1977)
Rat	theophylline	—		→	Schauder et al. (1977)
Rat/dog	glucagon + glucose	↑		↑	Schauder et al. (1977)
				↑	Patton et al. (1976)
Dog	glucagon		→	↑	Ipp et al (1977)
Rat/dog	α-ketoisocaproate	↑		↑	Schauder et al. (1977)
					Frerichs et al. (1977)
Dog	L-leucine	↑	↑	↑	Schauder et al. (1977)
					Ipp et al (1977)
					Frerichs et al. (1977)
Dog	L-arginine	↑	↑	↑	Pek et al. (1976)
Dog					Ipp et al. (1977)
Dog	tolbutamide	↑↑	↑↓		Samols and Harrison (1976)
	tolbutamide + amino acids	↑↑	↑↓		Samols and Harrison (1976)
	tolbutamide + amino acids + basal glucose	↑↑	↑↑		Samols and Harrison (1976)
	tolbutamide + basal glucose	↑→	↑→		Samols and Harrison (1976)
Dog	diazoxide	↑	→	→	Samols et al. (1977)
Dog, rat, man	FFA and ketones	↑	→		Edwards and Taylor (1970)
					Gerich et al. (1974b)
					Seyffert and Madison (1967)

Species	Agent				Reference
Man	biguanides		→	→	Stout et al. (1974)
					Bohannon et al. (1977)
Man (rat)	adrenalin		↓, ↑	→	Ipp et al. (1977)
		→			Sanderson and Dietel (1974)
					Iversen (1973a)
Man	dopamine		←	←	Gerich et al. (1974a)
Man	acetylcholine		←	←	Leblanc et al. (1977)
Man	atropine		→	→	Iversen (1973b)
					Henderson et al. (1976)
Man	vagotomy		→	→	Bloom et al. (1974)
					Bloom et al. (1974)
Man	glucagon		←	→	Håkanson et al. (1971)
		←			Patton et al. (1976)
Man	insulin		→	→	Ipp et al. (1977)
					Ipp et al. (1977)
Man	somatostatin		→	→	Dunbar et al. (1975)
Man (neonate)	insulin		→	→	Pek et al. (1976); text
Man (neonate)	somatostatin		—	—	Massi-Benedetti et al. (1974)
Guinea-pig	insulin		→	→	Sodoyez-Goffaux et al. (1977)
					Östenson et al. (1977)

Gastro-intestinal peptide (GIP) potentiates *in vivo* and *in vitro*, the glucose-mediated release of insulin, while maintaining basal glucagon levels (Brown et al., 1975; Taminato, Seino, Goto, Inoue, Kadowaki, Mori, Hazawa, Yajima and Imura, 1977); these effects are prevented by somatostatin (Pedersen, Drysburg and Brown, 1973). A transient elevation of GIP occurs 3 min after oral glucose and i.v. pentagastrin (Brown et al., 1975). In fasting man, exogenous GIP increases insulin levels only after i.v. glucose administration (Pedersen, Brown, Tobin and Andres, 1975; Cleator and Gourlay, 1975). Peak GIP levels after oral glucose, a standard meal or fat emulsion ingestion occur successively later, not always in phase with termination of gastric digestion (Brown et al., 1975) and are therefore probably related to intestinal absorption (Creutzfeldt, Ebert, Arnold, Frerichs and Brown, 1976). In human obesity, fasting and postprandial levels are doubled and correlate with the insulinaemia (Creutzfeldt, Ebert, Frerichs and Brown, 1978). Inhibition of GIP release by endogenous or exogenous insulin has been demonstrated (Brown et al., 1975; Cleator and Gourlay, 1975) but not consistently (Service, Go, Blix and Nelson, 1977a). GIP levels increase in insulinopaenia or mild pancreatitis (Creutzfeldt et al., 1975; Ebert, Creutzfeldt, Brown, Frerichs and Arnold, 1976), or diabetes (Brown et al., 1975; Eaton and Nye, 1973), or in obesity with B cell decompensation and delayed insulinaemia (Creutzfeldt et al., 1978). Overall evidence suggests that rates of gastric emptying, neural effects and nutrient absorption contribute to GIP and hence insulin levels; the latter in turn may suppress GIP release.

The location of gastrin in pancreatic islets is disputable. Antisera against antral preparations but not those against synthetic gastrin, demonstrated gastrin and somatostatin in the same cell type (Erlandsen, Hage, Parsons, McEvoy and Elder, 1976). Gastrin-producing cells occur in nesidioblastosis (Hollands, Giron, Leny, Accary and Rosi, 1976). Gastrin contribution to "incretin" after protein rich meals (Rehfeld, 1976) may be mediated by GIP (Friesen, Bolinger and Kyner, 1974), which however, can rise in the absence of gastrin after antrectomy (Creutzfeldt et al., 1976).

Elevation of endogenous cholecystokinin-pancreozymin (CCK-PZ) or i.v. use of highly purified preparations did not confirm the stimulatory effect of impure preparations on insulin release which was attributed to GIP contamination (Taminato et al., 1977). The physiological significance of the insulin response to pharmacological doses of the synthetic CCK octapeptide has been doubted (Bloom and Iversen, 1976).

Purified secretin does not cause insulin release in the rat (Ohara, 1976). Insulinaemia was observed in the portal but not in the peripheral circulation in the dog (Boden, Essa, Owen, Reichle and Sarago, 1974). Sensitivity to secretin is significantly increased in diabetes, although only large doses cause prompt release of insulin in normal man (Enk, 1976; Enk, Lund,

Schmidt and Deckert, 1976) and potentiate the response to glucose but not to arginine, tolbutamide or glucagon (Lerner, 1977; Czyzyk, Szadhowski, Kogela and Lawecki, 1973).

7. Neural Effects

Parts of the central nervous system, the ventromedial hypothalamic nuclei (Frohman and Bernardis, 1971) and cerebral lateral ventricles (Frohman Muller and Cocchi, 1973) are believed to suppress insulin release via the adrenal medulla. A direct neural inhibitory and stimulatory effect of hypothalamic stimulation on insulin release from the innervated, isolated rat pancreas has been demonstrated (Curry and Joy, 1974). A "ventrolateral hypothalamic factor" stimulates insulin release in the rat (Martin, Mok, Penfold, Howard and Crowne, 1973). Sympathetic and parasympathetic innervation of the islets has been demonstrated (Wood and Porte, 1974; Orci, 1974).

(a) Sympathetic nervous system

Sympathetic control may be mediated by nerves or through the adrenal medulla. Splanchnic innervation as well as the adrenomedullary catecholamines inhibit insulin (Bloom and Edwards, 1975; Sando, Miki and Kosaka, 1977) and augment glucagon release in the dog (Bloom and Edwards, 1975). Fasting insulin levels may not be controlled by the former route in man (Äärimaa, Slatis, Haapaniemi and Jeglinsky, 1974; Brodow, Pi-Sunyer and Campbell, 1974) but probably by the latter (Brodows et al., 1974). Adrenalin can depress fasting levels (Turner and Holman, 1976; Arnman, Carlström and Thorell, 1975; Turner and Hart, 1977a). This inhibition may be enhanced in diabetes since catecholamine levels can be high, and phentolamine, unlike in normal man, increases the fasting levels (Robertson, Halter and Porte, 1976; Efendic, Cerasi and Luft, 1973) not only by alpha blockade, which prevents catecholamine inhibition of release (Gerich, Langlois, Noacco, Schneider and Forsham, 1974; Robertson and Porte, 1973; Brandt, Kehlet, Faber and Binder, 1977; Hill, Sönksen and Brainbridge, 1974), but an accentuation of the beta effect (Wood and Porte, 1974) since catecholamines can prime rat islets in vitro (Burr, Slonin and Sharp, 1976) and in man (Massara, Camanni, Martelli and Molinatti, 1977) and increase the response to subsequent glucose stimulation. Also, they do not prevent glucose potentiation of the glucose-stimulated insulin release in man (Widström and Cerasi, 1973b). Hence the rebound insulin release in man after catecholamine infusion may be partly due to such a late beta-potentiation of release stimulated by the transient hyperglycaemia (Turner et al., 1977a; Cerasi, 1975b) and

D

partly due to increasing islet microcirculation (Bunnag, Bunnag and Werner, 1968).

Adrenalin is present in similar amounts in non-diabetic and diabetic human cadaver pancreas in higher amounts than in the other tissues tested (Christensen and Neubauer, 1976). Higher than normal levels were found in diabetic Chinese hamster islets (Feldman, Snyder and Gerritsen, 1977). Adrenalin inhibits, via the alpha-adrenergic receptors, insulin response to glucose, amino acids, tolbutamide, in the presence or absence of glucagon or theophylline (Wood and Porte, 1974; Iversen, 1973a; Malaisse, 1972). Inhibition of adenylcyclase and cAMP-dependent protein kinase activity in islet homogenates may involve direct effects (Montague and Howell, 1975). The glucose-inhibited calcium efflux (Brisson and Malaisse, 1973) and early calcium accumulation by the islets (Wollheim *et al.*, 1977), not yet correlated with cAMP changes, are also reversed. Adrenalin abolishes action potentials without altering the membrane potential set by glucose (Dean and Matthews, 1970a) or glucose oxidation in the islets (Herman and Deckert, 1977). In the obese mouse islets, with increased B:A cell ratio, oxidation is sensitive to adrenalin (Hellman *et al.*, 1969).

(b) Parasympathetic nervous system

This system mediates stimulation of insulin and glucagon release. Vagotomy partly abolishes this output (Frohman, Ezdinli and Javid, 1967; Kaneto, Miki and Kosaka, 1974). A "temporally related cooperativity" between sympathetic and parasympathetic systems in the control of insulin release with acetylcholine rather than glucose control of the first phase of insulin release has been proposed (Burr *et al.*, 1976). In man methacholine raises fasting insulin levels (Kajinuma, Kaneto, Kuzuya and Nakao, 1968) and atropine inhibits insulin response to oral but not i.v. glucose (Henderson, Jefferys, Jones and Stanley, 1976). Vagotomy impairs "incretin" effect in man (Hakanson, Liedberg and Lundquist, 1971), abolishes hyperphagia and islet hypertrophy of hypothalamic obesity in the rat (Powley and Opsahl, 1974), and prevents, like atropine, the "conditioned" hypoglycaemia in the dog and rat induced by the smell of food before ingestion (Wood, 1972; Wood and Porte, 1974). A similar cholinergic control of release has been demonstrated in man (Goldfine, Abraira, Grunewald and Goldstein, 1970; Parra-Cavarrubias, Rivera-Rodriguez and Almarez-Ugalde, 1971). Acetylcholine activates a guanyl cyclase (Montague and Howell, 1975) and causes atropine-sensitive insulin and glucagon release (Loubatieres-Mariani, Chapel, Alric and Loubatieres, 1973; Iversen, 1973b), the stimulatory effects being abolished by adrenalin (Montague and Howell, 1975; Kaneto *et al.*, 1974).

(c) Monoamines

Precursors are taken up, converted to monoamines probably in the insulin granule (Ericson, Håkanson and Lundquist, 1977; Lundquist, Sundler, Håkanson, Larsson and Heding, 1975) which is proposed to be a mechanism of catecholamine deactivation (Feldman and Chapman, 1974) and causes the inhibition of glucose and β-adrenergically stimulated release (Gylfe, Hellman, Sehlin and Täljedal, 1973; Feldman and Chapman, 1974; Wilson, Downs, Feldman and Lebowitz, 1974). Long-term treatment with monoamine precursors raises basal insulin levels and blunts the response to glucose *in vivo* and *in vitro* (Burr, Jackson, Culbert, Sharp, Felts and Olson, 1974). Extracellular dopamine effect is α-adrenergic (Wilson *et al.*, 1974). However, in man, dopamine infusion increases insulin, glucagon and blood glucose levels, but the glucagon depression normally occurring after a standard meal is enhanced by a subsequent dopamine infusion (Leblanc *et al.*, 1977). Antiserotoninergic treatment of potentially diabetic patients augments insulin response to glucose and tolbutamide (Lebovitz and Feldman, 1973; Baldridge, Quickel, Feldman and Lebovitz, 1975).

8. Prostaglandins

Prostaglandins may mediate neuro-endocrinological stimulation of islet function. Their effects *in vivo* and *in vitro* are not consistent. *In vitro* PGE_1, E_2 and E_{2k} augment insulin release from rat islets (Sacca, Perez, Ringo, Pascucci and Condorelli, 1975). Adenyl but not the guanyl cyclase is stimulated by PGE_1 and E_2 (Montague and Howell, 1975; Kuo, Hodgins and Kuo, 1974). In the dog, these can be stimulatory and inhibitory to insulin release (Lefebvre and Luyckx, 1973; Robertson, 1974). In man PGE_1 and E_2 depressed the glucose effect, but PGE_1 augmented release in the presence of adrenalin and PGE_2 did not modify the arginine effect (Robertson and Chen, 1977; Burr and Sharp, 1974). Salicylate infusion augmented the response to i.v. glucose in man and normalised the diabetic response (Robertson and Chen, 1977).

9. Drugs and Insulin Release

(a) Adrenergic and monoaminergic agents

Islet alpha- and beta-adrenergic receptors mediate, respectively, inhibition and facilitation of insulin release (Wood and Porte, 1974), through decreased and increased cAMP levels, respectively (Montague and Howell, 1975; Kuo *et al.*, 1974; Atkins and Matty, 1970). Catecholamines are predominantly α-adrenergic and α-blockade unmasks their beta effect, while L-isopropyl-noradrenaline is β-adrenergic (Wood and Porte, 1974; Leitner *et al.*, 1975; Wilson *et al.*, 1974; Gerich *et al.*, 1974a). In early diabetes beta-stimulation or alpha-blockade improved the response to stimuli (Robertson *et al.*, 1976; Efendic *et al.*, 1973). Beta-antagonist antihypertensives do not influence release when taken orally (Hedstrand and Aberg, 1974; Hasslacher *et al.*, 1976), but clonidine is strongly α-adrenergic (Metz, Halter, Porte and Robertson, 1977). After salbutamol, insulin levels slowly rise (Taylor, Gaddie, Madison and Palmer, 1976). Effects of i.v. propanolol on the insulin response to glucose is inconsistent (Cerasi, Luft and Efendic, 1972; Robertson and Porte, 1973b). It is a strong local anaesthetic (Manku and Horrobin, 1976; Browne and Duggan, 1974) and like other local anaesthetics (Tjälve, Popov and Slawina, 1974) has dose dependent effects on islets (Bressler, Vargas-Gordon and Brendel, 1969).

Antiserotoninergic cyproheptadine raises insulin levels in the nondiabetic, but not in diabetic acromegalics (Feldman, Birens, Skyler and Lebovitz, 1975). *In vitro* it inhibits insulin release and can lyse islet cells (Joost, Beckmann, Lenzen and Hasselblatt, 1976), and chronic administration depletes insulin stores reversibly (Rickert, Fischer, Burke, Redick, Erlandsen, Parsons and Carden, 1976). Metergolin inhibits the response to arginine in normal and diabetic subjects and the response to glucose in normals only (Pontiroli, Vibert, Tognetti and Pozza, 1975). Methysergide augments the mild diabetic response to tolbutamide and glucose (Lebovitz and Feldman, 1973; Baldridge *et al.*, 1975) and tranylcypromine is strongly beta-adrenergic in the mouse (Bressler, Vargas-Gordon and Lebovitz, 1968).

(b) Alkaloids, toxins and lectins

The alkaloid quinine potentiates the glucose effect *in vitro* at 1–50 μM dosage, above which it is reversibly inhibitory (Henquin, Horemans, Nanquin, Verniers and Lambert, 1975). Theophylline and caffeine are effective in the mM range (Montague and Howell, 1975; Ashcroft, 1976), and at increased glycolytic flux potentiate the glucose effect by increasing cAMP levels, amplify the effects of poorly metabolised sugars (Ashcroft, 1976) and increase calcium uptake (Malaisse *et al.*, 1976b). In hypocalcaemia, in man, response to OGTT is normalised (Gedik and Zileli, 1977) and in normal (Widström and Cerasi, 1973c; Peracchi, Cavagnini, Pinto, Bulgeroni and Panerai, 1975), but not in the diabetic man (Botha, Vinik, Blake and Jackson, 1976), glucose and arginine effects are potentiated, but hyperglycaemia is not decreased and can increase (Arman *et al.*, 1975).

Cholera toxin with its beta chain homologous to glycoprotein hormones like TSH (Kurosky, Markel, Peterson and Fitch, 1977), can potentiate

(Hellman *et al.*, 1974c; Cerasi, 1975a) more strongly than TSH (Malaisse, 1972) the glucose effect by activation of the adenyl cyclase (Henquin *et al.*, 1975). Hypoglycin (methylene-cyclopropyl-alanine), the toxic mediator of Jamaican vomiting sickness, is structurally similar to leucine and causes insulin release *in vitro* (Milner and Wirdham, 1977).

Two mushroom lectins stimulate insulin and glucagon release at very low concentrations (Ewart, Kornfeld and Kipnis, 1975). Concanavalin A blocks specifically the response to glucose (Maier, Schneider, Schatz and Pfeiffer, 1975).

Monoguanidine and derivatives, creatine, arginine and the diuretic Amiloride, stimulate insulin release, but other derivatives can be inhibitory (Aynsley-Green and Alberti, 1974).

(c) Sulphonylureas

Tolbutamide, carbutamide, metahexamide, chlorpropamide, glisoxepide, glibornuride, gliclazide, glibenclamide (Gotfredsen, 1976; Lazarus and Volk, 1959; Loubatieres, Mariani, Ribes and Alric, 1973; Brisson and Malaisse, 1971) stimulate insulin release independently of glucose. They associate with islet cell membranes, possibly at multiple sites (see Lenzen, 1978a) and perhaps like the sulphydryl reagents; and, the variety of intracellular effects ranging from lysosomal enzyme activation (Lundquist and Lördahl, 1975) to inhibition of insulin and RNA synthesis (Schatz, Maier, Hinz, Nierle and Pfeiffer, 1972; Puchinger and Wacker, 1972) are deemed secondary to their influence on membrane phenomena (Hellman and Täljedal, 1975). The avidity of sulphonylurea binding correlates with insulin releasing potency, the persistence of potentiation of glucose effect and the degree of stimulation of calcium uptake (Hellman and Täljedal, 1975; Malaisse, Mahy, Brisson and Malaisse-Lagae, 1972; Brisson and Malaisse, 1971). Cell surface modification influences tolbutamide and glucose effects on insulin release differently (Macchi and Zeytinoğlu, 1976; Hahn, Hellman, Lernmark, Sehlin and Täljedal, 1973). Also, increasing extracellular calcium, magnesium and sodium above the physiological levels, favours the binding (Hellman, Sehlin and Täljedal, 1976b), and the calcium excess enhances insulin release (Curry, Bennett and Grodsky, 1968). Hence, *in vivo* hypophosphataemia enhances response to glucose but hypercalcaemia after calcium administratration augments the tolbutamide effect (Harter, Santiago, Rutherford, Slatopolsky and Klahr, 1976).

In the absence of glucose, the insulin release is monophasic (Grodsky, Bennett, Smith and Nemecheck, 1967; Curry *et al.*, 1968; Basabe *et al.*, 1976) and occurs faster than with glucose (Bennett, Curry and Curry, 1973; Lenzen and Hasselblatt, 1974; Lenzen, 1978a), followed by a slow insulin leak (Meissner and Attwater, 1976). In parallel to these changes in insulin release, cells rapidly depolarise and continuous action potentials are fired with loss of burst pattern (Meissner and Attwater, 1976; Dean et al., 1975), when a continuous calcium leak ensues (Malaisse, Pipeleers and Mahy, 1973b). Increased calcium localisation occurs inside the cell membrane (Klöppel and Schäfer, 1976). Anoxia or iodoacetate does not abolish this electrical activity (Dean et al., 1975) and glucose antagonises the sulphonyl-urea-mediated calcium handling (Malaisse et al., 1973b) indicating independence of action (Lenzen, 1978a). In the presence of low glucose concentrations, theophylline and phentolamine potentiate the effect of tolbutamide and with glibenclamide a significant insulin leak is attained (Basabe et al., 1976). Sulphonylurea stimulation of adenylcyclase and augmentation of protein kinase activity has been shown (Montague and Howell, 1975), which suggests an ability to raise cAMP concentration and translocate intracellularly sequestered calcium (Malaisse et al., 1973b). This could explain the rapid depletion of islet glycogen also seen after exposure of islets to glucagon (Hellman et al., 1973) or theophylline (Malaisse et al., 1976b) and recovery of release from iodoacetate inhibition after exo-genous ATP supply (Georg et al., 1971; Basabe et al., 1976).

Tolbutamide does not stimulate insulin release from 12–16-week-old foetal pancreas (Los Monteros, Driscoll and Steinke, 1970). In normal man the tolbutamide effect is very rapid, dose dependent (Widström and Cerasi, 1973b; Ganda, Kahn, Soeldner and Gleason, 1975) and correlates in the individual patient with the insulin response to i.v. glucose Ganda et al., 1975). Conflicting results on the chronic use of sulphonylureas in man have been reviewed (Lauvaux, Mandart, Heymans and Ooms, 1972). As in animals (Altzuler, Moran and Hampshire, 1977; Blumenthal, 1977; Leichter and Galasky, 1977) extrapancreatic effects influence the glucose levels. With chlorpropramide these effects (Barnes, Garbian, Crowley and Bloom, 1974; Hecht, Gershberg and Hulse, 1973; Owens, Seldrup, Wragg, Shetty and Briggs, 1977) may correct the fasting hyperglycaemia, thereby restoring the monophasic response to glucose (Brunzell et al., 1976). Improvement in insulin binding of receptors has been shown (Olefsky and Reaven, 1976). Glibenclamide is hyperstimulatory to release but the hypoglycaemia is not proportionately deep (Owens et al., 1977).

Adrenalin, antimycin A, oligomycin, iodoacetate, anoxia, hypothermia, diazoxide (Hellman and Täljedal, 1975) and phenylbutazone (El-Denshary and Montague, 1976) but not propranolol (Widström and Cerasi, 1973a) inhibit, and acetylsalicylic acid, sulphadimidine, chlorpromazine (El-Denshary and Montague, 1976), and dihydroergotamine (Sirek, Sirek, and Policova, 1974) potentiate the sulphonylurea effect on insulin release. Phenylbutazone and sulphonamides may free the albumin-bound drugs, whereas chlorpromazine facilitates the binding to cells (Hellman and Täljedal, 1975; Hellman, 1974).

(d) *Therapeutic agents*

The thiazide diuretic diazoxide reversibly inhibits insulin, somatostatin and pancreatic polypeptide release *in vitro* (Levin, Reed, Ching, Davis, Blum and Forsham, 1973; Samols, Weir, Patel, Fernandez-Durango, Arimura and Loo, 1977) and counteracts tolbutamide (Basabe *et al.*, 1971) but not glibornuride (Brisson and Malaisse, 1971) effects. Glycolysis (Hellman *et al.*, 1974b), calcium accumulation (Malaisse-Lagae and Malaisse, 1971), and inhibition of protein kinases also occurs (Montague and Howell, 1975). It does not suppress release in infantile nesidioblastosis (Castro, Dyess, Buist and Potts, 1973; Heitz, Kloppel, Hachi, Polak and Everson-Pearse, 1977). Barbituric acid (Mennear, Schouwaller and Yan, 1976) and diltiazem (Taniguchi, Murakawi, Morita, Kazumi, Yoshino, Baeda and Baba, 1977) lower insulin response without changing glucose tolerance in rat, and are recommended as well as chlorpromazine (Federspil, Casara and Staufaccher, 1974) as alternatives to diazoxide. Dilantin and diuril slightly decrease and augment respectively, the peak response to glucose in late pregnancy (Spellacy, Farog, Buhi and Birk, 1975).

Diphenylhydantoin and mesantoin, the anticonvulsive agents, inhibit insulin release strongly and reversibly (Levin, Charles, O'Connor and Grodsky, 1975; Kizer, Vargas-Gordon, Brendel and Bressler, 1970) by stimulation of ion-transport pumps causing hyperpolarisation of the islet cell membrane (Somers *et al.*, 1976; Kizer *et al.*, 1970). In adults but not children, therapeutic serum levels of 13–22 µg/ml lowered the insulin response to glucose and arginine (Levin *et al.*, 1973; Cunningham, Rosenbloom, Kohler and Wilder, 1973).

The biguanides phenformin and metformin lower basal and the oral glucose mediated release but improve glucose tolerance (Stout, Brunzell, Bierman and Porte, 1974; Lütjens and Smit, 1976). Incretin may be suppressed (Czyzyk *et al.*, 1973) but a direct effect on islets has also been shown (Schatz, Katsilambros, Nierle and Pfeiffer, 1972).

Salicylates improve the early insulin response to glucose in mild diabetes (Robertson and Chen, 1977) and augment the tolbutamide effect *in vitro* (Frane, Ganguli, Christensen, Voina and Maddig, 1977). Indomethacin usage causes delay in early insulin release (Widström, 1977; Sylvälahti, 1975).

Clofibrate treatment lowers insulin and increases glucagon release in response to arginine (Eaton, 1973). Insulin response to oral glucose and basal levels in the diabetics are also lowered (Ferrari, Frezzati, Romuri, Bertazzani, Testori, Antonine and Peracchi, 1977).

Ethanol ingestion may cause potentiation of insulin release (Strauss, Urbach and Yalow, 1976). The delayed insulinaemia in obese and diabetic subjects after i.v. ethanol (Nikkila and Tashkinen, 1975) is attributed to its metabolite acetate (Shah, Wong, Surawat and Aran, 1977). Chronic ethanol ingestion lowers glucose tolerance (Nikkila and Tashkinen, 1975).

(e) Agents toxic to B cells

Alloxan, a disulphydryl reagent, causes B cell exhaustion with a dose-dependent time of onset (Fung and Mennear, 1974). Initially the cells are depolarised (Dean and Matthews, 1972) and glucose-mediated release is abolished (Tomita, Lacy, Matschinsky and McDaniel, 1974). Later, an insulin leak builds up (Fung and Mennear, 1974), and cell membrane composition is modified (Orci, Amherdt, Stauffacher, Like, Rouiller and Renold, 1972). Chronic alloxan diabetes increases the D cell areas seen in sections of islets (Hellman and Petersson, 1963). Glucose, other sugars and sugar derivatives (Battacharya, 1953; Tomita *et al.*, 1974; Padron, Sulman and Lewis, 1967), and theophylline and cytochalasin B (McDaniel and Lacy, 1975) protect against alloxan action.

Streptozotocin, the antibacterial, anti-tumour agent, causes oxidative B cell damage by generating the toxic product 1-methyl-1-nitrosourea (Golden, Basil, Melani, Malaisse-Lagae and Walker, 1976; Tjälve and Wilander, 1977). The sugar moiety of its structure may facilitate faster uptake by B cells (Golden *et al.*, 1976). Rapid depletion of NAD content, inhibition of proinsulin synthesis, and insulin release before any change in ATP levels (Maldonato, Truehart, Renold and Sharp, 1976) may be due to membrane damage (Howell and Whitfield, 1972) and can induce insulitis in the susceptible host (Rossini, Crick, Appl and Cahill, 1977). Chronic treatment greatly reduces B cell population and increases the number of D cells (Orci, Baetens, Rufener, Amherdt, Ravazzola, Studen, Malaisse-Lagae and Unger, 1975). Nicotinic acid, diazoxide, the antioxidant vitamin E, are protective (Tjälve and Wilander, 1977; Katada and Ui, 1977) but nicotinic acid may unmask oncogenic effects (Maldonato *et al.*, 1976). It has been used in treatment of islet cell tumours (Blackard, Garcia and Brown, 1970; Walter, Ensinck, Ricketts, Kendall and Williams, 1973; Alsever, Stjernholm, Sussman, Mako and Rubenstein, 1976).

Cytochalasin B (CYT-B) is a fungal metabolite which disrupts micro-filaments and inhibits cytokinetic functions like division, elongation or endocytosis. Previous exposure of islets to CYT-B at low concentration increases stimulus sensitivity of the islets (Lacy, Klein and Fink, 1973; Schauder and Frerichs, 1974; Obberghen, Somers, Devis, Vaughan, Malaisse-Lagae, Orci and Malaisse, 1973) despite resistance to glucose uptake

(McDaniel, King, Anderson, Fink and Lacy, 1974) indicating effects on the cell membrane. The presence of CYT-B during stimulation also amplifies the release, but the effect diminishes with increasing doses (Lacy et al., 1973). During amplified release, glycolysis and electric activity are altered (Pace and Matschinsky, 1974), with evidence of gross structural changes inside the cell membrane (Obberghen et al., 1973). It appears that facilitation of emiocytosis occurs with reduction of energy requirements.

The alkaloids vincristine, vinblastine (Devis, Obberghen, Somers, Malaisse-Lagae, Orci and Malaisse, 1974) and colchicine (Somers, Obberghen, Devis, Ravazzola, Malaisse-Lagae and Malaisse, 1974) have early facilitating and late inhibitory effects on glucose-stimulated release. Pretreatment with vinblastine overcomes the facilitative effect of CYT-B (Lacy et al., 1973) which is attributed to microtubule degeneration (Malaisse-Lagae, Greider, Malaisse and Lacy, 1971). After colchicine the early phase of release is less impeded (Somers et al., 1974; Lacy, Walker and Fink, 1972; Obberghen, Devis, Somers, Ravazzola, Malaisse-Lagae and Malaisse, 1974) suggesting this may corresponding to emiocytosis of already marginated granules (Malaisse, Obberghen, Devis, Somers and Ravazzola, 1974).

10. Comments

Current data suggest, but do not prove, that external calcium uptake, or a change in calcium bound at the plasma membrane, is related to initiation of insulin discharge, that this process is secondary to depolarisation, which in the case of glucose stimulated release, is dependent on glucose phosphorylation and that depolarisation in turn activates adenyl cyclase. Also, activation occurs at a specially controlled stage of glucose metabolism which may act as a "glucostat". These post-depolarisation events appear to be intimately related.

Since adrenalin can arrest discharge without repolarising, and, in conditions of glucose insensitivity, insulin release is improved by other stimuli than glucose (see Lenzen et al., 1976), the rate of granule discharge depends on a process beyond depolarisation, not always the same aspect of which fails in different conditions of diminished glucose effect. In hyperparathyroidism and diabetes, the early phase is reduced and the second phase delayed, but the former (Gedik and Zileli, 1977), not the latter (Botha et al., 1976) condition responds to theophylline, the diabetic response being slightly improved by gastro-intestinal factors (Botha et al., 1976; Enk, 1976; Enk et al., 1976) and glucagon (Simpson et al., 1968) or arginine (Seino et al., 1977). A "diabetic" response to glucose can also be elicited in vitro by exposing islets to moderately high potassium concentrations (Henquin and Lambert, 1974b; Dean and Matthews, 1970a), or by decreasing extracellular calcium levels (Charles *et al.*, 1975). In diabetes, therefore, changes in calcium handling and/or glucosensor adjustment or of cyclase activation may occur.

Regulation of the cyclic nucleotide generating systems in the islet cells appears to mediate the effects of physiological changes like feeding, starvation or pregnancy on the quantity of insulin stored and released by the B cells (Montague and Howell, 1975). B cell sensitivity to specific agents, e.g. gastro-intestinal factors, which increase cAMP levels may constitute the basis of the endocrinological control of B cell function (see also Sections D and F).

Islets are a paracrine system of cells (Orci, 1974; Orci and Unger, 1975) which share common stimuli and having direct hormonal effects on each other (Table 2). For example, during the less synchronised early phase of electrical activity (Meissner, 1976), depolarising stimulus may be relayed by cell–cell communication via the gap junctions between cells. The interspecies consistency in the relative distribution of cells implies a physiological significance (Erlandesen *et al.*, 1976). Glucagon release occurs ahead of insulin (Pek, Tai, Crowther and Fajans, 1976) which coming from within the islet can be inhibitory (Samols and Harrison, 1976; Östenson *et al.*, 1977). Equally possibly, when the stimulus is propagated inwards to the islets, glucagon can be stimulatory to D and B cells, while D cells are positioned to sustain the inhibitory effect both ways. Therefore, assuming, as has been done so far, that the effect of a stimulus is restricted to the particular cell type under investigation, may be misleading in the understanding of the co-ordinated function of that cell type within the islet as a whole. For example, in human diabetes, the islet D cell population increases (Fujita, 1966; Orci *et al.*, 1975). In this respect, and in the altered sensitivity to glucose and responsiveness to potentiators, it bears similarity to the foetal islet. Similar mechanisms for suppression of insulin release and augmentation of glucagon-release can be speculated.

D. ROLE OF INSULIN IN BLOOD GLUCOSE HOMEOSTASIS

Neither the mechanisms, nor the biological effects of the neuro-endocrinological control of blood glucose are well understood. Normally the blood glucose level is maintained within narrow margins, and the release of the hormones controlling it, i.e. insulin, glucagon, catecholamines, glucocorticoids, somatotrophin, is sensitive to changes of plasma glucose levels in either direction (Garber, Cryer, Santiago, Haymond, Pagliara and Kipnis,

1976; de Fronzo, Andres, Bledsoe, Boden, Faloona and Tobin, 1977; McCarthy, Harris and Turner, 1977).

1. Biological Effects of Insulin and Other Islet Hormones

(a) Insulin

In man, insulin is primarily anticatabolic, i.e. antilipolytic and antiglyco-genolytic, and at relatively higher levels favours glucose utilisation, e.g. synthesis of triglycerides and glycogen (Cheng and Kalant, 1970; Bomboy, Lewis, Sinclair-Smith and Lacy, 1977; Rushahoff, Matsenbaugh, Schultz, Gerich and Wallin, 1977).

Stimulation of the cell membrane transport of sugars, amino acids, ions and of nucleotide precursors, activation of membrane-bound and soluble enzymes, e.g. ATPases, cAMP-phosphodiesterase, inhibition of protein degradation, stimulation of protein, RNA and DNA synthesis, e.g. in fibro-blasts, are examples of the diverse cellular effects of insulin demonstrated *in vitro* (Goldfine, 1977). Alterations of cAMP metabolism in the liver (Pilkis and Park, 1974), activation of glycogen synthetase (Cohen, Antoni, Nimmo and Yeaman, 1976), and changes in protein phosphorylation in fat cells (Avruch, Leone and Martin, 1976) have been observed. All effects of insulin may be secondary to binding a specific receptor on the cell surface (see Section D.5). An intracellular messenger entity generated by this binding to mediate insulin effects has not been identified. Insulin entry into cells and its binding of receptors on cellular organelles (see Section E.1.*b*) as well as on the cell surface to initiate different effects have been postulated (Goldfine, 1977).

(b) Glucagon and other islet hormones

Glucagon is primarily glycogenolytic (Mackrell and Sokal, 1969; Mueller, Aoki, Egdahl and Cahill, 1977; Chiasson, Liljenquist, Sinclair-Smith and Lacy, 1977) and can be gluconeogenic (Mackrell and Sokal, 1969; Barnes, Bloom, Mashiter, Alberti, Smyth and Turner, 1977).

There is evidence that somatostatin influences nutrient absorption from the gut (Schusdziawa, Ipp and Unger, 1977), hepatic glucose output (Sachs, Waligona and Matthews, 1977; Koerker, Ruch, Chideckel, Palmer, Goodner, Ensinck and Gale, 1974) and ketogenesis (Schade and Eaton, 1977a). Pancreatic polypeptide responds to gut hormones and acetylcholine (Gingerich, 1977) and is extracted by the liver (Loo, Hirsch and Gabbay, 1977). The physiological significance of these is not known, and interpreta-tion of the control of glucose homeostasis by islet hormones is, therefore, restricted to insulin and glucagon.

2. Adaptation of B Cell Function to Peripheral Glucose Utilisation

Glucocorticoids, somatotrophin and thyroid hormones, which cooperate in peripheral energy production, mutually influence each others release (Evans, Simpson and Evans, 1958; Brauman and Corvilain, 1968; Müller, Sawano, Arimura and Schally, 1967; Fain, 1968) as well as pancreatic endocrine function, which ensures maintenance of normoglycaemia (see Section F.4.*e*).

Glucocorticoids are primarily gluconeogenic (Schade and Eaton, 1977b) and improve glucagon and lower insulin response to direct stimuli (Marco, Calle, Hedo and Villanueva, 1976; Billaudel and Sutter, 1977; Kalhan and Adam, 1975), render adipocytes sensitive to catecholamines (Fain, 1968), promote lipolysis and ketogenesis in insulinopaenia (Ginsberg, 1977; Schade and Eaton, 1977b) and reduce peripheral insulin effectiveness (Hjalmarson, 1968; Ginsberg, 1977). Excess glucocorticoids cause islet cell hypertrophy and prolonged excess brings about hyperplasia and later, degeneration (Lazarus and Bencosme, 1955; Bencosme and Lazarus, 1956; Lenzen, 1976).

Somatotrophin can be lipolytic and ketogenic in insulinopaenia (Schade and Eaton, 1976; Eaton, Schade and Peake, 1977; Fain, 1968; Goodman and Knobil, 1959), and reduces insulin effectiveness in liver and muscle (Cheng and Kalant, 1970; Hjalmarson, 1968). It may moderate glucocorticoid effects on hepatic gluconeogenesis (Schapiro, 1968) but in protein-energy malnutrition (Kwashiorkor) it may indirectly promote this (Lunn, Whitehead and Hay, 1973). Excessive somatotrophin causes islet hypertrophy (Martin, Akerblom and Garay, 1968).

In experimental hyperthyroidism, suppression of both phases of insulin release is dependent on the dose of thyroxine treatment (Lenzen, Panten and Hasselblatt, 1975; Lenzen, 1978b), and may be partially due to the decrease in islet cell insulin content (Lenzen *et al.*, 1975; Malaisse, Malaisse-Lagae and McCraw, 1967; Lenzen and Klöppel, 1978). Glucagon and somatotrophin as well as the insulin response to arginine, somatotrophin response to insulin hypoglycaemia, and hepatic glycogen content and glucose output in response to glucagon can be lowered (Brauman and Corrilain, 1968; Cavagnini, Peracchi, Raggi, Bana, Pontiroli, Malinverni and Pinto, 1974; Seino, Goto, Taminato, Ikeda and Imura, 1974; Imura, Seino, Ikeda, Taminato and Goto 1976; Shima, Sawazaki, Tanaka, Morishita, Tarui and Nishikawa, 1976), and insulin degradation increases (Orsetti, Collard and Jaffol, 1974). Prolonged excess of thyroid hormones causes islet cell degeneration (Houssay, 1944).

Diabetes ensues upon failure of B cell adaptation to increased insulin demand by glucocorticoid or somatotrophin excess (Sönksen, 1975; Reaven, Bernstein, Davis and Olefsky, 1976) or by the inhibition of B cell function as in thyroid hormone (see Malaisse et al., 1967; Cavagnini et al., 1974) or in catecholamine excess (see Table 6).

In deficiency of glucocorticoids (Serrano-Rios et al., 1974), somatotrophin (Riddick, Reissler and Kipnis, 1962; Merimee, Felig, Fineberg and Cahill, 1971; Parman, 1975a, 1975b), or thyroid hormones (Brauman and Corvilain, 1968; Cohn, Berger and Norton, 1968; Shah and Cerchio, 1973; Jolin and Montest, 1974; Andreani, Fallucca, Tamburranno, Iavicoli and Meninger, 1974), peripheral glucose utilisation, hepatic glucose output, B and A cell sensitivity to stimuli is reduced. In the former two conditions peripheral insulin sensitivity is increased. Delayed insulinaemia after hyperglycaemia can cause post-prandial hypoglycaemia in untreated adrenal cortical insufficiency or hypothyroidism (Hofeldt, Lufkin, Hagler, Block, Dippe and Davis, 1974).

3. Circadian Rhythms of Insulin Release and Peripheral Insulin Sensitivity

There is a characteristically overlapping diurnal rhythm to insulin, catecholamine, glucocorticoid and somatotrophin levels (Lakatua, Haus, Gold and Halberg, 1974; Turton and Deegan, 1974; Reinberg, Apfelbaum, Assan and Lacatis, 1971; Vernikos-Danellis, Leach, Wingot, Goodwin and Rambert, 1976), while that of glucagon is quite steady (Reinberg et al., 1971; Tasaka, Sekine, Wakatsuki, Ohgawara and Shizumel, 1975). Insulin falls during the night and rises early in the morning to a new basal level almost concurrently with the glucocorticoid peak (Turton and Deegan, 1974). Control of fasting insulin may not require intact adrenal medulla or splanchnic innervation (Brodows, Pi-Sunyer and Campbell, 1974).

Insulin response to stimuli is highest in late morning to midday in normal (Malharbe, Gasparo, Dettertogh and Hoet, 1969; Baker and Jarrett, 1972; Melani, Verillo, Marasco, Rivellese, Osorio and Bertolino, 1976; Owens et al., 1977) and diabetic man with residual B cell activity (Faber and Binder, 1977a; Lewis, Walleri, Kuzuya, Murray, Constan, Daane and Rubenstein, 1976), and diminishes in the afternoon. Peripheral insulin sensitivity in normal (Sensi and Capani, 1976; Gibson, Stimmler, Jarrett, Rutland and Shiu, 1975) and diabetic man (Mirouze, Selan, Pham and Cavadore, 1977) is also higher before midday. After midday, metabolic glucose clearance falls sharply (Sensi and Capani, 1976), skeletal muscle glucose uptake decreases (Mirouze et al., 1977) and fat utilisation increases (Gibson et al., 1977) which coincide with rising somatotrophin levels partly overlapping with the declining glucocorticoids (Turton and Deegan, 1974).

4. Control of Blood Glucose Level

(a) Physiological significance of the relative insulin and glucagon levels

The insulin:glucagon ratio in the peripheral circulation reflects the anabolic or catabolic regulation of glucose homeostasis (Unger, 1974). The ratio of the peripheral levels of the hormones is assumed to correlate with the portal levels (see Felig, Gusberg, Handler, Gump and Kinney, 1974; Horwitz et al., 1975b; Schultz et al., 1976) which is important in the regulation of hepatic glucose metabolism (Bomboy et al., 1977; Mackrell and Sokal, 1969).

In normal humans with regular eating and sleeping rhythms, and of moderate daily activity, the peripheral ratio was about 0·8–1·0 during meals, and 0·5 between meals and during sleep. Glucagon was slightly raised during meals, while insulin varied four to ten times (Santiago, Haymond, Clarke and Pagliara, 1977). Increase of the ratio positively correlates with the carbohydrate content of the meal (Reaven and Olefsky, 1974; Danforth, 1971; Unger, 1974), reduces hepatic gluconeogenesis and glucose output (Bomboy et al., 1977), which is probably facilitated by alteration of the direct control of glucose metabolism in the liver by the central nervous system (Szabo and Szabo, 1975), and also allows for increased peripheral insulin levels, and hence anabolic effects (Cheng and Kalant, 1970; Unger, 1974; see also Section E.1.c for hepatic clearance of insulin). Between meals, blood glucose may be maintained by basal levels of glucagon after reduction of insulin release (Felig, Wahren and Hendler, 1976; Porte, Smith and Ensinck, 1976).

In conditions of stress, the relative levels of the hormones controlling blood glucose homeostasis are adjusted according to the intensity or duration of stress, fuel requirements and state of repletion of glucose resources, and blood glucose is either maintained or raised. Primary adjustments involve maintenance of glucose supply to the central nervous system (CNS) and other tissues which may incur energy deficit, e.g. in ischaemia after shock or during wound repair after injury or surgery. When insulin levels are lowered, lipolysis is augmented. Mobilisation of free fatty acids provides an alternate fuel supply which minimises peripheral glucose utilisation and protein catabolism for hepatic gluconeogenesis (Newsholme, 1976).

(b) Insulin hypoglycaemia

Increased glucose utilisation and inhibition of its production associated with insulin-induced hypoglycaemia is reversed by increased glycogenolysis, despite high insulin levels, by catecholamines (Garber et al., 1976) the levels of which increase in plasma earlier than cortisol or somatotrophin (Garber et al., 1976; Feldman, Plonk and Birens, 1975). Catecholamines inhibit insulin release (see Section C.7) but the persistent endogenous hypoinsulinaemia after exogenous insulin (Horwitz et al., 1975) is also due to prolonged hypoglycaemia (McCarthy et al., 1977). Catecholamines are also lipolytic, ketogenic (Mueller et al., 1977), gluconeogenic (Kneer, Bosch, Clark and Lardy, 1974) and glycogenolytic (Garber et al., 1976), and antagonise insulin promoted muscle glycogenesis (Rushahoff et al., 1977).

(c) Exercise

Post absorptive moderate exercise lowers blood glucose (Pruett, 1970). Heavy exercise (Pruett, 1971) or lack of glucose replenishment in between exercise periods (Dahms, Atkinson, Golden, Whipp, Wasserman and Bray, 1977) increases glucagon and glucose levels. During exercise, muscle glucose utilisation is increased (Rennie, Park and Sulaiman, 1976) and depends on the rate of supply, i.e. by increased blood flow, as well as on insulin levels, whereas free fatty acid (FFA) uptake also increases but does not depend on insulin (Schultz, Lewis, Westbie, Wallin and Gerich, 1977; Berger, Halban, Muller, Renold and Vranic, 1977; Kalant, Lebovici and Rohan, 1977; Whichelow, Butterfield, Abrams, Sterky and Garrant, 1968). Hence lowered insulin levels may allow adjustment of glucose production to its utilisation, and also in extensive exercise, for FFA utilisation by the muscle (Dieterle, Birkmer, Gmeiner, Wagern, Erhardt, Hener and Dieterle, 1973; Rennie et al., 1976). During intensive exercise, the arterio-venous insulin difference is negative, indicating release of endothelially sequestered insulin which may be on account of increased utilisation of insulin (Dieterle et al., 1973; Rennie et al., 1976).

(d) Exsanguination

In the early stages of hypovolaemic shock, there is a venous insulin excess (Hiebert, McCormick and Egdahl, 1971) which is maintained despite lowered pancreatic flow and net insulin release (Lau, Taubenfliegel, Levenge, Farago, Chan, Koren and Ducker, 1972; Bor, 1975). Since anaesthesia and skin incision transiently lower fasting insulin (Lau et al., 1972) insulinaemia of circulatory shock overrides the catecholamine effect and delays the FFA rise (Skillman, Hedley-White and Palotta, 1971). This early hyperglycaemia and insulinaemia, which fails to suppress hepatic gluconeogensis (Long, Spencer, Kinney and Geiger, 1971), may be appropriate for maintenance of cardiac function (McNamara, Motot, Dunn and Stremple, 1972). The increase in acid ethanol-soluble nonsuppressible insulin-like activity (see Section E.2) in exercise (Couturier, Rasio and Coward, 1971) probably in association with somatotrophin (Rennie et al., 1976), and its unique equipotency with insulin on myocardial glucose utilisation (see Section E.2) also suggest a special control of cardiac metabolism, and merits investigation in early circulatory shock.

(e) Surgery

During surgery, maintenance (Nakao and Miyata, 1977) or lowering of insulin (Brandt et al., 1977) and glucagon levels and raised glucose levels (Giddings, O'Connor, Rowlands, Mangwald and Clark, 1976) may depend on the general anaesthetic and the nutritional state of the patient (Aynsley-Green, Biebuyck and Alberti, 1973) (see also Section F.3.q). Reduced insulin response to glucose is prevented by α-adrenergic block (Nakao and Miyata, 1977) and may be due to raised catecholamine levels (Wright, Henderson and Johnston, 1974), but hyperinsulinaemia does not overcome hyperglycaemia or suppress somatotrophin secretion, but prevents potassium and nitrogen depletion (Hill et al., 1974; Wright, 1973). Unlike in the dog (Sando et al., 1977), per-operative hypoinsulinaemia does not require intact splanchnic innervation (Äärimaa et al., 1974). Postoperative fasting insulinaemia (Giddings et al., 1976) despite increased catecholamine production may be relevant to wound repair (see Sections F.3.o and q). Its duration is reduced if cortisol is raised during prolonged surgery (Wright et al., 1974).

(f) Starvation

Chronic starvation lowers insulin and raises glucagon levels in plasma. After central nervous system adaptation to utilise ketone bodies, plasma glucagon is lowered and protein catabolism for hepatic gluconeogenesis is minimised (Unger, 1974; Newsholme, 1976). After six days of starvation, blood glucose levels of lean adults fell by 30% to 3·5 mmol/l (60 mg/dl) and free fatty acid levels rose by 200%. Glucose utilisation and insulin response to stimuli were low (Göschke, 1977).

(g) Birth

After cessation of placental nutrient supply, the neonate undergoes a cata-bolic starvation phase. In foetal rats, glycogen and fat is stored before term. At birth, stress lowers insulin and raises glucagon concentrations. Until the 12th day of life, when the amount of liver glycogen begins to rise, free fatty acids are used for fuel and the insulin response to glucose is suppressed. Normalisation occurs after high carbohydrate intake (Foa et al., 1976). In the human neonate, insulin and blood glucose levels fall and glucagon levels rise 15 min after birth, and in 3–6 hr glucagon synthesis and release and FFA levels are very high (Foa et al., 1976) which restores blood glucose to 3·3 mmol/l (60 mg/dl) on the second day (Sperling, De Lameter, Phelps, Fiser, Oh and Fisher, 1974). An insulin:glucagon ratio of 1:5 (Falorni, Massi-Benedetti, Gallo and Romizi, 1975a), low insulin and high glucagon response to gluconeogenic precursors (Sperling et al., 1974; Fiser, Williams, Fischer, De Lameter, Sperling and Oh, 1975; Falorni, Massi-Benedetti, Gallo and Trabalaza, 1975b), and reversal of this increased glucagon release after repletion of glucose resources and restoration of blood glucose (Massi-Benedetti, Falorni, Luyckx and Lefebvre, 1974; Fiser et al., 1975), but insuppressibility by somatostatin (Sodoyez-Goffaux, Sodoyez and Vos, 1977) indicates that gluconeogenesis is important for neonatal blood glucose homeostasis (Oka, Matsuda, Nambi, Nagai, Mitsuyama and Arashima, 1977).

Premature "appropriate-for-dates" babies have normal control of blood glucose levels, but "small for dates" babies with hepatic neoglucogenic insufficiency tend to go into hypoglycaemic crisis. The insulin:glucagon ratio is high, and glucose utilisation is increased but does not correlate with insulin levels (Falorni, Frecassini, Massi-Benedetti and Maffei, 1974; Falorni et al., 1975a; Salle and Ruitton-Uglienco, 1976; Salle and Uglienco, 1977). Neonates of diabetic mothers are similarly afflicted (Persson, Gentz, Kellum and Thorell, 1976).

(h) Toxaemia

Gram negative sepsis is associated with raised basal insulin, glucagon, cortisol and somatotrophin levels, a diminished insulin response to stimuli, inhibition of gluconeogenesis and an increased glucose requirement (Wilmore, 1976; Manny, Rabinovici and Schiller, 1977; Rayfield, Curnow, Reinnard and Kochicheril, 1977). Replacement with insulin and glucose may help to prevent death (Hinshaw, Peyton, Archer, Block, Coalson and Greenfield, 1974).

After hypoglycin (fruit toxin) ingestion, augmented insulin release may aggravate the hypoglycaemic trend, with inhibited gluconeogenesis and lipolysis (Milner and Wirdham, 1977).

(i) Diabetes

In the potentially diabetic, or the early diabetic subject, glucagon release is exaggerated after meals (Palmer et al., 1976; Gerich, Lorenzi, Karam, Schneider and Forsham, 1975) and is not suppressed by hyperglycaemia (Raskin, Fujita and Unger, 1975), but only after high doses of insulin (Raskin et al., 1975; Gerich, 1976). The potential diabetic also exhibits abnormalities of glucocorticoid or somatotrophin levels and of lipid metabolism in association with altered dynamics of insulin release (Tan, Williams, Soeldner and Gleason, 1977; Gottlieb, Soeldner, Kyner and Gleason, 1974).

In unstable diabetes complicated by neuropathy, cortisol elevation probably compensates for glucagon unresponsiveness to hypoglycaemia (Maher, Tannenberg, Greenberg, Hoffman, Doe and Goetz, 1977; Reynolds, Molnar, Horwitz, Rubenstein, Taylor and Jiang, 1977). In diabetic human liver, gluconeogenic enzymes are increased, glycolysis is suppressed (Belfiore, Romeo, Napoli and Lo Vecchio, 1974), and peak cortisol levels and glucose turnover are high (Moorhouse, 1969). In ketoacidosis associated with severe insulin resistance (Park, Soeldner and Gleason, 1974), insulin levels become undetectable, when cortisol levels correlate with the degree of hyperglycaemia (Ginsberg, 1977b). Fasting hyperglycaemia of diabetes is claimed to be appropriate for maintenance of basal insulinaemia required for cell growth (Turner and Holman, 1976).

5. Insulin Receptor and Insulin Resistance

Current evidence suggests that the biological effectiveness of insulin is secondary to its binding to specific receptors on the cell surface membrane.

Properties of the insulin receptor have been reviewed (Ginsberg, 1977a). In different species in which insulin has been characterised, the receptor has a remarkable identity of binding properties and antigenic cross-reactivity. Solubilised receptor is tetrameric and is non-homogenously distributed in the cell membrane (Kahn, 1976). Binding is driven by hydrophobic reactions (de Meyts and Wallbroeck, 1977) and the affinity of different insulins correlates with their biological potency (Ginsberg, 1977a). Binding displays a sharp pH optimum, is influenced by cations and the degree of receptor occupancy per cell determines the relative "high or low activity state" of the receptor population through negative site–site interactions (Ginsberg, Olefsky, Kimmerling, Crapo and Reaven, 1976b). Receptor numbers are directly and reversibly decreased by insulin and analogues in a dose-dependent fashion and with less specificity of structural requirements than for the initiation of receptor site–site interactions. The process is intracellular and partly protein synthesis dependent. The binding characteristics of remaining receptors are unaltered. Hence *in vivo* modified receptor affinity states or numbers can influence insulin dose effectiveness.

Indeed, changed basal insulin levels, metabolic alterations like acidosis, circulating insulin antagonists, hormones, age, and cell transformations, all influence tissue insulin sensitivity (Ginsberg, 1977a). Increased basal insulin levels with or without obesity cause reduction in the number of insulin receptors (Olefsky and Reaven, 1974a; Olefsky and Reaven, 1977) and probably thereby diminish peripheral insulin effectiveness (Harrison, Martin and Melick, 1976; Beck-Nielsen, Pedersen and Sprensen, 1977). Normal-isation of basal insulin levels and insulin-binding capacity of cells, as after long term diet control, is believed to underlie the improved glucose tolerance (Bar, Gordon, Roth, Kahn and Demoyl, 1976). Reduction in binding capacity per se does not adequately explain insulin insensitivity (Le Marchand, Jean-Renaud and Freychet, 1977a). Change in concentration per unit surface area may be more relevant (Amatruda, Livingstone and Lockwood, 1975; Olefsky, 1976b; Beck-Nielsden, Pedersen, Bagger and Sorensen, 1976). This may be a basic adaptive mechanism to regulate tissue metabolism in relation to hormone potency (Simon, Freychet and Rosselin, 1977) or availability (Goldfine, 1975; Davidson and Kaplan, 1977; Schoenle, Zapf and Froesch, 1977). Indeed, changes in surface receptors alter insulin uptake in parallel (Vigneri, Pliam, Cohen and Goldfine, 1977; Posner, Josefberg and Bergeron, 1977). Interestingly, glucocorticoids cause peripheral insulin resistance and can diminish receptor populations (Ginsberg, 1977a). However, in hypo-thalamic obesity, with basal hyperinsulinaemia and reduced receptors (Le Marchand et al., 1977a), or streptozotocin diabetes, with insulinopaenia and increased concentration of receptors (Schoenle et al., 1977) tissue glucose metabolism is insulin insensitive. Also, in non-obese, non-ketotic human diabetes with fasting hyperglycaemia insulin binding of cells is reduced by 45%. Correction of hyperglycaemia by sulphonylurea normalises binding. Fasting insulin levels remain at about twice that of normal control (Olefsky and Reaven, 1976) yet diminished insulin binding is also attributed to fasting hyperinsulinaemia (Olefsky and Reaven, 1977). The affinity of insulin receptor is different in the comparable basal hyperinsulinaemia of obesity and of acromegaly (Gorden, Gavin, Lesniak and Roth, 1973).

In congenital obesity an intracellular defect may resist the effect of insulin on glucose metabolism despite adaptive changes in receptor concentration after fasting or streptozotocin treatment (Cuendet, Loten, Jean-Renaud and Renold, 1976; Le Marchand, Loten, Assimacopoulas-Jeannet, Forgue, Freychet and Jean-Renaud, 1977b; Freychet, 1976). In acute fasting, there is similar resistance, with unaltered binding capacity, but increased binding affinity (Olefsky, 1976a; Kobayashi and Olefsky, 1977; Bar et al., 1976). Ageing increases insulin resistance without alteration of binding capacity, which is distinct from the increase or decrease of this capacity in insulinaemia or insulinopaenia (Schoenle et al., 1977; Olefsky, 1976c; Czech, 1976).

Mild glucose intolerance of metabolic acidosis (Guest, Mackler and Knowles, 1952; Weisinger, Swanson, Greene, Taylor and Reaven, 1972) may be partly due to ineffective insulin binding (Ginsberg, 1977a). Extreme insulin resistance occurs with polyclonal auto-antibodies against the insulin receptor (Kahn, Baird, Flier and Dano, 1977; Flier, Kahn, Jarrett and Roth, 1976).

E. DETERMINATION OF INSULIN IN BODY FLUIDS AND TISSUE EXTRACTS

Insulin is measured by its effectiveness on insulin sensitive indices of tissue metabolism, or by immunochemical methods designed to quantitate the hormone. Clinically, the aim is to assess the levels of the biologically effective hormone, the deviation of which from the normal range under particular physiological conditions such as fasting or food ingestion, would correlate with overt or imminent metabolic disorders and may indicate pancreatic disease. Therefore theoretically, estimation of the biological activity of insulin in blood is more relevant to accurate diagnosis. However, the immunochemical methods have been adopted for routine diagnosis because of their relatively higher specificity, sensitivity and reproducibility. This has imposed on clinical judgement the assumption that levels estimated under all conditions linearly correlate with the biological effectiveness *in vivo* (Suzuki, Ohsawa and Kosaka, 1976).

Insulin in blood displays molecular heterogeneity which is reflected in its biological potency. Tissue receptors modulate insulin effectiveness (see Section D.5), and immunochemically undetectable changes in biological effectiveness can occur (Freychet, Kahn, Roth and Neville, 1976). The recent development of sensitive insulin radioreceptor (or "radioceptor") assays may facilitate the correlation of changes in relative quantities of the immunoreactive hormone species to the biological effectiveness of the whole at the cellular level. Research application of the radioceptor assays may also reveal participation of other "insulin-like" constituents of blood, in the regulation of insulin-dependent cellular functions, e.g. in myocardium.

In this section, therefore, before outlining the methods of estimation, factors which would influence these estimations, i.e. the heterogeneity of insulin and its clinical significance, other insulin-like activity in the circulation, and the immunochemistry and antigenicity of insulin will be discussed.

1. Heterogeneity and Clinical Significance of Circulating Insulin

(a) Insulin and its precursors

The B cell secretory products in normal human serum consist predominantly of C-peptide (CP), insulin, and in less amounts, proinsulin (PRO) and intermediate products formed during conversion to insulin (De Häen, Little and May, 1977). C-peptide is the PRO connecting peptide less two basic dipeptides from either extremity cleaved from the A and B chains of insulin (Rubenstein, Steiner, Horwitz, Mako, Block, Starr, Kuzuya and Melani,

1977). After gel filtration of serum, insulin and CP are the major single fractions (Rubenstein *et al.*, 1977; Roth, Gorden and Pastan, 1968; Lazarus, Gutman, Penhos and Recant, 1972). Minor components, which show individual variation, can be demonstrated by disc-gel electrophoresis (De Häen *et al.*, 1977; Lazarus, Gutman and Recant, 1971). These consist mainly of two desdipeptides of PRO with CP still attached to either the B or the A chain, further split products of the former and minor quantities of insulin-like components (Chance, 1971; Steiner, Hallund, Rubenstein, Cho and Bayliss, 1968). The term "PRO-like component" or PLC as distinct from PRO is used to identify the measured constituents after separation from insulin and CP. The closer the conversion product in structure to that of insulin the closer are its biological and immunochemical properties (Lind, Gilmore and McClarence, 1975; Chance, 1971; Yu and Kitabchi, 1973; Rubenstein and Steiner, 1971) and the avidity of insulin receptor binding (Ginsberg, 1977a). The dose-response curve of biological activity of the intermediates *in vitro* are parallel to that of insulin (Gliemann and Sörensen, 1970; Gliemann and Gammeltoft, 1974); there is no mutual interference and CP is inactive (Yu and Kitabchi, 1973). Hypophysectomy or adrenalectomy sensitise tissues to insulin and PRO similarly (Rubenstein, Melani and Steiner, 1972). The biological potency of porcine PRO in man is 2·5% of that of porcine insulin (Sönksen, Tompkins, Srivasteva and Nabarro, 1973). Proinsulin stimulates glucose uptake in human forearm and causes a delayed but prolonged hypoglycaemia. Its peripheral conversion to insulin has not been unequivocally shown (Rubenstein *et al.*, 1972; Chance, 1971).

(b) Cellular uptake and degradation

Receptor binding of insulin results is apparently followed by transfer into the cell (Vigneri *et al.*, 1977; Posner *et al.*, 1977) and release of high and low molecular weight products into the circulation (Terris and Steiner, 1976; Kahn and Baird, 1977; Antoniades, Simon and Stathakos, 1973). Binding and degrading activities are separable (Terris and Steiner, 1976; Dial, Miyamoto and Arquilla, 1977; Flier, Marakos-Flier and Kahn, 1977). Insulin is degraded by "insulinase" and proteases (Thomas, 1973), which are widely distributed, including the pancreatic islets (Kohnert, Jahr, Schmidt, Hahn and Zühlke, 1976; Thomas, 1973). Insulinase parallels insulin levels (Varandani, 1974; Erwald, Hed, Nygren, Röjdmark, Sundblad and Wicchel, 1973). Insulin analogues, in inverse correlation to their biological potency, and glucagon increase insulin degradation, but PRO and CP do not interfere (Varandani, Nafz and Chandler, 1976).

(c) *Metabolic clearance*

Insulin disappearance *in vivo* is multiexponential (Sherman, Cramer, Tohin, Insol, Liljenquist, Berman and Andres, 1974; Berman, McGuire and Zelenik, 1977). The half disappearance time, $T_{\frac{1}{2}}$, for porcine insulin and PRO in man are, respectively, 4·3 and 25·6 min, and metabolic clearance rates (MCR) increased and decreased, respectively, with increasing concentration (possibly due to insulinase activity) (Sönksen *et al.*, 1973). After islet cell tumour, removal $T_{\frac{1}{2}}$ for endogenous insulin, PLC and CP were, respectively, 4·7, 17 and 11 min (Alsever *et al.*, 1976; Horwitz, Starr, Rubenstein and Steiner, 1973). Values of 9 and 20 min for endogenous insulin and CP, respectively, in normal individuals have also been reported (Kuzuya and Matsuda, 1976; Williams, Gleason and Soeldner, 1968). Insulin $T_{\frac{1}{2}}$ increased by 30% in old age, but not in diabetes (Ørskov and Christensen, 1969; Giron and Lestradet, 1973). Ageing does not change tissue:plasma distribution of insulin (McGuire, Tobin, Berman and Andres, 1977). An accelerated unusual mode of insulin degradation in the plasma of a juvenile diabetic has been reported (Paulsen, 1976).

In the dog 48% of insulin is extracted by the liver and this process is saturable (Navalesi, Pilo and Ferrannini, 1976). In man hepatic removal increases when portal levels exceed 300 µu/ml (Erwald *et al.*, 1973). Renal clearance is nonsaturable and at least 33% of any load is removed (Frankson and Ooms, 1973). In the rat MCR and renal clearance of exogenous insulin, PRO and CP are 16·4, 6·7 and 4·6 ml/min and 33, 55 and 70%, respectively, but the hepatic extraction of PRO and CP is very low (Katz and Rubenstein, 1973). Insulin is secreted as well as filtered into the proximal renal tubules, 98% of which is reabsorbed, less than 2% being excreted in the urine (Aun, Meguid, Soeldner and Stolf, 1975). Proximal tubular cells degrade the absorbed insulin as well as that provided in the extracellular fluid by the large permeability of peritubular capillaries (Frankson, Gassee, Ooms and Dubois, 1976), and hence the reason for the large (30–55%) renal arterio-venous insulin deficit.

(d) *Physiological and clinical significance of levels in blood and other body fluids*

In normal man, mean daily insulin excretion is 14–160 units (Aun *et al.*, 1975). The clearance during an oral glucose tolerance test (see Section F.1.*a*) repeated at weekly intervals varies not more than 1·7 times and urinary levels can be a good index of average serum levels over long periods (Ørskov and Johanson, 1972). Clearance varies between 0·23–0·87 ml/min (Rubenstein, Lowy, Wellbourne and Fraser, 1967). The fasting ratio, PLC:insulin in serum is four times higher than in urine (Constan, Mako, Juhn and Rubenstein, 1975). Glomerular filtration of PLC is low (Horwitz, Rubenstein and Katz, 1977; Kuzuya, Matsuda, Saito and Yoshida, 1976). However, CP:insulin urinary clearance is about 4·6:1, and urinary CP correlates with serum CP levels during oral or i.v. glucose tolerance tests (Kuzuya and Matsuda, 1976; Kaneko, Oka, Munemura, Oda, Suzuki, Yasuda, Yanaihara, Nakagawa and Makabe, 1975).

Only for 1–2 min after i.v. glucose are concentrations in the portal vein of insulin, CP and PLC within the range of pancreatic extracts. At all times the CP and PLC molar ratios to insulin in the general circulation are high on account of preferential hepatic extraction of insulin (Horwitz et al., 1975). Released insulin is also trapped by the vascular endothelium (Dieterle et al., 1973; Giron and Lestradet, 1973; Hammersten, Holm, Björntorp and Schersten, 1977). Peripheral CP starts to decline after the 2nd hour of an oral glucose tolerance test when normally insulin levels have become basal (Heding and Rasmussen, 1975). After oral glucose, the molar PLC:insulin ratio is below fasting level and starts rising by 90 min (Kitabchi, 1977). The fasting ratio is significantly elevated after the 4th decade of life (Duckworth and Kitabchi, 1976). In non-diabetic hyperinsulinaemic states, e.g. obesity (Kitabchi, 1977, Roth et al., 1968; Gutman, Lazarus and Recant, 1972) acromegaly, Cushing's syndrome, steroid therapy, myotonic dystrophy (Kitabchi, 1977) and pregnancy (Phelps, Bergenstahl, Freinkel, Rubenstein, Metzger and Mako, 1975; Kühl, 1976a), the PLC levels are high but the ratio to insulin is normal. This ratio tends to rise in mildly diabetic pregnancy (Persson and Lunnel, 1975) and diabetic obesity, but especially in insulin dependent diabetes (Table 3) (Phelps et al., 1975; Lewis et al., 1976; Kuzuya, Blix, Horwitz, Steiner and Rubenstein, 1977). Binding of PLC by insulin antibodies greatly prolongs its $T_{\frac{1}{2}}$ (Fink, Cresto, Gutman, Lavine, Rubenstein and Recant, 1974). In renal failure PLC catabolism is diminished and plasma levels are increased (Blackard et al., 1970). The molar PLC:insulin ratio exceeds 30% in islet cell tumours and tumour removal diminishes predominantly the PLC and relieves the hypoglycaemic symptoms (Alsever et al., 1976). The highest ratio (75–91%) was found in the rare condition of familial hyperproinsulinaemia accompanied with normoglycaemia (Gabbay et al., 1976).

Hence, the intrinsic biological activity of PLC becomes physiologically significant when levels are high. Both PLC and CP levels are of diagnostic significance in islet cell tumours (Turner and Heding, 1977; Service, Horwitz, Rubenstein, Kuzuya, Mako, Reynold and Molnar, 1977b). Since crystalline insulins are CP-free, endogenous levels of CP reflect residual B cell activity in insulin-dependent diabetes, and estimation is important for ascertaining correction of ketoacidosis (Block, Mako, Steiner and Rubenstein, 1972; Faber, Binder, Naithani and Heding, 1975) and for prognosis (Block,

Table 3

Insulin, C-peptide, proinsulin in serum and residual B cell function in diabetes. Abbreviations: CP—C-peptide; CPR—(CP + PLC); PLC—proinsulin-like component; IA—insulin antibodies (+bound IRI and PLC); IRI—immunoreactive insulin; TIR—(PLC + IRI); JOD—juvenile onset diabetes; MOD—maturity onset diabetes; IDM—insulin dependent diabetes; S.A.S.—Sepharose-bound antibody separation. From Heding and Rasmussen (1975)—A, Heding (1977)—B, Ludvigsson and Heding (1977)—C, Faber and Binder (1977b)—D, Hendricksen et al (1977)—E, and Block et al (1972)—F.

Subject (age)	Fasting levels (nmol/l)					Test levels 1 hr post-OGTT (nmol/l)					CP Assay
	CP	TIR	IRI	PLC	PLC:TIR	CP	TIR	IRI	PLC	PLC:TIR	
A											
Normal	0·37 ± 0·02 / 1·11 ± 0·06[a]		0·048 ± 0·009			2·53 ± 0·20		0·52 ± 0·077			S.A.S. and CP RIA
MOD	0·86 ± 0·17		0·110 ± 0·029			2·49 ± 0·30		0·49 ± 0·11			
JOD	0·37 ± 0·04		0·063 ± 0·009			0·49 ± 0·05		0·11 ± 0·014			
B											
Normal (15–65)	0·38	0·048		0·009	19%	1·67	0·45		0·053	8%	S.A.S. and CP RIA
MOD (24–72)	0·54	0·068		0·022	23%	1·84	0·48		0·046	11%	
IDM (JOD + MOD) (24–72)	0·24	0·048		0·010	16%	0·44	0·15		0·032	31%	
C						CP (min after i.v. glucagon)					
Normal (6–22)	0·22–0·73		0–31			—					S.A.S. and CP RIA
JOD (1976) (10–18)	0·03–0·13		13–2720			—					
JOD (1977) (11–19)	0·03–0·11		61–4000			0·13–0·18 (2–4) (increments above basals) / 0·05–0·08 (2–4) in three improved patients)					

D			
Normal (22–44) 0·26–0·63	0·03–0·15	0·36–1·28 (6)	S.A.S. and CP RIA
E			
IDM (13–49) 0–0·40 (> 0·07 good B cell reserve) (< 0·04 not functioning)		0–0·35 (4–6)	S.A.S. and CP RIA
IDM (1A) 0·06–0·94	(PLC interference when IA not removed, hence CPR and not CP values)		
F			
CP			
Normal 1·30 ± 0·3[a] (0·46 ± 0·1)		4·40 ± 0·80[a] (1·47 ± 0·26)	Biogel-P30 and CP RIA

[a] Elsewhere in the literature CPR has been expressed as ng/ml CP equivalents; therefore, CP values when provided in ng/ml (as well as nmol/l) have been included for comparison with CPR.

Rosenfield, Mako, Steiner and Rubenstein, 1973; Ludvigsson and Heding, 1976; Grajwer, Pildes, Horwitz and Rubenstein, 1977; Hendricksen, Faber, Dreger and Binder, 1977) (Table 3).

Insulin has been detected in body fluids other than plasma and urine, e.g. bile, lymph, cerebrospinal fluid, aqueous humour (Henderson, 1974) and human semen (Paz, Homonnai, Ayalon, Cordora and Kraicer, 1977), but only the changes of the levels in amniotic fluid have clinical significance (Draisey, Gagneja and Thibert, 1977). Elevation above 8 μu/ml during 34th–38th weeks of gestation prevents the normal increase of the lecithin:sphingomyelin ratio. Also, the complete absence of insulin during the last trimester is associated with intrauterine death (Rebuzzi, Bellati, Ghirlanda, Manna, Altomonte and Greco, 1977).

Unusual, non-precursor circulatory or storage forms of insulin in association with diabetes (Crossley and Elliott, 1975) and insulinoma (Permutt, Biesbroeck and Chyn, 1977; Arnold, Deutsch, Frerichs and Creutzfeldt, 1972) have been noted. Highly active complexed forms seen in islet adenoma cases (Nuñez-Correa, Lowy and Sönksen, 1974; Gorden, Freychet and Nankin, 1971) have been explained as gammaglobulin-entrapped insulin (Sramkova, Par and Engelberth, 1975). Protein-complexed, biologically inactive insulin, which can be freed by biotin, has also been demonstrated in human plasma (Guenther and McDonald, 1972).

2. Insulin-like Biological Activity in Circulation

The properties of "insulin antibody non-suppressible insulin-like activity" (NSILA) (Froesch, Zapf, Meuli, Mäder, Waldvogel, Kaufmann and Morell, 1975; Zapf, Mäder, Waldvogel and Froesch, 1975) and of related somatomedins (Chochinor and Daughaday, 1976) have been reviewed. Of the two species, the low mw form (6000), constituting 5% of the total, is, like insulin, acid ethanol soluble (NSILA-s) and the 90,000 dalton species is precipitable (NSILA-p) (Zapf et al., 1975; Rinderknecht and Humbel, 1976; Jacob, Hauri and Froesch, 1968; Poffenbarger, 1975). Both forms are carrier bound in serum (Froesch et al., 1975; Kauffmann, Zapf, Torroth and Froesch, 1977) and NSILA-s does not readily filter at the glomerulus hence interference with insulin biological activity in urine is low. In serum and urine, activity is equivalent to 10–35 μu/ml and 0–8 μu/ml insulin, respectively (El-Allawy, Humbel and Froesch, 1976). The serum levels are low in hypopituitarism (Megyesi, Kahn, Roth and Gorden, 1974), anorexia nervosa, diabetes; raised in acromegaly, pregnancy (Megyesi, Kahn, Roth and Gorden, 1975) and obesity (Megyesi, Gorden and Kahn, 1977), and also in fibrosarcomas, phaeochromocytoma, hepatomas; and normal in insulinomas (Megyesi et al., 1974), hence, correlating with insulin levels. Intravenous insulin lowers (Megyesi et al., 1974), and glucose raises the levels (Megyesi et al., 1975).

Probably on account of structural homology with insulin A and B chains (Rinderknecht and Humbel, 1976; Blundell, Bedarkar, Rinderknecht and Humbel, 1978), NSILA-s have about 2% of the biological activity of insulin on muscle and adipocyte metabolism (Zapf et al., 1975; Reckler, Podskalny, Goldfine and Wells, 1974), with parallel dose response curves with insulin (Morrell and Froesch, 1973; Zapf et al., 1975; Froesch et al., 1975; Schoenle Zapf and Froesch, 1977). However, on cardiac muscle (Froesch et al., 1975) and the fibroblasts (see Hall and Fryklund, this volume, Ch. V) NSILA-s and insulin are equipotent. They bind to a specific receptor on myocardium (Meuli and Froesch, 1976), fat cell (Schoenle et al., 1976), hepatocyte and the placenta; NSILA receptor binds insulin less avidly, and insulin receptor binds NSILA-s very weakly (Megyesi, Kahn, Roth, Neville and Nissley, 1973). In the diabetic rat, binding of insulin and NSILA-s to their respective receptors is reduced similarly (Schoenle et al., 1976). At physiological concentration, NSILA-s inhibits specific proteolysis of insulin at the hepatocyte membrane (Kahn, Megyesi and Roth, 1976; Burghen, Duckworth, Kitabchi, Solomon and Poffenbarger, 1976), and insulin potentiates the binding of NSILA-s to its receptor (Schoenle et al., 1976).

The identity of "bound insulin" on the grounds of its physicochemical properties including its electrophoretic mobility in the β-γ-globulin range, approximates to that of the NSILA-s and NSILA-p. "Bound insulin" prolongs insulin half life and is neutralised by potent, undiluted insulin antisera. It is ineffective on blood glucose and decreases after glucose infusion (Kitagawa and Aikawa, 1976).

3. Immunochemistry of Insulin and its Precursors

Insulin is weakly antigenic (Arquilla et al., 1972). Its precursors are relatively more (Kawazu, Kanazawa, Kajinuma, Miki, Kuzuya and Kosaka, 1975) and C-peptide is much less antigenic (Faber, Markussen, Naithani and Binder, 1976; Melani, Rubenstein, Oyer and Steiner, 1970a). Antibody production is genetically determined. Different species and strains within a species produce antibodies against different antigenic determinants of the insulin molecule. For example, guinea-pig but not rabbit anti-insulin antibodies neutralise insulin biological activity (Arquilla et al., 1972). The heterogeneity of antibody populations influences the relative binding specificities of insulin, PLC and CP in assay systems.

Different antigenic determinants of the insulin molecule are recognised in immune haemolysis (IH) and radioimmunoassay (RIA) methods, and PRO is virtually inactive in IH (Arquilla et al., 1972).

Cross-reactivity of PRO and its derivatives with RIA anti-insulin sera varies from about 30–98% on a molar basis (Arquilla *et al.*, 1972; Chance, 1972; Heding and Rasmussen, 1975; Markussen and Heding, 1976) but as a rule PRO is the least avid, while CP is non-reactive (Kitabchi, 1977; Yu and Kitabchi, 1973; Chance, 1972; Chance, 1971; Markussen and Heding, 1976). Therefore antisera must bind PLC and insulin equally when estimating insulin in samples of high PLC content.

Highly specific anti-PRO sera totally unreactive to insulin have been prepared (Chance, 1971). The CP region of PRO shows extensive interspecies heterogeneity (Snell and Smyth, 1975), and antibodies recognising this region are highly species-specific (Chance, 1971; Melani *et al.*, 1970a). Anti-CP antisera do not cross-react with homologous insulins (Yu and Kitabchi, 1973; Markussen and Heding, 1976; Melani *et al.*, 1970a), but reactivity with homologous PRO or PLC varies with the antiserum from 7–100% on a molar basis (Horwitz *et al.*, 1975; Faber and Binder, 1977a; Block, Mako, Steiner and Rubenstein, 1972; Kuzuya *et al.*, 1977; Markussen and Heding, 1976; Faber, Binder, Kuzuya, Blix, Horwitz and Rubenstein, 1977) but is significant even when low (Kuzuya *et al.*, 1976; Heding, 1977; Hendriksen *et al.*, 1977) so as to necessitate separation of PLC and CP for specificity. Binding of purified human PRO (h-PRO) by anti h-CP antisera was not equal to binding of endogenous PLC (Melani *et al.*, 1970). Hence, quantitation of endogenous PLC with homologous or heterologous PRO preparations is approximate. Endogenous h-CP may not be homogenous (Melani *et al.*, 1970). Fragments of purified h-CP cross-react with anti h-CP antisera (Block *et al.*, 1972; Yanaihara, Hashimoto, Yanaihara, Sakagami, Steiner and Rubenstein, 1974). Since h-CP is difficult to prepare (Melani *et al.*, 1970; Block *et al.*, 1972) synthetic h-CP (sh-CP) was prepared (Naithani, 1973) and characterised in RIA systems (Yanaihara *et al.*, 1974; Naithani, Dechesne, Markussen and Heding, 1975a); Kaneko, Oda, Yamashita, Suzuki, Yanaihara, Hashimoto and Yanaihara, 1974). Preparative procedures influenced sh-CP binding but two out of three preparations made available gave parallel dilution curves with h-CP. The identity of sh-CP and endogenous h-CP has yet to be demonstrated (Heding, 1975; Heding and Rasmussen, 1975).

One tyrosine residue has to be added to CP for iodination as a radiotracer in RIA (Melani *et al.*, 1970; Heding and Rasmussen, 1975; Naithani, Dechesne, Markussen and Heding, 1975b). The tyr-sh-CP binds antisera more avidly than sh-CP (Naithani *et al.*, 1975b). Patients' sera devoid of endogenous CP can interfere with ^{125}I-tyr-h-CP binding, according to the antiserum used. Hence there are many factors contributing to the variation of results in different assay systems (Heding, 1975). In comparison to the early antisera to h-CP (Melani *et al.*, 1970; Block *et al.*, 1972) the recent ones against sh-CP are considerably stronger (Faber *et al.*, 1976), with the lowest detection limit reaching 0·003 pmol, sh-CP equivalent per assay sample, which is comparable to the systems using other CP-recognising antisera (Heding and Rasmussen, 1975; Heding, 1975).

4. Insulin Antibodies in the Human Circulation

Purified insulin used therapeutically are antigenic (Chance, Root and Galloway 1976; Kerp and Kasemir, 1976; Kawazu *et al.*, 1975; Schlichtkrull, Brange, Christiansen, Hallund, Heding and Jorgensen, 1972). The problems associated with old and new insulins have been reviewed (Yue and Turtle, 1977). Antigenicity depends on the species of origin; for instance, purified porcine insulin is less antigenic than the bovine hormone in man (Chance *et al.*, 1976), although they are structurally very similar (Blundell and Wood, 1975). Impurities in commercial insulins (Schlichtkrull *et al.*, 1972) and antibodies to these (Kawazu *et al.*, 1975) have been demonstrated. Some impurities are unavoidable in insulin preparations (Kohnert, Schmidt, Zühlke and Fiedler, 1973). The physical state of the preparation is also contributory, and homologous insulins can therefore also be antigenic (Kerp and Kasemir, 1976).

Antibody formation is slower with purer preparations. Peak levels are reached in two to three months and then gradually decline to steady levels (Kerp and Kasemir, 1976). Young patients form more antibody than older patients (Andersen, 1972). Severe insulin resistance at all ages (Menczel, Levy and Bentwich, 1966; Burman, Cunningham, Klack and Burns, 1973) with short remission periods (Anderson, 1976; Hahn, Menzel, Gottschling, and Jahr, 1976; Ludvigsson and Heding, 1976) have been associated with high antibody titres which slightly delay the blood glucose nadir during treatment of ketoacidosis (Asplin and Hartog, 1977). Endogenous insulin is neutralised (Fink *et al.*, 1974) and inactivated (Antoniades and Simon, 1972). The PLC is bound less avidly and CP is not bound at all by insulin antibodies (Block *et al.*, 1972). Bound is degraded differently from free hormone (Frikke, Gingerich, Stranahan, Carter, Bauman, Greider, Wright and Lacy, 1974). All major classes of immunoglobulins participate in insulin binding (Fölling, 1976; Anderson, 1976). These are predominantly of IgG class and polyclonal (Christiansen and Kroll, 1973; Kawazu *et al.*, 1975). The IgM appears early and is correlated with insulin resistance. The type, as well as the titre of antibody relative to that of insulin determine the properties of the complex formed and the clinical picture (Kerp and Kasemir, 1976; Yue, Baxter and Turtle, 1976). High affinity–low capacity, and low affinity–high capacity species directed against different antigenic determinants of insulin molecule are described (Kerp and Kasemir, 1976; Baxter, Yue and Turtle, 1976; Yue, Baxter and Turtle, 1976).

Antibodies are complexed with insulin or have free sites available for reversible binding. The ratio of the insulin-binding capacity of both types of site to that of the free sites, but not the values of the binding capacity or the free sites alone, correlated with the total insulin immunoreactivity of serum (Jayarao, Faulk, Karam, Grodsky and Forsham, 1973). This ratio, calculated by the author from the very accurate data of Baxter, Yue and Turtle (1976) also positively correlated with the daily insulin requirement; an absolute increase in the high affinity sites also correlated with insulin dose (Baxter *et al.*, 1976; Kerp and Kasemir, 1976). Good control of glycaemia is more frequent when there is a relative abundance of low affinity sites (Shen, Yu and Singh, 1977; Dixon, Exon and Malins, 1975) and the insulin dose could be decreased when changing to monocomponent preparations (Moustaffa, Daggett and Nabarro, 1977). Indeed, these sites bind the less antigenic porcine insulins, whereas the complexing sites predominantly bind the more antigenic bovine insulins (Kerp and Kasemir, 1976). Therefore, routinely, an assessment of both types of site rather than measurement of total binding capacity of all or of one sub-class of antibodies may be more meaningful in relation to maintenance of free insulin levels.

Insulin antibodies cross the placental barrier (Block, Pildes, Mossaboy and Steiner, 1974) and cord blood levels are less than, but related to, the maternal levels (Martin, 1976). Monoclonal auto-antibodies of IgG class to endogenous insulin have been demonstrated in non-diabetic, but probably drug-sensitised patients (Ohneda, Matsuda, Sato, Yamagata and Sato, 1974).

5. Immunochemical Methods of Insulin Estimation

(a) *Total insulin immunoreactivity (TIR)*

In unfractionated serum or tissue extract TIR is measured by haemagglutination, immune haemolysis and radioimmunoassay (RIA) or enzyme-linked immunoassay methods. The first two methods involve inhibition by free insulin of the haemagglutination or haemolysis of insulin coated erythrocytes incubated with anti-insulin sera. The former method is semiquantitative. The latter has precision comparable to RIA but its sensitivity is two orders of magnitude lower on account of non-specific interference in biological fluids (Arquilla *et al.*, 1972). The more specific and sensitive RIAs have developed considerably since the first demonstration by Yalow and Berson in 1960. The techniques of antiserum raising, purification and characterisation, insulin iodination, details of incubation and counting have been described (Starr and Rubenstein, 1974). Also, factors contributing to accuracy and reproducibility with a new approach to optimisation of incubation conditions have been discussed (Albano, Ekins, Maritz and Turner, 1972).

A critical appraisal of the methods introduced between 1960 and 1968 with proposals (Zaharko and Beck, 1968) to avoid potential errors arising from impure radioligand or disturbance of the binding equilibrium have been outlined (Baxter *et al.*, 1976).

Estimation of hormone levels by the radioimmunoassays depends on the measurement of the radioactivity of labelled hormone, either that of the antibody-bound or of the unbound or the "free" component. Therefore, these methods are designed to separate the antibody-bound and unbound (or "free") components with minimal perturbation of the steady state equilibrium attained. The bound components has been selectively removed by electrophoresis (Yalow and Berson, 1960), paperwick chromatography (Ørskov, 1967; Ørskov and Johanson, 1972) or precipitated by sodium sulphite (Grodsky and Forsham, 1960), a second antibody, "the anti-anti-body" (Hales and Randle, 1963; Morgan and Lazarow, 1963; Zaharko and Beck, 1968; Soeldner and Slone, 1965), ethanol (Albano *et al.*, 1972; Wright, Makulu, Vichick and Sussman, 1971), polyethylene glycol (Desbuquois and Auerbach, 1971), zirconylphosphate gel (Coffey, Nagy, Lensky and Hanson, 1974) or fixation of the antibody on a plastic solid phase by polyacrylamide trapping (Updike, Simmons, Grant, Magnuson and Goodfriend, 1973) or sepharose binding (Velasco, Cole and Camerini-Davalos, 1974; Davis, Yoder and Adams, 1976). The free component has been removed by charcoal (Herbert, Lau, Gottlieb and Bleicher, 1965; Blanks and Gerritsen, 1974; Albano *et al.*, 1972; Updike *et al.*, 1973), silica (Velasco *et al.*, 1974), cellulose (Zaharko and Beck, 1968), resin (Malvano, Zucchelli, Quesada, Gandolfi and Piro, 1974) or enzymic destruction (Zaharko and Beck, 1968).

Two comparative studies on the assay of common standards and samples by groups of laboratories employing different methods has revealed significant variability despite agreement in ranking order of the results (Cotes, Mussett, Berryman, Ekins, Glover, Hales, Hunter, Lowy, Neville, Samols and Woodward, 1969; Costantini, Lostia, Malvano, Rolleri, Taggi and Zucchelli, 1975). A consistent difference in the results of the double antibody, paperwick chromatography and charcoal precipitation methods was noted (Ørskov and Seyer-Hansen, 1974) and confirmed (Malvano *et al.*, 1974). The double antibody method with damaged tracer lost from the bound component, or not bound, and chromatography with damaged unbound tracer contaminating the bound component gave higher and lower results, respectively, in comparison to the charcoal adsorption method which allows for individual correction of radioligand damage. The last method is advantageous in its manageability, accuracy, cheapness and applicability to capillary blood samples (Malvano *et al.*, 1974; Albano *et al.*, 1972). However, the double antibody method with pre-precipitated antibody (Hales and Randle, 1963) when carried out by back titration with radio-insulin (Wright *et al.*,

1971) offers excellent reproducibility with relatively short incubation times. Different filter materials for this method have been compared (Krause, Puchinger and Wacker, 1973) and an ultramicro adaptation described (Blanks and Gerritsen, 1974). Solid phase immunoassays exclude serum interference, especially proteolytic damage, allowing for use of high concentration of unlabelled insulin and quick equilibration, and possibly more specificity at the lower insulin concentration range than the double antibody methods (Davis *et al.*, 1976; Velasco *et al.*, 1974; Updike *et al.*, 1973) and are amenable to automation.

Haemolysis and clotting damages insulin (Feldman and Chapman, 1973; Ørskov and Seyer-Hansen, 1974) but reports on the influence of amino acids (Szabo and Mahler, 1970; Feldman and Quickel, 1973) or heparin (Soeldner and Slone, 1965; Henderson, 1970; Spellacy and Buhi, 1971; Thorell and Lanner, 1973; Crowley and Garbien, 1974) have been inconsistent. Extracted insulin-free blank serum has been found to alter insulin-binding characteristics (Silbert and Swain, 1975; Frayn, 1976).

For estimation of TIR in whole pancreatic tissue (Scott and Fisher, 1938; Best, Haist and Ridout, 1939; Taylor, Gardner, Parry and Jones, 1965), isolated islets (Morris and Korner, 1970), islet cell tumours (Steiner and Oyer, 1967; Hayashi, Floyd, Peks and Fajans, 1977) or injection sites on post mortem tissue in forensic investigations (Phillips, Webb and Curry, 1972) the material is extracted by acid ethanol and purified by gel chromatography, which also fractionates the insulin and PLC components. Preparation of urine for RIA of TIR and other components has been described (El-Allawy *et al.*, 1976; Constan *et al.*, 1975; Norwitz *et al.*, Kuzuya *et al.*, 1976; Kaneko *et al.*, 1975).

Two W.H.O. standard insulin preparations are available for quality control in RIA bioassays: insulin recrystallised from a mixture of 52% bovine and 48% porcine pancreas, with specific activity of 24 u/mg, established in 1958; and, the international human insulin standard for RIA, established in 1974 and consisting of human insulin recrystallised with sucrose, available in ampoules of 3u (Bulletin of the W.H.O.).

Normally TIR is representative of insulin, but in obesity, insulin-dependent diabetes with insulin antibodies and especially islet cell tumours, PLC is elevated. Unless assayed with antisera which bind insulin and PLC equally, TIR will be underestimated in an insulin immunoassay system (Melani *et al.*, 1970).

The preliminary data of an enzyme-linked immunoassay of insulin have appeared (Kitagawa and Aikawa, 1976). Insulin co-conjugated to *m*-maleimidobenzoyl *N*-hydroxy succinimide ester with β-D-galactosidase, EC 3.2.1.23, is immunoassayed with a double antibody technique. The bound and free conjugates are separated by centrifugation, and enzyme activity in both fractions is estimated spectrofluorimetrically. There is little non-specific binding of the conjugate, and very high sensitivity in the 0–2·5·0 μu/ml region of the total range of 0–20 μu/ml insulin assayed. Details of the preparative procedures in its application to plasma were not given.

(b) *"Free insulin"*

Free insulin immunoreactivity or FIR is that fraction of TIR which is in equilibrium with the insulin antibodies in diabetic serum at a particular time after insulin injection. It has been of clinical interest in relation to the control of diabetes after insulin antibody (IA) formation. Estimation by RIA is subsequent to the separation of FIR from the IA-bound fraction. Routine methods employing ethanol (Heding, 1972; Asplin, Goldie and Hartog, 1977) or polyethylene glycol (Rasmussen, Heding, Parbst and Volund, 1975; Gennaro and Van Norman, 1975; Lewis et al., 1976; Asplin et al., 1977) over-estimate FIR (Asplin et al., 1977). Accurate column fractionations are described (Asplin et al., 1977; Davidson and Deal, 1976) the ranking order of results of which agree better with that of the ethanol precipitation technique. Acidification and subsequent precipitation of IA allows for TIR estimation (Rasmussen et al., 1975; Lewis et al., 1976). The IA interferes with the RIA (Block et al., 1974; Gennaro et al., 1975; Martin, 1976).

(c) *Proinsulin-like component (PLC)*

Insulin and CP can be separated from PLC by gel chromatography using Sephadex G-50 or Biogel-P-30 (Rubenstein et al., 1977). Veronal buffer, pH 8·6, is best suited to the former (Lazarus et al., 1972) than acetic acid (Rubenstein and Steiner, 1971) and recoveries are about 83 % (Gutman et al., 1972). The labelled h-CP polymerises in alkaline buffers and elutes with PLC (Block et al., 1972). These methods are slow and require up to 10 ml serum (Melani et al., 1970).

A simpler method is selective degradation of insulin by insulin specific protease (Burr et al., 1976; Duckworth and Kitabchi, 1972). However, this method over estimated low PLC levels (Cresto, Lavine, Fink and Recant, 1974) and partial degradation of PLC also occurred (Starr, Juhn, Rubenstein and Kitabchi, 1975).

Solid phase-antibody has been used to separate PLC from CP (Heding, 1977) which allows for simultaneous CP assays with complete recovery of both components (Table 3.A, B).

Unless antisera bind PLC and insulin equally, PLC will be underestimated in an insulin RIA. Also, the use of PRO standards is necessary for the best approximation (Melani et al., 1970; Chance, 1971). The results are expressed

E

as PLC:TIR or, after chromatographic separation of insulin and PLC, as PLC:IRI.

(d) C-peptide estimation

Accurate CP estimation is only possible after PLC elimination, otherwise the estimated activity is a sum of CP and PLC and has been designated as CPR or CP-like reactivity. In diabetic sera with IA, PLC is very high and CPR is not representative of endogenous release (Table 3). There is considerable CP loss after acid ethanol extraction and subsequent gel fractionation of serum (Melani et al., 1970). After acidification and chromatography without extraction 70–75% CP recovery is obtained (Block et al., 1972). Similar losses also apply to solid phase-antibody separation of CP and PLC, since without acidification and removal of IA, PLC separation is not complete (Hendricksen et al., 1977) (Table 3.E). However, this is the most specific method available and is applicable on a routine basis. The main problems involve choice of antisera least influenced by the patients' sera (Faber et al., 1977) and the unproven identity of endogenous CP with s-hCP (Heding, 1975). Polyethylene glycol precipitates IA with the bound PLC with 88% recovery of the CPR in the supernatant (Kuzuya et al., 1977). When PLC interference is overlooked in CP assay the results are higher than the CP, and not of value in insulin-dependent diabetes (Table 3).

(e) Insulin antibodies (IA)

Serum IA activity is expressed either in terms of the serum dilution at which a set amount of radioinsulin tracer is bound (Jayarao et al., 1973) or as the insulin bound by the IA per unit volume of serum (Schlichtkrull et al., 1972; Baxter et al., 1976). The respective methods involve equilibration with a constant appropriate amount of tracer of the serially diluted or undiluted serum. The latter is preferred since serial dilution in the former influences the insulin:tracer ratio and tracer-IA association. Significant error arises from separation of bound and free tracer attempted by charcoal (Baxter et al., 1976; Jayarao et al., 1973; Dixon, 1974), double antibody precipitation (Moustaffa et al., 1977), or immunoelectrophoresis (Christiansen and Kroll, 1973). An elaborate gel filtration method achieving separation without perturbation of steady-state equilibrium, allowing accurate estimation of binding capacities and dissociation constants of IA has been described (Baxter et al., 1976). However, the routine methods described have been applied to the estimations of IA with different binding properties (Jayarao et al., 1973; Dixon et al., 1975).

6. Bioassays and Radioceptor Assays

Before the introduction of radioimmunoassays, insulin bioassays were in general use. The earliest methods estimated the blood sugar lowering potency of milligram quantities of purified insulins (Banting, Best, Collip, MacLeod and Noble, 1922; Young and Lewis, 1947). Later, methods were designed to estimate insulin-sensitive parameters of metabolism in isolated tissues like the rat diaphragm (Vallance-Owen, Hurlock and Please, 1955), rat fat pad (Renold, Martin, Dagenais, Steiner, Nickerson and Shaps, 1960; Liebermann, 1968) or the isolated fat cells (Gliemann, 1967). Technical details have been reviewed (Taylor, 1967).

With the description of the tertiary structure of insulin, investigation of the structure-activity relationships of purified insulins, precursors and analogues depended on the use of these methods *in vitro* (Gliemann and Sörensen, 1970; Gliemann and Gammeltoft, 1974; Yu and Kitabchi, 1973; Markussen and Heding, 1976) and *in vivo* (Chance, 1971; Markussen and Heding, 1976; Jones, Iron, Ellis, Sönksen and Brandenburg, 1976). Criticism of the rat diaphragm method (Hollands and Youson, 1973) developments in fat cell assay (Moody, Stan, Stan and Gliemann, 1974) and in the mouse blood sugar test (Markussen and Heding, 1976) have been reported. The limitations of the tests lie in the technical impossibility of standardisation of animal preparations. Using purified hormones, the dose-response is not identical with fat pad and adipocytes (Steiner *et al.*, 1968), *in vivo* and *in vitro* (Jones *et al.*, 1976) or on same parameters in different species. Use of biological fluids is precluded by the presence of non-specific interference with insulin action.

A sophisticated bioassay is the radioceptor assay. Insulin binding at its receptor to displace previously bound radioiodinated insulin is a function of insulin concentration (Ginsberg, 1977a). Using purified cell membranes from liver (Freychet, Brandenburg and Wollmer, 1974) and kidney (Suzuki *et al.*, 1976), or intact adipocytes and lymphocytes as templates, highly sensitive assays of the relative receptor binding potency of insulins, precursors or analogues have been set up (Ginsberg, 1977a). Application to human serum gave identical results with double antibody RIA, but the radioceptor assay gave consistently higher basal values which may be of greater physiological importance than given by the double antibody RIA (Suzuki *et al.*, 1976). An iodinated insulin preparation of full biological activity for use in radioceptor assay has been described (Schneider, Straus and Yalow, 1976).

F. INSULIN LEVELS IN BODY FLUIDS AND IN THE PANCREAS

1. B Cell Function Tests

Insulin levels are measured in body fluids during stimulatory or suppressive B cell function tests which assess the stimulus sensitivity, release capacity or the effectiveness of the response to maintenance homoestasis. In the account which follows the term "sugar" instead of "glucose" signifies that non-specific analytical methods have been used.

(a) Oral glucose tolerance test (OGTT)

Standard conditions of OGTT for patient preparation with attention to the state of health, nutrition, drug usage and ambulation, and the dose of glucose, blood sampling, analyses and evaluation of results have been proposed (Klimt, Prout, Bradley, Dolger, Fisher, Gastineau, Marks, Meinert and Schumacher, 1969). After oral glucose, peripheral insulin concentration varies directly with the portal concentration and can be estimated as an index of B cell stimulation (Schulz et al., 1976). The test of the true physiological capacity of islets, however, requires a standard meal of fat and protein, as well as carbohydrate (see Ebert et al., 1976). In the early or potentially diabetic state, B cells are highly responsive to gastro-intestinal factors (Enk, 1976; Enk et al., 1976; Vinik, Kalk, Keller, Beaumont and Jackson, 1973) and OGTT may not discriminate borderline defects of islet function. Gastro-intestinal disease influences results (see Table 7). Significant individual variation occurs in frequent tests of normal subjects (Olefsky and Reaven, 1974b). In a normal urban population, three distinct "types" of OGTT response were seen, irrespective of age and sex differences, and despite similar fasting blood "sugar", elevations of which decreased the insulin response (Szabo et al., 1974). Differences in timing of glucose response may partly arise by changing the glucose dose. Blood "sugar" levels may also contribute, and even be misleading (Reaven, Weisinger and Sorenson, 1974). For example, 2 hr after a 75 g OGTT, plasma glucose concentration best indicated the glucose tolerance status; plasma glucose above 9·4 mmol/l (169 mg/dl) marked the deterioration of insulin response in Pima Indians of mixed age, sex and weight (Savage, Dippe, Bennett, Gorden, Roth, Rushforth and Miller, 1975). In Jamaican rural populations the same critical values of the "blood sugar" in glucose equivalents occurred at 1 hr after a 100 g OGTT (Florey, Milner and Miall, 1977). Adherence to standard procedures, accurate estimation of plasma glucose (Marks and Alberti, 1976) and good selection of the control with respect to sex, age, weight and "type" (see Szabo *et al.*, 1974) of insulin and glucose response appear essential for a proper understanding of altered glucose tolerance.

(b) *Intravenous glucose tolerance test (IVGTT)*

0·33 g glucose/kg bw given within 2 min causes an optimal acute insulin response, "AIR" (Kruss-Jarres, Hilpert, Ross, Grohman and Kling Mullen, 1970; Fujita, Herron and Seltzer, 1975) which correlates with metabolic glucose clearance (Kg) (Lerner and Porte, 1971; Chen and Porte, 1976), but with increasing age, this correlation, despite apparent good health and undiminished "AIR", may deteriorate (Palmer and Ensinck, 1975). "AIR" and "Kg" do not correlate when fasting plasma glucose exceeds a critical limit of 6·3 mmol/l (115 mg/dl) (Brunzell *et al.*, 1976). In diabetes, "AIR" is diminished (Simpson *et al.*, 1968; Fujita *et al.*, 1975; Palmer and Ensinck, 1975). Peripheral "AIR" may not accurately reflect the portal pancreatic response (Horwitz *et al.*, 1975) due to variable rates of initial insulin extraction, independently of that of glucose, by the vascular endothelium (Riccardi, Heaf, Kaijser, Eklund and Carlson, 1976) especially in atherosclerosis (Hammersten *et al.*, 1977). Vascular disease (Hammersten *et al.*, 1977; Bylund, Hammersten, Holm and Schersten, 1976), regular physical activity (Björntorp, DeJounge, Sjöström and Sullivan, 1970; Dahlhof, Björntorp, Holm and Schersten, 1974) especially immediately before the test (Dieterle *et al.*, 1973), must be taken into account for accurate interpretation of the test, otherwise the coefficient of variation of the results of the tests is too high and reproducibility of "Kg" values is very low (Hedstrand and Boberg, 1975).

The insulin response in IVGTT with three times the recommended dose of glucose (1 g/kg bw) did not adequately discriminate latent or borderline diabetes of youth even when supplemented with i.v. glucagon or tolbutamide (Johnson, Guthrie, Murthy and Lang, 1973a). Glucagon, especially with tolbutamide, corrects a mildly diabetic response (Takeda, Usukura, Miwa, Nakabayashi, Kishitani and Yoshimitsu, 1977; Enk, 1977) and may not reduce the overlap between low normal and borderline responses. At the recommended dose of glucose (0·33 g/kg weight), combined with tolbutamide, adequate discrimination was found (Dujovna, Cresto, Sirco, Aparicio, Gimenez and De Majo, 1973). Detection of borderline glucose intolerance necessitates very strict age and sex matched control children (see Sections F.2.c and d), information which was not provided by Johnson *et al.* (1973a) and Dujovna *et al.* (1973).

Critical analysis of IVGTT parameters is more likely to detect B cell insensitivity than OGTT (Kawamori, Shichiri, Inoue and Hoshi, 1977). Results are qualitatively very similar to OGTT responses in genetically mixed (Fujita *et al.*, 1975) or homogenous populations (Aronoff, Bennett, Gorden, Rushforth and Miller, 1977). Insulin release within 3–6 min after the glucose pulse reflects B cell sensitivity to the stimulus, and that after 7–10 min reflects the peripheral insufficiency of the response (see Fujita *et al.*, 1975). In comparison with OGTT on the same subjects, results for mild glucose intolerance were 40% discordant (Olefsky, Farquhar and Reaven, 1973). Pulse glucose followed by infusion of glucose up to 1 hr, is better for overall assessment of B cell capacity and peripheral insulin sensitivity (Cerasi and Luft, 1967; Cerasi, 1975a), and is relevant to management during parenteral feeding (Dudl and Ensinck, 1977).

(c) *Intravenous tolbutamide test* (*IVTT*)

Response to IVTT has variable dose dependency and correlates with IVGTT on an individual basis (Ganda *et al.*, 1975; Marrigay, de Ruyter, Touber, Goughs, Schopman and Lequin, 1967). It is dangerous with a fasting blood glucose below 2·2 mmol/l and could not satisfactorily discriminate islet cell tumours from chronic hepatic disease (Marks and Samols, 1974).

(d) *Intravenous glucagon test*

The application and merits of this test have been reviewed (Marks and Samols, 1974; Marks and Alberti, 1976). In 84% of insulin dependent diabetics accurate prognosis is claimed on the basis of C-peptide response to glucagon (Hendricksen *et al.*, 1977; Faber and Binder, 1977b). Glucagon with IVTT increases the diabetic response to an OGTT (Vinik, Kalk, Botha, Jackson and Blake, 1976; Enk, 1977) or to an IVGTT (Takeda *et al.*, 1977) and allows for discrimination of insulin requiring, and diet and drug manageable cases. The test has caused hypotension in phaeochromocytoma (Lawrence, 1967).

(e) *Insulin suppression tests*

Fasting, diazoxide, porcine or fish insulin or adrenaline infusion are used to detect autonomous insulin release. Fasting is the most decisive test for islet cell tumours (Merimee and Tyson, 1977; Fajans and Floyd, 1976; Frerichs and Creutzfeldt, 1976). Diazoxide is not consistent (Heitz *et al.*, 1977; Castro, Builst, Grettie and Bartos, 1974; Castro and Grettie, 1973) and inhibition of insulin release is short-lived *in vitro* (Levin *et al.*, 1975). Insulins are useful for quick discrimination on the grounds of non-suppressible C-peptide (Horwitz, Rubenstein, Reynolds, Molnar and Yanaihara, 1975a; Service *et al.*, 1977b) or PLC release (Turner and Heding, 1977) (see

Section E.1.*d*). Adrenaline detects undifferentiated islet-cell tumours (Turner *et al.*, 1977b).

(*f*) Insulin tolerance test (ITT)

Intravenous insulin is employed to test peripheral insulin sensitivity but sites of action may depend on the dose (Sensi and Capani, 1976; Gibson *et al.*, 1975). It is stressful (Garber *et al.*, 1976) and potentially dangerous. The pancreatic suppression test (PST) is used as an alternative, by infusing 50–80 mu porcine insulin over one hour together with adrenalin, propranolol and glucose to attain about 100 μu/ml exogenous insulin levels and estimate steady state blood glucose response as an index of insulin resistance (IR). IR estimated by PST has been compared in the same subjects with the criteria of altered glucose tolerance in OGTT and IVGTT (Olefsky *et al.*, 1973) and applied in the diabetic (Reaven *et al.*, 1976) as well as in the normal subject (Kimmerling, Javorski and Reaven, 1977).

2. Physiological Variation of Insulin Levels

Basal and stimulated insulin release in normal man are dependent upon genetic factors, and insulin levels are influenced by sex, age, weight, nutrition, pregnancy and by long or short term stress. Stimulus sensitivity of release is adjusted diurnally by the central nervous system. When citing works on the influence of a particular variable on insulin levels, preference will be given to studies with good control of the other variables.

(a) Genetic and ethnic factors

The interrelationship between changes in blood glucose and insulin levels during a 2 hr IVGTT in a selected population of parent–offspring, mono-zygotic or dizygotic twins and siblings, has been shown, after correction for age, sex and weight, to display dependence on hereditary as well as common environmental factors (Lindsten, Cerasi, Luft, Morton and Ryman, 1976). Epidemiological studies of ethnic groups are not always well controlled with respect to age and sex (Florey *et al.*, 1977). However, differences show irrespective of traditional diet. For example, of the American population, the Navajo Indians have twice as high fasting insulin levels and 3–4 times as high early insulin response to OGTT, as do the Amish, who are hypo-insulinaemic. In hyperinsulinaemic "chemical diabetes", Amish resemble the Navajo, who show only a delay, but not further augmentation of the release (Rimoin, 1969). The Pima are obesity prone, and become diabetic in early middle age, but even the lean young are hyperinsulinaemic. The dynamics of the insulin response in normal and impaired glucose tolerance resembles that of the Caucasians (Aronoff *et al.*, 1977).

(b) Circadian rhythm

The circadian rhythm in insulin levels has been described in Sections D.3 and 4, F.2.*d.* and 3.*b.f.*

(c) Influence of age

In 2–18-month-old infants, the insulin response to a glucose–casein meal decreased with age. Fasting blood sugar, free fatty acids, and somatotrophin changed in parallel through the test and were highest in the youngest (Graham, Nakashima, Thompson and Blizzard, 1976). At 6, but not 12 months of age, rapid increase in body length positively correlated with a rapid and high response to IVGTT, but during slow growth, response was still neonatal, i.e. diminished and very delayed (Colle, Schiff, Andrew, Bauer and Fitzhardinge, 1976).

In children of up to 15 years of chronological age (Deschamp, Giron and Lestradet, 1977), or up to adult statural age (Rosenbloom, Wheeler, Bianchi, Chin, Tiwary and Orgic, 1975), fasting and stimulated insulin increased with age. Over the ages of 6–22 years, fasting C-peptide (0.45 ± 0.11 (S.D.) nmol/l) and insulin levels (11.3 ± 6.5 μu/ml) are higher than in adults (0.35 ± 0.10 nmol/l and 7.5 ± 4.3 μu/ml, respectively) (Ludvigsson and Heding, 1977a). Insulin content of pancreas increases during 0–3 years and 12–21 years of life (Haist, 1944). When fasting total insulin levels were increased after 30 years, plasma glucose remained similar to that at this age (Feldman and Plonk, 1976), but if insulin did not increase, blood "sugar" rose (Nolan, Stephan, Ghae, Vidalon, Gegick, Khurana and Danowski, 1973; see also Duckworth and Kitabchi, 1976).

Age-associated changes in insulin response are detected at 60 min after OGTT. Up to 50 years of age this may be insulin compensation for increased hyperglycaemic response (Duckworth and Kitabchi, 1976 and Table 4) but after 50 the increase may be predominantly PLC, which, being less effective on rapid glucose disposal (see Section E.1), may account for the increased glycaemia at, and after 60 min, and persistence of high TIR after 60 min (Duckworth and Kitabchi, 1976). Peak response to i.v. stimuli may diminish, remain nearly unchanged, or show relative persistence after the peak (Table 4), which may account for the decreased or maintained metabolic glucose clearance respectively. Hence, other causes than aging *per se* may alter insulin response. Lack of early B-cell compensation may lower glucose

Table 4

Influence of ageing on insulin release.

Sex	Age (years) Experimental	Age (years) Control	Test	Response—% of control (min after test)		References
F	30–49	20–29	oral glucose	insulin	100(0) $>$100(30+)	Nolan et al. (1973)
F	50–59	20–29	oral glucose	insulin	100(0) $\gg$100(30+)	
F + M	40–79	20–39	oral glucose	insulin	100(0) $>$100(30+)	Viberti et al. (1974)
F + M	40–79	20–39	i.v. arginine	insulin	100(0) $>$100(30+)	
F + M	30–69	20–29	basal	glucagon	$\gg$100(0) $\gg$100(30)	Berger et al. (1977a)
F + M	65–90	19–23	i.v. arginine	glucagon	$\gg$100(0) $\gg$100(30)	Marco et al. (1977)
F + M	65–90	19–23		insulin	— 40(30)	
M	65–88	20–31	i.v. glucose	insulin, glucose clearance	100(0) 100; $\ll$100(3–5)	Palmer and Ensinck (1975)
M	65–88	20–31	i.v. glucose	insulin, glucose clearance	100(0) $>$100; $\ll$100(0–10)	
M	65–88	20–31	i.v. arginine	insulin	100(0) 100(30)	Dudland and Ensinck (1977)
M	65–88	20–31	i.v. arginine	glucagon	100(0) 100(30)	
M	42–67	25	i.v. glucose	insulin, glucose clearance	$>$100(0) $>$100; 100(0–10)	Feldman and Plonk (1976)

clearance. In 97 non-obese, 64–98-year-old patients, insulin and glucose levels after OGTT were low or high in parallel, or altered in the opposite sense, and the insulinogenic index (incremental insulin: glucose ratio) varied inversely with triglyceridaemia (Woldow, Shapiro, Cohen and Kollman, 1972).

After 30 years of age, fasting glucagon (Table 4), and after 44, fasting and stimulated PLC (see Section E.1) levels increase (Duckworth and Kitabchi, 1976). Increased release or non-suppressibility of glucagon does not contribute to insulin resistance, but augments post-prandial hyperglycaemia during insulin release (Tiengo, Delprete, Nosadini, Betterle, Garotti and Bersani, 1977; Marco, Hedo and Villanueva, 1977). This may be necessary to meet peripheral glucose demand (Woldow et al., 1972) since arterial walls thicken with age when fractional extraction of glucose and, especially of insulin, may increase (see Hammersten et al., 1977).

(d) Influence of sex difference

In 715 children of 9–12 years of age, mean insulin release after 50 g OGTT was higher in girls (32 µu/ml/min) than in boys (25 µu/ml/min) with significant differences at 1 hr after glucose (Florey, Lowy and Uppal, 1976). Between the ages of 9·5–15·5 the mean fasting insulin of girls was 2 µu/ml higher than that of boys (Ballantyne, White, Stevens, Laurie, Lorimer, Anderson and Morgan, 1977). Women in the 3rd–7th decades of life (or when grouped according to blood sugar 1 hr after standard OGTT) had slightly higher fasting, but significantly higher stimulated insulin levels, than men grouped similarly. Mean 1 hr levels for all women were 70 µu/ml and 55 µu/ml for men after adjustment for adiposity (Florey et al., 1977).

Men on diets 1·5 times the energy content of those given to women have peak blood glucose higher at all meals, but the ratios of insulin: glucose were similar to those of women except in the morning (Haute-Couverture, Slama, Assan and Tchobroutsky, 1974). After diets of equal energy content, young men showed an insulin response equal to women in the morning, but blood glucose levels of women were lower. At midday, men and women had an equal blood glucose response, but insulin levels were less in men and fasting values were maintained between meals (Ahmed, Cannon and Nuttal, 1976).

During fasting for 72 hr, mean plasma glucose of women fell from 4·6 mmol/l to 3·5 and 2·7 mmol at 24 and 36 hr respectively, and remained almost constant thereafter. Corresponding mean insulin levels were 12, 6 and 4 µu/ml. In men, glucose decreased from 4·7 mmol/l to 4·3 and 4 mmol/l after 36 and 72 hr respectively. The mean insulin levels changed in parallel from 13·5–8·0 and 6 µu/ml (Merimee and Tyson, 1977). Relative increase in glucagon and free fatty acids over 72 hr was greater in men (Merimee and Fineberg, 1973). Hence men sustain a higher blood glucose in acute fasting, and insulin levels vary similarly, and after feeding there is less insulin response per unit of energy ingested.

(e) Influence of diet and response to parenteral feeding

Insulin response increases in proportion to the carbohydrate content of a diet (Reaven and Olesky, 1974; see also Pallotta and Kennedy, 1968). However, metabolic glucose clearance is not augmented, and triglyceride levels increase in proportion to insulin levels (Ginsberg et al., 1976b). After maintenance for two weeks on a diet of 80% fat and 20% protein, fasting insulin became undetectable. Peak insulin response to IVGTT and i.v. glucagon decreased by 50% and metabolic glucose clearance by 25%. Arginine hyperglycaemia and insulinaemia were attenuated, and the duration of hypoglycaemia after exogenous insulin was prolonged. Fasting somatotrophin levels were unchanged (Danforth, 1971). Diets of normal, but not of low or high carbohydrate content, maintain a constant pancreatic insulin content (Haist, 1944).

During parenteral feeding, in the absence of sepsis or shock, as glucose infusion is increased from 0–350 mg/min and subsequently to 500 mg/min, insulin levels were increased to 80 and 100 µu/ml. Initial stabilisation of insulin:blood glucose ratio took 4 hr and after cessation of the infusion, plasma insulin and glucose levels fell to their respective nadirs in 30 and 60 min (Sandersen and Dietel, 1974). In parenteral feeding glucose is the most effective nutrient in maintaining normal glucose homeostasis (Geser, Müller-Hess and Felber, 1973/74).

(f) Starvation

Prolonged fasting impairs glucose tolerance more in non-obese than in obese adults. Fasting insulin and glucose are lowered (Merimee and Tyson, 1977) and the early insulin response to stimuli is diminished followed by delayed and exaggerated hyperinsulinaemia (Göschke, 1977) (see also Lenzen, 1975). The insulin content of pancreas is lowered (Hairst, 1944).

(g) Menstrual cycle

During the follicular phase, fasting insulin levels were below 10 µu/ml, exceeding this at ovulation and in the luteal phase. Hyperglycaemia after OGTT also change similarly, but the insulin response was below 50 µu/ml at 1 hr around ovulation, when prolactin, cortisol and somatotrophin levels were high, and above 50 μu/ml during the other phases (Fioretti, Genazzani, Felber, Facchini, Onano, Romagnino, Facchinetti and Piras, 1975).

(h) Oral contraception and sex-hormone replacement

Six to twelve month trials with synthetic oestrogens and/or 17α-acetoxy-progesterones, with the exception of medroxyprogesterone, have been well tolerated whereas nortestosterone derivatives singly or in combination with oestrogens alter glucose tolerance (Beck, 1973) (Table 5). Oestrogens elevate somatotrophin levels, but counteract its insulinogenic action (Meri-mee and Pulkkinen, 1977). Nortestosterone derivatives prevent triglyceri-daemia due to oestrogen (Spellacy, Buhi, Birk and McReary, 1973b) but there is 10–11% incidence of deterioration of glucose tolerance (Beck, 1973). After six years of sequential mestranol and mestranol + chlormadi-none, or eight years of combined mestranol and norethindrone, the incidence of lowered glucose tolerance was 26 and 78% respectively. Exaggerated and persistent elevation of glucose and insulin levels occurred (Spellacy, Buhi, Spellacy, Moses and Goldzieher, 1970a). However, this exaggerated insulin release was suppressed after midday in contrast to obesity (Oakley, Monier and Wynn, 1973). Glucose tolerance of latent diabetics deteriorated within three months with these preparations, whereas chlormadinone given alone was relatively safer (Beck, 1973).

In post menopausal women, oestrogen replacement therapy slightly decreased glucose tolerance (Spellacy, Buhi and Birk, 1972a). Sylvälahti, Erkkola, Punnonen and Rauramo (1976a) found no change in blood glucose response to i.v. insulin after three to seven years therapy. Oophorectomy in the same age group slightly increased fasting insulin levels. Response to i.v. tolbutamide was elevated and persistent. Compensatory adrenal over-activity was postulated (Sylvälahti, Erkkola, Lisalao, Punnonen and Rauramo, 1975). When treated with oestradiol, midday premeal basal insulin level of men increased from 14·6 to 21·0 μu/ml, the peak at 1 hr shifted to 45 min after OGTT, and late levels were high (Haute-Couverture et al., 1974).

(i) Pregnancy

As pregnancy advances from 10–35 weeks, fasting insulin levels, early rate of increase and duration of insulin response are greater and peaks shift to later times during glucose tolerance tests (Lind, Billewicz and Brown, 1973; Kühl, 1975). Normally insulin is increased relative to PLC (Persson and Lunnel, 1975), suggesting that B cell hypertrophy of pregnancy is different from that of obesity (Kuhl, 1976a; Kitabchi, 1977). Fasting glucagon levels increase (Kühl, 1976b), but the insulin:glucagon ratio is unaltered relative to control levels estimated 6–12 weeks *post partum* (Metzger, Unger and Freinkel, 1977; Nitzan, Freinkel, Metzger, Unger, Faloona and Daniel, 1975). In the last trimester, 1 hr after a test meal (Metzger *et al.*, 1977) or OGTT (Nitzan *et al.*, 1975), glucagon is suppressed, increasing this ratio to three times the control value. This is presumably related to the lowered fasting gluconeogenesis and increased anabolism. In the rat, oestradiol blocks hepatic gluconeogenic enzymes, and progesterone, although increasing equally insulin and glucagon release (Mandour, Kissebah and Wynn, 1977; Costrini, Jacobson and Kalkhoff, 1969), favours glycogen deposition (Schillinger, Gerloff, Gerhards and Gunzel, 1974; Naismith and Fears, 1972). When administered together, these hepatic trends are further augmented (Matute and Kalkhoff, 1973). Progesterone also decreases glucocorticoid synthesis and release in rat (Naismith and Fears, 1972).

In the rat, oestrogen or progesterone only slightly augments cell function in response to direct stimuli (Howell, Tyhurst and Green, 1977; Lenzen, 1978b). Therefore, islet cell sensitivity to gastro-intestinal factors may have been increased, since cAMP generation is augmented during pregnancy (see Montague and Howell, 1975).

Fasting insulin levels at 30–40 weeks compared with levels at 6–12 weeks *post partum* are reported high (8 μu/ml cf. 6 μu/ml) (Lind *et al.*, 1973) or low (8–9 μu/ml cf. 11–12 μu/ml) (Metzger *et al.*, 1977; Nitzan *et al.*, 1975). Assay methodology contributes to apparent day to day variation of these levels (Campbell, Benther, Davidson and Sutherland, 1974). The nutritional state of the patients may also vary. After starvation for 48 hr fasting insulin level falls from 12 to 4 μu/ml; a similar fall occurs in 60 hr in the non-gravid control. With restricted gluconeogenesis, control of blood glucose may be altered. Release of chorionic somatomammotrophin (hCS) occurs during starvation. especially in early pregnancy (Tyson, Austin, Farinholt and Fiedler, 1976). In non-pregnant women, hCS has a hyperglycaemic effect without release of free fatty acids (Kalkhoff, Richardson and Beck, 1969). In rats, hCS opposes the insulinogenic effects of gestational hormones (Hager, Georg, Leitner and Beck, 1972). hCS is elevated in diabetic pregnancy (Persson and Lunnel, 1975).

(j) Childbirth

During childbirth, mean insulin levels at induction, cervical dilatation, delivery and 2–24 hr after delivery were 36, 25, 35 and 45–30 μu/ml respectively. With epidural analgesia the former two levels were 64–80% higher than the control without analgesia, and the other levels were higher by 15–18% (Jouppila, 1976).

Table 5

Insulin release in oral contraception.

Type	Dose/day	Duration of treatment (month)	Fasting insulin (μu/ml) Before treatment	After treatment	Test	Effect of treatment on insulin response	References
Oestrogens							
Premarin	1·25 mg	6	15·9	13·7	OGTT	unchanged	Spellacy et al. (1972a)
Mestranol	0·8 mg	6	13·3	11·9	OGTT	slight significant reduction in 1–3 hr insulin	Spellacy et al. (1972a)
Mestranol	0·1 mg	6	11·9	10·5	OGTT	slight significant reduction in 1–3 hr insulin	Spellacy et al. (1975a)
Ethyl oestradiol	0·05 mg	6	16·6	15·9	OGTT	slight non-significant	Spellacy et al. (1973a)
Ethyl oestradiol	0·05 mg	6	18·1	15·9	OGTT	reduction in 1 hr insulin	Spellacy et al. (1973a)
Ethyl oestradiol	0·5 mg	6	12·6	13·9	OGTT	slight increase in insulin	Spellacy et al. (1973a)
17α-Acetoxy progesterones							
Megestrol acetate	0·5 g	6	10·3	11·7	OGTT	slight significant increase in 2–3 hr insulin	Spellacy et al. (1973c)
Chlormadinone acetate	0·5 g	2·5	—	—	OGTT	variable total release probably some patients with increased levels	Beck (1973)
Medroxyprogesterone depot[a]		6	10·1	16·9	OGTT	20–50% progressive increase in 0·5–3 hr insulin	Spellacy et al. (1970b)
Medroxyprogesterone depot[b]		12	9·1	14·4	OGTT	20–93% progressive increase in 0·5–3 hr insulin (62% incidence of impaired glucose tolerance)	Spellacy et al. (1972c)

Nortestosterone derivatives

	Dose						Reference
Ethynodiol diacetate	0·25–0·5 mg	1	29·0	28·2	IVGTT	unchanged	Goldman and Eckerling (1971)
Ethynodiol diacetate	0·5 mg	6	18·0	17·7	IVGTT	unchanged	Goldman (1975)
Ethynodial diacetate	0·25 mg	6	10·6	13·1	OGTT	28% increase 0·5 and 3 hr insulin	
Ethynodiol diacetate	0·25 mg	6	11·2	13·9	OGTT	38% increase 1 and 2 hr insulin	Spellacy et al. (1972b)
Norethidrone	0·35 mg	6	11·4	17·6	OGTT	26–50% progressive increase in 0·5–3 hr insulin	Spellacy et al. (1973a)
							Spellacy et al. (1973b)
Combinations							
Mestranol + norethynodrel (enovid)	0·075 + 5·0 mg	6	21·0	22·8	IVGTT	peak insulin unchanged (15 min) and slight rise at 1 hr; 36% increase in glycaemia (15 min)	Goldman (1975)
Mestranol + norethynodrel (enovid)	0·075 + 5·0 mg	12	11·0	·15·0	OGTT	23–60% progressive increase in 0·25–2 hr insulin	Spellacy et al. (1968)

[a] 4 mg every six months.
[b] 150 mg every three months.

(k) Perinatal changes in insulin levels

During the first stage of labour followed by vaginal birth, response to maternal hyperglycaemia was slow, and insulin increments in fetal scalp vein plasma were low. A faster response correlated with maternal glucose intolerance and high birth weight (Feige, Kunzel and Mitzkat, 1977). Cord blood insulin at birth with Caesarian section correlated with duration of maternal hyperglycaemia, a rapid response occurring with infusion of leucine and glucose rather than of glucose alone (Grasso, Palumbo, Messina, Mazzarino and Reitano, 1976). At birth, the basal insulin level of 15 µu/ml was lowered to 6 µu/ml within 15 min and remained unchanged for two days until blood glucose was restored to 3·0 mmol/l (60 mg/dl) (Sperling et al., 1974). Mean cord plasma unsulin levels after vaginal birth with and without maternal glucose infusion were 8 and 7 µu/ml respectively, and after Caesarian section 8·3 µu/ml. In 10% of neonates, mean cord plasma insulin of 12µu/ml and in 6% mean values of 26 µu/ml or above were suspected to be associated with maternal glucose intolerance or diabetes (Lind et al., 1975).

(l) Exercise

Plasma insulin levels fall by 60–67% in the first minute of exercise and remain low irrespective of oxygen supply (Dahms et al., 1977) and the initial insulin levels (Pruett, 1970). During exercise arteriovenous insulin difference becomes negative indicating mobilisation of endothelially trapped insulin (Dieterle et al., 1973) (see also Section D.4.c).

(m) Psychological stress

After a written examination of less than 1 hr duration, mean insulin levels increased by 200% in young people of both sexes. After longer examinations, insulin levels were raised by 140% and somatotrophin was significantly higher (Sylvälahti, Lammin, Tausta and Pekkarinen, 1976b).

3. Pathological Variation of Insulin Levels

(a) Glucose intolerance and diabetes mellitus

Prospective (Pildes, 1973; Strauss and Hales, 1974; Rosenbloom et al., 1975; Ganda, Soeldner, Gleason, Smith, Kilo and Williamson, 1977) and retrospective studies with potentially or overtly diabetic patients as well as an epidemiological survey of the Pima Indians (Aronoff et al., 1977) indicate a consistent pattern of deterioration of glucose tolerance (GT) (Fujita et al.,

1975; Reaven *et al.*, 1976). At all stages of impaired oral GT there is insufficient early insulin release to maintain glycaemia normal for age at 30–60 min after oral glucose, and the hyperglycaemia increases until appropriate rates of insulin release are attained; glucose then falls to normal peak levels and release declines. If the stimulus sensitivity and/or secretory capacity is greatly deranged, this may not occur during the oral glucose tolerance test (Fujita *et al.*, 1975; Reaven *et al.*, 1976). The deficient early insulin response after i.v. glucose is associated with exaggeration of second phase release to return glycaemia to normal (Fujita *et al.*, 1975; Aronoff *et al.*, 1977). However ineffective in reducing glycaemia, retention of a rapid early release is advantageous and prognosis is good (Fajans, Floyd, Tattersall, Williamson, Pek and Taylor, 1976). Insulin-dependent diabetes (IDM) presents in the juvenile when discrepancy between B cell capacity and increased insulin and glucose requirement is exaggerated by growth (Rosenbloom *et al.*, 1975).

Reduced secretory capacity is associated with genetic and environmental factors (Rosenthal, Goldfine and Siperstein, 1976; Pyke, Theophanides and Tattersall, 1976). Two different broad genotypes have been suggested. The juvenile onset type of diabetes (JOD) correlates with the incidence of histocompatibility antigens which may be of predisposing (Nerup, Platz, Anderson, Christy, Lyngsoa, Poulsen, Kyder, Nielsen, Tomsen and Svejgaard, 1974; Nelson, Pyke, Cudworth, Woodrow and Batchelor, 1975; Cudworth and Woodrow, 1975) or of moderating significance (Baker, Shin, Burgess, Kilo and Miller, 1977; Illeni, Pellegris, Del Guercio, Tarantino, Bursetto, Di Pietro, Clerici, Garotta and Chinmella, 1977; Ganda *et al.*, 1977) in viral insulitis and autoimmune islet cell destruction (Nerup *et al.*, 1974; Botazzo, Florin-Christensen and Doniach, 1974; Del Prete, Betterle, Bersani, Romano and Tiengo, 1976). For example, incidence of HLA-BW15 and B8 antigens correlate with islet cell antibodies (ICA), low residual C-peptide reserve, and high titre of insulin antibodies, while coincidence with B7 moderates these features (Ludvigsson, Safwenberg and Heding, 1977b). Subclinical infections may be responsible for the development of islet cell antibodies (ICA) (Botazzo, Doniach and Pouplard, 1976) and for insulinopaenia and glucose intolerance in prediabetic JOD before overt DM (Pildes, 1973; Ganda *et al.*, 1977) which would usually follow a severe infection (Ganda *et al.*, 1977; Dacou-Voutetakis, Constantinidis, Moschos, Vlachon and Metsaniotis, 1974; John, 1949; Block, Berk, Friedlander, Steiner and Rubenstein, 1973), and B cell destruction (Orci *et al.*, 1975). The ICA persist in 20% of JOD for up to five years, and 19% of "chemical diabetes" (CDM) patients under the age of 35 are also ICA positive (Del Prete, Betterle, Padovan, Erle, Toffol and Bersani, 1977). In "CDM" fasting glucose is normal, insulin levels are high and response to stimuli is very variable in adults (Fajans *et al.*, 1976; Reaven *et al.*, 1976; Tiengo *et al.*, 1977) and in children (Rosenbloom, 1970; Rosenbloom *et al.*, 1975) whose breakfast and lunch insulin levels are low and high respectively (Rayfield, Gorelkin, Curnow and Jahrling, 1976). In borderline glucose intolerance mild hyperinsulinaemia is accompanied by ICA (Tiengo *et al.*, 1977). Twins with early JOD are slightly hyperinsulinaemic especially compared with the offspring of parents with maturity onset (MOD) type of mild diabetes (Gottlieb *et al.*, 1974). These are comparable to stages of the much severer and more rapidly developing experimental viral insulitis in mice (Rayfield *et al.*, 1976; Jansen, Munteferring and Schmidt, 1977).

Incidence of ICA is rare in MOD (Del Prete *et al.*, 1977; Lendrum, Walker, Cudworth, Woodrow and Gamble, 1976) which is usually associated with a family history of diabetes (Fajans *et al.*, 1976). In the offspring of MOD the immediate and 1 hr total insulin responses in IVGTT are reduced by 50–70% and 20–50% respectively, indicating delayed sensitivity or reduced early capacity. Metabolic glucose clearance is less than in offspring of JOD parents (Tan *et al.*, 1977) but less insulin delay occurs after OGTT compared with that of twins with early JOD (Gottlieb *et al.*, 1974), but insulin fails to increase when glucose is above 9·4 mmol/l (170 mg/dl) (Tan *et al.*, 1977) which is the limit of hyperglycaemia detected in epidemiological surveys above which insulin response deteriorates (Savage *et al.*, 1975; Florey *et al.*, 1977). Hence despite improvement of glucose sensitivity after oral stimulation, there remains a limitation to secretory capacity which in addition to reduced glucose sensitivity there is also a limited secretory capacity. This limitation to secretory capacity may underlie the deterioration of glucose tolerance after challenge, e.g. by obesity (Strauss and Hales, 1974) of increased B cell function, in association with family history of DM. In obesity, hyperinsulinaemia is not more effective against hyperglycaemia than in the non-obese mild DM (Fujita *et al.*, 1975). Control of diet (Göschke, Denes, Girard, Collard and Berger, 1974) or weight reduction (Savage *et al.*, 1977) to reduce blood glucose or exercise therapy (Björntorp *et al.*, 1970) to increase glucose utilisation improves fasting and stimulated insulin levels, but the delayed response persists. In MOD, diminished glucose sensitivity may be due to increased α-adrenergic activity (Lebovitz and Feldman, 1973; Baldridge *et al.*, 1975; Feldman *et al.*, 1975; Robertson *et al.*, 1976; Robertson and Chen, 1977) or perhaps increased sensitivity of islets to this activity. There is increased sensitivity to gastro-intestinal (Botha *et al.*, 1976; Deckert, Lauridsen, Madsen and Deckert, 1972) and other stimuli which potentiate the glucose effect (Baker and Jarrett, 1972; Cerasi, 1975a; Palmer *et al.*, 1976; Vinik *et al.*, 1976; Seino *et al.*, 1977).

The relative PLC and CP levels are nearly normal in mild MOD, but not in severe MOD (Table 3, A, B), when CP response is delayed (Faber and

Binder, 1977a) or lost (Rasmussen *et al.*, 1975). Improvement in CP and TIR in JOD can occur temporarily (Table 3, C cf. D, E). This also occurs in mild diabetes or in "CDM" (Rosenbloom, 1970; Floyd *et al.*, 1976) and may be due to lowering of blood glucose (see Section C.9.c), which improves early insulin response (Brunzell *et al.*, 1976), and also improvement of insulin binding at receptor (Olefsky and Reaven, 1976). Insulin resistance may be an aetiological factor in hyperinsulinaemic hyperglycaemic "CDM" and obesity-associated DM (Reaven *et al.*, 1976). It is increased in ketoacidosis when endogenous insulin release is undetectable (Ginsberg, 1977) but improves after therapy (Block *et al.*, 1972; Faber *et al.*, 1975). During sulphonyl-urea therapy, diurnal insulin, glucose and lipid peaks may become very exaggerated necessitating moderation by diet control (Göschke *et al.*, 1974).

(b) *Gestational diabetes and diabetic pregnancy*

In gestational diabetes, GDM, increased early insulin release and hence efficient glucose disposal is lost, resulting in hyperglycaemia and late insulin-aemia (Botella, Llusia, Delolmo, Parache, Catalan, Vila and Alberto, 1973; Kühl, 1975; Gillmer, Beard, Brooke and Oakley, 1975), especially after midday (Phelps *et al.*, 1975), which causes hypertriglyceridaemia (Persson and Lunnel, 1975). In late pregnancy, and 4–6 weeks *post partum*, the insulin: glucagon ratio is higher than normal (2·3 cf. 1·8) (Kühl, 1976b), and the PLC: TIR ratio tends to (see Sections E.1 and E.5) increase (Persson and Lunnel, 1975; Phelps *et al.*, 1975). In Natal subjects of Indian origin, GDM is common with apparent loss of sensitivity to ingested, as compared with parental stimuli (Notelowitz and James, 1974; Notelowitz and James, 1977). Infant mortality is higher when fasting blood glucose regularly exceeds 5·5 mmol/l (100 mg/dl) (Ledward, Paterson and Turner, 1974) and amniotic fluid insulin levels are high (Rebuzzi *et al.*, 1977; see also Section E.1.d). Increased fasting blood glucose, fasting insulin levels (except in the non-obese GDM) (Turner *et al.*, 1977a) and early response to IVGTT (Ledward *et al.*, 1974) correlate with infant birth weight. In the obese and older GDM, vitamin B6 improves glucose tolerance (Spellacy, Buhi and Birk, 1977).

(c) *Neonatal diabetes*

This can present as non-ketotic hyperosmolar hyperglycaemic coma within 30 hr of birth. Over 55 cases have been described. Patients either remained permanently diabetic, or the insulin requirement was transient (Cole, Kim, Zelson and Velasco, 1973; Gentz and Cornblath, 1969; Sodoyez-Goffaux and Sodoyez, 1977).

One case of permanent diabetes with a history of transient neonatal diabetes has been reported (Campbell, Fraser and Duncan, 1978). Most cases of neonatal diabetes are small-for-dates, and 33% are secondary to infections, with one case of mumps. Islet morphology is normal or shows excess, or paucity of islets (Gentz and Cornblath, 1969). In one transient type, diabetes was associated with greatly delayed (2 hr) and about 20 µu/ml response to 22 mmol/l (400 mg/dl) blood glucose. Prompt biphasic response to 7 mmol/l (140 mg/dl) glucose occurred at 7 months of age when insulin replacement was discontinued (Sodoyez-Goffaux and Sodoyez, 1977).

(d) Islet cell tumours and hyperplasia

The literature on insulinomas has been reviewed (Frerichs and Creutzfeldt, 1976; Marks and Samols, 1974; Fajans and Floyd, 1976). Mean daily insulin and glucagon levels are high and blood glucose levels are low (Nelson, Go and Service, 1977). A survey of case reports showed that the serum PLC:TIR (total insulin immunoreactivity) ratio is mostly above normal (20%) reaching 78% (Alsever et al., 1976; Kitabchi, 1977). Six minutes after i.v. tolbutamide, 44% of TIR was PLC (Lindall, Steffes and Wong, 1974). Tumour removal or chemotherapy corrects PLC levels, and abolishes hypoglycaemic symptoms (Alsever et al., 1976). Tumour cells with normal or atypical insulin granules have been identified. The latter are found in islet cell carcinoma and contain low TIR (0·01–0·2 u/g), but PLC released is not always maximal (Creutzfeldt et al., 1973). Tumour and serum insulin, PLC and glucagon levels in adenomas, adenomatosis, nesidioblastosis and carcinomas have been estimated and compared with normal levels (Hayashi et al., 1977).

Insulin (TIR) release is episodic; levels can vary from 118 to 10 µu/ml within 1 hr (Fajans and Floyd, 1976). After overnight fasting the ratio of TIR to the glucose increment over the lowest basal level (usually 1·7 mmol/l or 30 mg/dl) is high in most cases (Frerichs and Creutzfeldt, 1976). After 72 hr this ratio exceeds the upper normal limit of 50 (Fajans and Floyd, 1976). The TIR:blood glucose is also higher than those of lean normal or obese subjects. (Merimee and Tyson, 1977). Porcine insulin (140 µu/ml in serum) failed to suppress CPR (largely PLC) in 11 of 12 cases (Service et al., 1977b). After fish insulin, CP overlapped with the upper normal range and PLC was more discriminatory (Turner and Heding, 1977). Secretion from un-differentiated tumours was not suppressed by adrenaline (Turner et al., 1977b).

Islet cell hyperplasia is extremely rare in the adult, and occurs secondarily to pancreatitis. One such case of insulin-dependent diabetes with hyper-plasia, excess CPR (see Section E.5.d) and impaired glucose tolerance is reported (Sandler, Horwitz, Rubenstein and Kuzuya, 1975).

Nesidioblastosis can present on the first day of life. Fasting insulin levels are high in infants, e.g. 30–63 µu/ml (Heitz et al., 1977), but lower in children

(13–20 μu/ml) (Castro *et al.*, 1973), and are not suppressed in the former, by diazoxide (Heitz *et al.*, 1977; Castro *et al.*, 1973), somatostatin or propranolol (Weber, Pi-Sunyer, Woda, Zimmerman, Derehoncourt, Hardy, Price and Reemtsma, 1976). Tumour insulin concentration varies (30–200 cf. 1·1–1·3 u/g, normal). Lesions range from proliferation of ducts to solitary adenoma, but the relative number of islet cells is unaltered (Heitz *et al.*, 1977). In one case serum PLC:TIR was normal (Hayashi *et al.*, 1977).

(e) Endocrinopathies and hormone replacement (Table 6)

(1) Pituitary dysfunction. In isolated somatotrophin deficiency (ISD), as in panhypopituitarism, and in idiopathic short stature, the insulin response to i.v. arginine is low (Sizonenko, Rabinovitch, Schneider, Pannier, Wolheim and Zahn, 1975). The response to oral stimuli (Larson, Mimoun, Josefberg, Zadic and Doron, 1977) and i.v. glucagon is lower in ISD and corrected by somatotrophin replacement (August and Hung, 1976).

In acromegaly, the dynamics of the insulin to OGTT is normal, but resembles obesity or diabetes if glucose tolerance fails, as when there is a family history of diabetes (Schandellari, Casera, Zaccaria, Sirotich, Zago, Sicolo and Federspil, 1974). Leucine stimulation can be diagnostic in the active phases (Johnson, Karam, Lenn, Grodsky and Forsham, 1973b). Metabolic insulin clearance and insulin distribution in various compartments have been studied (Manecchi, Pilo, Citti and Navalesi, 1977). Prolactin releasing tumours were associated with hyperinsulinaemia after OGTT (Table 6).

(2) Disorders of the adrenal cortex. Treatment of primary adrenal insufficiency increases sensitivity to oral stimulation and gastro-intestinal factors (Serrano-Rios, Hawkins, Escobar, Mato, Larrodera, de Oya and Rodriguez-Minon, 1974). In hyperactivity of the adrenal cortex with or without obesity, the response is delayed and diabetic in dynamics (Duran, Maranon and Romano, 1974; Karam, Grodsky and Forsham, 1965).

In primary aldosteronism, insulin levels are low, which is attributed to potassium depletion and hypokalaemia, and 50% of the patients have lowered glucose tolerance (Conn, 1965). The findings are similar in secondary aldosteronism (Helge and Merken, 1968).

(3) Chromaffin and argentaffin cell tumours. In phaeochromocytoma, insulinopaenia accompanies raised serum catecholamine levels. In the carcinoid syndrome, reduction in 5-hydroxy indole acetic acid excretion correlates with improved glucose tolerance. The adrenal medulla, or splanchnic innervation, may exert slight suppressive control of basal insulin levels (Table 6).

(4) Disorders of the thyroid. In adult myxoedema, blood glucose depression

Table 6

Insulin release in different endocrinopathies.

Condition	Test	Fasting insulin (% control)	Peak insulin response (% control)	References
Pituitary tumours				
Somatotrophin (active)	oral glucose	200–600	≥200–600	Karam et al. (1965)
Somatotrophin (active)	oral leucine	—	≥200	Scandellari et al. (1974)
Somatotrophin (inactive)	oral glucose	≥100	200	Johnson et al. (1973b)
Prolactin (active)	oral glucose	100	150–200	Karam et al. (1965)
Prolactin (bromocriptine)	oral glucose	100	100	Landgraf et al. (1977)
Prolactin (residual?)	oral glucose	300	300	Landgraf et al. (1977)
Prolactin (residual?)	i.v. tolbutamide	—	200	Costin et al. (1977)
Craniopharyngioma (post-op)	oral glucose	100	120	Costin et al. (1976)
Craniopharyngioma (post-op)	i.v. tolbutamide	—	100	Costin et al. (1976)
Adrenocortical insufficiency				
Untreated	oral glucose	100	67	Serrano-Rios et al. (1974)
Treated	oral glucose	100	130	Serrano-Rios et al. (1974)
Untreated	pancreozymin	<100	80	Hawkins-Carranza et al. (1976)
Treated	pancreozymin	100	130	Hawkins-Carranza et al. (1976)
Untreated	secretion	100	100	Hawkins-Carranza et al. (1976)
Treated	secretion	100	100	Hawkins-Carranza et al. (1976)
Adrenomedullary insufficiency				
Adrenolectomised (on cortisone)	i.v. glucose	133	108–130 (90–100% total response; hence, augmented 1st phase)	Brodows et al. (1974)
Cervical transection	i.v. glucose	126	100 (116–120% total response)	Brodows et al. (1974)
Phaechromocytoma				
Phaechromocytoma (pre-op)	oral glucose	60 (of post-treatment)	50 (of post-treatment)	Passwell et al. (1977)
Phaechromocytoma (post-op)	oral glucose	100	100	Passwell et al. (1977)
Carcinoid tumours	oral glucose	50–100 (of post-treatment)	33–50 (of post-treatment)	Feldman et al. (1972)
Carcinoid tumours (after streptozotocin)	oral glucose	50–100 (of post-treatment)	33–50 (of post-treatment)	Feldman et al. (1972)

Condition	Test			Reference
Hypothyroidism	i.v. arginine	100	135–161	Savage et al. (1977)
Hypothyroidism	i.v. arginine	128	500	Andreani et al. (1974)
Hypothyroidism	oral glucose	100	153	Andreani et al. (1974)
Hypothyroidism (off therapy)	oral glucose	—	220 (delayed)	Hofeldt et al. (1974)
Hypothyroidism (on therapy)	oral glucose	—	180	Hofeldt et al. (1974)
Hypothyroidism (after hyperthyroidism)	i.v. glucose	100 (of euthyroid)		Shah and Cerchio (1973)
Euthyroid (after hyperthyroidism)	i.v. glucose	100	100	Shah and Cerchio (1973)
Hyperthyroidism	i.v. arginine	100	30 (single peak)	Seino et al. (1974)
Hyperthyroidism	i.v. arginine	100	60, 40 (1st peak, 2nd peak)	Imura et al. (1976)
Hypothyroidism	i.v. arginine + glucose	100	72, 55	Imura et al. (1976)
Hyperthyroidism	i.v. arginine + xylitol	100	45, 70	Imura et al. (1976)
Hyperthyroidism	i.v. arginine + theophylline	100	67, 47	Imura et al. (1976)
Hyperthyroidism	i.v. arginine	—	43	Cavagnini et al. (1974)
Hyperthyroidism	oral glucose	—	70	Cavagnini et al. (1974)
Hyperthyroidism	oral glucose	150	130	Andersen et al. (1977)
Hyperthyroidism (pre-treatment)	oral glucose	187	166	Andersen et al. (1977)
Hyperthyroidism (post-treatment)	i.v. glucose	100	130	Andersen et al. (1977)
Hyperthyroidism (pre-treatment)	i.v. glucose	130	145	Andersen et al. (1977)
Hyperthyroidism (post-treatment)	i.v. tolbutamide	140	200	Andersen et al. (1977)
Hyperthyroidism (pre-treatment)	i.v. tolbutamide	180	200	Andersen et al. (1977)
Hypoparathyroidism				
Hypoparathyroidism (before vit. D)	oral glucose	75	50 (delayed)	Gedik and Zileli (1977)
Hypoparathyroidism (before vit. D)	oral glucose + i.v. theophylline	177	83 (normal)	Gedik and Zileli (1977)
Hypoparathyroidism (after vit. D)	oral glucose + i.v. theophylline	107	102 (delayed)	Gedik and Zileli (1977)

after i.v. insulin can be less than normal, and the early insulin response to IVGTT and OGTT is decreased, while the late phase is increased (Brauman and Corvilain, 1968; Andreani *et al.*, 1974), as shown in experimental hypothyroidism (Lenzen, Joost and Hasselblatt, 1976a). It is further exaggerated if there is coincidence of mild diabetes (Andreani *et al.*, 1974). In hyperthyroidism, peripheral insulin sensitivity is increased (Shima *et al.*, 1976; Andersen, Friis and Ottesen, 1977). The apparent inconsistency in B cell response to stimuli in hyperthyroidism (see Table 6; Andersen *et al.*, 1977) may be due to the severity of the disease. In experimental hyperthyroidism, B cell response to i.v. stimuli decreases with increasing doses of thyroid hormones (Lenzen, 1978c) and gradual B cell atrophy occurs (see Section D.2). Early during treatment with low doses, the first phase of insulin release may become prominent, especially during potentiation of the glucose effect (Lenzen *et al.*, 1975), which may explain the occasional observation of increased early insulin response in human hyperthyroidism. Increased early response to OGTT may also be due to rapid absorption of glucose from the gut (Andersen *et al.*, 1977) before the onset of extensive B cell atrophy. Decreased insulin levels may be partly due to increased insulin destruction (Orsetti *et al.*, 1974) and increased catecholamine inhibition of release has also been postulated (Cavagnini *et al.*, 1974).

(5) *Disorders of the parathyroid.* In hypoparathyroidism (Table 6) and hyperparathyroidism (Yasuda, Harukawa, Okuyama, Kikuchi and Yoshinaga, 1975), insulin response to OGTT parallels serum calcium levels. In secondary hyperparathyroidism, lack of factors other than calcium, e.g. phosphate, may reduce B cell function (Yasuda *et al.*, 1975).

(*f*) *Obesity*

The causes of glucose intolerance in obesity are not understood. Hyperinsulinaemia is correlated with adiposity (Deschamp *et al.*, 1977) and may be accompanied by exaggerated GIP release (Creutzfeldt *et al.*, 1978). Maintenance of near normal blood glucose during OGTT (Santiago *et al.*, 1977; Nolan *et al.*, 1973) or IVGTT (Karam *et al.*, 1965; Santiago *et al.*, 1977) depends on rapid insulin release at 2–3 times the normal throughout the test. The mean peak insulin response to 4·4 mmol/l (85 mg/dl) and 11·1 mmol/l (200 mg/dl) plasma glucose is about 100 and 1220 μu/ml respectively, compared with 80 and 490 μu/ml in suitable control subjects (Karam, Grodsky, Ching, Schmid, Burrill and Forsham, 1974). The insulin response to arginine is exaggerated, while glucagon and somatotrophin release are lowered (Fallucca, Menzinger, Gambardella, Tamburrano and Andreani, 1975; Santiago *et al.*, 1977). The afternoon suppression of insulin release (see Section D.3) is less marked (Santiago *et al.*, 1977). In obese children, peaks after the midday meal are exaggerated while the normal insulinaemia after breakfast is absent (Di Natale, Deretta, Rossi, Carlashi, Caccamo, Del Guarcio and Chiamello, 1973). In adults, daily insulin:glucagon ratio and peak insulin values between and during meals are twice the normal; the times of nadir are delayed by at least 1 hr (Santiago et al., 1977). Low energy diets reduce insulin peaks by a third and the diurnal insulin rhythm shifts forward (Reinberg et al., 1974). Urinary insulin excretion is greatly increased and falls during starvation, but increases upon resuming food ingestion (Aun et al., 1975).

Prolonged fasting in obese subjects causes less alteration of insulin response to oral glucose than in the lean (Göschke, 1977) but before (Santiago et al., 1977) and after fasting (Göschke, 1977) metabolic clearance of glucose is less than normal. Reduced insulin sensitivity in tissue biopsies has been reported in obesity (Vondra, Rath, Bass, Slabochova, Teisinger and Vitek, 1977; Burns, Terry, Langley and Robison, 1977; Nestel, Austin and Foxman, 1969; see also Section C.5.c). During 72 hrs of fasting, insulin and blood glucose levels do not fall below 10 µu/ml and 3·0 mmol/l (50 mg/dl) respectively. Sex-dependent differences in insulin levels (Merimee and Tyson, 1977) and age dependent blood glucose differences are abolished by obesity, but total insulin response to stimuli is significantly decreased after the second decade of life (Nolan et al., 1973). The insulin response is augmented in obese children (Deschamp et al., 1977), but unlike the young adult, blood glucose response to exogenous insulin and insulin disappearance times are unaltered (Giron and Lestradet, 1973). The concentration of insulin receptors may also not be reduced (see Section D.5).

(g) Malnutrition

If in infants serum albumin concentration is above 35 g/l, plasma insulin is above the normal for age (e.g. 6–22 µu/ml at 2 months, and 20–32 µu/ml at 12–16 months). When albumin levels fall below 30 g/l, insulin levels fall, cortisol levels rise and glucose tolerance decreases. At 22 g/l, somatotrophin levels rise and mark the development of Kwashiorker (Lunn et al., 1973). The PLC:TIR ratio before (0–41%) and after (4–30%) treatment is very variable, and is not related to plasma insulin or the insulinogenic index (Becker, Murray, Hanson and Pimstone, 1973). Early potassium replacement (Mann, Becker, Pimstone and Hansen, 1975) or alanine infusion (Becker, Pimstone, Kronheim and Weinkove, 1975) improves the insulin response, but not glucose tolerance. Metabolic glucose clearance returns to normal with a peak insulin response of 20–60 µu/ml to IVGTT when the weight starts to increase (Haist, 1944). Good insulin responders usually have high fasting insulin levels (Graham et al., 1976).

(h) *Anorexia nervosa*

In anorexia nervosa there is a diminished fasting insulin level and diminished and delayed response to oral glucose (Harrower, Yap, Nairn, Walton, Strong and Craig, 1977) and to i.v. arginine and OGTT (Sizonenko et al., 1975).

(i) *Pancreatitis and gastro-intestinal influences on insulin release*

Glucose sensitivity of insulin release in chronic pancreatitis with normal or nearly normal glucose tolerance was not altered, but the maximal response to glucose with and without theophylline was 45% of the normal control, and returned to normal by pancreozymin perhaps due to gastro-intestinal peptide (GIP) contamination. Fasting insulin was raised, with slight glucose intolerance (Botha et al., 1976). The insulin response to a standard meal decreased in proportion to the severity of exocrine insufficiency, leading to impaired glucose tolerance (Ebert et al., 1976).

In hypergastrinaemic disorders uncomplicated by previous surgery, insulin response to OGTT is normal or high, and in hypogastrinaemic conditions normal or low (Table 7). In coeliac disease, low response is not due to diminished hyperglycaemia response, but GIP levels are low. However, GIP status alone does not explain the insulin response. Glucagon release was not augmented during OGTT in patients with duodenal ulcer (Table 7).

(j) *Kidney disease*

In chronic renal failure (CRF), acute renal failure, and during recovery, the Fanconi syndrome, or cadmium nephropathy, but not during primary glomerular disease or the nephrotic syndrome, urinary insulin loss in increased (Amatruda et al., 1975). In CRF, the plasma half life of insulin is increased by 150%. More than 50% of uraemic patients have lowered metabolic glucose clearance, which may be due to secondary hyperparathyroidism, azotaemia, potassium depletion or toxaemia. However, early insulin response to IVGTT (Reaven et al., 1974), OGTT or i.v. arginine were normal, but the peak periods were prolonged. Elevated CPR (see Section E.1) after 120 min suggested reduced degradation of insulin due to renal damage (Jaspan, Mako, Kuzuya, Blix, Horwitz and Rubenstein, 1977).

(k) *Liver disease*

In chronic and viral hepatitis, and obstructive jaundice, the mean insulin response 1 hr after oral glucose was 133, 200 and 220% of the normal control respectively, and the insulinogenic index in the latter two conditions was significantly increased (Gündoğdu, Bağriaçik, Alemdaroğlu, Basri, Biyal and Korugan, 1977).

Table 7

Insulin release in gastro-intestinal disorders.

Disorder	Fasting values gastrinaemia (basal)	Peak response after oral or i.v. glucose as % of control				References
		Oral glucose Insulin	GIP	i.v. glucose Insulin	i.v. tolbutamide Insulin	
Pernicious anaemia	hyper	135	—	>100	—	Rehfeld (1976)
Zollinger-Ellison syndrome	hyper	≫100	—	—	—	Rehfeld (1976)
Gastrinoma	hyper	100	—	≪100	—	Massara (1974)
Duodenal ulcer	hyper	>100	—	—	—	Lager et al. (1976)
Pernicious anaemia	hypo	100	17	40	>100	Rehfeld (1976)
Coeliac disease	hypo	≪100	—	—	—	Creutzfeldt et al. (1976)
Post Whipple operation	hypo	>100 (faster)	—	<100 (delayed)	—	Rehfeld et al. (1975)
Post Whipple operation	hypo	67 (delayed)	450	—	—	Creuzfeldt et al. (1976)
Chronic pancreatitis	hypo	47	150	—	—	Creuzfeldt et al. (1976)

In confirmed cirrhosis, glucose tolerance (GT), said to be normal, was associated with faster early release than control, and impairment was associated with a late shift of hyperinsulinaemia (Megyesi, Samols and Marks, 1967) and increased relative PLC release (Toccafondi, Rotella, Tanini and Arcangeli, 1977). The insulinogenic index was diabetic after IVGTT (Greco, Ghirlanda, Patrono, Fedeli and Mann, 1974). Insulin release was lowered when there was hepatic decompensation (Podolsky and Burrows, 1977) and potassium replacement improved the response to glucose (Podolsky, Zimmerman, Burrows, Cardarelli and Pattavina, 1973). Glucagon and somatotrophin were raised unexpectedly after IVGTT (Greco et al., 1974; Podolsky et al., 1973). Portacaval shunting raises peripheral insulin levels by 67% (Schurberg, Resnick, Ros, Baum and Pallotta, 1977).

In haemochromatosis, iron pigment is selectively deposited in B cells (Hartroft, 1956) and leads to diabetes, probably in relation to a positive family history (Dymock, Cassar, Pyke, Oakley and Williams, 1972), when it is typical of the maturity onset type (Passa, Rousselei, Gauville and Canivet, 1977). Long term repeated transfusion therapy in thalassaemia major leads to hyperinsulinaemia during fasting and after OGTT, and thereby maintenance of normal glucose levels.

(l) Reactive hypoglycaemia

These conditions, which have been thoroughly reviewed (Permutt, 1976), are predominantly idiopathic (62%), but also associate with diabetes (24%) and alimentary (7%) and hormonal disorders (7%) (Hofeldt et al., 1974) and also with alcohol and glucose intake (Marks and Alberti, 1976). Compared with appropriate controls, after oral glucose there was consistent delayed hyperinsulinaemia at 18–72 min instead of the normal 8–26 min after the glucose peak; this is inappropriate in relation to blood glucose, which became subnormal at 3–4 hr.

(m) Lipid disorders and atherosclerosis

Insulin release during OGTT in Type II and Type IV lipidaemias is increased by 60 and 130% respectively (Ballantyne et al., 1977); type IV is associated with an increased incidence (73 cf. 10% in normal population) of impaired glucose tolerance (GT) in those patients who had a myocardial infarct two years previously (Enger and Rutland, 1973). Insulin levels correlate with very low density lipoprotein levels and serum triglycerides (TG) (Olefksy, Farquhar and Reaven, 1974). A linear relationship: insulinogenic index = 0·6 TG + 0·25 can be calculated from the data in Table 8 which persists as long as there is an adequate insulin response to maintain normal glucose levels after OGTT.

Table 8

Glucose tolerance in triglyceridaemia and cardiovascular disease. Response 0 and 1 + 2 hr after oral glucose. (From Sorgé, Schwartz-kopf and Neuhans, 1976.)

Groups	\[Normal\] TG mg/dl (mmol/l) 0	Insulin (μu/ml) 0	Insulin 1 + 2	Blood glucose mg/dl (mmol/l) 0	Blood glucose 1 + 2	II[b] 1 + 2	\[Impaired\] TG mg/dl (mmol/l) 0	Insulin (μu/ml) 0	Insulin 1 + 2	Blood glucose mg/dl (mmol/l) 0	Blood glucose 1 + 2	II[b] 1 + 2
Control	97	15–18	145	77	198	0·78	143	20	243	85	321	0·78
Lean	107	15–18		4·3	11·0		158			4·7	18	
MI, PVD[a]	157	15–18	260	80	217	1·16	200	18·5	377	99	395	1·03
Lean	173			4·4	12·2		222			5·5	22	
Control	160	24	252	79	212	1·18	206	27	342	89	358	0·97
Obese	176			4·4	12·1		231			5·0	19·9	
MI, PVD[a]	174·5	28	317	86	217	1·49	283	32·5	480	98	405	1·27
Obese	193			4·8	12·1		312			5·5	22·5	

[a] MI = myocardial infarction; PVD = peripheral vascular disease. The values for MI and PVD groups being very close have been combined.

[b] II = insulinogen index, i.e. insulin response: glucose response.

When GT is impaired because of the persistence of hyperglycaemia despite delayed hyperinsulinaemia, the insulinogenic index is low, and TG increases disproportionately (Table 8; see also Marukama, Ohneda, Tadaki, Ohtsuki, Yaube, Abe and Yamagata, 1975). In vascular disease (atherosclerosis), fractional uptake of insulin by the vascular endothelium is increased above that of glucose (Hammersten *et al.*, 1977) perhaps aggravating early atherosclerosis (Stout, 1977); therefore the extra insulin may be necessary to maintain normal peripheral function (see Bylund *et al.*, 1976).

In lipodystrophy, fasting free fatty acid levels are increased, and only increased insulin response after OGTT can suppress these. In partial lipodystrophy type V, and in complete lipodystrophy Type IV lipoproteinaemias can occur (Boucher, Cohen, Frenkel, Maron and Broadley, 1973) and are associated with exaggerated insulinaemia with virtual absence of PLC (Sövik, Oseid and Oyasreten, 1973) until B cell decompensation occurs in the latter part of the second decade. Between eight and ten years of age, before the decline of GT occurs, fasting insulin is 25–125 μu/ml, and 1000–2000 μu/ml peak response to tolbutamide and IVGTT rapidly restores to normal the glycaemia as high as 20 mmol/l (Oseid, 1973).

(n) Angina and acute myocardial infarction (MI)

Stress of comparable severity may occur in angina or MI with normal or high (7–14 mmol/l, 120–240 mg/dl) blood glucose, with insulin levels below or above 30 μu/ml (Prakash and Chhablani, 1974). Within 12 hr of the onset of precordial pain insulin levels above 30 μu/ml were associated with higher metabolic glucose clearance, less plasma catecholamines and fat mobilisation, and patients with lower insulin levels maintained low metabolic glucose clearance at follow-up (Christensen and Videback, 1974). In the young, obese and hyperinsulinaemic patients insulin response to OGTT fell for one day after MI, but in the older, leaner patients with normal insulin levels the insulin response was slightly higher during the first week after MI compared with the response three weeks after MI; the insulin:glucose ratio was about 30% of that observed in the younger group throughout the three weeks after MI. Despite these differences in the insulin response urinary catecholamine increases were similar in both groups of patients, who were also similarly hyperglycaemic compared with normal control subjects given the OGTT (Kurt, Genton, Chidsey, Bech and Sussman, 1973).

(o) Injury

In rats up to 24 hr after 20% total body surface (TBS) burns, blood glucose is doubled and insulin response to various stimuli lowered by 80%. After 24 hr to six days fasting or stimulated insulinaemia exceeds the control levels, but growth rate was low for three weeks (Turinsky, Saba, Scovill and Chestnut, 1977). In humans, 30 hr after a 40–75 % TBS burn, insulin, glucagon and plasma glucose is 200, 1000 and 150% of the controls respectively with elevated free fatty acids and triglyceride levels (Shuck, Eaton, Shuck, Wachtel and Schaden, 1977). With cardiac arrest and resuscitation, insulin release was lowered (Wilmore, Long, Mason, Skreen and Pruitt, 1974). Six–16 days after injury patients were hypermetabolic with raised basal (150%) and stimulated (200%) insulin levels which returned to normal when nitrogen balance became positive at wound closure (Wilmore, Mason and Pruitt, 1976; Wilmore et al., 1974). During burn trauma, urinary insulin clearance can be doubled (Meguid, Ann and Soeldner, 1976).

(p) Toxic shock

Bacterial toxins cause high basal but low stimulated insulin levels (see D.4.h) and depressed hepatic neoglucogenesis and tendency to hypoglycaemia (Hinshaw et al., 1974). After burns with sepsis due to Gram negative organisms blood glucose is variable (3·6–15·6 mmol/l) and glucose utilisation and insulinogenic index remain low even after treatment (Wilmore, 1976).

(q) Surgery

In surgery general anaesthesia but not epidural analgesia is associated with hyperglycaemia, and surgical incision is invariably accompanied by lowered insulin release (Brandt et al., 1977). During general anaesthesia fasting insulin levels remain unaltered or are lowered (see Section D.4.e). In rats, the effect of halothane on insulin and blood glucose levels depends on the nutritional state (Aynsley-Green et al., 1973). In man, thiopental can cause slight glucose intolerance without altering insulin levels (Kaniaris, Katsilambros, Castanas and Theophanidis, 1975). During, and post surgery, the insulin response to stimuli is lowered in inverse proportion to catecholamine release. Post-surgery fasting insulin levels are high for up to three days (Wright et al., 1974; Giddings et al., 1976). Intravenous immunosuppressive drugs contribute to the postoperative hyperinsulinaemia of the renal transplant patients (Buckingham, Service, Palumbo, Aguilo, Woods and Zincke, 1976).

(r) Hypovolaemic shock

Haemorrhage is associated with increased insulin levels despite raised catecholamines (Skillman et al., 1971). In animals in circulatory shock there is an early tendency to maintain high blood glucose levels with a negative arteriovenous difference of insulin levels (see Section D.4.d) despite diminished pancreatic blood flow and net insulin release (Hiebert, McCormick and Egdahl, 1971; Bor, 1975)

(s) Erythroblastosis foetalis

High (32 µu/ml) and low (24 µu/ml) fasting insulin levels, and similarly high and low responses to stimuli, correlate directly with haemoglobin concentration and inversely with bilirubin levels within 3 hr of birth. The islets are hyperplastic without eosinophilia, unlike in the infants of diabetic mothers (Molsted-Pedersen, Trantner and Jorgensen, 1973).

(t) Exchange transfusion

Exchange transfusion is associated with hypoinsulinaemia (Skillman et al., 1971; Cser and Milner, 1975). In the infant, transfusion via the umbilical artery causes greater stress and lower insulin levels than via the vein (Cser and Milner, 1975), perhaps because of a different degree of involvement of the carotid baroreceptors (Järhult and Holst, 1977).

(u) Various hereditary and other disorders which influence insulin release

Investigation of B cell function and glucose tolerance in inherited or congenital disorders is scant and incomplete, since not only are the patients rare, but also the interest is recent. Examples cited here indicate that these investigations are rewarding.

In hyperproinsulinaemia, in a single kindred of three generations, 80–90% of insulin, both during fasting (38 µu/ml cf. 1–18 µu/ml control) and stimulation, consisted of PLC with normoglycaemia and normal metabolic glucose clearance (Gabbay et al., 1976). In homocystinuria there is elevation of serum methionine levels with a raised fasting insulin level (20–45 µu/ml cf. 5–25 µu/ml control) and high-normal, or excessive response to OGTT (Holmgren, Falkmer and Hambraelis, 1973). In familial dysautonomia, fasting insulin levels and the response to IVGTT are reduced by 18 and 60% respectively (Cole, 1973a). In Turner's syndrome, fasting levels are normal, but response to IVGTT is delayed. Islet hyperplasia can occur, and an increased incidence of diabetes does not correlate with the family history (Lindsten, Cerasi, Luft and Hultquist, 1967). In Kleinefelter's syndrome, four of six patients had severely insulinopaenic diabetes (Serrano-Rios, Hawkins, Escobar, Mato, Larrodera and Rodriguez-Miñon, 1973). Most cystic fibrosis patients have low normal fasting insulin and halved insulin response to IVGTT, i.v. arginine or glucagon (Stahl, Girar, Rachtshausen, Nars and Zappinger, 1974; Redmund, Buchanan and Timble, 1977). In psoriasis, there is reduced early and persistent late insulinaemia after OGTT, irrespective of a family history of diabetes (Jucci, Vignini, Pelfini, Criffo and Fratino, 1977). In Down's syndrome, the insulin response was either very low or low normal; in the lean patients, insulin response to glucose was normal, but sub-normal after arginine, except in the obese patients when it was exaggerated (Raitini, Lifschitz, Trias and Sigman, 1974).

(v) Neuropathies and myopathies

The incidence of diabetes is high in hereditary ataxias, e.g. telangiectasia, amyotropic lateral sclerosis, muscular dystrophy, late onset myopathy, myotonic dystrophy, and chronic peripheral neuropathy (see Schubotz, Hausmann, Kaffarnik, Zehner and Oepen, 1976). In Friedrich's ataxia, 60% of patients had lowered glucose tolerance (GT) and 20% of the patients had overt diabetes with fasting insulin levels of 2 $\mu u/ml$ or less, and a flat or delayed insulin response to OGTT (Schapcott, Melancon, Butterworth, Khoury, Colk, Breton, Geoffrey, Lemleux and Barbeau, 1976). Lowered GT occurs with a normal fasting insulin level, but there was a delayed release after OGTT in 32% of patients with Huntingdon's chorea (Schubotz et al., 1976). In myotonic dystrophy, the fasting insulin level was three times the normal after OGTT; there was severe hypoglycaemia with insulin levels up to 1000 $\mu u/ml$ in 30 min (Huff, Horton and Lebovitz, 1967; Tewaarwerk and Hudson, 1977). The insulin response to IVGTT was twice normal in malignant hyperpyrexia (Denborough, Warne, Mould, Tse and Martin, 1974).

CONCLUSION

An attempt has been made in this section to emphasise briefly the necessity of good control and standardisation, and the limitations to the interpretation of the B cell function tests. Although investigation of endocrine pancreatic function is at its early stages, its importance in the minute by minute regulation of blood nutrient levels emerges from the data in Sections C, D and F. However, the control of this function, as well as that of the biological effects of islet hormones, is complicated, and further investigations, especially in different pathological conditions, is necessary for the better understanding of the underlying mechanisms. For example, endocrinological control of insulin release may involve changes in the B cell sensitivity to gastro-intestinal factors, or in the rates of nutrient absorption and release of these factors, together with alteration in the sensitivity of target cells to islet hormones. Recently expanding research in endocrinopathies and the initial findings in various conditions of stress and hereditary disorders are indeed promising. Studies in drug abuse, e.g. heroin addiction (Ghodse, 1977) or suicidal phenothiazine poisoning and alcoholism (Dobrzanski and Pieschl, 1976) with highly exaggerated changes of islet cell function, also merit continuation.

REFERENCES

Äärimaa, M., Slatis, P., Haapaniemi, L. and Jeglinsky, B. (1974). *Ann. Surg.* **179**, 926.
Ahmed, M., Cannon, M. C. and Nuttall, K. W. (1976). *Diabetologia*, **12**, 61.
Akhtar, M. I., Verspohl, E., Hegner, D. and Ammon, H. P. T. (1977). *Diabetes*, **26**, 857.
Albano, J. D. M., Ekins, R. P., Martiz, G. and Turner, R. G. (1972). *Acta endocr., Copnh.* **70**, 487.
Albert, S., Chyn, R., Goldford, M. and Permutt, M. A. (1977) *Diabetes*, **26**, (Suppl. 1), 378A.
Alsever, R. N., Stjernholm, M. R., Sussman, K. E., Mako, M. E. and Rubenstein, A. H. (1976), *Diabetologia*, **12**, 527.
Altzuler, N., Moran, E. and Hampshire, J. (1977). *Diabetes*, **26** (Suppl. 1), 386A.
Amatruda, J. M., Livingstone, J. N. and Lockwood, D. H. (1975). *Science*, **188**, 264.
Andersen, O. O. (1972). *Acta endocr., Copnh.* **71**, 126.
Andersen, O. O. (1976). *Acta endocr., Copnh.* **83** (Suppl. 205), 231.
Andersen, O. O., Friis, Th. and Ottesen, B. (1977). *Acta endocr., Copnh.* **84**, 576.
Andreani, D., Fallucca, F., Tamburranno, G., Iavicoli, M. and Menzinger, G. (1974). *Diabetologia*, **10**, 7.
Antoniades, H. N. and Simon, J. D. (1972). *Diabetes*, **21**, 930.
Antoniades, H. N., Simon, J. D. and Stathakos, D. (1973). *Biochem. Biophys. res. Commun.* **53**, 182.
Arnman, K., Carlström, S. and Thorell, J. I. (1975) *Horm. metab. Res.* **7**, 437.
Arnold, R., Deutsche, U., Frerichs, H. and Creutzfeldt, W. (1972). *Diabetologia*, **8**, 250.
Aronoff, S. L., Bennett, P. H., Gordon, P., Rushforth, N. and Miller, M. (1977). *Diabetes*, **26**, 827.
Arquilla, E. R., Miles, P. V. and Morris, J. W. (1972). *In* "Handbook of Physiology", (D. F. Steiner, N. Freinkel, eds), Vol. 1, p. 159. Williams and Wilkins, Baltimore.
Ashcroft, S. J. H. (1976). *In* "Polypeptide Hormones· Molecular and Cellular Aspects", p. 117. Ciba Foundation Symposium 41 (New Series). Excerpta Medica, Amsterdam.
Ashcroft, S. J. H., Bassett, J. M. and Randle, P. J. (1972). *Diabetes*, **21** (Suppl, 2), 538.
Ashcroft, S. J. H., Chatra, L., Weerasinghe, C. and Randle, P. J. (1973). *Biochem. J.* **132**, 223.
Asplin, C. M., Goldie, D. J. and Hartog, M. (1977). *Clin. chim. Acta*, **75**, 393.
Asplin, C. M. and Hartog, M. (1977). *Diabetologia*, **13**, 475.
Atkins, T. and Matty, A. J. (1970). *In* "Diabetes" (R. R. Rodriguez, F. J. G. Ebling, I. Henderson and R. Assan, eds), p. 45. Proc. VII Cong. Int. Diabetes Federation. Excerpta Medica, Amsterdam
Attwater, E. and Meissner, H. P. (1975). *J. Physiol.* **247**, 56.
August, G. P. and Hung, W. (1976). *J. clin. Endocr. Metab.* **43**, 1029.
Aun, F., Meguid, M. M., Soeldner, J. S. and Stolf, N. A. (1975). *Postgrad. med. J.* **51**, 622.
Avruch, J., Leone, G. R. and Martin, D. B. (1976). *J. biol. Chem.* **352**, 1735.
Aynsley-Green, A. and Alberti, K. G. M. M. (1974). *Horm. metab. Res.* **6**, 115.

Aynsley-Green, A., Biebuyck, J. F. and Alberti, K. G. M. M. (1973). *Diabetologia*, **9**, 274.

Baker, B., Shin, D. H., Burgess, D., Kilo, G. and Miller, W. V. (1977). *Diabetes*, **26**, 997.

Baker, I. A. and Jarrett, R. J. (1972). *Lancet*, ii, 945.

Baker, P. G. B. and Mottram, R. F. (1973). *Clin. Sci.* **44**, 479.

Balasse, E. and Ooms, H. A. (1968). *Diabetologia*, **3**, 488.

Balasse, E. and Ooms, H. A. (1973). *Diabetologia*, **9**, 145.

Baldridge, J. A., Quickel, K. E., Feldman, J. M. and Lebovitz, H. E. (1975). *Diabetes*, **23**, 21.

Ballantyne, D., White, C., Stevens, E. A., Laurie, T. D. V., Lorimer, A. R., Manderson, N. G. and Morgan, H. G. (1977). *Clin. chim. Acta*, **78**. 323.

Banting, F. G. and Best, C. H. (1921–1922). *J. Lab. clin. Med.* **7**, 251.

Banting, F. G., Best, C. H., Collip, J. B., MacLeod, J. J. R. and Noble, E. C. (1922). *Am. J. Physiol.* **62**, 162.

Bar, R. S., Gorden, P., Roth, J., Kahn, C. R. and De Meyts, P. (1976). *J. clin. Invest.* **58**, 1123.

Barnes, A. J., Bloom, S. R., Mashiter, K., Alberti, K. G. M. M., Smyth, P. and Turner, D. (1977). *Diabetologia*, **13**, 71.

Barnes, A. J., Garbian, K. J. T., Crowley, M. T. and Bloom, A. (1974). *Lancet*, ii, 68.

Basabe, J. C., Farina, J. M. S. and Chieri, R. A. (1976). *Horm. metab. Res.* **8**, 413.

Basabe, J. C., Lopez, N., Victora, J. and Wollf, F. (1971). *Diabetes*, **20**, 449.

Battacharya, G. (1953). *Science*, **117**, 230.

Baxter, R. C., Yue, D. K. and Turtle, J. R. (1976). *Clin. Chem.* **22**, 1089.

Beck, P. (1973). *Metabolism*, **22**, 841.

Becker, D. J., Murray, P. J., Hansen, J. D. L. and Pimstone, B. L. (1973). *Br. J. Nutr.* **30**, 345.

Becker, D. J., Pimstone, B. L., Kronheim, S. and Weinkove, E. (1975). *Metabolism*, **24**, 953.

Beck-Nielsen, H., Pederson, O., Bagger, J. and Sörensen, N. S. (1976), *Acta endocr., Copnh.* **83**, 565.

Beck-Nielsen, H., Pedersen, O. and Sprensen, N. S. (1977). *Diabetologia*, **13**, 381A.

Belfiore, F., Romeo, F., Napoli, E. and Lo Vecchio, L. (1974). *Diabetes*, **23**, 293.

Bencosme, S. A. and Lazarus, S. S. (1956). *A.M.A. Arch. Path.* **62**, 285.

Bennett, L. L., Curry, D. L. and Curry, K. (1973). *Proc. Soc. exp. Biol. Med.* **144**, 436.

Berger, D., Crowther, R., Floyd, J. C., Pek, S. and Fajans, S. S. (1977a). *Diabetes*, **26** (Suppl. 1), 381A.

Berger, H., Halban, P., Müller, W. A., Renold, A. E. and Vranic, M. (1977b). *Diabetes*, **26** (Supp. 1), 357A.

Berger, W., Dahl. G. and Meissner, H. P. (1975). *Cytobiologie*, **12**, 119.

Berger, W., Geissner, H., Moppert, J. and Künzli, H. (1973). *Horm. metab. Res.* **5**, 4.

Berman, M., McGuire, E. A. and Zelenik, A. J. (1977). *Diabetes*, **26**, 387A.

Best, C. H., Haist, R. E. and Ridout, J. H. (1939). *J. Physiol.* **97**, 107.

Bhathena, S. J., Perrino, P. V., Voyles, N. R., Smith, S. S., Wilkins, S. D., Coy, D. H., Schally, A. V. and Recant, L. (1976). *Diabetes*, **25**, 1031.

Billaudel, B. and Sutter, B. C. J. (1977). *Diabetologia*, **13**, 382A.

Björntorp, P., De Jounge, K., Sjöström, L. and Sullivan, L. (1970). *Metabolism*, **19**, 631.

Blackard, W. G., Garcia, A. R. and Brown, C. L. (1970). *J. clin. Endocr. Metab.* **31**, 215.

Blanks, M. C. and Gerritsen, G. C. (1974). *Proc. Soc. exp. Biol. Med.* **146**, 448.

Block, M. B., Berk, E., Friedlander, L. S., Steiner, D. F. and Rubenstein, A. H. (1973a). *Ann. int. Med.* **78**, 663.

Block, M. B., Mako, M. E., Steiner, D. F. and Rubenstein, A. H. (1972). *Diabetes,* **21**, 1013.

Block, M. B., Pildes, R. S., Mossaboy, N. A. and Steiner, D. F. (1974). *Paediatrics,* **53**, 923.

Block, M. B., Rosenfield, R. L., Mako, M. E., Steiner, D. F. and Rubenstein, A. H. (1973b). *New Engl. J. Med.* **288**, 1444.

Bloom, S. R. and Edwards, A. V. (1975). *J. Physiol.* **253**, 157.

Bloom, S. R. and Iverscn, J. (1976). *Metabolism,* **26** (Suppl. 1), 457.

Bloom, S. R., Iversen, J., Polak, J. M., Hermanson, K. and Adrian, T. E. (1977). *Diabetologia,* **13**, 383A.

Bloom, S. R., Vaughan, N. J. S. and Russell, R. C. G. (1974). *Lancet,* **ii**, 546.

Blumenthal, S. A. (1977). *Diabetes,* **26**, 485.

Blundall, T. L., Bedarkar, S., Rinderknecht, E. and Humbel, R. E. (1978). *Proc. Natn. Acad. Sci. USA,* **75**, 180.

Blundell, T. L., Dodson, G. G., Hodgkin, D. C. and Mercola, D. A. (1972). *Adv. Prot. Chem.* **26**, 279.

Blundell, T. L. and Wood, S. P. (1975). *Nature, Lond.* **257**, 197.

Boden, G., Essa, N., Owen, O., Reichle, F. A. and Sarago, W. (1974). *J. clin. Invest.* **53**, 1185.

Bohannon, N. V., Karam, J. H., Lorenzi, M., Gerich, J. E., Martin, S. B. and Forsham, P. H. (1977). *Diabetologia,* **13**, 503.

Brodows, R. G., Pi-Sunyer, F. X. and Campbell, R. G. (1974). *J. clin. Endocr. Metab.* **38**, 1103.

Bomboy, J. D., Lewis, S. B., Sinclair-Smith, B. C. and Lacy, W. W. (1977). *J. clin. Endocr. Metab.* **44**, 474.

Bor, N. M. (1975). *New Istanbul Contrib. clin. Sci.* **11**, 70.

Botazzo, G. F., Doniach, D. and Pouplard, A. (1976). *Acta endocr., Copnh. (Suppl.* 205), 55.

Botazzo, G. F., Florin-Christensen, A. and Doniach, D. (1974). *Lancet,* **ii**, 1279.

Botella Llusia, J., Del Olmo, J., Parache, J., Catalan, E., Vila, T. and Alberto, J. C. (1973). *J. reprod. Med.* **11**, 59.

Botha, J. L., Vinik, A. I., Blake, K. C. H. and Jackson, W. P. U. (1976). *Eur. J. clin. Invest.* **6**, 365.

Boucher, B. J., Cohen, R. D., Frankel, R. J., Maron, A. S. and Broadley, G. (1973). *Clin. Endocr.* **2**, 111.

Bowen, V. and Lazarus, N. R. (1974). *Biochem. J.* **142**, 385.

Bradbury, J. H. and Brown, L. R. (1977). *Eur. J. Biochem.* **76**, 573.

Brandt, M. R., Kehlet, H., Faber, O. and Binder, C. H. R. (1977). *Clin. Endocr.* **6**, 167.

Brauman, H. and Corvilain, J. (1968). *J. clin. Endocr. Metab.* **28**, 301.

Bressler, R., Vargas-Cordon, M. and Brendel, K. (1969). *Diabetes,* **18**, 262.

Bressler, R., Vargas-Cordon, M. and Lebovitz, H. E. (1968). *Diabetes,* **17**, 617.

Brinn, J. E., Owen, J. and Schweisthal, M. (1976). *Diabetes,* **26** (Suppl. 1), 389A.

Brisson, G. R. and Malaisse, W. J. (1971). *Can. J. physiol. Pharmacol.* **49**, 536.

Brisson, G. R. and Malaisse, W. J. (1973). *Metabolism,* **22**, 455.

Brodows, R. G., Pi-Sunyer, F. C. and Campbell, R. G. (1974). *J. clin. Endocr. Metab.* **38**, 1103.

Brown, J. G., Drysburgh, J. R., Ross, S. A. and Dupre, J. (1975). *Rec. Prog. Horm. Res.* **31**, 487.

Browne, S. and Duggan, P. F. (1974). *Biochem. Soc. Trans.* **2**, 1383.

Brunzell, J. D., Robertson, R. P., Lerner, R. L., Hazzard, W. L., Ensinck, J. N., Bierman, E. L. and Porte, D. (1976). *J. clin. Endocr. Metab.* **42**, 222.

Buckingham, J. M., Service, F. J., Palumbo, P. J., Aguilo, J. J., Woods, J. E. and Zincke, H. (1976). *Urology*, **8**, 210.

Bunnag, S. C., Bunnag, S. and Werner, N. E. (1968). *Anat. Res.* **196**, 117.

Burghen, G. A., Duckworth, W. C., Kitabchi, A. E., Solomon, S. and Poffenbarger, P. L. (1976). *J. clin. Invest.* **57**, 1089.

Burman, K. D., Cunningham, E. J., Klacko, D. M. and Burns, T. W. (1973). *Mo. Med.* **70**, 363.

Burns, T. W., Terry, B., Langley, P. E. and Robison, G. A. (1977). *Diabetes*, **26**, 657.

Burr, I. M., Jackson, A., Culbert, S., Sharp, R., Felts, P. and Olson, W. (1974). *Endocrinology*, **94**, 1072.

Burr, I. M. and Sharp, R. (1974). *Endocrinology*, **94**, 835.

Burr, I. M., Slonim, A. E. and Sharp, R. (1976). *J. clin. Invest.* **58**, 230.

Burr, I. M., Staufacher, W., Balant, L., Renold, A. E. and Grodsky, G. M. (1969). *Lancet*, **ii**, 882.

Bylund, A. G., Hammersten, J., Holm, J. and Schersten, T. (1976). *Eur. J. clin. Invest.* **6**, 425.

Campbell, D. M., Benther, P. D., Davidson, J. M. and Sutherland, H. W. (1974). *J. Obstet. Gynaec. Br. Commonw.* **81**, 615.

Campbell, I. W., Fraser, D. M. and Duncan, L. J. P. (1978). *Br. med. J.* **2**, 174.

Castro, A., Buist, N., Grettie, D. and Bartoss, F. (1974). *Biochem. Med.* **10**, 208.

Castro, A., Dyess, K., Buist, N. and Potts, J. (1973). *Clin. Biochem.* **6**, 211.

Cavagnini, F., Peracchi, M., Raggi, U., Bana, R., Pontiroli, A. E., Malin-Verni, A. and Pinto, M. (1974). *Eur. J. clin. Invest.* **4**, 71.

Cerasi, E. (1975a). *Diabetologia*, **11**, 1.

Cerasi, E. (1975b). *Acta endocr., Copenh.* **79**, 502.

Cerasi, E., Fick, G. and Rudemo, M. (1974). *Eur. J. clin. Invest.* **4**, 267.

Cerasi, E. and Luft, R. (1967). *Acta endocr., Copenh.* **55**, 278.

Cerasi, E., Luft, R. and Efendic, S. (1972). *Acta endocr., Copenh.* **69**, 333.

Chan, S. J., Keim, P. and Steiner, D. F. (1976). *Proc. natn. Acad. Sci. USA*, **73**, 1964.

Chance, R. E. (1971). *In* "Proceedings of the 7th Congress of International Diabetes Federation" (R. R. Rodriguez and J. Vallance-Owen, eds), p. 292. Excerpta Medica, Amsterdam.

Chance, R. E. (1972). *Diabetes*, **21** (Suppl. 1), 461.

Chance, R. E., Root, M. A. and Galloway, J. A. (1976). *Acta endocr., Copenh.* **83** (Suppl. 205), 185.

Charles, M. A., Lawecki, J., Pictet, R. and Grodsky, G. M. (1975). *J. biol. Chem.* **250**, 6134.

Chen, M. C. and Porte, D. (1976). *J. clin. Endocr. Metab.* **42**, 1168.

Cheng, J. S. and Kalant, N. (1970). *J. clin. Endocr. Metab.* **31**, 647.

Chiasson, J. L., Liljenquist, J. E., Sinclair-Smith, B. C. and Lacy, W. W. (1977). *Diabetes*, **26**, 574.

Chin, H. P., Hamashiro, P. K., Khan, A. H. and Blankenhorn, D. H. (1974). *Steroids Lipids Res.* **5**, 2000.

Chochinor, R. H. and Daughaday, W. H. (1976). *Diabetes*, **25**, 994.

Christensen, N. J. and Neubauer, B. (1976). *Acta endocr., Copenh.* **82**, 753.

Christensen, N. J. and Videbaek, J. (1974). *J. clin. Invest.* **54**, 278.

Christiansen, A. H. and Kroll, J. (1973). *Scand. J. Immunol.* **2** (Suppl. 1), 133.

Claro, A., Grill, V., Efendic, S. and Luft, R. (1977). *Acta endocr., Copenh.* **85**, 374.

Cleator, I. G. M. and Gourlay, R. H. (1975). *Am. J. Surg.* **130**, 128.

Coffey, J. W., Nagy, C. F., Lensky, R. and Hansen, H. J. (1974). *Biochem. Med.* **9**, 54.

Cohen, P., Antoni, J. F., Nimmo, H. J. and Yeaman, S. J. (1976). *In* "Polypeptide Hormones. Molecular and Cellular Aspects", p. 281. Ciba Foundation Symposium 41 (New Series), Excerpta Medica, Amsterdam.

Cohn, C., Berger, S. and Norton, M. (1968). *Diabetes*, **17**, 72.

Cole, H. S. (1973). *Paediatrics*, **52**, 137.

Cole, H. S., Kim, H. S., Zelson, C. and Velasco, C. A. (1973). *Acta diabet. lat.* **10**, 283.

Colle, E., Schiff, D., Andrew, G., Bauer, C. B. and Fitzhardinge, P. (1976). *Paediatrics*, **57**, 363.

Conn, J. W. (1965). *New Engl. J. Med.* **273**, 1135.

Constan, L., Mako, M., Juhn, D. and Rubenstein, A. H. (1975). *Diabetologia*, **11**, 119.

Costantini, A., Lostia, O., Malvano, R., Rolleri, E., Taggi, F. and Zucchelli, G. C. (1975). *J. nucl. biol. Med.* **19**, 164.

Costin, G., Kogut, M. D., Phillips, L. S. and Daughaday, W. H. (1976). *J. clin. Endocr.* **42**, 370.

Costrini, N. V., Jacobson, M. and Kalkhoff, R. K. (1969). *Diabetes*, **18** (Suppl. 1), 322A.

Cotes, P. M., Mussett, M. V., Berryman, I., Ekins, R. P., Glover, R., Hales, C. N., Hunter, W. M., Lowy, G., Neville, R. W. J., Samols, E. and Woodward, P. M. (1969). *J. Endocr.* **45**, 557.

Couturier, E., Rasio, L. and Coward, V. (1971). *Horm. metab. Res.* **3**, 382.

Crespin, S. R., Greenoghn, W. and Steinberg, D. (1973). *J. clin. Invest.* **48**, 1934.

Cresto, J. C., Lavine, R. L., Fink, G. and Recant, L. (1974). *Diabetes*, **23**, 505.

Creutzfeldt, W., Arnold, R., Creutzfeldt, C., Deuticke, U., Frerichs, H. and Tracks, N. S. (1973). *Diabetologia*, **9**, 217.

Creutzfeldt, W., Ebert, R., Arnold, H., Frerichs, H. and Brown, J. C. (1975). *Diabetologia*, **12**, 279.

Creutzfeldt, W., Ebert, R., Frerichs, H. and Brown, J. C. (1978). *Diabetologia*, **14**, 15.

Crossley, J. R. and Elliott, R. B. (1975). *Diabetes*, **24**, 609.

Crossley, M. F. and Garbien, K. J. T. (1974). *Clin. chim. Acta*, **51**, 345.

Cser, A. and Milner, R. D. G. (1975). *Biol. Neonate*, **27**, 61.

Cudworth, A. G. and Woodrow, J. G. (1975). *Diabetes*, **24**, 345.

Cuendet, G. S., Loten, E. G. Jeanrenaud, B. and Renold, A. E. (1976). *J. clin. Invest.* **58**, 1078.

Cunningham, N. P., Rosenbloom, A. L., Kohler, W. G. and Wilder, B. J. (1973). *Paediatrics*, **51**, 1091.

Curry, D. L. and Joy, R. M. (1974) *Endocr. Res. Commun.* **1**, 229.

Curry, D. L., Bennett, L. L. and Grodsky, G. M. (1968). *Am. J. Physiol.* **214**, 174.

Curry, D. L., Joy, R. M., Holley, D. and Bennett, L. L. (1977). *Endocrinology*, **101**, 203.

Czech, M. P. (1976). *J. clin. Invest.* **57**, 1523.

Czyzyk, A., Szadhowski, M., Kogela, H. and Lawecki, J. (1973). *Diabetes*, **22**, 932.

Dacou-Voutetakis, C., Constantinidis, M., Moschos, A., Vlachon, C. and Metsaniotis, N. (1974). *Am. J. Dis. Child.* **127**, 890.

Dahlhöf, A. G., Björntorp, P., Holm, J. and Schersten, T. (1974). *Eur. J. clin. Invest.* **4**, 9.

Dahms, W. T., Atkinson, R. L., Golden, M., Whipp, B., Wasserman, K. and Bray, G. A. (1977). *Diabetes*, **26**, 393A.

Davidson, M. B. and Deal, R. B. (1976). *J. Lab. clin. Med.* **87**, 1050.

Davidson, M. B. and Kaplan, S. A. (1977). *J. clin. Invest.* **59**, 22.

Danforth, E. (1971). *Diabetes*, **20**, 843A.

Davis, B. and Lazarus, N. R. (1972). *Biochem. J.* **129**, 373.

Davis, B. and Lazarus, N. R. (1975). *J. Memb. Biol.* **20**, 301.

Davis, B. and Lazarus, N. R. (1976). *J. Physiol., Lond.* **256**, 709.

Davis, J. W., Yoder, J. M. and Adams, E. C. (1976). *Clin. chim. Acta*, **66**, 379.

Dean, P. M. and Matthews, K. E. (1970a). *J. Physiol.* **210**, 255.

Dean, P. M. and Matthews, K. E. (1970b). *J. Physiol.* **210**, 265.

Dean, P. M. and Matthews, K. E. (1972). *Diabetologia*, **8**, 173.

Dean, P. M., Matthews, K. E. and Sakomoto, Y. (1975). *J. Physiol.* **246**, 459.

Deckert, T., Lauridsen, U. B., Madsen, S. N. and Deckert, M. (1972). *Horm. metab. Res.* **4**, 229.

Deconinck, J. F., Potvliege, P. R. and Gepts, W. (1971). *Diabetologia*, **7**, 266.

Deconinck, J. F., Van Assche, F. A., Potvliege, P. R. and Gepts, W. (1972). *Diabetologia*, **8**, 326.

De Fronzo, R. A., Andres, R., Bledsoe, T. A., Boden, G., Faloona, G. A. and Tobin, J. D. (1977). *Diabetes*, **26**, 445.

De Häen, C., Little, S. A. and May, J. M. (1977). *Diabetes*, **26** (Suppl. 1), 376A.

Del Prete, G. F., Betterle, C., Bersani, G., Romano, M. and Tiengo, A. (1976). *Lancet*, **ii**, 1090.

Del Prete, G. F., Betterle, C., Padovan, D., Erle, G., Toffol, A. and Bersani, G. (1977). *Diabetes*, **26**, 909.

De Meyts, P. and Waelbroeck, M. (1977). *Diabetes*, **26** (Supp. 1), 354A.

Denborough, M. A., Warne, G. L., Moulds, R. F. W., Tse, P. and Martin, F. I. R. (1974). *Br. med. J.* **3**, 493.

Desbuquois, B. and Auerbach, G. D. (1971). *J. clin. Endocr. Metab.* **33**, 732.

Deschamp, I., Giron, B. and Lestradet, H. (1927). *Diabetes*, **26**, 89.

Devis, G., Obberghen, E. C., Somers, G., Malaisse-Lagae, F., Orci, L. and Malaisse, W. J. (1974). *Diabetologia*, **10**, 53.

Dial, L. K., Miyamoto, S. and Arquilla, E. R. (1977). *Biochem. biophys. Res. Commun.* **74**, 545.

Dieterle, P., Birkmer, B., Gmeiner, K. H., Wagner, P., Erhardt, F., Haner, J. and Dieterle, C. (1973). *Horm. Metab. Res.* **5**, 316.

Di Natale, B., Deretta, M., Rossi, L., Carlashi, C., Caccamo, A., Del Guarcio, M. and Chiumello, G. (1973). *Helv. paediatr. Acta*, **28**, 591.

Dixon, K. (1974). *Clin. Chem.* **20**, 1275.

Dison, K., Exon, P. D. and Malins, J. M. (1975). *Quart. J. Med.* **44**, 543.

Dobrzanski, T. and Pieschl, D. (1976). *J. Stud. Alcohol*, **37**, 327.

Dormer, L., Kerbey, A. L., McPherson, M., Marley, S., Ashcroft, S. J. H., Schofield, J. G. and Randle, P. J. (1973). *Biochem. J.* **140**, 135.

Dorn, V. A., Lorenz, D. and Koch, G. (1977). *Acta histochem., Jena*, **58**, 364.

Draisey, T. F., Gagneja, G. L. and Thiebert, R. J. (1977). *Obstet. Gynecol.* **50**, 197.

Duckworth, W. C. and Kitabchi, A. E. (1972). *Am. J. Med.* **53**, 418.

Duckworth, W. C. and Kitabchi, A. E. (1976). *J. Lab. clin. Med.* **88**, 359.

Dudl, R. J. and Ensinck, J. W. (1977). *Metabolism*, **26**, 33.

Dujovna, I. L., Cresto, J. C., Sires, J. M., Aparicio, N., Gimenez, H. and De Majo, S. F. (1973). *In* "International Congress Series" (P. J. Hoet, P. Lefebvre, W. J. H. Butterfield and J. Vallance-Owen, eds), Vol. 280, p. 32A. Excerpta Medica, Amsterdam.

Dunbar, J. C., McLaughlin, W. J., Walsh, M. F. J. and Foa, P. P. (1975). *Horm. metab. Res.* **8**, 1.

Dunlop, M. and Court, J. M. (1974). *Clin. chim. Acta* **52**, 353.
Duran-Garcia, S., Jarrousse, C. and Rosselin, G. (1976). *J. clin. Invest.* **57**, 230.
Duran, S., Maranon, A. and Romano, E. (1974). *Rev. clin. Esp.* **132**, 41.
Dymock, I. W., Cassar, J., Pyke, D. A., Oakley, W. C. and Williams, R. (1972). *Am. J. Med.* **52**, 203.
Eaton, R. P. (1973). *Metabolism*, **23**, 763.
Eaton, R. P. and Nye, W. H. R. (1973). *J. lab. clin. Med.* **81**, 682.
Eaton, R. P., Schade, D. S. and Peake, G. T. (1977). *Diabetes*, **26**, 395A.
Ebert, R., Creutzfeldt, W., Brown, J. C., Frerichs, H. and Arnold, R. (1976). *Diabetologia*, **12**, 609.
Edwards, J. C. and Taylor, K. W. (1970). *Biochim. biophys. Acta*, **215**, 310.
Efendic, S., Cerasi, E. and Luft, R. (1973). *Acta endocr., Copenh.* **74**, 542.
Efendic, S., Cerasi, E. and Luft, R. (1974a). *Diabetes*, **23**, 161.
Efendic, S., Claro, A. and Luft, R. (1976). *Acta endocr., Copenh.* **81**, 753.
Efendic, S., Lins, P. E., Sigurdsson, G., Ivemark, B., Granberg, P. D. and Luft, R. (1971). *Acta endocr., Copenh.* **81**, 525.
Efendic, S. and Luft, R. (1975). *Acta endocr., Copenh.* **78**, 516.
Efendic, S., Luft, R. and Grill, V. (1974b). *FEBS Letts*, **42**, 169.
El-Allawy, R. M. M., Humbel, R. E. and Froesch, E. R. (1976). *Diabetologia*, **12**, 523.
El Denshary, E. S. and Montague, W. (1976). *Biochem. Pharmacol.* **25**, 1451.
Emdin, S. O., Gammeltoft, S. and Gliemann, J. (1975). *Diabetologia*, **11**, 340A.
Enger, S. C. and Rutland, S. (1973). *Acta med. scand.* **194**, 97.
Enk, B. (1976). *Acta endocr., Copenh.* **82**, 312.
Enk, B. (1977). *Acta endocr., Copenh.* **85**, 559.
Enk, B., Lund, B., Schmidt, I. and Deckert, T. (1976). *Acta endocr., Copenh.* **82**, 306.
Ericson, L. E., Håkanson, R. and Lundquist, I. (1977). *Diabetologia*, **13**, 117.
Erlandsen, S. L., Hage, O. D., Parsons, J. A., McEvoy, R. C. and Elder, F. (1976). *J. Histochem. Cytochem.* **24**, 883.
Erwald, R., Hed, R., Nygren, A., Rödjmark, S., Sundblad, L. and Wiechel, K. L. (1973). *Acta med. scand.* **194**, 103.
Evans, E. S., Simpson, M. E. and Evans, H. M. (1958). *Endocrinology*, **63**, 836.
Ewart, R. B. L., Kornfeld, S. and Kipnis, D. M. (1975). *Diabetes*, **24**, 705.
Faber, O. K. and Binder, C. (1977a). *Diabetologia*, **13**, 263.
Faber, O. K. and Binder, C. (1977b). *Diabetes*, **26**, 605.
Faber, O. K., Binder, C., Naithani, V. K. and Heding, L. G. (1975). *Diabetologia*, **11**, 340A.
Faber, O. K., Binder, C., Kuzuya, H., Blix, P., Horwitz, D. and Rubenstein, A. H. (1977). *Diabetologia*, **13**, 392A.
Faber, O. K., Markussen, J., Naithani, V. K. and Binder, C. (1976). *Hoppe Seyler's Z. physiol. Chem.* **357**, 751.
Fain, J. N. (1968). *Endocrinology*, **82**, 825.
Fajans, S. S. and Conn, J. W. (1961). *Diabetes*, **10**, 63.
Fajans, S. S. and Floyd, J. C. (1972). *In* "Handbook of Physiology and Endocrinology", (R. O. Greep, E. B. Astwood, eds), Vol. 1, Sect 7, pp. 473. Am. Physiol. Soc., Washington, DC.
Fajans, S. S. and Floyd, J. C. (1976). *New Engl. J. Med.* **294**, 766.
Fajans, S. S., Floyd, J. C., Tattersall, R. B., Williamson, J. R., Pek, S. and Taylor, C. I. (1976). *Arch. int. Med.* **136**, 194.
Falkmer, S. and Östberg, Y. (1976). *In* "The Evolution of Pancreatic Islets (T. A. Grillo, L. Leibson and A. Epple, eds), p. 141. Pergamon Press, London.

Fallucca, F., Menzinger, G., Gambardella, S., Tamburranno, S. and Andreani, D. (1975). *Acta diabet. lat.* **12**, 239.

Falorni, A., Frecassini, F., Massi-Benedetti, F. and Maffei, S. (1974). *Diabetes*, **23**, 172.

Falorni, A., Massi-Benedetti, F., Gallo, S. and Romizi, S. (1975a). *Pediatr. Res.* **9**, 55.

Falorni, A., Massi-Benedetti, F., Gallo, G. and Trabalza, N. (1975b). *Biol. Neonate*, **27**, 271.

Federici, G., Dupre, S., Barboni, E., Fiori, A. and Costa, M. (1973). *FEBS Letts.*, **32**, 27.

Federspil, G., Casara, D. and Staufaccher, W. (1974). *Diabetologia*, **10**, 188.

Feige, A., Künzel, W. and Mitzkat, H. J. (1977). *J. perinat. Med.* **5**, 84.

Feldman, J. M., Birens, C. H., Skyler, J. S. and Lebovitz, H. E. (1975). *Horm. metab. Res.* **7**, 279.

Feldman, J. M. and Chapman, B. A. (1973). *Clin. Chem.* **19**, 1250.

Feldman, J. M. and Chapman, B. A. (1974). *Diabetes*, **23**, 754.

Feldman, J. M., Marecek, R. L., Quickel, K. E. and Lebovitz, H. E. (1972). *J. clin. Endocr. Metab.* **35**, 307.

Feldman, J. M. and Plonk, J. W. (1976). *J. Am. Geriatr. Soc.* **24**, 1.

Feldman, J. M., Plonk, J. W. and Birens, C. H. (1975). *Horm. metab. Res.* **7**, 378.

Feldman, J. M. and Quickel, K. E. (1973). *Diabetes*, **22**, 9.

Feldman, J. M., Snyder, J. H. and Gerritsen, G. C. (1977). *Diabetes*, **26** (Suppl. 1), 396A.

Felig, P., Gusberg, R., Handler, R., Gump, F. E. and Kinney, J. M. (1974). *Proc. Soc. exp. Biol. Med.* **147**, 88.

Felig, P., Wahren, J. and Handler, R. (1976). *J. clin. Invest.* **58**, 761.

Ferrari, C., Frezzati, S. Romuni, M., Bertazzani, A., Testori, G. P., Antonine, S. and Peracchi, A. (1977). *Metabolism*, **26**, 120.

Fink, G., Cresto, J. C., Gutman, R. A., Lavine, R. L., Rubenstein, A. H. and Recant, L. (1974). *Horm. metab. Res.* **6**, 439.

Fioretti, P., Genazzani, A. R., Felber, J. P., Facchini, V., Onano, A. M., Romagnino, S., Facchinetti, F. and Pira, G. L. (1975). *Acta Eur. Fertil.* **6**, 63.

Fiser, R. H., Williams, P. R., Fisher, D. A., De Lameter, P. V., Sperling, M. A. and Oh, W. (1975). *Paediatrics*, **56**, 78.

Flier, J. S., Kahn, C. R., Jarrett, D. B. and Roth, J. (1976). *J. clin. Invest.* **58**, 1142.

Flier, J. S., Marakos-Flier, E., Baird, K. and Kahn, C. R. (1977). *Diabetes*, **26** (Suppl. 1), 357A.

Florey, C. Du V., Lowy, C. and Uppal, S. (1976). *Diabetologia*, **12**, 313.

Florey, C. Du V., Milner, R. D. G. and Miall, W. E. (1977). *J. chron. Dis.* **30**, 49.

Foa, P. P., Blazquez, E., Sodoyez, J. and Sodoyez-Goffaux, F. (1976). *In* "The Evolution of Pancreatic Islets" (T. A. Grillo, L. Leibson and A. Epple, eds), p. 7. Pergamon Press, London.

Fölling, I. (1976). *Acta endocr., Copenh.* **83** (Suppl. 205), 199.

Frane, C. M., Ganguli, S., Christensen, R., Voina, R., Maddig, C. (1977). *Diabetes*, **26** (Suppl. 1), 397A.

Frank, B. H., Veros, A. J. and Pekar, A. H. (1972). *Biochemistry*, **11**, 4926.

Frankson, J. R. M., Gassee, J. P., Ooms, H. A. and Dubois, R. (1976). *Curr. Prob. clin. Biochem.* **6**, 233.

Frankson, J. R. M. and Ooms, H. A. (1973). *Postgrad. med. J.* **49**, 931.

Frayn, K. N. (1976). *Horm. metab. Res.* **8**, 102.

Frerichs, H. and Creutzfeldt, W. (1976). *Clin. Endocr. Metab.* **5**, 747.

Frerichs, H., Schauder, P., McIntosh, C., Panten, U. and Creutzfeldt, W. (1977). *Diabetes*, **26** (Suppl. 1), 397A.

Freychet, P. (1976). *Diabetologia*, **12**, 83.

Freychet, P., Brandenburg, D. and Wollmer, A. (1974). *Diabetologia*, **10**, 1.

Freychet, P., Kahn, C. R., Roth, J. and Neville, D. M. (1976). *J. biol. Chem.* **247**, 3953.

Friesen, S. R., Bolinger, R. E. and Kyner, J. L. (1974). *Surgery*, **76**, 804.

Frikke, M. J., Gingerich, R. L., Stranahan, P. D., Carter, G., Baumer, A. K., Greider, M. H., Wright, P. H. and Lacy, P. E. (1974). *Diabetologia*, **10**, 345.

Froesch, E. R., Zapf, J., Meuli, C., Mäder, M., Waldvogel, M., Kaufmann, U. and Morell, B. (1975). *In* "Advances in Metabolic Disorders" (R. Luft and K. Hall, eds), p. 211. Academic Press, New York and London.

Frohman, L. A. and Bernardis, L. L. (1971). *Am. J. Phys.* **221**, 1896.

Frohman, L. A., Ezdinli, E. Z. and Javid, R. (1967). *Diabetes*, **16**, 443.

Frohman, L. A., Muller, E. E. and Cocchi, D. (1973). *Horm. metab. Res.* **5**, 21.

Fujita, T. (1966). *Z. Zellforsch.* **69**, 363.

Fujita, Y., Herron, A. L. and Seltzer, H. S. (1975). *Diabetes*, **24**, 17.

Fung, W. and Mennear, J. H. (1974). *Proc. Soc. exp. Biol. Med.* **146**, 949.

Gabbay, K. H., Korff, J. and Schneeberger, E. E. (1975). *Science*, **187**, 177.

Gabbay, K. H., De Luca, K., Fisher, J. N., Mako, M. E. and Rubenstein, A. H. (1976). *New Engl. J. Med.* **294**, 911.

Gabbay, K. H., Wolff, J., Bergenstahl, R., Mako, M. E. and Rubenstein, A. H. (1977). *Diabetes*, **26** (Suppl. 1), 376A.

Ganda, O. P., Kahn, C. P., Soeldner, J. S. and Gleason, R. E. (1975). *Diabetes*, **24**, 354.

Ganda, O. P., Soeldner, S., Gleason, R. E., Smith, T. M., Kilo, C. and Williamson, J. R. (1977). *Diabetes*, **26**, 469.

Garber, A. J., Cryer, P. E., Santiago, J. V., Haymond, J. W., Pagliara, A. S. and Kipnis, D. M. (1976). *J. clin. Invest.* **58**, 7.

Garcia-Hermida, O. and Gomez-Acebo, J. (1974). *Biochem. biophys. Res. Commun.* **57**, 209.

Gedik, O. and Zileli, M. S. (1977). *Diabetes*, **26**, 813.

Gennaro, W. D. and Van Norman, J. U. (1975). *Clin. Chem.* **21**, 873.

Gentz, J. C. H. and Cornblath, M. (1969). *Adv. Pediatr.* **16**, 345.

George, R. H., Sussman, K. E., Leitner, J. W. and Kirsch, W. M. (1971). *Endocrinology*, **89**, 169.

Gerich, J. E. (1976). *Metabolism*, **25** (Suppl. 1), 1513.

Gerich, J. E., Langlois, M., Noacco, C., Schneider, V. and Forsham, P. H. (1974a). *J. clin. Invest.* **53**, 1441.

Gerich, J. E., Langlois, M., Schneider, V., Karam, J. H. and Noacco, C. (1974b). *J. clin. Invest.* **53**, 1284.

Gerich, J. E., Lorenzi, M., Karam, J. H., Schneider, V. and Forsham, P. H. (1975). *J. Am. med. Assoc.* **234**, 159.

Geser, C. A., Müller-Hess, R. and Felber, J. P. (1973/74). *Infusionstherapie*, **1**, 483.

Ghodse, A. H. (1977). *Pahlavi med. J.* **8**, 141.

Gibson, T., Stimmler, L., Jarrett, R. J., Rutland, P. and Shiu, M. (1975). *Diabetologia*, **11**, 83.

Giddings, A. E. B., O'Connor, K. J., Rowlands, B. J., Mangwall, D. and Clark, R. G. (1976). *Br. J. Surg.* **63**, 612:

Gillmer, M. D. G., Beard, R. W., Brooke, F. M. and Oakley, N. W. (1975). *Br. med. J.* **3**, 399.

Gingerich, R. L. (1977). *Diabetes*, **26**, 375A.

Ginsberg, H. (1977a). *In* "Biochemical Actions of Hormones" (G. Litwack, ed.), Vol. IV, p. 313. Academic Press, London and New York.

Ginsberg, H. (1977b). *Metabolism*, **26**, 1135.

Ginsberg, H., Kahn, R. C., Roth, J. and De Meyts, P. (1976a). *Biochem. Biophys. Res. Commun.* **73**, 1068.

Ginsberg, H., Olefsky, J. M., Kimmerling, G., Crapo, P. and Reaven, G. M. (1976b). *J. clin. Endocr. Metab.* **42**, 729.

Giron, B. J. and Lestradet, H. (1973). *In* "IRCS No. 280" (J. J. Hoet, P. Lefebvre, W. J. H. Butterfield and J. Vallance-Owen, eds), p. 17, 38A. Excerpta Medica, Amsterdam.

Gliemann, J. (1967). *Diabetologia*, **3**, 382.

Gliemann, J. and Gammeltoft, S. (1974). *Diabetologia*, **10**, 105.

Gliemann, J. and Sörensen, H. H. (1970). *Diabetologia*, **6**, 499.

Goberna, R., Tamarit, J., Osoria, J., Fussgänger, R., Tamarit, J. and Pfeiffer, E. F. (1974). *Horm. metab. Res.* **6**, 256.

Golden, P., Basil, L., Melani, W. J., Malaisse-Lagae, F. and Walker, R. M. (1976). *Diabetologia*, **12**, 207.

Goldfine, I. D. (1975). *Endocrinology*, **97**, 948.

Goldfine, I. D. (1977). *Diabetes*, **26**, 148.

Goldfine, I. D., Abraira, C., Grunewald, D. and Goldstein, M. S. (1970). *Proc. Soc. exp. Biol. Med.* **133**, 274.

Goldfine, I. D., Roth, J. and Birnbaumer, L. (1972). *J. biol. Chem.* **247**, 1211.

Goldman, J. A. (1975). *Diabetologia*, **11**, 45.

Goldman, J. A. and Carpenter, F. H. (1974). *Biochemistry*, **13**, 4566.

Goldman, J. A. and Eckerling, B. (1971). *Isr. J. Med.* **8**, 1724.

Goodman, H. M. and Knobil, E. (1959). *Endocrinology*, **65**, 451.

Gorden, P., Freychet, P. and Nankin, H. (1971). *J. clin. Endocr. Metab.* **33**, 983.

Gorden, P., Gavin, J. R., Lesniak, M. A. and Roth, J. (1973). *J. clin. Endocr. Metab.* **36**, 627.

Göschke, H. (1977). *Metabolism*, **26**, 1147.

Göschke, H., Denes, A., Girard, J., Collard, F. and Berger, W. (1974). *Horm. metab. Res.* **6**, 386.

Gotfredsen, C. F. (1976). *Diabetologia*, **12**, 339.

Gottlieb, M. S., Soeldner, S., Kyner, J. L. and Gleason, R. E. (1974). *Diabetes*, **23**, 684.

Graham, G., Nakashima, J., Thompson, R. G. and Blizzard, R. M. (1976). *Pediatr. Res.* **10**, 832.

Grajwer, L. A., Pildes, R. S., Horwitz, D. L. and Rubenstein, A. H. (1977). *J. Paediat.* **90**, 42.

Grasso, S., Palumbo, G., Messina, A., Mazzarino, C. and Reitano, G. (1976). *Diabetes*, **25**, 545.

Greco, A. V., Ghirlanda, G., Patrono, C., Fedeli, G. and Manna, R. (1974). *Acta diabetol. lat.* **11**, 330.

Grodsky, G. M. (1975). *Handb. exp. Pharmacol.* **32**, 1.

Grodsky, G. M. and Forsham, P. H. (1960). *J. clin. Invest.* **39**, 1070.

Grodsky, G. M., Bennett, L. L., Smith, D. and Nemechek, K. (1967). *In* "Tolbutamide, After Ten Years" (W. J. H. Butterfield and W. V. Westering, eds), p. 11. Excerpta Medica, Amsterdam.

Guenther, H. L. and McDonald, J. H. (1972). *Prep. Biochem.* **2**, 397.

Guest, G. M., Mackler, B. and Knowles, H. C. (1952). *Diabetes*, **1**, 276.

Gutman, R. A., Lazarus, N. R. and Recant, L. (1972). *Diabetologia*, **8**, 136.
Gündoğdu, S., Bağriaçik, N., Hatemi, H., Alemdaroğlu, N., Basri, M., Biyal, F. and Korugan, U. (1977). *Diabetologia*, **13**, 397A.
Gylfe, E. (1974). *Biochim. biophys. Acta* **343**, 584.
Gylfe, E., Hellman, B., Sehlin, J. and Täljedal, I. B. (1973). *Endocrinology*, **93**, 932.
Hager, D., Georg, R. H., Leitner, J. W. and Beck, P. (1972). *Endocrinology*, **91**, 977.
Hahn, H. J., Hellman, B., Lernmark, A., Sehlin, J. and Taljedal, I. B. (1973). *J. biol. Chem.* **249**, 5275.
Hahn, H. J., Menzel, R., Gottschling, H. D. and Jahr, D. (1976). *Acta endocr., Copenh.* **83**, 123.
Haist, R. E. (1944). *Physiol. Rev.* **24**, 409.
Håkanson, R., Liedberg, G. and Lundquist, I. (1971). *Experentia*, **27**, 461.
Hales, C. N. and Randle, P. J. (1963). *Biochem. J.* **88**, 137.
Hammersten, J., Holm, J., Björntorp, P. and Schersten, T. (1977) *Metabolism*, **26**, 883.
Harrison, L. C., Martin, F. I. R. and Melick, R. A. (1976). *J. clin. Invest.* **58**, 1435.
Harrower, A. D. B., Yap, P. L., Nairn, I. M., Walton, H. J., Strong, J. A. and Craig, A. (1977). *Brit. med. J.* **2**, 156.
Harter, H. R., Santiago, J. V., Rutherford, W. E., Slatopolsky, E. and Klahr, S. (1976). *J. clin. Invest.* **58**, 359.
Hartroft, W. S. (1956). *Diabetes*, **5**, 98.
Hasslacher, C., Wahl, P. and Riemer, G. (1976). *Acta diabetol. lat.* **13**, 77.
Haute-Couverture, H., Slama, C., Assan, R. and Tchobroutsky, G. (1974). *Diabetologia*, **10**, 725.
Hawkins, R. A., Alberti, K. G. M. M., Houghton, C. R. I., Williamson, D. H. and Krebs, H. A. (1973). *Biochem. J.* **125**, 541.
Hawkins-Carranza, F. G., Larrodera, L. and Schutter, A. (1976). *Horm. metab. Res.* **8**, 237.
Hayashi, M., Floyd, J. C., Pek, S. and Fajans, S. S. (1977). *J. clin. Endocr. Metab.* **44**, 681.
Hecht, A., Gershberg, H. and Hulse, M. (1973). *Metabolism*, **22**, 723.
Heding, L. G. (1972). *Diabetologia*, **8**, 260.
Heding, L. G. (1975). *Diabetologia*, **12**, 541.
Heding, L. G. (1977). *Diabetologia*, **13**, 467.
Hedstrand, H. and Aberg, H. (1974). *Acta med. scand.* **196**, 39.
Hedstrand, H. and Boberg, J. (1975). *Scand. J. lab. Invest.* **35**, 331.
Heding, L. G. and Rasmussen, M. A. (1975). *Diabetologia*, **11**, 201.
Heitz, P. U., Klöppel, G., Hacht, W. H., Polak, J. M. and Everson-Pearse, A. G. (1977). *Diabetes*, **26**, 632.
Helge, H. and Merker, H. J. (1968). *Helv. paediatr. Acta*, **23**, 509.
Hellman, B. (1970). *Diabetologia*, **6**, 110.
Hellman, B. (1974). *Metabolism*, **23**, 839.
Hellman, B. (1975). *FEBS Letts* **54**, 343.
Hellman, B. and Idahl, L. A. (1970). *In* "The Structure and Metabolism of the Pancreatic Islets" (S. Falkmer, B. Hellman and I. B. Täljedal, eds), p. 253. Pergamon Press, London.
Hellman, B., Idahl, L. A., Lernmark, A., Sehlin, J. and Täljedal, I. B. (1973). *Biochem. J.* **132**, 775.
Hellman, B., Idahl, L. A., Lernmark, A., Sehlin, J. and Täljedal, I. B. (1974a). *In* "Diabetes" (W. J. Malaisse and J. Pirart, eds), Proc. 8th Cong. Int. Diabetes Fed. p. 65. Excerpta Medica, Amsterdam.

Hellman, B., Idahl, L. A., Lernmark, A. and Täljedal, I. B. (1974b). *Biochem. J.* **138**, 33.

Hellman, B., Idahl, L. A., Lernmark, A. and Täljedal, I. B. (1974c). *Proc. natn. Acad. Sci. USA*, **71**, 3405.

Hellman, B., Idahl, L. A., Sehlin, J. and Täljedal, I. B. (1975a). *Diabetologia*, **11**, 495.

Hellman, B., Lernmark, A., Sehlin, J. and Täljedal, I. B. (1972a). *Biochem. Pharmacol.* **21**, 659.

Hellman, B. and Petersson, B. (1963). *Endocrinology*, **72**, 238.

Hellman, B., Sehlin, J., Söderberg, M. and Täljedal, I. B. (1975b). *J. Physiol.* **252**, 701.

Hellman, B., Sehlin, J. and Täljedal, I. B. (1969). *Med. exp.* **19**, 351.

Hellman, B., Sehlin, J. and Täljedal, I. B. (1971). *Am. J. Physiol.* **221**, 1795.

Hellman, B., Sehlin, J. and Täljedal, I. B. (1972b). *Endocrinology*, **90**, 335.

Hellman, B., Sehlin, J. and Täljedal, I. B. (1976a). *J. Physiol.* **254**, 639.

Hellman, B., Sehlin, J. and Täljedal, I. B. (1976b). *Horm. metab. Res.* **2**, 427.

Hellman, B. and Täljedal, I. B. (1975). *Handbuch exp. Pharm.* **32**, 175.

Henderson, J. R. (1970). *Lancet*, **ii**, 545.

Henderson, J. R. (1974). *Physiol. Rev.* **54**, 1.

Henderson, J. R., Jefferys, D. B., Jones, R. H. and Stanley, D. (1976). *Acta endocr., Copenh.* **83**, 772.

Hendricksen, C., Faber, O. K., Drejer, J. and Binder, C. (1977). *Diabetologia*, **13**, 615.

Henquin, J. C., Horemans, B., Nanquin, M., Verniers, J. and Lambert, A. E. (1975). *FEBS Letts*, **57**, 280.

Henquin, J. C. and Lambert, A. E. (1974a). *Diabetologia*, **10**, 788.

Henquin, J. C. and Lambert, A. E. (1974b). *Diabetes*, **23**, 933.

Henquin, J. C. and Lambert, A. E. (1975). *Am. J. Physiol.* **228**, 1669.

Herbert, V., Lau, K. S., Gottlieb, G. W. and Bleicher, W. (1965). *J. clin. Endocr. Metab.* **25**, 1375.

Herman, L., Sato, T. and Hales, C. N. (1973). *J. Ultrastruct. Res.* **42**, 298.

Hermann, L. S. and Deckert, T. (1977). *Acta endocr., Copenh.* **84**, 105.

Hicks, B. H., Taylor, C. I., Vij, S. K., Pek, S., Knopf, R. F., Floyd, J. C. and Fajans, S. S. (1977). *Metabolism*, **26**, 1011.

Hiebert, J. M., McCormick, J. M. and Egdahl, R. H. (1971). *Ann. Surg.* **176**, 296.

Hill, B. (1971). *J. gen. Physiol.* **58**, 599.

Hill, D. G., Sönksen, P. H. and Brainbridge, M. V. (1974). *J. thorac. cardiovasc. Surg.* **67**, 712.

Hinshaw, L. B., Peyton, M. D., Archer, L. T., Block, M. K., Coalson, J. J. and Greenfield, L. J. (1974). *Surg. Gynaecol. Obstet.* **145**, 198.

Hirsch, J. I., Fratkin, M. J., Wood, J. H. and Thomas, R. B. (1977). *Am. J. Hosp. Pharm.* **34**, 583.

Hjalmarson, A. (1968). *Acta endocr., Copenh.* **57** (Suppl. 126), 1.

Hofeldt, F. D., Lufkin, E. G., Hagler, L., Block, M. B., Dippe, S. E. and Davis, J. N. (1974). *Diabetes*, **23**, 589.

Hollands, E., Giron, B., Leny, T., Accary, J. P. and Rosi, C. (1976). *Gastroenterology*, **71**, 255.

Hollands, T. R. and Youson, J. H. (1973). *Anal. Biochem.* **54**, 413.

Holmgren, C., Falkmer, S. and Hambraeus, L. (1973). *Upsala J. med. Sci.* **78**, 215.

Horino, M., Machlin, L., Hertelendy, F. and Kipnis, D. M. (1968). *Endocrinology*, **83**, 118.

Horwitz, D. L., Rubenstein, A. H. and Katz, A. (1977). *Diabetes*, **26**, 30.

Horwitz, D. L., Rubenstein, A. H., Reynolds, C., Molnar, G. D. and Yanaihara, N. (1975a). *Horm. metab. Res.* **7**, 449.

Horwitz, D. L., Starr, J. I., Mako, M. E., Blackard, W. G. and Rubenstein, A. H. (1975b). *J. clin. Invest.* **54**, 1278.

Horwitz, D. L., Starr, J. I., Rubenstein, A. H. and Steiner, D. F. (1973). *Diabetes,* **22** (Suppl. 1), 298A.

Houssay, B. A. (1944). *Endocrinology,* **35**, 158.

Howell, S. L., Hellerström, C. and Tyhurst, M. (1974). *Horm. metab. Res.* **6**, 267.

Howell, S. L., Tyhurst, M. and Green, I. C. (1977). *Diabetologia,* **13**, 579.

Howell, S. L. and Whitfield, M. (1972). *Horm. metab. Res.* **4**, 349.

Huff, T. A., Horton, E. S. and Lebovitz, H. E. (1967). *New Engl. J. Med.* **277**, 837.

Humbel, R. E., Bosshard, H. R. and Zahn, H. (1972). *In* "Handbook of Physiology" (D. F. Steiner and N. Freinkel, eds.), Vol. 1, p. 159. Williams and Wilkins, Baltimore.

Illeni, M. T., Pellegris, G., Del Guercio, M. J., Tarantino, A., Bursetto, F., Di Pietro, C., Clerici, E., Garotta, G. and Chiumello, G. (1977). *Diabetes,* **26**, 870.

Imura, H., Seino, Y., Ikeda, M., Taminato, T., Miyamoto, Y. and Goto, Y. (1976). *Diabetes,* **25**, 961.

Ipp, E., Patton, G., Dobbs, R., Harris, E., Vale, W. and Unger, R. H. (1977). *Diabetes,* **26** (*Suppl.* 1), 359A.

Iversen, J. (1973a). *J. clin. Invest.* **52**, 2102.

Iversen, J. (1973b). *Diabetes,* **22**, 381.

Jacob, A., Hauri, C. and Froesch, E. R. (1968). *J. clin. Invest.* **47**, 2678.

Jain, K. and Logothetopoulos, J. (1977). *Diabetes,* **26**, 650.

Jansen, F. K., Munteferring, H. and Schmidt, W. A. K. (1977). *Diabetologia,* **13**, 545.

Jaspan, J. B., Mako, M. E., Kuzuya, H., Blix, P. M., Horwitz, D. L. and Rubenstein, A. H. (1977). *J. clin. Endocr. Metab.* **45**, 441.

Jayarao, K. S., Faulk, W. P., Karam, J. H., Grodsky, G. M. and Forsham, P. H. (1973). *J. immunol. Methods,* **3**, 337.

Jarhült, J. and Holst, J. J. (1977). *Experentia,* **33**, 236.

Jeffrey, P. D. (1974). *Biochemistry,* **13**, 4441.

Jeffrey, P. D., Milthorpe. B. K. and Nichol, L. W. (1972). *Biochemistry,* **15**, 4660.

John, H. J. (1949). *J. Paediatr.* **35**, 723.

Jolin, T. and Montes, A. (1974). *Horm. metab. Res.* **5**, 199.

Johnson, R. L., Guthrie, R. A., Murthy, D. Y. N. and Lang, J. (1973a). *Metabolism,* **22**, 247.

Johnson, S., Karam, J. H., Lenn, S. R., Grodsky, G. M. and Forsham, P. H. (1973b). *J. clin. Endocr. Metab.* **37**, 431.

Jones, R. H., Iron, D. I., Ellis, M. J., Sönksen, P. H. and Brandenburg, D. (1976). *Diabetologia,* **12**, 601.

Joost, H. G., Beckmann, J., Lenzen, S. and Hasselblatt, A. (1976). *Acta endocr., Copenh.* **82**, 121.

Jouppila, R. (1976). *Ann. chirur. gynaecol.* **65**, 398.

Jucci, A., Vignini, M., Pelfini, C., Criffo, A. and Fratino, P. (1977). *Arch. derm. Res.* **257**, 239.

Kahn, C. R. (1976). *J. Cell. Biol.* **70**, 261.

Kahn, C. R. and Baird, L. (1974). *Diabetes,* **26** (Suppl. 1), 354A.

Kahn, C. R., Baird, K., Flier, J. S. and David, B. (1977). *J. clin. Invest.* **60**, 1094.

Kahn, C. R., Megyesii, K. and Roth, J. (1976). *J. clin. Invest.* **57**, 526.

Kajinuma, H., Kaneto, A., Kuzuya, T. and Nakao, K. (1968). *J. clin. Endocr. Metab.* **28**, 1384.

Kalant, N., Lebovici, T. and Rohan, I. (1977). *Diabetes,* **26** (Suppl. 1), 357A.

Kalhan, S. C. and Adam, A. J. (1975). *J. clin. Endocr. Metab.* **41**, 600.

Kalkhoff, R. K., Richardson, B. L. and Beck, P. (1969). *Diabetes*, **18**, 153.

Kaneko, T., Oka, H., Munemura, M., Oda, T., Suzuki, S., Yasuda, H., Yanaihara, S., Nakagawa, S. and Makabe, K. (1975). *Endocr. jap.* **22**, 207.

Kaneko, T., Oda, T., Yamashita, K., Suzuki, S., Yanaihara, N., Hashimoto, T. and Yanaihara, C. (1974). *Endocr. jap.* **21**, 141.

Kaneto, A. (1977). *Metabolism*, **26**, 781.

Kaneto, A., Miki, E. and Kosaka, K. (1974). *Endocrinology*, **95**, 1005.

Kaniaris, P., Katsilambros, N., Castanas, E. and Theophanidis, C. (1975). *Anaesthes. Analges.* **54**, 718.

Karam, J. H., Grodsky, G. M. and Forsham, P. H. (1965). *Ann. N.Y. Acad. Sci.* **131**, 374.

Karam, J. H., Grodsky, G. M., Ching, K. N., Schmid, F., Burrill, K. and Forsham, P. H. (1974). *Diabetes*, **23**, 763.

Karamanos, B., Butterfield, W. J. H., Asmal, A. C. and Cox, B. D. (1971). *Postgrad. med. J.* (Suppl.), 440.

Karl, R. C., Zawalich, W. S., Ferrendelli, J. A. and Matschinsky, F. M. (1975). *J. biol. Chem.* **250**, 4575.

Katada, T. and Ui, M. (1977). *Diabetologia*, **13**, 521.

Katz, A. I. and Rubenstein, A. H. (1973). *J. clin. Invest.* **52**, 1113.

Kauffmann, U., Zapf, J., Torretti, B. and Froesch, E. R. (1977). *J. clin. Endocr. Metab.* **44**, 160.

Kawamori, K., Shichiri, M., Inoue, M. and Hoshi, M. (1977). *Diabetes*, **26** (Suppl. 1), 404A.

Kawazu, S., Kanazawa, Y., Kajinuma, H., Miki, E., Kuzuya, T. and Kosaka, K. (1975). *Diabetologia*, **11**, 169.

Kerp, L. and Kasemir, H. (1976). *Acta endocr., Copenh.* **83** (Suppl. 205), 211.

Kiang, D. T., Bauer, G. E. and Kennedy, B. J. (1973). *Cancer*, **31**, 801.

Kimmerling, G., Javorski, W. C. and Reaven, G. M. (1977). *J. Am. Geriatr. Soc.* **25**, 349.

Kitabchi, A. E. (1970). *J. clin. Invest.* **49**, 879.

Kitabchi, A. E. (1977). *Metabolism*, **26**, 547.

Kitagawa, T. and Aikawa, T. (1976). *J. biochem.* **79**, 233.

Kizer, J. S., Vargas-Cordon, M., Brendel, K. and Bressler, R. (1970). *J. clin. Invest.* **49**, 1942.

Klimt, C. R., Prout, T. E., Bradley, R. F., Dolger, H., Fisher, G., Gastineau, C. F., Marks, H., Meinert, C. L. and Schumacher, O. P. (1969). *Diabetes*, **18**, 299.

Klöppel, G. and Schäfer, H. J. (1976). *Diabetologia*, **12**, 227.

Kneer, N. M., Bosch, A. L., Clark, M. G. and Lardy, H. A. (1974). *Proc. natn. Acad. Sci. USA*, **71**, 4523.

Knopf, R. F., Conn, J. W., Floyd, J. C., Fajans, S. S., Rull, A. J., Guntsche, E. M. and Thiffault, C. A. (1966). *Am. J. Physicians*, **79**, 312.

Kobayashi, M. and Meck, J. G. (1977). *Diabetologia*, **13**, 251.

Kobayashi, M. and Olefsky, J. M. (1977). *Diabetes*, **26** (Suppl. 1), 405A.

Koerker, D. J., Ruch, W., Chideckel, E., Palmer, J., Goodner, C. J., Ensinck, J. and Gale, C. C. (1974). *Science*, **184**, 482.

Kohnert, K. D., Jahr, H., Schmidt, S., Hahn, H. J. and Zuhlke, H. (1976). *Biochim. biophys. Acta*, **422**, 2115.

Kohnert, K. D., Schmidt, E., Zühlke, H. and Fiedler, H. (1973). *J. Chromatogr.* **76**, 263.

Krause, U., Puchinger, H. and Wacker, A. (1973). *Horm. metab. Res.* **5**, 140.

156   U. A. PARMAN

Kruss-Jarres, J. D., Hilpert, C., Ross, H. J., Grohman, K. and Kling Müller, V. (1970).
    In "International Congress Series", Vol. 209, p. 159. Excerpta Medica, Amsterdam.
Kühl, C. (1975). *Acta endocr., Copenh.* **79**, 709.
Kühl, C. (1976a). *Diabetologia,* **12**, 295.
Kühl, C. (1976b). *Diabetes,* **25**, 16.
Kühl, C., Jensen, S. L. and Nielsen, O. V. (1976). *Endocrinology,* **99**, 1667.
Kuo, W., Hodgins, D. S. and Kuo, J. F. (1974). *Biochem. Pharmacol.* **23**, 1387.
Kurosky, A., Markel, D. E., Peterson, J. W. and Fitch, W. M. (1977). *Science,* **195**, 299.
Kurt, T. L., Genton, E., Chidsey, C., Beck, P. and Sussman, K. E. (1973). *Chest,* **64**, 21.
Kuzuya, H., Blix, P. M., Horwitz, D. L., Steiner, D. F. and Rubenstein, A. H. (1977).
    Diabetes, **26**, 22.
Kuzuya, T. and Matsuda, A. (1976). *Diabetologia,* **12**, 519.
Kuzuya, T., Matsuda, A., Saito, Y. and Yoshida, S. (1976). *Diabetologia,* **12**, 511.
Lacy, P. E. (1970). *Diabetes,* **19**, 895.
Lacy, P. E., Klein, N. J. and Fink, C. J. (1973). *Endocrinology,* **92**, 1458.
Lacy, P. E., Walker, M. M. and Fink, C. J. (1972). *Diabetes,* **21**, 987.
Lager, I., Lundquist, G. and Dotevall, G. (1976). *Scand. J. Gastroent.* (Suppl. 41), p. 18.
Lakatua, D. J., Haus, E., Gold, E. M. and Halberg, F. (1974). *In* "Chronobiology".
    (L. E. Schering, F. Halberg and J. E. Pawley, eds.), p. 88. Georg Thieme, Stuttgart.
Lambert, A. E., Henquin, J. C. and Malvaux, P. (1974a). *Endocrinology,* **95**, 1069.
Lambert, A. E., Henquin, J. C. and Malvaux, P. (1974b). *Horm. metab. Res.* **6**, 470.
Landgraf, R., Landgraf-Leurs, M. M. C., Weissman, A., Horl, R., von Werder, K.
    and Scriba, P. C. (1977). *Diabetologia,* **13**, 99.
Laron, Z., Mimoun, M., Josefberg, Z., Zadic, Z. and Doron, M. (1977). *Diabetologia,*
    13, 447.
Lau, T. S., Taubenfligel, W., Levenge, R., Farago, L. G., Chan, H., Koren, I. and
    Drucker, W. R. (1972). *J. Trauma,* **12**, 880.
Lauvaux, J. P., Mandart, G., Heymans, G. and Ooms, H. A. (1972). *Horm. metab. Res.*
    4, 58.
Lawrence, A. M. (1967). *Ann. int. Med.* **66**, 1099.
Lazarus, N. R., Gutman, R. A., Penhos, J. C. and Recant, L. (1972). *Diabetologia,* **8**,
    131.
Lazarus, N. R., Gutman, R. A. and Recant, L. (1971). *Anal. Biochem.* **40**, 241.
Lazarus, S. S. and Bencosme, S. A. (1955). *Proc. Soc. exp. Biol. Med.* **89**, 114.
Lazarus, S. S. and Volk, B. W. (1959). *Proc. Soc. exp. Biol. Med.* **102**, 67.
Leblanc, H., Lachelin, G. C., Abu-Fadl, S. and Yen, S. S. G. (1977). *J. clin. Endocr.
    Metab.* **44**, 196.
Lebovitz, H. E. and Feldman, J. M. (1973). *Fed. Proc.* **32**, 1797.
Ledward, R. S., Paterson, F. J. and Turner, R. L. (1974). *J. Obstet. Gynaecol. Brit.
    Cmwlth* **81**, 545.
Lefebvre, P. and Luyckx, A. S. (1973). *Biochem, Pharmacol.* **22**, 1773.
Leichter, S. B. and Galasky, S. P. (1977). *Diabetes,* **26**, 406A.
Leitner, J. W., Sussman, K. E., Vatter, A. E. and Schneider, V. (1975). *Endocrinology,*
    96, 662.
Le Marchand, T., Jean-Renaud, B. and Freychet, P. (1977a). *Diabetes,* **26**, 355A.
Le Marchand, Y., Loten, E. G., Assimacopoulos-Jeannet, F., Forgue, M. E., Freychet,
    P. and Jean-Renaud, B. (1977b). *Diabetes,* **26**, 582.
Lendrum, R., Walker, G., Cudworth, A. G., Woodrow, J. C. and Gamble, D. R. (1976).
    Br. med. J. **1**, 1565.
Lenzen, S. (1976). *Endokrinologie,* **68**, 189.

Lenzen, S. (1978a). *Diabetes*, **27**, 234.

Lenzen, S. (1978b). *J. Endocr.* **77**, 11.

Lenzen, S. (1978c). *Metabolism*, **27**, 81.

Lenzen, S. and Hasselblatt, A. (1974). *Naunyn-Schmiedeberg's Arch. Pharmacol.* **282**, 317.

Lenzen, S., Joost, H. G. and Hasselblatt, A. (1976a). *Endokrinologie*, **99**, 125.

Lenzen, S., Joost, H. G. and Hasselblatt, A. (1976b). *Diabetologia*, **12**, 495.

Lenzen, S. and Klöppel, G. (1978). *Endocrinology*, **103**, 1546.

Lenzen, S., Panten, U. and Hasselblatt, A. (1975). *Diabetologia*, **11**, 49.

Lerner, L. (1977). *J. clin. Endocr. Metab.* **45**, 1.

Lerner, L. and Porte, D. (1971). *J. clin. Endocr. Metab.* **33**, 409.

Lernmark, A., Chen, S. I., Choy, R., Nathans, A., Carroll, R., Tager, H. S., Rubenstein, A. H., Swift, H. H. and Steiner, D. F. (1976). *In* "Polypeptide Hormones: Molecular and Cellular Aspects." Ciba Foundation Symposium 41 (New Series), p. 7, Excerpta Medica, Amsterdam.

Lernmark, A., Parman, A. and Tahjedal, I. B. (1977). *Biochem. J.* **166**, 181.

Levin, S., Charles, M. A., O'Connor, M. and Grodsky, G. M. (1975). *Am. J. physiol.* **229**, 49.

Levin, S., Reed, J. W., Ching, K., Davis, J. W., Blum, M. K. and Forsham, P. H. (1973). *Diabetes*, **22**, 194.

Lewis, S. B., Waller, J. D., Kuzuya, H., Murray, W. R., Constan, D. R., Daane, T. A. and Rubenstein, A. H. (1976). *Diabetologia*, **12**, 343.

Lieberman, L. L. (1968). *Lancet*, **1**, 148.

Lin, B. J. (1977). *Diabetologia*, **13**, 77.

Lind, T., Billewicz, W. Z. and Brown, G. (1973). *J. Obstet. Gynaecol. Brit. Cwlth*, **80**, 1033.

Lind, T., Gilmore, E. A. and McClarence, M. (1975). *Br. J. Obstet. Gynaecol.* **82**, 562.

Lindall, A. W., Steffes, M. W. and Wong, E. T. (1974). *Metabolism*, **23**, 249.

Lindsten, J., Cerasi, E., Luft, R. and Hultquist, G. (1967). *Acta endocr., Copenh.* **56**, 107.

Lindsten, J., Cerasi, E., Luft, R., Morton, N. and Ryman, N. (1976). *Clin. Genet.* **10**, 125.

Long, C. L., Spencer, J. L., Kinnery, J. M. and Geiger, J. W. (1971). *J. appl. Physiol.* **31**, 110.

Loo, S. W., Hirsch, H. J. and Gabbay, K. H. (1947). *Diabetes*, **26** (Suppl. 1), 407A.

Los Monteros, E., Driscoll, S. G. and Steinke, J. (1970). *Science*, **168**, 1111.

Loubatières, A. L., Mariani, M. M., Ribes, G. and Alrich, R. (1973a). *Acta diabet. lat.* **10**, 261.

Loubatières-Mariani, M. M., Chapal, J., Alric, R. and Loubatières, A. (1973b). *Diabetologia*, **9**, 439.

Low, B. W., Fullerton, W. W. and Rosen, L. S. (1974). *Nature, Lond.* **248**, 339.

Lowe, D. A., Richardson, B. P., Donatsch, P. and Buchelli, E. (1976). *Diabetologia*, **12**, 407A.

Ludvigsson, J. and Heding, L. G. (1976). *Diabetologia*, **12**, 627.

Ludvigsson, J. and Heding, L. G. (1977). *Acta endocr., Copenh.* **85**, 364.

Ludvigsson, J., Safwenberger, J. and Heding, L. G. (1977). *Acta paediatr. Scand.* **66**, 177.

Lundquist, I. and Lördahl, R. (1975). *Horm. metab. Res.* **7**, 6.

Lundquist, I., Sundler, F., Håkanson, R., Larsson, L. I. and Heding, L. G. (1975). *Endocrinology*, **97**, 137.

Lunn, P. G., Whitehead, R. G., Hay, R. W. and Baker, B. A. (1973). *Br. J. Nutr.* **29**, 399.

Lütjens, A. and Smit, J. L. J. (1976). *Helv. paediatr. Acta*, **31**, 473.

Macchi, I. A. and Zeytinoğlu, F. N. (1976). *Horm. metab. Res.* **8**, 92.

Mackrell, D. J. and Sokal, J. E. (1969). *Diabetes*, **18**, 724.

Madison, L. L., Mebane, R., Unger, R. H. and Lochrer, H. (1964). *J. clin. Invest.* **43**, 408.

Maher, T. D., Tannenberg, R. J., Greenberg, B. Z., Hoffman, J. E. and Doe, R. P. (1977). *Diabetes*, **26**, 196.

Maier, V., Schneider, C., Schatz, H. and Pfeiffer, E. (1975). *Hoppeseyler's Z. physiol. Chem.* **356**, 887.

Malaisse, W. J. (1972). *In* "Handbook of Physiology and Endocrinology" (R. O. Greep and E. B. Astwood, eds.), Vol. I, Section 7, p. 237. Am. Physiol. Soc., Washington, D.C.

Malaisse, W. J., Brisston, W. G. R. and Baird, L. E. (1973a). *Am. J. Physiol.* **224**, 389.

Malaisse, W. J., Mahy, M., Brisson, G. R. and Malaisse-Lagae, F. (1972). *Eur. J. clin. Invest.* **2**, 85.

Malaisse, W. J., Malaisse-Lagae, F. and King, S. (1968). *Diabetologia*, **4**, 370.

Malaisse, W. J., Malaisse-Lagae, F. and McCraw, E. F. (1967). *Diabetes*, **16**, 643.

Malaisse, W. J., Obberghen, E. V., Devis, G., Somers, G. and Ravazzola, M. (1974). *Eur. J. clin. Invest.* **4**, 313.

Malaisse, W. J., Pipeleers, D. G. and Mahy, M. (1973b). *Diabetes*, **19**, 1.

Malaisse, W. J., Sener, A., Devis, G. and Somers, G. (1976a). *Horm. metab. Res.* **8**, 434.

Malaisse, W. J., Sener, A., Kawazu, S. and Boschero, A. C. (1977). *Diabetologia*, **13**, 416.

Malaisse, W. J., Sener, A., Koser, M., Ravazzola, M. and Malaisse-Lagae, F. (1976b). *Diabetologia*, **12**, 408A.

Malaisse-Lagae, F., Greider, M. H., Malaisse, W. J. and Lacy, P. E. (1971). *J. cell. Biol.* **49**, 530.

Malaisse-Lagae, F. and Malaisse, W. J. (1971). *Endocrinology*, **88**, 72.

Malaisse-Lagae, F., Ravazzola, M., Amherdt, M., Gutzeit, A., Stauffacher, W., Malaisse, W. J. and Orci, L. (1975). *Diabetologia*, **10**, 71.

Maldonato, A., Truehart, P. A., Renold, A. E. and Sharp, G. W. G. (1976). *Diabetologia*, **12**, 471.

Malharbe, C., de Gasparo, M., Dettertogh, R. and Hoet, J. J. (1969). *Diabetologia*, **5**, 379.

Malvano, R., Zucchelli, G. C., Quesada, T., Gandolfi, C. and Piro, M. A. (1974). *J. nucl. Biol. Med.* **18**, 80.

Mandour, T., Kissebah, A. H. and Wynn, V. (1977). *Eur. J. clin. Invest.* **7**, 181.

Manecchi, F., Pilo, A., Citti, L. and Navalesi, R. (1977). *Diabetologia*, **13**, 417A.

Manku, M. S. and Horrobin, D. F. (1976). *Lancet*, **ii**, 1115.

Mann, M. D., Becker, D., Pimstone, B. L. and Hansen, D. L. (1975). *Br. J. Nutr.* **33** 55.

Manny, J., Rabinovici, N. and Schiller, M. (1977). *Surg. Gynaecol. Obstet.* **145**, 198.

Marco, J., Calle, C., Hedo, J. A. and Villanueva, M. L. (1976). *Diabetologia*, **12**, 307.

Marco, J., Hedo, J. A. and Villanueva, M. L. (1977). *Diabetes*, **26** (Suppl. 1), 381A.

Marks, V. and Alberti, K. G. M. M. (1976). *Clin. Endocr. Metab.* **5**, 805.

Marks, V. and Samols, E. (1974). *Clin. Gastroent.* **3**, 559.

Markussen, J. and Heding, L. G. (1976). *Int. J. Peptide Protein, Res.* **8**, 597.

Marrigay, D., de Ruyter, H. A., Touber, J. L., Croughs, R. J. M., Schopman, W. and Lequin, R. M. (1967). *Lancet*, **i**, 361.

Martin, F. I. R. (1976). *Am. J. Obstet. Gynecol.* **125**, 71.

Martin, J. M., Akerblom, H. K. and Garay, G. (1968). *Diabetes*, **77**, 661.

Martin, J. M., Mok, C. C., Penfold, J., Howard, N. J. and Crowne, D. (1973). *J. Endocr.* **58**, 681.

Massara, F., Camanni, F., Martelli, S. and Molinatti, G. M. (1977). *Diabetologia*, **13**, 417A.

Massara, R. P. (1974). *Gastroenterology*, **66**, 1058.

Massi-Benedetti, F., Falorni, A., Luyckx, A. and Lefebvre, P. (1974). *Horm. metab. Res.* **6**, 392.

Matschinsky, F. M. and Ellerman, J. (1973). *Biochem. Biophys. Res. Commun.* **50**, 193.

Matthews, E. K. (1970). *Acta diabetol. lat.* **7** (Suppl. 1), 83.

Matute, M. L. and Kalkhoff, R. K. (1973). *Endocrinology*, **92**, 762.

McCarthy, S. T., Harris, E. and Turner, R. C. (1977). *Diabetologia*, **13**, 93.

McDaniel, M. L., King, S., Anderson, S., Fink, J. and Lacy, P. E. (1974). *Diabetologia*, **10**, 303.

McDaniel, M. L. and Lacy, P. E. (1975). *Diabetes*, **24** (Suppl. 1), 400A.

McGuire, E. A., Tobin, J., Berman, M. and Andres, P. (1977). *Diabetes*, **26** (Suppl. 1), 408A.

McIntyre, N., Holdsworth, C. D. and Turner, D. S. (1964). *Lancet*, **ii**, 201.

McNamara, J. J., Motot, M. D., Dunn, R. A. and Stremple, J. F. (1972). *Ann. Surg.* **176**, 247.

Meguid, M. M., Aun, F. and Soeldner, J. (1975). *Surg. Forum*, **26**, 37.

Meguid, M. M., Aun, F. and Soeldner, J. S. (1976). *Surgery*, **79**, 177.

Megyesi, K., Gordon, P. and Kahn, C. R. (1977). *J. clin. Endocr. Metab.* **45**, 330.

Megyesi, K., Kahn, C. R., Roth, J. and Gorden, P. (1974). *J. clin. Endocr. Metab.* **38**, 931.

Megyesi, K., Kahn, C. R., Roth, J. and Gorden, P. (1975). *J. clin. Endocr. Metab.* **41**, 475.

Megyesi, K., Kahn, C. R., Roth, J., Neville, D. M. and Nissley, S. P. (1973). *J. biol. Chem.* **250**, 8990.

Megyesi, K., Samols, E. and Marks, V. (1967). *Lancet*, **ii**, 1051.

Meissner, H. P. (1976). *Diabetologia*, **12**, 409A.

Meissner, H. P. and Attwater, E. (1976). *Horm. metab. Res.* **8**, 11.

Melani, F., Rubenstein, A. H., Oyer, P. E. and Steiner, D. F. (1970). *Proc. natn. Acad. Sci. USA*, **67**, 148.

Melani, F., Verillo, A., Marasco, M., Rivellese, A., Osorio, J. and Bertolini, M. G. (1976). *Horm. metab. Res.* **8**, 85.

Menczel, J., Levy, M. and Bentwich, Z. (1966). *Isr. J. Med.* **2**, 764.

Mennear, J. H., Schouwaller, C. and Yan, E. T. (1976). *Diabetologia*, **12**, 263.

Merimee, T. J. and Fineberg, S. E. (1973). *J. clin. Endocr. Metab.* **37**, 698.

Merimee, T. J. and Pulkkinen, A. J. (1977). *J. clin. Endocr. Metab.* **45**, 232.

Merimee, T. J. and Tyson, J. E. (1977). *Diabetes*, **26**, 161.

Metz, S., Halter, J., Porte, D. and Robertson, R. P. (1977). *Diabetes*, **26** (Suppl. 1), 378.

Metzger, B. E., Unger, R. A. and Freinkel, N. (1977). *Metabolism*, **26**, 151.

Meuli, C. and Froesch, E. R. (1976). *Arch. Biochem. Biophys.* **177**, 31.

Milner, R. D. G. and Wirdham, P. K. (1977). *Diabetologia*, **13**, 636.

Mirouze, J., Selan, J. L., Pham, T. C. and Cavadore, D. (1977). *Diabetologia*, **13**, 273.

Molsted-Pedersen, L., Trantner, H. and Jorgensen, K. R. (1973). *Acta paediatr. Scand.* **62**, 11.

Montague, W. and Howell, S. L. (1975). *In* "Advances in Cyclic Nucleotide Research" (P. Greengard and G. A. Robison, eds), Vol. 6, p. 201. Raven Press, New York.

Montague, W. and Taylor, K. W. (1969). *Biochem. J.* **115**, 257.

Moody, A. J., Stan, M. A., Stan, M. and Gliemann, J. (1974). *Horm. metab. Res.* **6**, 12.

Moorhouse, J. A. (1969). *Diabetologia*, **5**, 269A.

Morgan, C. K. and Lazarow, A. (1963). *Diabetes*, **12**, 114.

Morrell, B. and Froesch, E. R. (1976). *Arch. Biochem. Biophys.* **177**, 31.

Morris, G. E. and Korner, A. (1970). *Biochim. biophys. Acta*, **208**, 404.

Moustaffa, B. E., Daggett, P. R. and Nabarro, J. D. N. (1977). *Diabetologia*, **13**, 311.

Müller, W. A., Aoki, T. T., Egdahl, R. E. and Cahill, G. F. (1977). *Diabetologia*, **13**, 55.

Müller, E. E., Sawano, S., Arimura, A. and Schally, A. V. (1967). *Acta endocr., Copenh.* **56**, 499.

Naber, S. P., McDaniel, M. L. and Lacy, P. E. (1976). *Diabetes*, **25** (Suppl. 1), 346A.

Naismith, D. J. and Fears, R. B. (1972). *Proc. Nutr. Soc.* **31**, 79A.

Naithani, V. K. (1973). *Hoppe Seyler's Z. physiol. Chem.* **354**, 659.

Naithani, V. K., Dechesne, M., Markussen, J. and Heding, L. G. (1975a). *Hoppe Seyler's Z. physiol. Chem.* **356**, 987.

Naithani, V. K., Dechesne, M., Markussen, J. and Heding, L. G. (1975b). *Hoppe Seyler's Z. physiol. Chem.* **356**, 1305.

Nakao, K. and Miyata, M. (1977). *Eur. J. clin. Invest.* **7**, 41.

Navalesi, R., Pilo, A. and Ferrannini, E. (1976). *Am. J. Physiol.* **230**, 1630.

Nelson, K. L., Go, V. L. and Service, F. J. (1977). *Diabetes*, **26**, 410A.

Nelson, P. G., Pyke, D. A., Cudworth, A. G., Woodrow, J. C. and Batchelor, J. R. (1975). *Lancet*, **ii**, 193.

Nerup, J., Platz, P., Anderson, O. O., Christy, M., Lyngsoe, J., Poulsen, J. E., Kyder, L. P., Nielsen, L. S., Tomsen, M. and Svejgaard, A. (1974). *Lancet*, **ii**, 864.

Nestel, P. J., Austin, W. and Foxman, C. (1969). *J. Lipid Res.* **10**, 383.

Newsholme, E. A. (1976). *Clin. Endocr. Metab.* **5**, 543.

Niki, A. and Niki, H. (1976). *In* "Endocrine Gut and Pancreas" (T. Fujita, ed.), p. 225. Elsevier, Amsterdam

Nikkila, E. and Tashkinen, M. (1975). *Diabetes*, **24**, 933.

Nitzan, M., Freinkel, N., Metzger, B. E., Unger, R. H., Faloona, G. R. and Daniel, R. R. (1975). *Isr. J. med. Sci.* **11**, 617.

Nolan, S., Stephan, T., Chae, S., Vidalon, C., Gegick. C., Khurana, R. C. and Danowski, T. S. (1973). *J. am. Geriatr. Soc.* **21**, 106.

Notelowitz, M. and James, S. (1974). *Obstet. Gynaecol.* **48**, 268.

Notelowitz, M. and James, S. (1977). *Horm. metab. Res.* **9**, 105.

Nuñez-Correa, J., Lowy, C. and Sonksen, P. H. (1974). *Lancet*, **i**, 837.

Oakley, N. W., Monier, D. and Wynn, U. (1973). *Diabetologia*, **9**, 235.

Obberghen, E. V., Devis, G., Somers, G., Ravazzola, M., Malaisse-Lagae, F. and Malaisse, W. J. (1974). *Eur. J. clin. Invest.* **4**, 307.

Obberghen, E. V., Somers, G., Devis, G., Vaughan, G. D., Malaisse-Lagae, F., Orci, L. and Malaisse, W. J. (1973). *J. clin. Invest.* **52**, 1041.

O'Connor, M. D. L., Landahl, H. D. and Grodsky, G. M. (1977). *Endocrinology*, **101**, 85.

Ohara, H. (1976). *In* "Endocrine Gut and Pancreas" (T. Fujita, ed.), p. 321. Elsevier, Amsterdam.

Ohneda, A., Matsuda, K., Sato, M., Yamagata, S. and Sato, T. (1974). *Diabetes*, **23**, 41.

Oka, T., Matsuda, I., Nambu, H., Nagai, B., Mitsuyama, T. and Arashima, S. (1977). *Eur. J. Pediatr.* **125**, 191.

Olefsky, J. M. (1967a). *J. clin. Invest.* **58**, 1450.

Olefsky, J. M. (1976b). *J. clin. Invest.* **57**, 1165.

Olefsky, J. M. (1976c). *J. clin. Invest.* **57**, 842.

Olefsky, J. M., Farquhar, J. W. and Reaven, G. M. (1973). *Diabetes*, **22**, 202.

Olefsky, J. M., Farquhar, J. W. and Reaven, G. M. (1974). *Am. J. Med.* **57**, 551.

Olefsky, J. M. and Reaven, G. M. (1974a). *J. clin. Invest.* **54**, 1323.

Olefsky, J. M. and Reaven, G. M. (1974b). *Diabetes*, **23**, 449.

Olefksy, J. M. and Reaven, G. M. (1976). *Am. J. Med.* **60**, 89.

Olefsky, J. M. and Reaven, G. M. (1977). *Diabetes*, **26**, 680.

Orci, L. (1974). *Diabetologia*, **10**, 163.

Orci, L., Amherdt, M., Malaisse-Lagae, F., Rouiller, C. and Renold, A. E. (1973a). *Science*, **179**, 82.

Orci, L., Amherdt, M., Stauffacher, W., Like, A. A., Rouiller, C. and Renold, A. E. (1972). *Diabetes*, **21** (Suppl. 1), 326A.

Orci, L., Baetens, D., Rufener, C., Amherdt, M., Ravazzola, M., Studer, P., Malaisse-Lagae, F. and Unger, R. (1975). *Proc. natn. Acad. Sci. USA*, **73**, 1338.

Orci, L., Malaisse-Lagae, F., Ravazzola, M., Amherdt, M. and Renold, A. E. (1973b). *Science*, **181**, 561.

Orci, L. and Unger, R. H. (1975). *Lancet*, **ii**, 1243.

Orsetti, A., Collard, F. and Jaffiol, C. (1974). *Acta diabetol. lat.* **11**, 486.

Ørskov, H. (1967). *Scand. J. clin. Lab. Invest*, **20**, 297.

Ørskov, H. and Christensen, N. J. (1969). *Diabetes*, **18**, 653.

Ørskov, H. and Johansen, K. (1972). *Acta endocr., Copenh.* **71**, 697.

Ørskov, H. and Seyer-Hansen, K. (1974). *Eur. J. clin. Invest.* **4**, 207.

Oseid, S. (1973). *Acta endocr., Copenh.* **72**, 475.

Östenson, C. G., Anderson, A., Brolin, S. E., Petersson, B. and Hellerstrom, C. (1977). *In* "Glucagon: its role in Physiological and Clinical Medicine", p. 243. Springer-Verlag, Berlin.

Ostlund, R. E. (1977). *Diabetes*, **26**, 245.

Owens, D. R., Seldrup, J., Wragg, K. G., Shetty, K. J. and Biggs, P. I. (1977). *Horm. metab. Res.* **9**, 347.

Pace, C. S. and Matschinsky, F. M. (1974). *Biochim. biophys. Acta*, **354**, 188.

Pace, C. S., Matschinsky, F. M., Lacy, P. E. and Conant, S. (1977). *Biochim. biophys. Acta*, **497**, 408.

Pace, C. S. and Price, S. (1972). *Biochem. Biophys. Res. Commun.* **46**, 1557.

Padron, J. L., Hunt, C. and Lewis, N. (1972). *Japan. J. med. Sci. Biol.* **25**, 57.

Padron, J. L., Sulman, M. and Lewis, N. R. (1967). *Nature, Lond.* **213**, 1254.

Pallotta, J. A. and Kennedy, P. J. (1968). *Metabolism*, **17**, 901.

Palmer, J. P., Benson, J. W., Walter, K. M. and Ensinck, J. (1976a). *J. clin. Invest.* **58**, 565.

Palmer, J. P. and Ensinck, J. (1975). *J. clin. Endocr. Metab.* **41**, 498.

Palmer, J. P., Walter, R. M. and Ensinck, J. W. (1976b). *Diabetes*, **24**, 735.

Panten, U. and Christians, J. (1973). *Naunyn-Schmiedeberg's Arch. Pharmacol.* **276**, 55.

Park, B. N., Soeldner, J. S. and Gleason, R. E. (1974). *Diabetes*, **23**, 616.

Parman, U. A. (1975a). *J. Endocr.* **67**, 1.

Parman, U. A. (1975b). *J. Endocr.* **67**, 19.

Parra-Cavarrubias, A., Rivera-Rodriguez, I. and Almaraz-Ugalde, A. (1971). *Diabetes*, **20**, 800.

Passa, P., Rousselie, F., Gauville, C. and Canivet, J. (1977). *Diabetes*, **26**, 113.

Passwell, J., Boichis, H., Lotan, D., David, R., Theodor, R., Cohn, B. E. and Many, M. (1977). *Am. J. Dis. Child.* **131**, 1011.

Patton, G. S., Dobbs, R., Orci, L., Vale, W. and Unger, R. H. (1976). *Metabolism*, **25** (Suppl. 1), 1499A.

Paulsen, E. P. (1976). *Diabetes*, **25** (Suppl. 1), 334A.

Paz, G., Homonnai, Z. T., Ayalon, D., Cordora, T. and Kraicer, P. F. (1977). *Fertil. Steril*, **28**, 836.

Pedersen, D. C., Brown, J. C., Tobin, J. D. and Andres, R. (1975). *Clin. Res.* **24**, 455A.

Pedersen, A., Drysburg, J. R. and Brown, J. C. (1973). *Can. J. Pharm.* **53**, 1200.

Pek, S., Tai, T. Y., Crowther, R. and Fajans, S. S. (1976). *Diabetes*, **25**, 764.

Pekar, A. H. and Frank, B. H. (1972). *Biochemistry*, **11**, 4013.

Pelletier, G. (1977). *Diabetes*, **26**, 749.

Peracchi, M., Cavagnini, F., Pinto, M., Bulgeroni, P. and Panerai, E. (1975). *Horm. metab. Res.* **7**, 437.

Permutt, M. A. (1976). *Diabetes*, **25**, 719.

Permutt, M. A., Biesbroeck, J. and Chyn, R. (1977). *J. clin. Endocr. Metab.* **44**, 536.

Permutt, M. A., Biesbroeck, J., Chyn, R., Buime, I., Szcziesna, E. and McWilliams, D. (1976). *In* "Polypeptide Hormones: Molecular and Cellular Aspects", Ciba Foundation Symposium 41 (New Series), p. 97. Exerpta Medica, Amsterdam.

Permutt, M. A. and Kipnis, D. M. (1975). *Fed. Proc.* **34**, 1549.

Persson, B., Gentz, J., Kellum, M. and Thorell, J. (1976). *Acta paediat. Scand.* **65**, 1.

Persson, B. and Lunnel, N. O. (1975). *Am. J. Obstet. Gynaecol.* **122**, 737.

Peterson, J. D., Coulter, C. L. and Steiner, D. F. (1974). *Nature, Lond.* **251**, 239.

Peterson, J. D., Steiner, D. F., Emdin, S. O. and Falkmar, S. (1975). *J. biol. Chem.* **250**, 5183.

Pfeiffer, E. and Telib, M. (1968). *Acta diabetol. Lat.* **5** (Suppl. 1), 30.

Phelps, R. L., Bergenstahl, R., Freinkel, N., Rubenstein, A. H., Metzger, B. E., Mako, M. E. (1975). *J. clin. Endocr. Metab.* **41**, 1085.

Phillips, A. P., Webb, B. and Curry, A. S. (1972). *J. for. Sci.* **17**, 460.

Pildes, R. S. (1973). *Metabolism*, **22**, 307.

Pilkis, S. and Park, R. (1974). *Ann. Rev. Pharmacol.* **14**, 365.

Pimstone, B. L., Kronheim, S. and Berkowitz, M. (1977). *Diabetes*, **26** (Suppl. 1), 359.

Podolsky, S. and Burrows, B. A. (1977). *Diabetes*, **26**, 411A.

Podolsky, S., Zimmerman, H. J., Burrows, B. A., Cardarelli, J. A. and Pattavina, C. G. (1973). *New Engl. J. Med.* **288**, 644.

Poffenbarger, P. L. (1975). *J. clin. Invest.* **56**, 1455.

Pontiroli, A. E., Vibert, G. C., Tognetti, A. and Pozza, G. (1975). *Diabetologia*, **11**, 165.

Porte, D., Smith, P. H. and Ensinck, J. W. (1976). *Metabolism*, **25** (Suppl. 1), 1453.

Posner, B. I., Josefberg, Z. and Bergeron, J. J. M. (1977). *Diabetes*, **26** (Suppl. 1), 368.

Powley, T. L. and Opsahl, C. A. (1974). *Am. J. Physiol.* **226**, 25.

Prakash, R. and Chhablani, R. (1974). *Chest*, **65**, 408.

Price, S. (1973). *Biochim. biophys. Acta*, **318**, 459.

Pronina, T. S. and Sapronova, A. Ya. (1976). *In* "The Evolution of Pancreatic Islets" (T. A. Grillo, L. Leibson and A. Epple, eds), p. 25. Pergamon Press, London.

Pruett, E. D. R. (1970). *J. appl. Physiol.* **28**, 199.

Pruett, E. D. R. (1971). *Diabetologia*, **7**, 398A.

Puchinger, H. and Wacker, A. (1972). *FEBS Letts*, **21**, 14.

Pullen, R. A., Lindsay, D. G., Wood, S. P., Tickle, J., Blundell, T. L., Willmer, A.,

Krail, G., Brandenburg, D., Zahn, H., Gliemann, J. and Gammeltoft, S. (1976). *Nature, Lond.* **259**, 369.

Pyke, D. A., Theophanides, C. G. and Tattersall, R. (1976). *Lancet*, **ii**, 464.

Rabinowitz, D., Spitz, I., Gonen, B. and Paran, E. (1973). *J. clin. Endocr. Metab.* **36**, 901.

Raitini, S., Lifschitz, F., Trias, E. and Sigman, B. (1974). *Acta endocr., Copenh.* **76**, 506.

Raptis, S., Dollinger, H. C., Schröder, K. E., Schleyer, M., Rothenburger, G. and Pfeiffer, E. (1975). *New Engl. J. Med.* **288**, 1199.

Raskin, P., Fujita, Y. and Unger, R. H. (1975). *J. clin. Invest.* **56**, 1132.

Rasmussen, S. M., Heding, L. G., Parbst, E. and Volund, A. (1975). *Diabetologia*, **11**, 151.

Ravazzola, M., Malaisse-Lagae, F., Amherdt, M., Perrelet, A., Malaisse, W. J. and Orci, L. (1976). *J. cell. Sci.* **27**, 107.

Rayfield, E. J., Curnow, R. T., Reinhard, D. and Kochicheril, N. M. (1977). *J. clin. Endocr. Metab.* **45**, 513.

Rayfield, E. J., Görelkin, L., Curnow, R. T. and Jahrling, P. B. (1976). *Diabetes*, **25**, 623.

Reaven, G. M., Bernstein, R., Davis, B. and Olefsky, J. M. (1976). *Am. J. Med.* **60**, 80.

Reaven, G. M. and Olefsky, J. M. (1974). *J. clin. Endocr. Metab.* **38**, 151.

Reaven, G. M., Weisinger, J. R. and Swenson, R. S. (1974). *Kidney int.* (Suppl. 1), 63.

Rebuzzi, A. G., Bellati, U., Ghirlanda, G., Manna, R., Altomonte, L. and Greco, A. V. (1977). *Diabetologia*, **13**, 427A.

Reckler, M. M., Podskalny, J., Goldfine, I. D. and Wells, C. A. (1974). *J. clin. Endocr. Metab.* **39**, 512.

Redmond, A., Buchanan, K. D. and Timble, E. R. (1977). *Acta paediatr. Scand.* **66**, 199.

Rehfeld, J. E. (1976). *J. clin. Invest.* **58**, 41.

Rehfeld, J. E., Lauritsen, K. B. and Stadil, F. (1976). *Scand. J. Gastroent.* **11** (Suppl. 37), 63.

Rehfeld, J. E., Stadil, F., Boden, H. and Fischerman, K. (1975). *Diabetologia*, **11**, 207.

Reinberg, A., Apfelbaum, M., Assan, R. and Lacatis, D. (1974). *In* "Chronobiology" (L. E. Schering, F. Halberg and J. E. Powley, eds), p. 88. Georg Thieme, Stuttgart.

Rennie, M. J., Park, D. M. and Sulaiman, W. R. (1976). *Am. J. Physiol.* **231**, 967.

Renold, A. E., Martin, D. B., Dagenais, Y. M., Steiner, J., Nickerson, R. J. and Sheps, M. C. (1960). *J. clin. Invest.* **39**, 1487.

Reyes-Leal, B., Castro, A., Bernal, E. and Guardiola, O. (1973). *Sem. Hop. Paris*, **22**, 1611.

Reynolds, C., Molnar, G. D., Horwitz, D. L., Rubenstein, A. H., Taylor, W. F. and Jiang, W. (1977). *Diabetes*, **26**, 36.

Riccardi, G., Heaf, D., Kaijser, L., Eklund, B. and Carlson, L. A. (1976). *Diabetologia*, **12**, 589.

Rickert, D. E., Fischer, L. J., Burke, J. P., Redick, J. A., Erlandsen, S. L., Parsons, S. A. and Carden, L. (1976). *Horm. metab. Res.* **8**, 430.

Riddick, F. A., Reissler, D. M. and Kipnis, D. M. (1962). *Diabetes*, **11**, 171.

Rimoin, D. L. (1969). *Arch. int. Med.* **124**, 695.

Rinderknecht, E. and Humbel, R. E. (1976). *Proc. natn. Acad. Sci., USA*, **73**, 2365.

Robertson, R. P. (1974). *Prostaglandins*, **6**, 501.

Robertson, R. P. and Chen, M. (1977). *J. clin. Invest.* **60**, 747.

Robertson, R. P., Halter, J. and Porte, D. (1976). *J. clin. Invest.* **57**, 791.

Robertson, R. P. and Porte, D. (1975a). *Diabetes*, **22**, 1.

Robertson, R. P. and Porte, D. (1973b). *J. clin. Invest.* **52**, 870.

Rocha, D., Faloona, G. R. and Unger, R. H. (1972). *J. clin. Invest.* **51**, 2346.

Rosenbloom, A. L. (1970). *New Engl. J. Med.* **282**, 1228.

Rosenbloom, A. L., Wheeler, L., Bianchi, K., Chin, F. T., Tiwary, C. M. and Grgic, A. (1965). *Diabetes*, **24**, 820.

Rosenthal, M. B., Goldfine, I. D. and Siperstein, M. D. (1976). *Lancet*, **ii**, 250.

Rossini, A. A., Crick, H. L., Appl, K. and Cahill, G. F. (1977). *Proc. natn. Acad. Sci., USA*, **74**, 2485.

Rossini, A. A. and Soeldner, J. S. (1976). *J. clin. Invest.* **57**, 1083.

Roth, J., Gorden, P. and Pastan, I. (1968). *Proc. natn. Acad. Sci., USA*, **61**, 138.

Rubenstein, A. H., Lowy, C., Wellbourne, T. A. and Fraser, T. R. (1967). *Metabolism*, **16**, 234.

Rubenstein, A. H., Melani, F. and Steiner, D. F. (1972). *In* "Handbook of Physiology Endocrinology" (D. F. Steiner and N. Freinkel, eds) Vol. I, p. 515. Williams and Wilkins, Baltimore.

Rubenstein, A. H. and Steiner, D. F. (1971). *Ann. Rev.* **22**, 1.

Rubenstein, A. H., Steiner, D. F., Horwitz, D. L., Mako, M. E., Block, M. B., Starr, J. I., Kuzuya, H. and Melani, F. (1977). *Rect. Prog. Horm. Res.* **33**, 435.

Rushahoff, R. J., Matsenbaugh, S. L., Schultz, T. A., Gerich, J. E. and Wallin, J. D. (1977). *Diabetes*, **26** (Suppl. 1), 414A.

Ryle, A. P., Sanger, F., Smith, L. F. and Kitai, R. (1955). *Biochem. J.* **60**, 541.

Sacca, L., Perez, G., Ringo, F. Pascucci, I. and Condorelli, M. (1975). *Acta endocr., Copenh.* **79**, 626.

Sachs, H., Waligora, K. and Matthews, J. (1977). *Diabetes*, **26** (Suppl. 1), 358A.

Salle, B. L. and Ruitton-Uglienco, A. (1976). *Biol. Neonate*, **29**, 1.

Salle, B. L. and Uglienco, A. (1977). *Pediatr. Res.* **11**, 108.

Samols, E. and Harrison, J. (1976). *Metabolism*, **25** (Suppl. 1), 1443.

Samols, E., Weir, G. G., Patel, Y. C., Fernandez-Durango, B., Arimura, A. and Loo, S. W. (1977). *Diabetes*, **26** (Suppl. 1), 375A.

Sandek, C. D., Hemm, R. M. and Peterson, C. M. (1977). *Metabolism*, **26**, 43.

Sandersen, I. and Dietel, M. (1974). *Ann. Surg.* **179**, 387.

Sandler, R., Horwitz, D. L., Rubenstein, A. H. and Kuzuya, H. (1975). *Am. J. Med.* **59**, 730.

Sando, H., Borg, J. and Steiner, D. F. (1972). *J. clin. Invest.* **51**, 1476.

Sando, H., Miki, E. and Kosaka, K. (1977). *Am. J. Physiol.* **232**, 237.

Santiago, J. V., Haymond, M. W., Clarke, W. L. and Pagliara, A. S. (1977). *Metabolism*, **26**, 1115.

Savage, P. J., Brannison, L. J., Flock, E. V. and Bennett, P. H. (1977). *Diabetes*, **26**, 414A.

Savage, P. J., Dippe, S. E., Bennett, P. H., Gordon, P., Roth, J., Rushtworth, W. B. and Miller, M. (1975). *Diabetes*, **24**, 36.

Scandellari, C., Casara, D., Zaccaria, M., Sirotich, G., Zago, E., Sicolo, M. and Federspile, G. (1974). *Acta diabet. lat.* **11**, 61.

Schade, D. S. and Eaton, R. P. (1976). *J. clin. Endocr. Metab.* **56**, 1340.

Schade, D. S. and Eaton, R. P. (1977a). *Diabetes*, **26**, 596.

Schade, D. S. and Eaton, R. P. (1977b). *J. clin. Endocr. Metab.* **44**, 1038.

Schafer, H. J. and Kloppel, G. (1974). *Virchows Arch. Path. Anat. Histol.* **362**, 231.

Schafer, L. D., Wilder, M. L. and Williams, R. H. (1973). *Proc. Soc. exp. Biol. Med.* **143**, 314.

Schapcott, D., Melancon, S., Butterworth, R. F., Khoury, K., Collu, R., Breton, G., Geoffrey, G., Lemieux, B. and Barbeau, A. (1976). *Can. J. Neurol. Sci.* **3**, 361.

Schapiro, S. (1968). *Endocrinology*, **83**, 475.

Schatz, H., Katsilambros, N., Nierle, C. and Pfeiffer, E. (1972a). *Diabetologia*, **8**, 402.

Schatz, H., Maier, V., Hinz, M., Nierle, C. and Pfeiffer, E. (1972b). *FEBS Letts*, **26**, 237.

Schatz, H. and Pfeiffer, E. (1977). *J. Endocr.* **74**, 243.

Schauder, P., Arends, J., Schindler, B., Ebert, R. and Frerichs, H. (1977a). *Diabetologia*, **13**, 171.

Schauder, P. and Frerichs, H. (1974). *Diabetologia*, **10**, 85.

Schauder, P., McIntosh, C., Frerichs, H. and Creutzfeldt, W. (1977b). *Diabetes*, **26** (Suppl. 1) 359A.

Schebalin, M., Said, S. and Makhlouf, G. M. (1977). *Am. J. Physiol.* **232**, E 197.

Schlichtkrull, J., Brange, J., Christiansen, A. H., Hallund, O., Heding, L. G. and Jorgensen, K. H. (1972). *Diabetes*, **21**, 649.

Schillinger, E., Gerloff, C., Gerhards, E. and Gunzel, P. (1974). *Acta endocr., Copenh.* **75**, 305.

Schneider, B., Straus, E. and Yalow, R. S. (1976). *Diabetes*, **25**, 260.

Schoenle, E., Zapf, J. and Froesch, E. R. (1976). *FEBS Letts*, **67**, 175.

Schubotz, R., Hausmann, L., Kaffarnik, H., Zehner, J. and Oepen, H. (1976). *Res. exp. Med.* **167**, 203.

Schultz, T. A., Lewis, S. B., Westbie, D. K., Wallin, J. D. and Gerich, J. E. (1977). *Am. J. Physiol.* **233**, E514.

Schulz, B., Michaelis, D., Ziegler, M., Teichmann, W., Nowak, W., Albrecht, G. and Bibergeil, H. (1976). *Endokrinologie*, **68**, 309.

Schurberg, E., Resnick, R. H., Koff, R. S., Ros, E., Baum, R. A. and Pallotta, J. A. (1977). *Gastroenterology*, **72**, 301.

Schusdziawa, V., Ipp, E. and Unger, R. H. (1977). *Diabetes*, **26** (Suppl. 1), 359A.

Scott, A. and Fisher, A. M. (1938). *Am. J. Physiol.* **121**, 253.

Scurol, A., Le Cercio, V., Adam, S., Gawannini, G., Bianchi, I., Cominacini, L. and Corgnati, A. (1976). *Metabolism*, **25**, 603.

Sehlin, J. and Tahjedal, I. B. (1974). *J. Physiol.* **242**, 505.

Seino, Y. (1976). *J. clin. Endocr. Metab.* **42**, 736.

Seino, Y., Goto, Y., Taminato, T., Ikeda, M. and Imura, H. (1974). *J. clin. Endocr. Metab.* **38**, 1136.

Seino, Y., Ikeda, M., Nakane, K., Nakahara, H., Seino, S. and Imura, H. (1977). *Metabolism*, **26**, 911.

Selawry, H. (1973). *Diabetes*, **22**, 295A.

Sener, A. and Malaisse, W. J. (1977). *Diabetologia*, **13**, 125.

Sensi, S. and Capani, F. (1976). *J. clin. Endocr. Metab.* **43**, 462.

Serrano-Rios, M., Hawkins, F., Escobar, F., Mato, J. M., Larrodera, L., de Oya M., Rodriguez-Miñon, J. L. (1974). *Horm. Metab. Res.* **6**, 17.

Serrano-Rios, M., Hawkins, F., Escobar, F., Mato, J. M., Larrodera, L., de Oya, M. and Rodriguez-Miñon, J. L. (1973). *Diabetologia*, **9**, 89A.

Service, F. J., Go, V. L., Blix, P. and Nelson, R. L. (1977a). *Diabetes*, **26** (Suppl. 1), 374A.

Service, F. J., Horwitz, D. L., Rubenstein, A. H., Kazuya, H., Mako, M. E., Reynold, C. and Molnar, G. D. (1977b). *J. Lab. clin. Med.* **90**, 180.

Seyffert, W. A. and Madison, L. L. (1967). *Diabetes*, **16**, 765.

Shah, J. H. and Cerchio, G. M. (1973). *Arch. int. Med.* **132**, 657.

Shah, J. H., Wong Surawat, N. and Aran, P. P. (1977). *Diabetes*, **26**, 375A.

Shen, S. W., Yu, S. S. and Singh, S. P. (1977). *Diabetes*, **26**, 416A.

Sherwin, R. C., Cramer, K. J., Tobin, J. D., Insel, P. A., Liljenquist, J. E., Berman, M. and Andres, R. (1974). *J. clin. Invest.* **53**, 1482.

Shima, K., Sawazaki, N., Tanaka, R., Morishita, S., Tarui, S. and Nishikawa, M. (1976). *Acta endocr., Copenh.* **83**, 114.

Shuck, J. M., Eaton, R. P., Shuck, L. W., Wachtel, T. L. and Schade, D. S. (1977). *J. Trauma*, **17**, 706.

Sieradzki, J., Schatz, A., Nierle, C. and Pfeiffer, E. F. (1975). *Horm. metab. Res.* **7**, 284.

Silbert, C. K. and Swain, C. T. (1975). *Clin. Chem.* **21**, 1520.

Simon, J., Freychet, P. and Rosselin, G. (1977). *Diabetologia*, **13**, 219.

Simpson, R. G., Benedetti, A., Grodsky, G. M., Karam, J. H. and Forsham, P. H. (1968). *Diabetes*, **17**, 684.

Sirek, A., Sirek, O. V. and Policova, Z. (1974). *Diabetologia*, **10**, 267.

Sizonenko, P. C., Rabinovitch, A., Schneider, P., Pannier, L., Wollheim, C. B. and Zahnd, G. (1975). *Paediatr. Res.* **9**, 733.

Skillman, J. J., Hedley-Whyte, J. and Pallotta, J. A. (1971). *Ann. Surg.* **174**, 911.

Slonim, A. E., Sharp, R., Page, D. and Burr, I. M. (1977) *Diabetes*, **26** (Suppl. 1), 417A.

Snell, C. R. and Smyth, D. C. (1975). *J. biol. Chem.* **250**, 6291.

Sodoyez-Goffaux, F. and Sodoyez, J. C. (1977). *J. Pediatr*, **9**, 395.

Sodoyez-Goffaux, F., Sodoyez, J. C. and de Vos, C. (1977). *Diabetes*, **26** (Suppl. 1), 399A.

Soeldner, J. I. and Slone, D. (1965). *Diabetes*, **14**, 771.

Somers, G., Devis, G., Van Obberghen, E. and Malaisse, W. J. (1976). *Pflügers Archiv.* **365**, 21.

Somers, G., Obberghen, E. V., Devis, G., Ravazzola, M., Malaisse-Lagae, F. and Malaisse, W. J. (1974). *Eur. J. clin. Invest.* **4**, 299.

Sorge, F., Schwartzkopf, W. and Neuhans, G. A. (1976). *Diabetes*, **25**, 586.

Sönksen, P. N. (1975). *Proc. R. Soc. Med.* **68**, 707.

Sönksen, P. H., Tompkins, C. V., Srivastava, M. C. and Nabarro, J. D. N. (1973). *Clin. Sci. mol. Med.* **45**, 633.

Sövik, O., Oseid, S. and Oyasreten, S. (1973). *Acta endocr., Copenh.* **72**, 731.

Spellacy, W. N. and Buhi, W. C. (1971). *Lancet*, **ii**, 87.

Spellacy, W. N., Buhi, W. C. and Birk, S. A. (1972a). *Am. J. Obstet. Gynecol.* **114**, 378.

Spellacy, W. N., Buhi, W. C. and Birk, S. A. (1972b). *Acta endocr., Copenh.* **70**, 373.

Spellacy, W. N., Buhi, W. C. and Birk, S. A. (1977). *Am. J. Obstet. Gynecol.* **127**, 599.

Spellacy, W. N., Buhi, W. C., Birk, S. A. and Cabal, R. (1973a). *Fertil. Steril.* **24**, 178.

Spellacy, W. N., Buhi, W. C., Birk, S. A. and McReary, S. A. (1973b). *Fertil. Steril.* **24**, 419.

Spellacy, W. N., Buhi, W. C., Spellacy, C. E., Moses, L. E. Goldzieher, J. W. (1970a). *Am. J. Obstet. Gynecol.* **106**, 173.

Spellacy, W. N., Carlson, K. L., Birk, S. A. and Schade, S. L. (1968). *Metabolism*, **17**, 496.

Spellacy, W. N., Farog, M. D., Buhi, W. C. and Birk, S. A. (1975). *Obstet. Gynecol.* **45**, 159.

Spellacy, W. N., McLeod, A. G. W., Buhi, W. C. and Birk, S. A. (1972c). *Fertil. Steril.* **23**, 239.

Spellacy, W. N., McLeod, A. G. W., Buhi, W. G., Birk, S. A. and McReary, S. A. (1970b). *Fertil. Steril.* **21**, 457.

Spellacy, W. N., Newton, R. E., Buhi, W. C. and Birk, S. A. (1973c). *Am. J. Obstet. Gynecol.* **116**, 1074.

Sperling, M. A., De Lameter, P. V., Phelps, D., Fiser, R. H., Oh, W. and Fisher, D. A. (1974). *J. clin. Invest.* **53**, 1159.

Sramkova, J., Par, J. and Engelberth, O. (1975). *Diabetes,* **24**, 214.

Stahl, M., Girar, J., Rachtshausen, M., Nars, P. W. and Zappinger, K. (1974). *J. Paediatr.* **84**, 821.

Starr, J. I., Juhn, N. J., Rubenstein, A. H. and Kitabchi, A. E. (1975). *J. clin. Lab. Med.* **86**, 631.

Starr, J. I. and Rubenstein, A. H. (1974). *In* "Methods of Hormone Radioimmunoassay" (B. M. Jaffe and H. R. Behrman, eds), p. 289. Academic Press, London and New York.

Steiner, D. F. (1977). *Diabetes,* **26**, 322.

Steiner, D. F., Hallund, O., Rubenstein, A. H., Cho, S. and Bayliss, C. (1968). *Diabetes,* **17**, 725.

Steimer, D. F., Kemmler, W., Clark, J. L., Oyer, P. E. and Rubenstein, A. H. (1972). *In* "Handbook of Physiology" (D. F. Steiner and N. Freinkel, eds), Vol. I, p. 175. Williams and Wilkins, Baltimore.

Steiner, D. F. and Oyer, P. E. (1967). *Proc. natn. Acad. Sci., USA,* **57**, 473.

Stout, R. W. (1977) *Atherosclerosis,* **27**, 1.

Stout, R. W., Brunzell, J. D., Bierman, E. L. and Porte, D. (1974). *Diabetes,* **23**, 624.

Strauss, E., Urbach, H. J. and Yalow, R. S. (1976). *New Engl. J. Med.* **293**, 1031.

Strauss, W. T. and Hales, C. N. (1974). *Diabetologia,* **10**, 237.

Sugden, M. C. and Ashcroft, S. J. H. (1977). *Diabetologia,* **13**, 467.

Sussman, K. E. and Leitner, J. W. (1976). *Diabetes,* **25** (Suppl. 1), 386A.

Suzuki, K., Ohsawa, N. and Kosaka, K. (1976). *J. clin. Endocr. Metab.* **42**, 399.

Sylvälahti, E. (1975). *Acta pharmac. tox.* **37**, 336.

Sylvälahti, E., Erkkola, R., Lisalao, E., Punnonen, R. and Rauramo, L. (1975). *Horm. metab. Res.* **7**, 438.

Sylvälahti, E., Erkkola, R., Punnonen, R. and Rauramo, L. (1976a). *Acta pharmac. tox.* **38**, 177.

Sylvälahti, E., Lammin Tausta, R. and Pekkarinen, A. (1976b). *Acta pharmac. toxic.* **38**, 344.

Szabo, A. J. and Szabo, O. (1975). *Diabetes,* **24**, 328.

Szabo, O. and Mahler, R. J. (1970). *Horm. metab. Res.* **2**, 125.

Szabo, O., Oppermann, W., Victor, C. and Camerini-Davalos, R. A. (1974). *Acta diabet. lat.* **11**, 265.

Taborsky, G. J. and Smith, P. H. (1977). *Diabetes,* **26**, 419A.

Tager, H. S., Markese, J., Kramer, K. J., Speirs, R. D. and Childs, N. S. (1976). *Biochem. J.* **156**, 515.

Takeda, R., Usukura, N., Miwa, U., Nakabayashi, H., Kishitani, M. and Yoshimitsu, K. (1977). *A.L.A.J. med. Sci.* **14**, 125.

Taminato, F., Seino, Y., Goto, Y., Inoue, Y., Kadowaki, S., Mori, K., Nozawa, M., Yajima, H. and Imura, H. (1977). *Diabetes,* **26**, 480.

Tan, M. H., Williams, R. F., Soeldner, J. S. and Gleason, R. E. (1977). *Diabetes,* **26**, 490.

Taniguchi, H., Murakawi, K., Morita, S., Kazumi, T., Yoshino, G., Maeda, M. and Baba, S. (1977). *Lancet,* **ii**, 501.

Tasaka, Y., Sekine, M., Wakatsuki, M., Ohgawara, H. and Shizume, K. (1975). *Horm. metab. Res.* **7**, 205.

Taylor, K. W. (1967). *In* "Hormones in Blood" (C. H. Gray and A. L. Bacharach, eds), p. 47. Academic Press, London and New York.

Taylor, K. W., Gardner, G., Parry, D. G. and Jones, V. E. (1965). *Biochim. biophys. Acta* **100**, 521.
Taylor, M. W., Gaddie, J., Madison, L. E. and Palmer, K. H. V. (1976). *Br. med. J.* **1**, 22.
Terris, S. and Steiner, D. F. (1976). *J. clin. Invest.* **57**, 885.
Tewaarwerk, G. J. M. (1977). *J. clin. Endocr. Metab.* **44**, 491.
Thomas, J. H. (1973). *Postgrad. med. J.* **49**, 940.
Thorell, J. I. and Lanner, A. (1973). *Scand. J. clin. Lab. Invest.* **31**, 187.
Tiengo, A., Del Prete, G. F., Nosadini, R., Betterle, C., Garotti, C. and Bersani, C. (1977). *Diabetologia*, **13**, 451.
Tjälve, H., Popov, D. and Slawina, P. (1974). *Horm. metab. Res.* **6**, 106.
Tjälve, H. and Wilander, E. (1977). *Diabetologia*, **13**, 521.
Toccafondi, R., Rotella, C. M., Tanini, A. and Arcangeli, P. (1977). *Horm. metab. Res.* **9**, 101.
Tomita, T., Lacy, P. E., Matschinsky, F. M. and McDaniel, M. (1974). *Diabetes*, **23**, 517.
Trueheart, P. A. and Herrera, M. G. (1971). *Diabetes*, **20**, 46.
Trueheart, P. A., Maldonato, A., Kaelin, D., Renold, A. E. and Sharp, G. W. G. (1976). *Diabetologia*, **12**, 463.
Turinsky, J., Saba, T. M., Scorill, W. A. and Chestnut, T. (1977). *J. Trauma*, **17**, 344.
Turner, R. C. and Cohen, N. M. (1974). *Dev. Med. Child. Neurol.* **16**, 371.
Turner, R. C., Harris, E., Bloom, S. R. and Uren, C. (1977a). *Diabetes*, **26**, 166.
Turner, R. C., Hart, G. and London, D. R. (1977b). *Diabetologia*, **13**, 19.
Turner, R. C. and Heding, L. G. (1977). *Diabetologia*, **13**, 571.
Turner, R. C. and Holman, R. R. (1976). *Lancet*, **i**, 1272.
Turton, M. B. and Deegan, T. (1974). *Clin. chim. Acta* **55**, 389.
Tyson, J. E., Austin, K., Farinholt, J. and Fiedler, J. (1976). *Am. J. Obstet. Gynecol.* **125**, 1073.
Unger, R. H. (1974). *Metabolism*, **23**, 581.
Updike, S. J., Simmons, J. D., Grant, D. H., Magnuson, J. A. and Goodfriend, T. L. (1973). *Clin. Chem.* **18**, 1339.
Vallance-Owen, J., Hurlock, B. and Please, N. W. (1955). *Lancet*, **ii**, 583.
Van Noorden, S. and Pearse, A. G. E. (1976). *In* "The Evolution of Pancreatic Islets" (T. A. Grillo, L. Leibson and A. Epple, eds), p. 141. Pergamon Press, London.
Varandani, P. T. (1974). *Diabetes*, **23**, 117.
Varandani, P. T., Nafz, M. A. and Chandler, M. (1976). *Biochim. biophys. Acta*, **422**, 2115.
Velasco, C. A., Cole, H. S. and Camerini-Davalos, R. A. (1974). *Clin. Chem.* **20**, 700.
Vernikos-Danellis, J., Leach, C. S., Winget, C. M., Goodwin, A. L. and Rambert, P. C. (1976). *Aviat. Space environ. Med.* **47**, 583.
Viberti, G., Pontiroli, A. E., Mignani, E., Tognetti, A., Marigo, S. and Pozza, G. (1974). *Acta diabetol. lat.* **11**, 432.
Vigneri, R., Pliam, N. B., Cohen, D. G. and Goldfine, I. D. (1977). *Diabetes*, **26** (Suppl. 1), 355A.
Vinik, A. I., Kalk, W. J., Botha, J. L., Jackson, W. P. U. and Blake, K. C. H. (1976). *Diabetes*, **25**, 11.
Vinik, A. I., Kalk, W. J., Keller, P., Beumont, P. and Jackson, W. P. U. (1973). *Lancet*, **i**, 183.
Vondra, K., Rath, R., Bass, A., Slabochova, Z., Teisinger, J. and Vitek, V. (1977). *Diabetologia*, **13**, 527.

Walter, R. M., Ensinck, J. C., Ricketts, H., Kendall, J. W. and Williams, R. H. (1973). *Am. J. Med.* **55**, 667.

Watari, N. and Hotta, Y. (1976). *In* "Endocrine Gut and Pancreas" (T. Fujita, ed.), p. 179. Elsevier, Amsterdam.

Weber, C. J., Pi-Sunyer, F. X., Woda, B. A., Zimmerman, E., Derehoncourt, F., Hardy, M. A., Price, J. B. and Reemtsma, K. (1976). *Diabetes*, **26**, 423A.

Weisinger, J., Swenson, R. S., Greene, W. G., Taylor, J. B. and Reaven, G. M. (1972). *Diabetes*, **21**, 1109.

Weitzel, G., Bauer, F. and Eisele, K. (1976). *Hoppe Seyler's Z. physiol. Chem.* **357**, 187.

Whichelow, M. J., Butterfield, W. J. H., Abrams, M. E., Sterky, G. and Garrant, C. J. (1968). *Metabolism*, **17**, 84.

Widström, A. (1977). *Horm. Metab. Res.* **9**, 172.

Widström, A. and Cerasi, E. (1973a). *Acta endocr., Copenh.* **72**, 506.

Widström, A. and Cerasi, E. (1975b). *Acta endocr., Copenh.* **72**, 519.

Widström, A. and Cerasi, E. (1973c). *Acta endocr., Copenh.* **72**, 532.

Williams, R. F., Gleason, R. E. and Soeldner, J. S. (1968). *Metabolism*, **17**, 1025.

Wilmore, D. W. (1976). *Clin. Endocr. Metab.* **5**, 731.

Wilmore, D. W., Long, J. M., Mason, A. D., Skreen, R. W. and Pruitt, B. A. (1974). *Ann. Surg.* **180**, 653.

Wilmore, D. W., Mason, A. D. and Pruitt, B. A. (1976). *Ann. Surg.* **183**, 314.

Wilson, J. P., Downs, R. W., Feldman, J. M. and Lebovitz, H. E. (1974). *Am. J. Physiol.* **227**, 305.

Woldow, A., Shapiro, B., Cohen, J. J. and Kollman, G. (1972). *J. Am. Geriatr. Soc.* **20**, 515.

Wollheim, C. B., Kikuchi, M., Renold, A. E. and Sharp, G. W. G. (1977). *J. clin. Invest.* **60**, 1165.

Wood, S. C. (1972). *Am. J. Physiol.* **223**, 1424.

Wood, S. C. and Porte, D. (1974). *Physiol. Rev.* **54**, 596.

Wood, S. P., Blundell, T. L., Wollmer, A., Lazarus, N. R. and Neville, R. W. J. (1975). *Eur. J. Biochem.* **55**, 531.

Wright, P. D. (1973). *J.R. Coll. Surg. Edinb.* **18**, 284.

Wright, P. D., Henderson, K. and Johnston, I. D. A. (1974). *Br. J. Surg.* **61**, 5.

Wright, P. H., Makulu, D. R., Vichick, D. and Sussman, K. E. (1971). *Diabetes*, **20**, 33.

Yalow, R. S. and Berson, S. A. (1960). *J. clin. Invest.* **39**, 1157.

Yanaihara, N., Hashimoto, T., Yanaihara, C., Sakagami, M., Steiner, D. F. and Rubenstein, A. H. (1974). *Biochem. biophys. Res. Commun.* **59**, 1124.

Yasuda, K., Harukawa, Y., Okuyama, M., Kikuchi, M. and Yashinaga, K. (1975). *Diabetes*, **24**, 1066.

Young, D. M. and Lewis, A. H. (1947). *Science*, **105**, 368.

Yu, S. S. and Kitabchi, K. E. (1973). *J. biol. Chem.* **248**, 3753.

Yue, D. K., Baxter, R. C. and Turtle, J. R. (1976). *Biochim. biophys. Acta*, **444**, 231.

Yue, D. K. and Turtle, J. R. (1977). *Diabetes*, **26**, 341.

Zaharko, D. S. and Beck, L. V. (1968). *Diabetes*, **17**, 444.

Zahn, H. and Smith, L. F. (1972). *Diabetes*, **21** (suppl. 2), 457.

Zapf, J., Mäder, M., Waldvogel, M. and Froesch, E. R. (1975). *Isr. J. Med.* **11**, 664.

Zawalick, W. S., Karl, R. C., Ferrendelli, J. A. and Matschinsky, F. M. (1975). *Diabetologia*, **11**, 231.

Zermatten, A., Heptner, W., DeLahoye, D., Se chaud, R. and Feiber, J. P. (1977). *Diabetologia*, **13**, 85.

Zühlke, H., Steiner, D. F., Lernmark, A. and Lipsey, C. (1976). *In* "Polypeptide Hormones; Molecular and Cellular Aspects". Ciba Foundation Symposium 41 (New Series), p. 183, Excerpta Medica, Amsterdam.

III. Glucagon

P. J. LEFEBVRE and A. S. LUYCKX

A. CHEMICAL AND PHYSICAL PROPERTIES

Porcine glucagon has been isolated and crystallised by Staub, Sinn and Behrens (1953, 1955). It consists of a single chain polypeptide comprising

NH₂
|
His–Ser–Glu–Gly–Thr–Phe–Thr–Ser–Asp–Tyr–Ser–Lys–Tyr–Leu–Asp →

NH₂   NH₂   NH₂
| | |
→Ser–Arg–Arg–Ala–Glu–Asp–Phe–Val–Glu–Try–Leu–Met–Asp–Thr

Fig. 1. Primary structure of porcine glucagon.

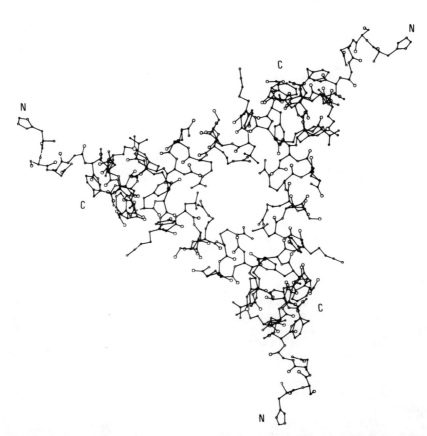

Fig. 2. A view of a glucagon trimer resulting from heterologous contacts between hydrophobic residues; the region around the 3 fold axis of symmetry in the centre comprises hydrophyllic residues including arginines and aspartates. Reproduced from Sasaki *et al.* (1975a), with kind permission of the authors and the copyright holders.

29 amino acid residues (Fig. 1) and having a molecular weight of 3485 (Bromer, Sinn, Staub and Behrens, 1957). Porcine, bovine (Bromer, Boucher and Koffenberger, 1971) and human (Thomsen, Kristiansen, Brunfeldt and Sundby, 1972) glucagons have identical sequences. The amino acid composition, crystal form and electrophoretic behaviour of rabbit, camel and rat glucagon strongly indicate their identity with porcine glucagon (Sundby, 1976*). In contrast, guinea-pig glucagon appears larger: it contains 40 amino acid residues and gel filtration indicates a molecular weight of 4000–5000. Bird glucagon differs from porcine glucagon in having one or two amino acid substitutions. For instance, duck glucagon has threonine instead of serine in position 16 and serine instead of asparagine in position 28 (Sundby, Frandsen, Thomsen, Kristiansen and Brunfeldt, 1972), turkey glucagon differs from porcine glucagon in having one more serine residue and one less Asp/Asn residue (Markussen, Frandsen, Heding and Sundby, 1972). According to Pollock and Kimmel (1975), the amino acid composition of chicken glucagon is identical with that of turkey glucagon.

Anglerfish (Trakatellis, Tada, Yamaji and Gardiki-Kouidou, 1975) and shark (Sundby, 1976) glucagons have 29 amino acid residues but differ in their composition from porcine glucagon. Porcine glucagon crystallises without metals in the pH range 5–8, appearing as rhombic dodecahedra that conform to the cubic system. Sasaki, Dockerill, Adamiak, Tickle and Blundell (1975a), using X-ray analysis, have shown that the structure in the crystals is largely helical, with molecules associated in a complex arrangement of trimers (Fig. 2). The evidence in favour of the existence of such helical trimers in the α-granules of the islets of Langerhans and the formation of helical conformers at the receptor sites has been recently reviewed by Blundell, Dockerill, Sasaki, Tickle and Wood (1976). The complete synthesis of glucagon has been achieved in the late sixties by Wünsch and his associates (Wünsch and Weinges, 1972*).

B. SITES OF ORIGIN

1. The Islets of Langerhans

The A-cells (sometimes called A_2-cells) of the islets of Langerhans of the pancreas represent the main and longest known source of glucagon (Munger, 1972*). Glucagon-producing cells can be identified by histochemistry, immunofluorescence techniques or electron microscopy. Phylogenetically,

---

* Indicate review articles in this chapter.

G

glucagon-producing A-cells occur in the pancreas of mammals, birds, reptiles, amphibia, bony fish and in cartilaginous fish. Typical A-cells have not been observed, so far, in the islet parenchyma of jawless fish, nor in the hepatopancreas of lower chordates, protochordates or protostomian invertebrates (Falkmer and Marques, 1972*). Ontogenetically, A-cells appear in embryonic life as early as B-cells and acinar parenchyma; they develop from the primitive pancreatic cords and later from the ducts (Falkmer and Marques, 1972*). Recently, much interest has been devoted to the microanatomy of the islets of Langerhans (Orci and Unger, 1975; Unger and Orci, 1976; Orci, 1976a, b). In most animal species studied, including human, a rim of glucagon-secreting A-cells tends to surround a nest of insulin-producing B-cells, which make up approximately 60% of the islet cell population (Fig. 3). D-cells (former A$_1$-cells) manufacturing and secreting somatostatin are almost

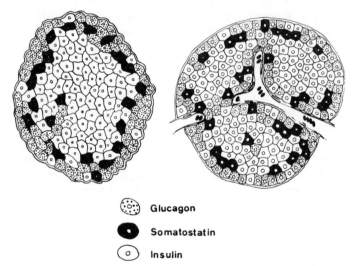

⦂⦂⦂ Glucagon

● Somatostatin

◯ Insulin

Fig. 3. Left: schematic representation of the number and distribution of insulin-, glucagon- and somatostatin- containing cells in the normal rat islet. Note the characteristic position of most glucagon- and somatostatin-containing cells at the periphery of the islet, surrounding the centrally located insulin-containing cells. Cell types in the islet for which a characteristic function and/or morphology is not defined are intentionally omitted.

Right: schematic representation of the number and distribution of insulin-, glucagon- and somatostatin-containing cells in the normal human islet. Large vascular channels penetrate the islet and are followed by glucagon- and somatostatin-containing cells. This pattern divides the total islet mass into smaller subunits, each of which contains a centre formed mainly of insulin-containing cells and surrounded by glucagon- and somatostatin-containing cells. Cell types for which definite functions and morphologies have not yet been determined are intentionally omitted. Reproduced from Orci (1977), with kind permission of the author and the copyright holders.

always found in juxtaposition to the A-cells. Orci and Unger (1975) have developed hypothetical functional implications of such a deposition. Since somatostatin inhibits the secretion of both insulin and glucagon, it has been suggested that "the presence of D-cells between A- and B-cells may signify an inhibitory role upon secretion of these last cells. According to this hypothesis, the function of the D-cells would be to turn off the release of glucagon from adjacent A-cells and of insulin from adjacent B-cells. The respective positions of A-, B-, and D-cells make it evident that the impact of locally released somatostatin would be considerably greater on glucagon than on insulin secretion" (Unger and Orci, 1976).

As shown by Orci and his co-workers (Orci, Malaisse-Lagae, Amherdt, Ravazzola, Weisswange, Dobbs, Perrelet and Unger 1975a; Orci, Malaisse-Lagae, Ravazzola, Rouiller, Renold, Perrelet and Unger, 1975b) specialised junctional complexes exist not only between B-cells and B-cells and between A-cells and A-cells, but also between B-cells and A-cells. These complexes, revealed by conventional electron microscopy and freeze-fracturing techniques, consists of "gap junctions" and "tight junctions". These junctions may be implied in electrical and metabolic coupling of adjacent cells ("gap junctions") or in compartmentalization of the intra-islet intercellular space ("tight junctions"). As hypothesised by Unger and Orci (1976), "cell-to-cell communication (through gap junctions) could influence the total secretory response of an individual islet, making possible a given net bihormonal output from asynchronously secreting individual cells, whereas compartmentalization of intercellular spaces (by tight junctions) may separate outgoing secretory products from incoming signals". Morphological studies have demonstrated the presence of autonomic nerve terminals within the islets (Munger, 1972*) thus giving support to the physiologic investigations demonstrating a control of A-cell function by both the cholinergic and the adrenergic systems (see later, p. 183). The morphological events associated with glucagon release are still poorly known. Intracytoplasmic dissolution of secretory granules as well as extrusion of granules by exocytosis have been described. Combining biochemical measurements, morphometric quantification of thin-section preparations and freeze fracturing, Carpentier, Malaisse-Lagae, Muller and Orci (1977) have shown that arginine-stimulated glucagon release was associated with a significant increase of morphological events linked to exocytosis. By contrast, the paradoxical release of glucagon provoked by calcium deprivation, although accompanied by a significant loss of granule stores was not associated with an increase of morphologically detectable exocytosis, suggesting the possibility of other mechanisms of release. There is a great need for similar morphologic investigations of other conditions of stimulation of glucagon release (hypoglycemia, neural stimulation, etc.).

2. Extrapancreatic Glucagon

Sutherland and De Duve (1948) were the first to suggest that glucagon may be present, outside the pancreas, in the gastro-intestinal tract. Since then, various groups have reported that the oxyntic glandular mucosa of the canine stomach contains cells resembling pancreatic A-cells (Orci, Forssmann, Forssmann and Rouiller 1968; Cavallero, Solcia, Vassallo and Capella, 1969; Cavallero, Capella, Solcia, Vassallo and Bussolati, 1970; Solcia, Vassallo and Capella, 1970; Kubes, Jirasek and Lomsky, 1974). The existence of A-cells in the dog gastric fundus and corpus is now firmly established on the basis of immunohistological, immunocytological and ultrastructural studies (Larsson, Holst, Håkanson and Sundler, 1975; Sasaki, Rubalcalva, Baetens, Blazquez, Srikant, Orci and Unger, 1975b; Baetens, Rufener, Srikant, Dobbs, Unger and Orci, 1976). Similar observations were made on the oxyntic gland area of the stomach of the cat (Larsson *et al.*, 1975). The presence of A-cells in the human gastro-intestinal tract is still a matter of discussion. Sasagawa, Kobayashi and Fujita (1974) reported the existence of A-cells in the human duodenum; Orci (1976a) has described A-cells in the gastric fundus of a human foetus and, finally, Munoz-Barragan, Rufener, Srikant, Dobbs, Shannon, Baetens and Unger (1977) demonstrated glucagon-containing cells in one of eight human gastric fundi that they examined. An excellent review on extrapancreatic glucagon has been given by Holst (1978)*. Although the presence of glucagon has been reported in the salivary glands of some animal species (mouse, rat and to a lesser extent man and rabbit) by Lawrence, Tan, Hojvat and Kirsteins (1976), the presence of typical A-cells in these glands has not yet been established (Orci, 1976).

C. BIOSYNTHESIS

Pulse-labelling studies with labelled tryptophan have been performed, using anglerfish islets, by Noe and Bauer (1971, 1975). These authors suggested that the biosynthetic precursor of glucagon would be a polypeptide with a molecular weight near 12,000. This precursor is rapidly converted to an intermediate peptide having a molecular weight near 9000. More recent studies by Noe (1976), on the same material, have indicated that the microsomal fraction is the site of synthesis for the 12,000 molecular weight component. Portions of the 12,000 and 9000 molecular weight components are transported to the secretory granule fractions before cleavage to smaller products: another intermediate with a molecular weight of about 4900 and, finally, glucagon (about 3500). According to Trakatellis *et al.* (1975) the anglerfish proglucagon is a 78-amino acid single chain polypeptide from which glucagon is liberated by tryptic cleavage. On the other hand, Tager and Steiner (1973) isolated from crystalline mammalian glucagon a strongly basic 37-amino acid residue acid fragment of proglucagon containing the 29-amino acid primary sequence of bovine glucagon. This fragment is apparently similar, or identical, to the 4900 intermediate identified by Noe and Bauer (Noe, 1976). Factors affecting the biosynthesis of glucagon are still unknown.

D. EFFECTS OF GLUCAGON

Among the many effects attributed to glucagon some are likely to be considered as physiological, others are more probably pharmacological. Among the physiological effects of glucagon, we will consider the action of the hormone on liver carbohydrate metabolism, adipose tissue lipolysis and hepatic ketogenesis. Effects on insulin secretion, lipoprotein metabolism and kidney function will be summarised without attempting to consider them as physiological or pharmacological. Other actions (heart, adrenal medulla, gastric and gut mobility, etc.) will be considered as pharmacological.

1. Liver Carbohydrate Metabolism

The liver is the first organ encountered by glucagon after its secretion by the pancreas (and, at least in certain animal species, the stomach). As abundantly demonstrated, the action of glucagon on the liver results in increased glucose production (Park and Exton, 1972*). Such an effect observed on isolated hepatocytes, isolated perfused liver or in animal experimentation has been unequivocally demonstrated in man by Bomboy, Lewis, Sinclair-Smith, Lacy and Liljenquist (1977). These authors showed that net splanchnic glucose production increased 2·3 fold after i.v. infusion of glucagon (5 ng/kg/min). Similar results were obtained by Felig, Wahren and Hendler (1976) who, in addition, showed that the effect of exogenous hyperglucagonemia on splanchnic glucose output was evanescent: despite ongoing infusion of glucagon (3 ng/kg/min), splanchnic glucose output returned to baseline by 30 min.

The stimulation of hepatic glucose output by glucagon involves inhibition of liver glycogen synthesis, stimulation of liver glycogenolysis and stimulation of gluconeogenesis (Park and Exton, 1972*; Hanoune, 1976* and Hers, 1976*). The following steps are likely to be involved in the stimulation by glucagon of liver glucose output (Fig. 4):

(i) binding of glucagon to its receptor sites on the hepatocytes;
(ii) activation of adenylate cyclase;

  (iii) synthesis of cAMP;

  (iv) activation of the cAMP-dependent protein kinase (or histone-kinase);

  (v) phosphorylation of glycogen synthetase, with transformation of the enzyme from its active form (*a*) to its inactive form (*b*);

  (vi) subsequent inhibition of glycogen synthesis; also

  (vii) activation of phosphorylase-kinase;

 (viii) phosphorylation of phosphorylase, with transformation of the enzyme from its inactive form (*b*) to its active form (*a*);

  (ix) subsequent stimulation of glycogenolysis.

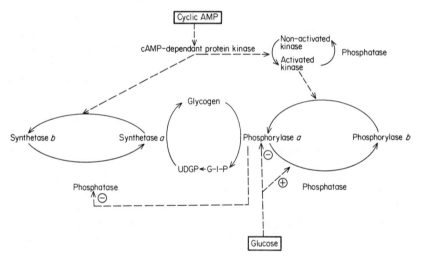

Fig. 4. Glycogen synthesis and breakdown according to Hers (1976).

In this system, phosphorylase *a* also inhibits glycogen synthetase phosphatase, and therefore contributes to the inhibition of glycogen synthesis (Stalmans *et al.*, 1971). Thus inhibition of glycogen synthesis and stimulation of glycogenolysis are two processes largely interdependent and controlled by the intracellular concentration of cAMP in such a way that there is no futile recycling of glucose to glycogen and vice-versa.

The mechanisms whereby glucagon exerts its stimulation on gluconeogenesis is still under discussion. Recent investigations, however, have suggested that it may also be cAMP-dependent: according to Ljungström, Hjhelmquist and Engström (1974) and to Feliu, Hue and Hers (1976), the cAMP-dependent protein kinase would phosphorylate pyruvate-kinase and thereby inactivate it; this would interrupt the "futile pyruvate–phosphoenolpyruvate cycle" and, therefore, redirect phosphoenolpyruvate (and pyruvate) towards gluconeogenesis.

2. Adipose Tissue Lipolysis

Glucagon stimulates the hydrolysis of adipose tissue triglycerides into glycerol and free fatty acids (lipolysis). The main characteristics of glucagon-induced lipolysis, the factors which modify it and the physiologic importance of these observations have been reviewed in detail (Lefebvre, 1972*, 1975*).

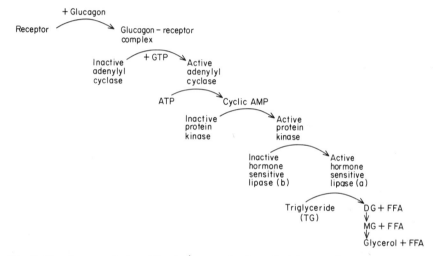

Fig. 5. The glucagon-induced lipolytic cascade; from Steinberg and Huttunen (1972). GTP = guanosine triphosphate; ATP = adenosine triphosphate; DG = digly-ceride; MG = monoglyceride; FFA = free fatty acid. Reproduced from Lefebvre (1975) with permission of the copyright holders.

The mechanism involved includes a sequence of events known as the "lipo-lytic cascade" (Fig. 5). If little doubt persists concerning the physiological relevance of glucagon-induced lipolysis in certain animal species like the rodents, such a role is challenged in other species like dog or man. In dog, for instance, infusion of physiological quantities of glucagon into the portal vein has been reported to be associated with an increase in plasma FFA levels (Lefebvre, 1966), a finding which has not been confirmed by Muller, Aoki, Egdahl and Cahill (1977) who infused glucagon in the systemic circula-tion thus suggesting the possibility that intraportal glucagon may promote lipolysis from hepatocytes (instead of adipocytes) or alter the uptake and/or metabolism of free fatty acids in the liver.

In man, the presence of insulin (or the insulin response to an infusion of glucagon, see below) may inhibit the lipolytic response to glucagon. In insulin-dependent diabetics, relatively high concentrations of glucagon are capable of stimulating lipolysis (Liljenquist, Bomboy, Lewis, Sinclair-Smith, Felts, Lacy, Crofford and Liddle, 1974; Schade and Eaton, 1975).

In studies involving administration of exogenous hormone during suppression of endogenous hormone secretion with somatostatin, Gerich, Lorenzi, Bier, Tsalikian, Schneider, Karam and Forsham (1976c) clearly showed that physiological levels of glucagon in man can stimulate lipolysis but that this effect was effectively antagonised by relatively small plasma concentrations of insulin (25–35 μu/ml, evaluated, unfortunately not measured).

3. Ketogenesis

Experiments performed in rats led McGarry, Wright and Foster (1975b) to suggest that the development of ketosis involves metabolic changes occurring in both the adipose tissue and the liver, which are governed largely by insulin and glucagon. Accelerated lipolysis favoured by insulin deficiency (and glucagon excess as we have just seen) results in mobilisation of free fatty acids (FFA) to the liver. At the latter site, glucagon excess induces an activation of the carnitine acyltransferase system of enzymes with the result that the fatty acids are taken up by the liver cells and oxidised with the production of acetoacetic and β-hydroxybutyric acids (McGarry, Robles-Valdes and Foster, 1975a). The increase in ketone body plasma levels observed in man during glucagon infusion is in agreement with such a role for glucagon (Liljenquist et al., 1974; Schade and Eaton, 1975; Gerich et al., 1976c).

4. Insulin Secretion

Samols, Marri and Marks (1965) were the first to establish firmly that glucagon had a direct stimulatory effect on insulin secretion by the B-cells of the islets of Langerhans. On the basis of this and other investigations, these authors (Samols, Tyler and Marks, 1972) attempted to analyse the glucagon–insulin interactions on the basis of an "insulin–glucagon negative feedback system" in which insulin suppresses glucagon while glucagon stimulates insulin secretion. This concept has received relatively little experimental support over the succeeding 10 years during which the insulinogenic effect of glucagon has been widely used as a pharmacological tool for investigating B-cell function as proposed by Marks and Samols (1968).

Recent careful analyses of the microanatomy of the islets of Langerhans and of the junctional complexes between A- and B-cells, as observed with conventional electromicroscopy and freeze-fracturing technics, have shed new light on the phenomenon discovered by Samols *et al.* (1965) and led Unger and Orci (1976) to hypothesise new mechanisms involved in the response of the islets of Langerhans under certain conditions (see p. 174).

5. Lipoprotein Metabolism

A plasma hypolipemic action of glucagon was first described by Amatuzio, Grande and Wada (1962). The physiologic significance of this effect in normal man and the implications for lipoprotein regulation during pathologically altered glucagon secretion are still not clear (Eaton, 1977). A role for glucagon in the physiologic regulation of plasma lipids in the rat is suggested on the basis of the observations of Gey, Georgi and Buhler (1977). A basic function of glucagon may consist in augmenting FFA availability to the liver while simultaneously "shifting" hepatic fatty acid metabolism towards oxidative pathways of ketogenesis and away from synthetic pathways of lipoprotein production (Eaton, 1977). This suggestion is supported by the recent observation that during perfusion of rat liver with oleate, pharmacologic doses of glucagon induce a significant decrease in triglyceride and an increase in β-hydroxybutyrate output (Tiengo, Nosadini, Garotti, Fedele, Muggeo and Crepaldi, 1977).

6. Kidney Function

Glucagon has a moderate but definite diuretic effect due to increased glomerular filtration rate and increased urinary excretion of electrolytes (Avioli, 1972*). In normal man, glucagon infusion, resulting in a 4 fold increase in plasma glucagon concentration, induced a significant increase in glomerular filtration rate ($+9\%$), filtration fraction ($+9\%$) and urinary β_2-microglobulin excretion rate ($+32\%$); these findings suggest that glucagon may contribute to the reversible alterations of kidney function typically found in poorly controlled juvenile diabetes, a state with relative or absolute hyperglucagonemia (Parving, Noer, Kehlet, Mogensen, Svendsen and Heding, 1977).

7. Other Actions of Glucagon

The pharmacology and clinical use of glucagon has been reviewed by Galloway (1972). Some of the clinical indications of glucagon are derived from its effects previously summarised in the present chapter: treatment of hypoglycemia, investigation of glycogen storage diseases, studies of insulin secretion in organic hyperinsulinism, etc.

In addition, other properties of glucagon have led to extensive clinical uses:

(i) inotropic positive effect on the heart (Parmley and Sonnenblick, 1971*; Glick, 1972*);

(ii) stimulation of adrenal medulla catecholamine release, a property used for the diagnosis of phaeochromocytoma (Lefebvre and Luyckx, 1972*; Sebel, Hull, Kleerkoper and Stokes, 1974*);

(iii) stimulation of growth hormone secretion, a tool for the investigation of pituitary disorders (Anonymous, 1973*);

(iv) inhibition of gastro-intestinal motility (Whalen, 1974*; Miller, Chernisch, Brunelle and Rosenak, 1978*).

E. FACTORS CONTROLLING GLUCAGON SECRETION

Reviewing in detail the numerous factors affecting glucagon secretion is beyond the scope of the present contribution. In this section, we will briefly survey the methods available for investigating glucagon secretion, the stimulants and inhibitors of glucagon secretion and the mechanisms involved in the control of glucagon secretion. Specific references can be found in Lefebvre and Unger (1972), Luyckx (1974), Unger and Orci (1976), Unger, Srere, Bromer and Felig (1976), Gerich, Charles and Grodsky (1976a), Foà, Bajaj and Foà (1977) and Unger, Dobbs and Orci (1978).

1. Methods for Studying Glucagon Secretion

Glucagon secretion can be investigated using isolated tissues, isolated perfused organs, *in situ* organs or entire organisms. Isolated tissues include pancreas slices as such (an inadequate procedure because of the damage caused to glucagon by the proteolytic enzymes simultaneously released) or slices from a duct-ligated pancreas (to obviate the preceding artefact), and isolated islets of Langerhans prepared either by microdissection or by collagenase digestion of pancreatic pieces (using this last procedure caution must be taken to avoid damage to the A-cells which in species such as the rat are located at the periphery of the islets). Isolated organ systems use isolated rat or dog pancreas or stomach, preparations which are perfused by artificial media or blood. Appropriate catheterizations permit simultaneous measurements of blood flow and net pancreatic or gastric glucagon production in large animals such as the dog or the pig. Finally, at the level of the whole organism, samples can be taken at the portal vein or peripherally; in this last instance, one should remember that liver glucagon uptake may represent 30–85% of the liver glucagon inflow (see Section F).

2. Stimulants and Inhibitors of Glucagon Secretion

Table 1 lists those factors demonstrated to stimulate glucagon secretion. The increase in plasma glucagon levels observed during or after muscular exercise results from adrenergic stimulation in mild-to-moderate exercise (Luyckx, Dresse, Cession-Fossion and Lefebvre 1975a) but in more severe exercise is also due to glucose lack since it is markedly inhibited and delayed when glucose is simultaneously given (Luyckx, Pirnay and Lefebvre, 1978).

Table 1

Stimulants of glucagon secretion.

Substrates	Hypoglycemia or cytoglycopenia (2-deoxyglucose)
	Low circulating levels of free fatty acids (FFA)
	Most amino acids
	Fumarate and glutamate
Neural factors	Stimulation of adrenergic and cholinergic nervous systems; stimulation of the ventro-medial hypothalamic structures
Local transmitters or factors	Adrenaline, noradrenaline, acetylcholine, dopamine, vasoactive intestinal peptide (VIP), neurotensin, substance P, prostaglandins, bombesin, (cyclic nucleotides?)
Hormones	Gastrin, cholecystokinin-pancreozymin, gastric inhibitory peptide (GIP), growth hormone
Ions	Total absence of calcium; lack of phosphate
Situations	Starvation, exercise, stress, balanced meal

Species differences appear to be important in relation to the mechanisms of exercise-induced glucagon rise: in rats, for instance, adrenergic stimulation seems to be prominent (Luyckx and Lefebvre, 1974; Luyckx *et al.*, 1975a) while, in man, β-adrenergic blockade does not inhibit exercise-induced glucagon rise (Galbo, Holst, Christensen and Hilsted, 1976). The rise in circulating glucagon levels after a balanced meal is probably due mainly to amino acid-induced glucagon release. The factors and conditions inhibiting glucagon release are listed in Table 2.

Table 2

Inhibitors of glucagon secretion.

Substrates	Hyperglycemia (also fructose and xylitol)
	High circulating levels of FFA (and ketone bodies?)
Local transmitters or factors	Serotonin, somatostatin
Hormones	Secretin, oestrogens (insulin)
Pharmacological agents	Atropine, β-receptor blocking agents, procaine, diazepam, phenformin, diazoxide (?), sulphonylureas (?)
Situations	Carbohydrate meal, pregnancy

3. Mechanisms Involved in the Control of Glucagon Secretion

The detailed mechanisms which control the release of glucagon are still poorly understood. Some studies seem to indicate that the mechanisms controlling glucagon release are somehow linked to substrate availability at the level of the A-cell. When energy substrates are lacking (hypoglycemia, starvation . . .) glucagon is released, when they are abundant (glucose administration, FFA infusion . . .) glucagon secretion is inhibited.

Numerous investigations have suggested that glucose-induced glucagon inhibition may be an insulin-requiring process. There is evidence that glucose entry into the A-cell may require insulin and, indeed, Östenson, Anderson, Brolin, Petersson and Hellerström (1977) using "A-cell rich guinea-pig islets" (prepared by streptozotocin destruction of most of the B-cells) have recently demonstrated that insulin simultaneously increases glucose utilisation by the A-cells, augments their ATP formation and permits glucose to inhibit glucagon secretion.

This concept that the amount of energy substrates within the A-cell plays a crucial role in the control of glucagon secretion is further supported by earlier observations of Edwards and Taylor (1970) which demonstrated that various metabolic inhibitors stimulate glucagon secretion. A role for cyclic nucleotides in the control of glucagon secretion has been suggested but not yet proved (Weir, Knowlton and Martin, 1975a; Wollheim, Blondel, Renold and Sharp, 1976). Some reports indicate that calcium ions and the microfilamentous microtubular system of the A-cells might be involved (Leclercq-Meyer, Marchand and Malaisse, 1974). The role of calcium in glucagon secretion appears complex: small amounts of calcium are normally required for glucagon secretion but glucagon suppression by glucose is a calcium-requiring process. In the total absence of calcium, a paradoxical stimulation of glucagon release by glucose has been reported (Leclercq-Meyer, Rebolledo, Marchand and Malaisse, 1975). There is an urgent need for careful histological investigations of the A-cells under various stimulatory or inhibitory conditions. The most recent investigations of Carpentier et al. (1977) have started to fill this gap. In their study, arginine-stimulated glucagon release was associated with a significant increase in morphological events linked to exocytosis. In contrast, the paradoxical release of glucagon observed in the presence of glucose and the absence of calcium, although accompanied by a significant decrease in granule stores, was not associated with an increase in morphologically detectable exocytosis. Thus, the release of similar quantities of glucagon in different conditions is not accompanied by similar morphological events, suggesting that different mechanisms are involved, and that our search for a unitary concept explaining the control of glucagon release might be in vain.

F. METABOLISM OF GLUCAGON

The metabolism of glucagon has been recently reviewed (Jaspan and Rubenstein, 1977*).

1. Metabolic Clearance Rate and Half Life in Plasma

The metabolic clearance rate (MCR) of glucagon in normal man has been reported to be 537 ± 27 ml/m^2/min by Fischer, Sherwin, Hendler and Felig (1976) and 9.0 ± 0.6 ml/kg/min by Alford, Bloom and Nabarro (1976). The MCR of glucagon is similar for plasma concentrations ranging from 200–600 pg/ml. The half life of glucagon in circulating plasma is about 5 min.

2. Hepatic Catabolism of Glucagon

The liver is the first organ encountered by glucagon after its secretion from the A-cells and it is indeed a major site of removal of glucagon from the circulation. The uptake of glucagon by the liver was first demonstrated by bioassay procedures (Goldner, Jauregui and Weisenfeld, 1954; Lefebvre and Luyckx, 1965) and has been confirmed by various investigators using a radioimmunoassay for the hormone (Buchanan, Solomon, Vance, Porter and Williams, 1968; Assan, 1972; Blackard, Nelson and Andrews, 1974; and others). In rats, Jaspan, Huen, Morley, Moossa and Rubenstein (1977), reported a portal-peripheral ratio of immuno-reactive glucagon (IRG) of 2.80 ± 0.55, a portal-peripheral difference of 124 ± 15 pg/ml and a percentage extraction of 58 ± 3 but showed that if the liver is a major site of metabolism of the 3500 dalton glucagon, it does not extract a significant amount of the other circulating immunoreactive glucagon components (see below). Thus, portal-peripheral ratios based on direct assay of plasma IRG will vary depending on the percentage glucagon immunoreactivity in each fraction. The greater the combined contribution of fractions other than the 3500-dalton component to total plasma IRG levels, the lower will be the ratio.

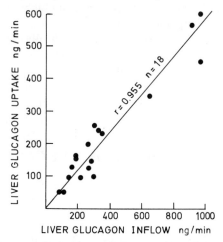

Fig. 6. Correlation between liver glucagon inflow in the portal vein and liver glucagon uptake. Eighteen determinations were performed in five overnight fasted anesthetised dogs. Reproduced from Lefebvre *et al.* (1978a) with permission of the copyright holders.

In overnight-fasted anaesthetised dogs, we reported (Lefebvre, Fischer, Jutzi, Hommel and Luyckx, 1978a) a highly statistically significant correlation between uptake and inflow of liver glucagon (Fig. 6). The percentage liver extraction (total IRG) was $61 \cdot 5 \pm 3 \cdot 8 \%$ (18 measurements in five dogs). A lower hepatic extraction has recently been reported by Röjdmark, Bloom, Chou and Field (1978).

3. Renal Handling of Glucagon

Narahara, Everett, Simons and Williams (1958) were the first to demonstrate an uptake of ^{131}I-glucagon by the rat kidney tubules. More precise data on the renal handling of glucagon were provided using dog kidneys either transplanted to the neck vessels of a perfusing anaesthetised dog or completely isolated and perfused *in vitro* using whole blood. Kidney glucagon uptake is linearly correlated with arterial plasma glucagon levels at all concentrations investigated between 26 and 1184 pg/ml, with a renal clearance rate of glucagon of about 0·5 ml/min/g kidney. The urinary clearance of glucagon represented less than 5% of the total kidney glucagon clearance (Lefebvre, Luyckx and Nizet, 1974; 1976b). The kidney thus appears as a major site of glucagon catabolism. However, Emmanouel, Jaspan, Kuku, Rubenstein and Katz (1976) have elegantly demonstrated that the renal handling of the various circulating IRG components may entail different mechanisms: it was suggested that the 3500 dalton-component is handled by both glomerular filtration and tubular secretion, while the metabolism of the 9000 dalton-fraction was mainly dependent on tubular secretion. The influence of interruption or impairment of kidney function on peripheral plasma glucagon levels will be described later (p. 211–212).

G. ASSAY OF GLUCAGON

If for the chemist, glucagon is a well defined compound (see Section A), for the physiologist (or the clinician) it is still a poorly characterised concept as recently emphasised by Unger (1976). It is accepted that glucagon is a circulating polypeptide hormone originating mainly, but not exclusively, from the A-cells of the islets of Langerhan. It is usually detected in plasma and tissues by radioimmunoassay and the term "immunoreactive glucagon" or IRG should be used. The bioassay of glucagon retains some limited, but important, applications.

1. Radioimmunoassay of Glucagon

The radioimmunoassay of glucagon has always been a problem (Luyckx, 1972; Luyckx and Lefebvre, 1976), not only due to the difficulties in obtaining appropriate antisera and the lability of the iodinated glucagon tracer, but mainly because of the presence in the digestive tract of a family of poly-peptides which possess different physicochemical, immunological and bio-logical properties than glucagon but which cross-react with many of the antisera raised against this hormone. These polypeptides are usually referred to as "glucagon-like immunoreactive material" (GLI) or, erroneously, as "enteroglucagon"; they have obscured for many years the whole field of glucagon research. It is now accepted that an antiserum which is to be used in a glucagon radioimmunoassay should not (or at most very poorly) cross-react with gut-GLI: the 30 K antibody raised by Dr Unger in Dallas is a world-wide accepted example of an antiserum "specific" for glucagon.

(a) Preparation of labelled glucagon

The usual technique by which glucagon is iodinated is based on the method described by Greenwood, Hunter and Glover (1963) for the iodination of growth hormone. At first, ^{131}I was employed by most investigators but it has now been increasingly replaced by [125]I. Improvements in the radio-iodination of glucagon have been introduced by Jorgensen and Larsen (1972). Holohan, Murphy, Buchanan and Elmore (1973), Desbuquois, Krug and Cuatrecasas (1974), Desbuquois (1975) and Von Schenk, Larsson and Thorell (1976). In this last method, iodination at pH 10 with an average of 0·3 g-atom of iodine per mole of glucagon resulted in ^{125}I-labelled glucagon with higher immunoreactivity and stability than that produced at the more conventional pH 7·5 or 8·5.

Procedures for purification, or repurification, of labelled glucagon solution can be found in Leclercq-Meyer, Miahle and Malaisse (1970), Heding (1971), Luyckx (1972) or Luyckx and Lefebvre (1976).

A fundamental advance in the development of the glucagon assay was made by Eisentraut, Whissen and Unger (1968) who demonstrated that incubation of labelled glucagon with plasma results in marked damage to the labelled molecule, leading to a decrease in the percentage bound and falsely elevated values of plasma glucagon. The presence of Trasylol® (500 to 1000 u/tube) in the assay mixture inhibits incubation damage almost completely and gives lower values for plasma glucagon which are probably closer to the true glucagon level in the plasma. Since it is well established that the destruction of glucagon by plasma varies with species (Mirsky, Perisutti and Davis, 1959), the adequacy of the amount of Trasylol® to be added must be tested by checking the binding to origin and the immuno-reactivity of the labelled preparation after its incubation with the plasma of the species under study. Ensinck, Shepard, Dudl and Williams (1972) reported the advantages of replacing Trasylol® by benzamidine as a proteolytic inhibitor in the radioimmunoassay of glucagon in plasma.

(b) Preparation of glucagon standards

Five mg of twice-crystallized pork-glucagon are dissolved in 10 ml 0·02 M HCl. A 10 μg/ml solution is prepared by dilution with the assay diluent (p. 196) or with "glucagon free plasma (p. 189). Aliquots of this stock solution can be deep frozen and stored for up to six months. In our laboratory (Luyckx, 1972), fresh working standards (0, 31·25, 62·5, 125, 250, 500, 1000 pg/ml) are prepared for each assay series. Sets of standards can be stored at − 20° for up to three months and thawed once.

(c) Preparation of plasma samples

The instability of circulating glucagon necessitates great care in the sampling of plasma. The blood sample must be placed in chilled tubes containing 1·2 mg Na_2EDTA and 0·1 ml (500 u) of Trasylol®/ml of blood. Blood specimens must be centrifuged immediately at 4°, and plasma frozen and stored at −20° until the time of assay. Storage for up to several months does not appear to be associated with loss of glucagon immunoreactivity. Plasma has been used as is in the assay procedure but gamma globulins can inhibit the binding of labelled glucagon by certain antibodies (Unger and Eisentraut, 1967). In order to avoid possible interference with the enzymes and gamma globulins present in the plasma, an extraction procedure was proposed by Heding (1971). The method consists in direct precipitation of all high-mw proteins in the plasma by ethanol at neutral pH, leaving the GLI in the supernatant. A final ethanol concentration of 61% gives a satisfactory and reproducible recovery of GLI in plasma. The extract, evaporated to dryness, is dissolved in the immunoassay buffer. The current availability of antisera that are highly specific for glucagon and that give results proportional to dilution of plasma samples would seem to make this step unnecessary in routine determinations. Recently, Alford, Bloom and Nabarro (1977) described a procedure to avoid the problem of the "non-specific plasma effects" that may produce errors in the estimation of true plasma glucagon concentrations by radioimmunoassay. In this procedure the glucagon content of each plasma is measured against a standard curve made up in an aliquot of the same plasma made free of glucagon by prior extraction with a specific glucagon immunoabsorbent. This sophisticated procedure involves the preparation of an antibody–sepharose complex and a subsequent affinity chromatography technique. However, it is no longer believed that glucagon circulates as a single component with a mw of 3500. Plasma IRG, undoubtedly exists in a number of different forms in both normal subjects and patients with various disorders (Jaspan and Rubenstein, 1977*). In these conditions, it is quite possible that extraction of plasma by ethanol or measurements against a "glucagon-free" plasma result in glucagon determinations that do not take into account some circulating components of still unknown biological importance (p. 199–200).

(d) Production and evaluation of antiglucagon antibodies

The techniques of immunization have been reviewed by Heding (1972) and Luyckx and Lefebvre (1976). The antisera are usually produced in rabbits or guinea-pigs using as antigen crystalline glucagon emulsified in adjuvant (Unger, Eisentraut, Keller, Lanz and Madison, 1959; Unger, Eisentraut, McCall and Madison, 1961; Baum, Simmons, Unger and Madison, 1962; Kologlu, Wiesell, Positano and Anderson, 1963; Assan, Rosselin, Drouet, Dolais and Tchobroutsky, 1965; Lawrence, 1966; Schopman, Hackeng and Steendijck, 1967; Hazzard, Crockford, Buchanan, Vance, Chen and Williams, 1968; Senyk, Nitecki and Goodman, 1971), glucagon bound to polyvinylpyrrolidone (Unger *et al.*, 1961; Assan *et al.*, 1965; Shima and Foà, 1968; Edwards, Howell and Taylor, 1970), glucagon polymerised by carbodiimide activation (Heding, 1969), or glucagon conjugated to serum albumin, ovalbumin or hemocyanin using bis-diazotized benzidine (Senyk, Nitecki, Spitler and Goodman, 1972), diethylmalonimidate (Grey, McGuigan and Kipnis, 1970) or carbodiimide (Unger *et al.*, 1961). Recently, Tager, Hohenboken and Markese (1977) reported production of high titre glucagon antisera with glucagon conjugated to albumin using difluorodinitrobenzene and McEvoy, Madson and Elde (1977) reported the value of using as antigenic conjugates homopolymer (glucagon to glucagon) or heteroconjugate (glucagon to keyhole limpet hemocyanin). A given antiserum is characterised by its titre, its affinity, and its specificity. The titre is reflected by the final dilution at which the antiserum can be used in the immunoassay procedure. The affinity is characterised as low, medium, high, or extremely high according to the slope of the standard curve. The specificity depends upon the degree of reactivity toward gut GLI, glucagon fragments, and with gamma globulins. In order to determine simultaneously the binding capacity and the binding affinity of the antiserum, the antibody dilution curve is determined both in the absence of unlabelled glucagon and in the presence of the glucagon concentrations corresponding to the desirable standard curve. The antiserum dilutions that bind 25–50% of the tracer can be used for the assay, if a suitably small quantity of unlabelled glucagon concentration causes a sufficient decrease in the percentage of tracer bound to antibody. The optimal conditions for a given sensitivity must be established by using different amounts of tracer to determine the optimal amount (e.g. 45, 20, and 15 pg/tube). Typical screening studies of various antiglucagon antisera can be found in Heding (1972), Luyckx (1972) and Luyckx and Lefebvre (1976). Before a given antiserum is used for plasma glucagon determination, its cross-reactivity with gut GLI, glucagon fragments and gamma globulins must be determined.

(*1*) *Immunoreactivity of gut GLI toward glucagon antibodies.* The gastrointestinal tract contains several peptides reacting with many of the antisera raised against pancreatic glucagon, they are usually referred to as gut GLI. "Gut GLI peptides" possess different physicochemical, immunological and biological properties than "glucagon" originating either from the A-cells of the islets of Langerhans or, at least in some species, from other similar cells also found in the gastro-intestinal tract (p. 176). An antiserum to be used in a glucagon radioimmunoassay should exhibit no, or very little, cross-reaction with a crude gut extract, or with one of the gut GLI peptides thus far purified from porcine small intestine and called "glycentin" (Sundby, Jacobsen and Moody, 1976).

Unger's 30K antibody is considered to be specific for glucagon: it measures less than 3% of the immunoreactivity present in crude or purified gut extract and evaluated with a "non-specific" antiserum.

(2) *Immunoreactivity of glucagon fragments.* The immunological and biological activities of the glucagon molecule are definitely not associated with the same portion of the polypeptide. For example, Sundby (1970) has observed that a glucagon molecule lacking the N-terminal histidine loses all its biological activity, while its immunologic activity is only slightly, if at all, altered. The extensive studies of Heding, Frandsen and Jacobsen (1976) have shown that the antigenic site in glucagon is located within the 24–29 section of the molecule but have also shown that biologically-inactivated glucagon may retain immunoreactivity in spite of the loss of receptor-binding activity.

Heding (1972) has investigated the residual immunoreactivity of labelled and unlabelled glucagon after incubation in plasma. At room temperature the plasma enzymes degraded the ^{125}I glucagon into different fragments, several of which could be bound to excess glucagon antibodies. As with gut GLI, glucagon fragments reacted differently with different antibodies. These findings could explain the differences among laboratories in the levels of plasma pancreatic glucagon in normal subjects despite the use of antisera devoid of cross-reactivity with gut GLI. After column chromatography (p. 199) small amounts of glucagon immunoreactivity with a mw of less than 2000 are found in plasma from control subjects (Jaspan and Rubenstein, 1977*). Preliminary evidence suggests that its concentration may increase in plasma in which proteolytic activity has not been fully inhibited, in which case it would represent an *in vitro* degradation product. It is however possible that this component represents a circulating fragment derived from the glucagon molecule during its *in vivo* catabolism (Jaspan and Rubenstein, 1977*).

(3) *"The interference factor".* Weir, Turner and Martin (1973) investigated the existence of non-specific factors interfering with the glucagon assay performed with antiserum 30K. Assuming that charcoal treatment was able to remove the glucagon in a given plasma sample, these authors demonstrated that charcoal-pretreated plasma still depresses the binding of labelled glucagon to the 30K antibody. The interfering factors appear to be neither pancreatic glucagon nor an enteric factor with glucagon-like immunoreactivity. When a correction factor was used, the mean fasting glucagon level has altered from 131 to 43 pg/ml. The persistence of a substance interfering with the glucagon assay (30K antiserum) was also demonstrated after treating plasma from a normal subject or pancreatectomised patient with charcoal (Muller, Brennan, Tan and Aoki, 1974). Using G-200 Sephadex, the interference factor was estimated to have a mw of approximately 160,000 (Weir, Knowlton and Martin, 1975b). It is now recognised that the "inter-

ference factor" is probably identical with the "big plasma glucagon" (BPG) described by Valverde, Villanueva, Lozano and Marco (1974). The physiological significance of BPG is still unknown.

(4) *Other possible interferences*

(i) *Gamma globulins.* Unger and Eisentraut (1967) have shown that human gamma globulin interferes with the reaction between ^{131}I-glucagon and some glucagon antibodies. It is therefore necessary to investigate the reaction with pure gamma globulins before using any glucagon antiserum.

(ii) *Antiglucagon antibodies.* The presence of endogenous glucagon antibodies in the plasma of diabetics receiving insulin therapy or treated by glucagon for insulin reactions may interfere with the glucagon radioimmunoassay (Stahl, Nars, Herz, Baumann and Girard, 1972; Cresto, Lavine, Perrino, Recant, August and Hung, 1974; Weir, Knowlton and Martin, 1975b; Villalpando and Drash, 1976). As analysed by Weir (1977), increased glucagon-binding by the plasma of significant numbers of diabetics is important because of possible interference in the radioimmunoassay: artefactually high values may be obtained in a double-antibody system but low values with adsorption techniques, such as charcoal or talc.

(iii) *Benzamidine.* Benzamidine has been proposed, in lieu of Trasylol®, to protect against the degradation of glucagon in human plasma (Ensinck *et al.*, 1972). No significant perturbation of the reaction of glucagon with the antibody 30K was encountered with benzamidine concentrations up to 0·025 M. Nevertheless, at concentrations between 0·05 and 0·01 M benzamidine, inhibition of the reaction was observed. In addition, the susceptibility of glucagon antisera to interference by benzamidine varied, since in two of the four guinea-pig antisera tested by Ensinck and associates, the affinity of the antibody for glucagon was significantly inhibited by 0·01 M benzamidine.

(e) *Separation of free- from antibody-bound glucagon*

As in the radioimmunoassay of other polypeptide hormones, several techniques for separating free- from antibody-bound hormone have been described (chromatoelectrophoresis, chromatography, immunoprecipitation, salt or ethanol precipitation of bound hormone, and charcoal, amberlite, talc or cellulose adsorption of free hormone).

Chromatography on Whatman 3 MM filter-paper strips was used in the first glucagon radioimmunoassay by Unger *et al.* (1961). Although this time-consuming method has become less popular for the assay itself, it remains highly suitable for use as a control procedure for the quality of labelled glucagon after iodination, for the estimation of damage to labelled hormone by plasma, and for the determination of the percentage of immunoreactive glucagon in the presence of an excess of antibody. Whatman 3 MM or 3 MC paper may be used for separation, but the property of retaining intact labelled hormone at the origin varies considerably from one batch of paper to the next. Only a few batches have proved suitable for separation. Chromatoelectrophoresis (0·05 M barbital buffer, pH 8·6, 750 v, 1 hr) increases the velocity of the migration (Assan, Rosselin and Dolais, 1967).

Descending chromatography on Ecteola paper (Lawrence, 1966; Assan et al., 1967; Luyckx and Lefebvre, 1970), although a very easy method to use, has two drawbacks: damaged labelled glucagon binds to the origin of Ecteola paper, and the paper itself is very fragile when wet. The glucagon–antibody complex may be precipitated by Na_2SO_4 (Unger et al., 1963), immunoprecipitation (Hazzard et al., 1968; Shima and Foà, 1969; Chesney and Schofield, 1969), or ethanol. The suitable final ethanol concentrations have been found to be 67 % (Edwards et al., 1970) or 80 % (Heding, 1971).

Cellulose powder, amberlite G 400, and dextran-coated charcoal when added to a mixture of free- and antibody-bound glucagon have the property of adsorbing the free hormone almost instantaneously, leaving the antibody-bound fraction in the supernatant. Details of these methods have been reported by Nonaka and Foà (1969) for cellulose powder and by Weinges (1968) for amberlite G 400. The dextran-coated charcoal method originally described by Herbert, Kam-Seng, Gottlieb and Bleicher (1965) for insulin and used for the glucagon assay by Aguilar-Parada, Eisentraut and Unger (1969), Leclercq-Meyer et al. (1970) and Luyckx (1972), will be described here in full. In theory, charcoal coated with molecules of appropriate size and configuration may be used for a virtually instantaneous separation of any free agent from the same agent bound to a carrier, provided there is a significant difference in molecular size and configuration between the agent alone and the agent when complexed with its carrier (Herbert et al., 1965).

We currently employ a dextran-coated charcoal suspension prepared by mixing 100 ml of a dextran T 70 solution (2·5 gm/100 ml) with 900 ml of the charcoal suspension (12·5 gm/900 ml). The mixture is shaken and stored for 4–6 weeks at 4°. A much less concentrated dextran-charcoal suspension, prepared by mixing equal volumes of 1 % Norit-A and 0·5 % dextran 70 in 0·2 M glycine buffer, pH 8·8, is used in Unger's laboratory (Aguillar-Parada et al., 1969).

In order to obtain adequate separation between free- and antibody-bound labelled glucagon, the quantity of charcoal which will adsorb the total amount of free hormone must be determined.

As shown in Fig. 7, for a given batch of ^{131}I-glucagon, the radioactivity bound to charcoal increases with the amount of dextran-coated charcoal suspension up to 2·5 ml/tube. For a given batch of labelled glucagon, the percentage bound by charcoal may be regarded as an index of tracer quality.

This parameter, F'/T (radioactivity bound to charcoal in the absence of antibody, F', divided by total radioactivity in each tube T), ranges between 90 and 97% for ^{131}I-glucagon and between 86 and 99% for ^{125}I-glucagon. Occasionally, for some batches of ^{125}I-glucagon, it will fall to 75%. Figure 8 illustrates the changes in the standard curve when a partially degraded tracer is used.

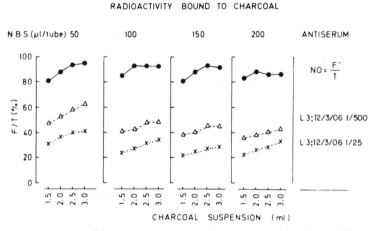

Fig. 7. Influence of the amount of charcoal suspension and of normal bovine serum (NBS) added to each tube on the fraction of labelled glucagon bound to charcoal (F'/T) (●——●) in the absence and in the presence (F/T) of two dilutions of antiglucagon serum (1 to 500, △---△; 1 to 25, ×----×). Reproduced from Luyckx and Lefebvre (1976) with permission of the copyright holders.

Another problem is that a relatively large amount of antibody-bound labelled hormone may be adsorbed on charcoal if the incubation medium does not contain the optimal concentration of protein. Figure 7 shows that, for a given antibody dilution (1/25), the radioactivity bound to charcoal apparently corresponding to free tracer decreases when 50, 100 or 150 μl of normal bovine serum is added to each tube before the dextran-charcoal suspension. The decrease in the F'/T ratio when 200 μl normal serum is added before the charcoal indicates that an excessive protein concentration might prevent the adsorption of free tracer on charcoal.

Such a preliminary study enables one to select the optimal quantities of normal serum and dextran-charcoal suspension to be used in the assay. It is essential to adjust the protein concentration in all tubes to the same value before adding the dextran-charcoal suspension. When artificial media are being assayed, this adjustment can be achieved by preparing standard

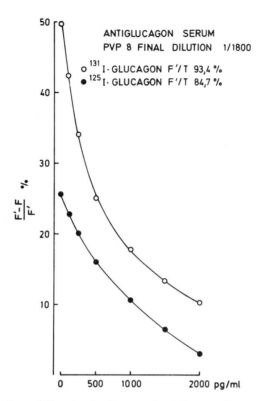

Fig. 8. Modification of the standard curve through use of a partially degraded labelled glucagon. Reproduced from Luyckx and Lefebvre (1976) with permission of the copyright holders.

glucagon solutions in the medium to be used for the *in vitro* experiments and adding the appropriate amount of normal serum at the end of the incubation period immediately before the dextran charcoal.

When assaying unextracted plasma by comparison with standards in 0·25% albumin buffer; it is necessary to add normal plasma to the standard curve tubes and buffer to the unknown tubes in order to adjust the protein concentration to the same optimal value in all tubes of the assay series.

(*f*) *Details of the procedure*

We provide hereafter the details of the basic materials, equipment and procedures used in our laboratory for the assay of glucagon in plasma:

Materials: Crystalline beef–pork glucagon (Eli Lilly Co., Indianapolis, Indiana) or crystalline pork glucagon (Novo Industri AS, Copenhagen,

Denmark); Norit-A (Pfanstiehl Laboratories, Inc., Waukegan, Illinois); Dextran 80 or T70 (Pharmacia, Uppsala, Sweden); Trasylol® (Bayer, Leverkusen, Germany).

Equipment: 13 × 78 mm disposable polyethylene tubes; standard volumetric glassware; automatic dispensing unit (0 to 1000 µl); refrigerated centrifuge; autogamma counter.

Assay diluent: the dilutions of labelled glucagon, antiserum, plasma samples, and glucagon standards are made in 0·2 M glycine buffer (pH 8·8) containing 0·25% human albumin and 1% normal bovine serum.

METHOD A

Incubation volumes. The following are added consecutively to the incubation tubes: 0·4 ml of the selected dilution of antiserum, 0·2 ml (1000 u) of Trasylol®, 0·2 ml of standard or plasma sample, 0·4 ml of tracer—^{125}I or ^{131}I glucagon, 15 pg. The standard curves and the unknown incubations are prepared in duplicate. Four control tubes (T) are prepared for the standard curve and two or more for each series of plasma from each patient (P). In these tubes the antiserum is omitted and replaced by the assay diluent. Three tubes containing only 0·4 ml of the tracer solution are prepared to be used as counting standards.

The tubes are covered with parafilm and incubated at 4° for four days. It has been well established that the whole incubation procedure and all manipulations during assay should be performed at 4°, since dissociation of the glucagon–antibody complex occurs if the tubes are allowed to stand at 25 or 37° (Heding, 1971).

Separation. The dextran-coated charcoal suspension (equal volumes of 1% Norit plus 0·5% dextran T70, both in 0·2 M glycine, pH 8·8) is kept in an ice bath with continuous stirring on a magnetic stirrer. Normal bovine serum and assay diluent are also chilled and kept in crushed ice.

To the tubes containing the glucagon standards is added 0·2 ml of the normal bovine serum and to the tubes containing plasma 0·2 ml of diluent is added in order to bring the protein concentration to approximately the same value in all tubes. Immediately after the bovine serum or the diluent, 0·5 ml of the dextran-charcoal suspension is added to each tube. The rack of tubes is left in an ice bath for 45 min and shaken four or five times during that period.

METHOD B

Incubation volumes. The following are added consecutively to the incubation tubes: 0·1 ml of the selected dilution of antiserum, 0·2 ml (1000 u) of Trasylol®, 0·1 ml of standard or plasma sample, 0·1 ml of tracer—^{125}I or

[131]I glucagon, 45 pg. Control incubations and counting standard are prepared as in method A. Incubations last four days at $4°$.

Separation. The dextran-coated charcoal suspension prepared by mixing 100 ml of 2·5 % dextran T70 and 900 ml of Norit (12·5 gm/900 ml) in 0·2 M glycine, pH 8·8, is kept at $4°$ under continuous stirring. To all tubes of the standard curve, 0·15 ml of normal bovine serum is added. To the tubes containing plasma, 0·15 ml of a mixture made with 10 ml of assay diluent and 5 ml of bovine serum are added. Lastly, 2·5 ml of the dextran-coated charcoal suspension are added to all tubes. In this case we have found it best to centrifuge the tubes not later than 20 min after the dextran-charcoal addition. Incubation for a further 60 min in the presence of charcoal results in dissociation of the tracer–antibody complex with an increase of about 5 % in the free form.

Centrifugation, counting and calculations. For both methods A and B, all tubes except the counting standards are centrifuged for 30 min at 2800 rpm at 4–6°. The supernatants are decanted by gentle inversion, and the tubes containing the charcoal pellets are ready for automatic gamma counting. Let us review the following symbols, which we have used earlier: T = cpm in counting standards (aliquot fraction of tracer solution kept without manipulation); F'_t = radioactivity bound to charcoal (in cpm) in the absence of antibody and corresponding to the control incubations of the standard curve; F'_p = radioactivity bound to charcoal (in cpm) in the absence of antibody, but in the presence of the plasma to be assayed, corresponding to the control incubations of a series of plasma from the same patient; F_{0-1000} = radioactivity bound to charcoal (in cpm) in the presence of antiserum and a given concentration (0–1000 pg/ml) of crystalline glucagon; F_p = radioactivity bound to charcoal (in cpm) in the presence of antiserum and a given plasma; $(F'_t \times 100)/T$ gives an index of the quality of the tracer: F'_p/T is most often close to F'_t/T; it gives an index of degrading activity of the plasma.

A moderate but significant reduction of the binding of the tracer to charcoal after incubation in the presence of human plasma may be observed. Incubation of the tracer with rat plasma leads to slight but significant reduction of its binding to charcoal. In the presence of dog plasma, this reduction never reaches the level of statistical significance.

The standard curve is obtained by plotting the ratio $(F'_t - F)/F'$ as a function of the concentrations of the glucagon standards (Fig. 8). Each plasma is characterised by its ratio $(F_p - F)/F'p$, which permits, by reference to the standard curve, determination of its glucagon content.

The sensitivity, precision, and reproducibility of the glucagon immunoassay are indicated in Table 3. The lowest concentration of glucagon detectable for plasma samples is 10 pg/ml.

Table 3

Details of 14 successive standard curves for glucagon assay with antiserum 30 K.

Glucagon concentration (pg/ml)	(^{131}I) glucagon bound to antibody (%) (M. ± S.E.M.)	Precision of points on standard curves (%)	Sensitivity of individual curves (%) ($p < 0.05$)	Equivalent glucagon concentration (pg/ml)
0	46·1 ± 0·8	1·0	0·52	10
62·5[a]	41·7 ± 1·1	1·7	1·20	15
125	37·0 ± 0·6	0·8	0·42	10
250	28·8 ± 0·6	0·9	0·47	15
500	18·3 ± 0·5	0·7	0·37	10
1000	9·6 ± 0·5	1·0	0·56	40
1500[b]	5·8 ± 0·6	1·0	0·80	300
2000	4·7 ± 0·5	0·9	0·45	250

[a] n = 8.
[b] n = 6.

2. Bioassays of Glucagon

In vivo and *in vitro* bioassays for glucagon are available (Sokal, 1972*; Luyckx and Lefebvre, 1976*). *In vivo* methods (Rowlinson and Lesford, 1951; Staub and Behrens, 1954; Bromer, 1961) have mainly an historical interest although they are still in use for assay of purified pharmaceutical glucagon concentrates or for measurements of the glucagon content of commercial insulin preparations. They will not be considered here.

In vitro procedures include the use of liver slices (Vuylsteke and De Duve, 1957), isolated perfused rat liver (Sokal and Weintraub, 1966; Sokal, 1970; Mortimore, 1973), isolated chicken fat cells (Langslow and Hales, 1970) and isolated rat liver cell membranes (Solomon, Londos and Rodbell, 1974; Holst, 1975). Among these techniques, the most used are the isolated perfused rat liver and the isolated rat liver cell membranes.

The isolated perfused rat liver is *par excellence* the reference method since it is based on the most widely accepted physiological effect of glucagon (p. 177). For the purpose of glucagon bioassay (Sokal, 1970), phosphorylase activation and hepatic glucose release were used as parameters. This method allowed Sokal and Ezdinli (1967) to demonstrate that plasma glucagon values determined by various immunoassays available at that time had been grossly overestimated. Analyses of the discrepancies between the results of the immunoassay and the isolated liver bioassay led Unger et al. (1968) to discover the damage that plasma proteolytic enzymes can cause to the labelled tracer (p.188) and its prevention by Trasylol®. More recently, the isolated perfused rat liver has permitted the characterisation of the properties of the various immunoreactive glucagon fractions of canine stomach and pancreas (Srikant, McCorckle and Unger, 1977).

Procedures for isolation of rat liver cell membranes have been described by Solomon *et al.* (1974), and Lesko, Donlon, Marinetti and Hare (1973), and their use for a glucagon radioreceptor assay by Rosselin, Freychet, Bataille and Kitabgi (1974) and Holst, 1975. As recently emphasised by Holst (1978) "in radioreceptor assay as in radioimmunoassay, anything which interferes with the binding of the labelled ligand will be recognised as if a substance were bound to the glucagon receptor; the radioreceptor assay being quite sensitive to such non-specific interference, its use has been restricted to assays of plasma and tissue extracts only after gel filtration".

H. CIRCULATING GLUCAGON

This section will be restricted to a brief survey of the *data available in man*, and thus pertinent to human physiology and pathology.

1. Human Physiology

(a) *Basal levels*

The high values published up to 1966 (Luyckx and Lefebvre, 1976) resulted from (i) the absence of Trasylol® or benzamidine in the incubation medium, leading to degradation of the tracer and over-estimation of the glucagon concentration (p. 189) and (ii) the side use of antisera cross-reacting with gut-GLI (p. 190). Artefactual plasma glucagon readings may result from inappropriate handling of the samples such as blood coagulation, freezing and thawing, and inappropriate temperature.

Using the 30K antiserum glucagon concentration in the plasma of fasting normal persons is about 50–150 pg/ml. Data of our own laboratory are illustrated by Table 4. Using a specific immunoabsorbent step in their radioimmunoassay, Alford *et al.* (1977) reported lower values: 24 ± 3 (S.E.M.) pg/ml ($n = 18$; range 4–52).

(b) *Heterogeneity*

The heterogeneity of plasma IRG in healthy individuals has been described by Valverde *et al.* (1974), Weir *et al.* (1975b), Kuku, Zeidler, Emmanouel, Katz, Rubenstein, Levin and Tello (1976), and Jaspan and Rubenstein (1977*). Biogel P30 column chromatography of plasma samples and subsequent

Table 4

Plasma glucagon values in fasting normal controls: data obtained with antiserum 30 K.

Mean value (pg/ml)	Standard deviation	Number of determinations	Upper limit of normals at the 95% level (pg/ml)	References
65	38	23	145	Luyckx and Lefebvre (1976)
80	37	6	157	Lefebvre and Luyckx (1976a)
72	34	7	139	Quabbe et al., (1977)
72	37	7	147	Quabbe et al., (1977)
68	39	7	157	Quabbe et al., (1977)
81	48	10	176	Luyckx et al., (1978)

measurements of IRG on the fractionated samples permitted the identification of four components in the plasma IRG of normal humans (Jaspan and Rubenstein, 1977; Valverde, 1977). Table 5 gives the basal plasma 30K immunoreactive components as found by Valverde (1977). As already discussed (p. 191), the high mw component corresponds to the "interference factor" described by Weir et al. (1973), or to the big plasma glucagon or BPG, described by Valverde et al. (1974). It represents the highest percentage of immunoreactivity recovered from the column. The 9000 dalton component was not initially detected in the plasma of normal subjects by Kuku et al. (1976) but was subsequently found in low concentrations by the same authors (Jaspan and Rubenstein, 1977); it was present in 75% of normal humans by Valverde (1977) and is likely to be a glucagon precursor (p. 176). The 3500 dalton component is thought to represent "true" circulating glucagon; its mean concentration represents 17% only of the total immunoreactivity found in basal plasma of normal humans. Small amounts of glucagon immunoreactivity are found in the 2000 dalton region; they probably correspond to in vivo (or in vitro) degradation products (p. 191).

Table 5

Basal plasma 30 K immunoreactive components-Biogel P-30; mean of 20 samples from normal humans (from Valverde, 1977).

	Total plasma (pg/ml)	160,000 mw (pg/ml)	9000 mw (pg/ml)	3500 mw (pg/ml)	2000 mw (pg/ml)
M.	155	91	19	27	19
S.D.	96	54	17	25	16
% of total (range)		28–100	0–31	0–39	0–33

(c) *Some factors affecting basal plasma IRG in normal subjects*

(1) *Age.* No effect of age on basal plasma glucagon was detected by Dudl and Ensinck (1977), but a significant rise after the third decade was reported by Berger, Crowther, Floyd, Pek and Fajans (1977). A hyperglucagonism of the elderly was also reported by Marco, Hedo and Villanueva (1977).

(2) *Sex.* No sex difference in basal plasma glucagon has been reported. Beck, Eaton, Arnett and Alsever (1975) reported that glucagon secretion in response to i.v. arginine was blunted in normal women taking contraceptive steroids (mestranol plus norethidrone as well as ethinyl-estradiol).

(3) *Pregnancy.* A moderate increase in basal plasma glucagon during the second trimester of human pregnancy has been observed by Luyckx, Gerard, Gaspard and Lefebvre (1975b) while no significant change compared with nongravid nullipara was found by Daniel, Metzger, Freinkel, Faloona, Unger and Nitzan (1974). Plasma glucagon is more readily suppressed after oral or i.v. glucose during pregnancy than in the non-pregnant state (Daniel *et al.,* 1974; Luyckx *et al.,* 1975b; Kuhl and Holst, 1976). The rise in plasma glucagon after a protein meal is less compared with the rise observed in the same conditions during the post-partum period (Kuhl, Homnes and Klebe, 1977). The glucagon response to insulin-induced hypoglycaemia is reduced by about 60% during the last month of pregnancy; furthermore it is completely abolished by raising plasma FFA to about 1500 μmol/l (Luyckx, Gaspard and Lefebvre, 1978).

(4) *Neonatal period.* The presence of glucagon in the portal plasma of human neonates has been reported by Luyckx, Massi-Benedetti, Falorni and Lefebvre (1972) and Bloom and Johnston (1972). Intraportal administration of glucose did not suppress plasma glucagon in infants of diabetic mothers; concomitant intraportal administration of both glucose and insulin permitted glucagon suppression in infants born from normal mothers (Massi-Benedetti, Falorni, Luyckx and Lefebvre, 1974). These findings support the concept that the human A-cell is sensitive to insulin (p. 184). Further data on the control of glucagon secretion in the normal newborn have been provided by Sperling, Delamater, Phelps, Fiser, Oh and Fisher (1974).

(d) *Physiological changes in plasma glucagon levels*

(1) *Starvation.* During starvation, normal individuals usually exhibit a rise in plasma glucagon concentration to an average of 50–100% of their usual overnight fasting level (Muller, Faloona and Unger, 1971). A similar rise was reported after three days of starvation in obese patients (Marliss, Aoki, Unger, Soeldner and Cahill, 1970; Fisher, Sherwin, Hendler and Felig, 1976) but was followed by a fall to a plateau sometimes above the post-

absorptive level (Marliss *et al.*, 1970) and sometimes not (Fisher *et al.*, 1976).

(*2*) *Exercise.* Plasma glucagon rises in man in response to exercise (Böttger, Schlein, Faloona, Knochel and Unger, 1972; Felig, Wahren, Hendler and Ahlborg, 1972). The exercise-induced rise in glucagon is greater in prolonged exercise than in graded short-time exercise (Galbo, Holst and Christensen, 1975) and is delayed and reduced by the ingestion (Ahlborg and Felig, 1976; Luyckx, Pirnay and Lefebvre, 1978) or the infusion (Galbo, Christensen and Holst, 1977) of glucose. In contrast with the results obtained in rats (Luyckx and Lefebvre, 1974), beta-receptor blockade do not diminish, in man, the glucagon response to exercise (Galbo, Holst, Christensen and Hilsted, 1976). Training results in a marked reduction in the magnitude of the rise in exercise-induced plasma glucagon (Gyntelberg, Rennie, Hickson and Holloszy, 1977).

(*3*) *Changes in blood glucose.* Elevation of blood glucose reduces plasma glucagon levels, while hypoglycemia, on the contrary, stimulates glucagon secretion (Unger and Lefebvre, 1972*). The possible permissive role of insulin on the glucose-induced glucagon suppression has already been discussed (p. 184); it is supported by various clinical observations (Massi-Benedetti, Falorni, Luyckx and Lefebvre, 1974; Raskin, Aydin and Unger, 1976; Aydin, Raskin and Unger, 1977; Hatfield, Banasiak, Driscoll, Kim and Kalkhoff, 1977).

The rise in glucagon in the insulin-tolerance test is illustrated by Fig. 9. Its role in the correction of blood glucose after insulin injection has been challenged by Garber, Cryer, Santiago, Haymond, Pagliara and Kipnis (1976) who presented arguments suggesting that adrenergic mechanisms, rather than glucagon, play a major role in the initiation of counter-regulatory responses to insulin-induced hypoglycemia in man.

(*4*) *Changes in plasma FFA.* Elevation of plasma FFA is usually accompanied by a fall in circulating glucagon concentrations in normal man (Gerich, Langlois, Schneider, Karam and Noacco, 1974; Andrews, Lopez and Blackard, 1975) or normal pregnant women (Luyckx, Gerard, Gaspard and Lefebvre, 1975b). This effect, however, has not been found by Hicks, Taylor, Vij, Pek, Knopf, Floyd and Fajans (1977). On the other hand, a fall in plasma FFA due to nicotinic-acid infusion induces an unequivocal rise in plasma glucagon (Gerich *et al.*, 1974; Quabbe, Ramek and Luyckx, 1977; Hicks *et al.*, 1977); this fall can be completely reversed by glucose infusion (Quabbe *et al.*, 1977).

(*5*) *Changes in plasma amino acids.* Ingestion or infusion of amino acids markedly stimulate glucagon secretion and, thus, increase plasma glucagon circulating levels (Assan, Rosselin and Dolais, 1967; Fajans, Floyd, Knopf and Conn, 1967; Unger, Aguilar-Parada, Müller and Eisentraut, 1970).

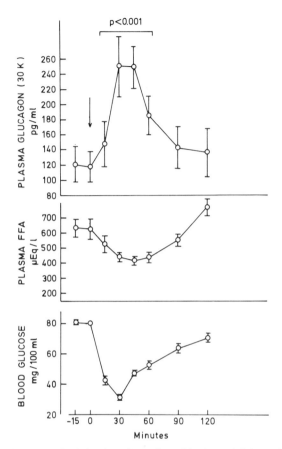

Fig. 9. Effect of i.v. insulin injection (0·1 u/kg of body weight) on blood glucose, plasma-free fatty acids (FFA), and glucagon concentrations in 12 normal subjects (M. ± S.E.M.; paired comparisons *vs* basal values). Reproduced from Luyckx *et al.* (1978) with permission of the copyright holders.

The arginine-infusion test, as originally proposed by Unger *et al.* (1970) is now used as a standard test of alpha-cell function. As recently demonstrated by Valverde (1977), the 3500 dalton fraction of circulating IRG is mainly responsible for the rise observed after arginine infusion. Recently, tryptophan ingestion (10 gm) has been reported to increase significantly IRG plasma levels in man (Hedo, Villanueva and Marco, 1977).

(6) *Carbohydrate feeding.* The ingestion of a glucose load or a carbo-hydrate meal promptly lowers plasma glucagon by about 20 pg/ml (Müller, Faloona, Aguilar-Parada and Unger, 1970), a diminution corresponding to

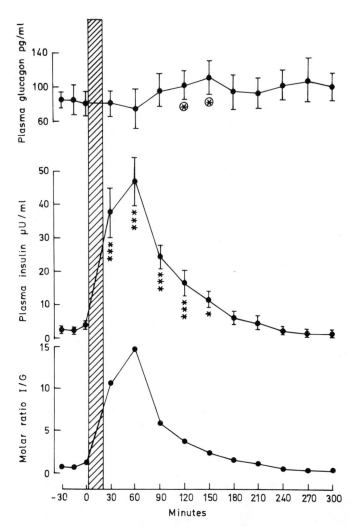

Fig. 10. Effect of the ingestion of a standardised breakfast (hatched area) on plasma glucagon and insulin levels, and on the mean insulin: glucagon molar ratio in a groups of six normal subjects. Results are indicated as M. ± S.E.M. *** and * correspond to *p* values less than 0·01 or 0·05 respectively (non-paired comparison). * corresponds to a *p* value less than 0·05 (paired comparison *vs* sample collected at time 0). Reproduced from Lefebvre and Luyckx (1976a) with permission of the copyright holders.

an almost complete disappearance of the 3500 dalton circulating fraction (Valverde, 1977; see also p. 200).

(7) *Fat feeding.* The ingestion of a pure fat meal by man causes a modest but significant rise in plasma glucagon (Böttger, Faloona, Dobbs and Unger, 1973), an observation which has been reproduced by the instillation of fat into the duodenum of dogs (Böttger *et al.*, 1973). The mechanism of this effect, and its physiological relevance, are still discussed (Unger and Orci, 1976).

(8) *Protein feeding.* The ingestion of a protein meal, protein hydrolysates, amino acid mixtures or even single amino acids elicits a prompt rise in plasma glucagon (Assan *et al.*, 1967; Fajans *et al.*, 1967; Unger *et al.*, 1970). The function of this aminogenic glucagon secretion has been analysed by Unger, Ohneda, Aguilar-Parada and Eisentraut (1969) and Unger and Orci (1976) and is believed to prevent hypoglycemia that might result from insulin secretion stimulated by the amino acids. Recent observations made on the isolated perfused dog stomach suggest that intraluminal arginine may directly stimulate the gastric A-cell (Lefebvre and Luyckx, 1978). The relevance of this last observation to human physiology or pathology is probably limited.

(9) *Mixed meal.* Ingestion of a mixed meal may result in a rise, a fall or no change in plasma glucagon depending upon the relative amounts of carbohydrates that tend to reduce plasma glucagon levels and of lipids, and mainly proteins, that tend to increase them. A standard breakfast (Fig. 10), for instance, has been reported to increase slightly, but significantly, plasma glucagon concentrations (Lefebvre and Luyckx, 1976a).

2. Human Pathology

(a) Diabetes

Since the availability of a radioimmunoassay for glucagon, numerous investigators attempted to define a possible role for glucagon in the aetiology and/or physiopathology of diabetes. Major references on this topic can be found in Lefebvre and Unger (1972), Luyckx (1974, 1975), Unger and Orci (1976), Unger, Srere. Bromer and Felig (1976). Glucagon secretion in human diabetes has been reviewed by Gerich (1977). A relative or absolute hyperglucagonemia has been reported in most forms of diabetes mellitus. In some instances, the hyperglucagonemia is *absolute*; by this it is meant that the glucagon plasma concentrations found in diabetics exceed those found in normal controls and this regardless of the blood glucose level. In most cases, however, the hyperglucagonaemia is *relative*, i.e. relatively high in relation to a high blood glucose concentration (which normally inhibits

H

glucagon secretion and depresses plasma glucagon levels, (p. 184). A classical example of the relative hyperglucagonemia of diabetes is the lack of suppression of plasma glucagon during oral or i.v. glucose loading in diabetic patients (Müller, Faloona, Aguilar-Parada and Unger, 1970). Frequently, diabetic subjects exhibit a *paradoxical* rise in plasma glucagon after glucose administration (Buchanan and McCarroll, 1972). The mechanism of this paradoxical rise is still unknown. The question of determining if the abnormalities in glucagon secretion observed in diabetes are secondary to the absolute or relative insulin lack or if there is an intrinsic defect of A-cell function in diabetes is still open. In both cases, however, there is much evidence that both insulin deficiency and glucagon excess contribute to the metabolic abnormalities associated with diabetes mellitus (bihormonal abnormality hypothesis of Unger and Orci, 1975), even if diabetic keto-acidosis can develop in the absence of glucagon (see below).

Extremely high concentrations of circulating glucagon have been reported in diabetic keto-acidosis (Assan, Hautecouverture, Guillemant, Dauchy, Protin and Derot, 1969; Unger et al., 1970) as well as in hyperosmolar hyperglycemia (Lindsey, Faloona and Unger, 1974). As demonstrated by Gerich, Lorenzi, Bier, Schneider, Tsalikian, Karam and Forsham (1975), infusion of somatostatin prevents both the rise in glucagon and the development of keto-acidosis which normally occurs after acute cessation of i.v. insulin in insulin-dependent diabetics, thus suggesting an essential role of glucagon in the development of human diabetic keto-acidosis. This conclusion was challenged by Barnes, Bloom, Alberti, Smythe, Alford and Chisholm (1977) who showed that keto-acidosis can develop in the pancreactomised man deprived of insulin, without any detectable increase in plasma glucagon. However, the rise in blood glucose and plasma ketones was much less rapid in the pancreatectomised than in the non-pancreatectomised subjects, thus demonstrating that glucagon may accelerate the onset of ketonemia and hyperglycemia in conditions associated with insulin deficiency. Insulin administration in diabetic keto-acidosis induces a rapid fall in circulating levels of plasma glucagon (Assan et al., 1970; Unger et al., 1970). Somatostatin, a potent glucagon suppressing agent, may improve diabetic control in insulin-requiring diabetics (Gerich, 1977*) although its use in maturity-onset diabetes is, on the contrary, deleterious because it also inhibits residual insulin function (Tamborlane, Sherwin, Hendler and Felig, 1977). Sulphonylureas have been reported to reduce (Ohneda, Ishii, Horigome and Yamagata, 1975; Loreti, Sugase and Foa, 1974; Telner, Taylor, Pek, Crowther, Floyd and Fajans, 1977; Falucca, Iavicoli, Menzinger, Mirabella and Andreani, 1978) or not affect (Pek, Fajans, Floyd, Knopf and Conn, 1972; Marco and Valverde, 1973; Podolsky and Lawrence, 1977; Lecomte, Luyckx and Lefebvre, 1977) plasma glucagon levels in normal man or in diabetic patients. Dimethylbiguanide (Carpentier, Luyckx and Lefebvre, 1975) and butylbiguanide (Lefebvre, Luyckx, Mosora, Lacroix and Pirnay, 1978b) did not modify basal, stimulated or inhibited plasma glucagon levels in maturity-onset diabetics, while phenformin has been recently reported to suppress postprandial hyperglucagonemia (Tsalikian, Dunphy, Bohannon, Lorenzi, Gerich, Matin and Forsham, 1976; Bohannon, Karam, Lorenzi, Gerich, Matin and Forsham, 1977).

(b) Glucagon and haemochromatosis

Enhanced glucagon secretion in response to i.v. arginine and non-suppressibility of glucagon by oral glucose were reported in patients with idiopathic haemochromatosis (Passa, Luyckx, Carpentier, Lefebvre and Canivet, 1977). Glucagon hypersecretion in response to arginine was confirmed by Gonvers, Henchoz, Hoffstetter and Muller (1977).

(c) Glucagon and the pancreatectomised man

True A-cells are present outside the pancreas in several animal species like dog, cat or rat but the presence of such extrapancreatic A-cells in man is still a matter of controversy (p. 176). Table 6 reports the data available for measurements of glucagon in the peripheral plasma of pancreatectomised humans. To 1977, measurements had been performed in 16 pancreatectomised subjects; significant amounts of glucagon were found in 10 of them with a rise after arginine infusion in two and a paradoxical rise in the oral glucose tolerance test in another two. Apparent absence of glucagon in some patients may be due to incomplete insulin deprivation or, in some cases, to simultaneous partial gastrectomy. However, as stated earlier, moderate hyperglycemia and hyperketonemia can develop unequivocally in the pancreatectomised man deprived of insulin without any significant rise in plasma glucagon (Barnes et al., 1977).

(d) Glucagonoma

Although possible cases had been reported before (Lawrence, 1972*; Mallinson, Bloom, Warin, Salmon and Cox, 1974*) it is usually accepted that the first documented case of a primary glucagon-secreting tumour was reported by McGavran, Unger, Recant, Polk, Kilo and Levin (1966). Mallinson et al. (1974) gave a full description of the "glucagonoma syndrome" based on the observation of nine patients: all nine had necrolytic migratory erythema, stomatitis, weight loss and seven had diabetes. Since then, several similar cases were reported (Bloom, 1977*). Plasma glucagon levels

Table 6

Glucagon and pancreatectomy in man.

Number of patients	Assay standard	Insulin deprivation (hr)	Plasma glucagon (pg/ml)	Response to arginine	Remarks	References
2	30 K	12	before charcoal: 80–85 after charcoal: 35	no rise	—	Muller et al. (1974)
1	30 K	12	80–110	no rise	40–80% "big plasma glucagon"	Marco et al. (1975)
5	C-terminal reacting; standard curve in "glucagon-free plasma"	12	5 ± 2 (not different from zero)	no rise	—	Barnes and Bloom (1976)
1	30 K	24	zero	no rise	—	Gerich et al. (1976b)
3	30 K; acetone extraction		35–60	rise in 2 patients	—	Palmer et al. (1976)
1	AGS 18	?	100		rise in OGTT	Foà (1976)
1	30 K	?	"normal"		—	Vranic (1976)
1	30 K	18	0–200	no rise	—	Miyata et al. (1976)
1	30 K	24	before charcoal: 80–100 after charcoal: 35–45 after affinity chromatography: 35–45	no rise	rise in OGTT	Botha et al. (1977)

are usually extremely high: 850–3500·pg/ml in four of the patients reported by Mallinson *et al.* (1974). Only a few cases have been described where the initial value was below 1000 pg/ml (Bloom, 1977). In five patients with glucagonoma, higher plasma concentrations of the 9000 dalton fraction of IRG (p. 200) have been reported, suggesting that, like insulinomas which secrete proinsulin, A-cells of glucagonomas may secrete increased amounts of a possible glucagon precursor (Weir, Horton, Aoki, Slovik, Jaspan and Rubenstein, 1977). Finally, Boden and Owen (1977) reported that they found elevated basal immunoreactive glucagon levels in four of nine asymptomatic relatives of a patient with glucagonoma. Most intriguing is that gel filtration of plasma revealed that over 85% of the IRG of the four relatives had a molecular size greater than 9000 daltons whereas two-thirds of the IRG of the patients with the glucagonoma had a molecular weight of 3500 daltons, with the remaining one-third (as in the cases of Weir *et al.*, 1977) corresponding to 9000 daltons. The data of Boden and Owen (1977) suggest an autosomal dominant transmission of hyperglucagonemia in the family that they have studied. A similar observation has been made by Ensinck and Palmer (1976) in three generations of a family where so far no glucagonoma has been found.

(e) Glucagon deficiency

As reviewed by Lawrence (1972), attempts to isolate a glucagon deficiency syndrome have been disappointing. Glucagon deficiency has been suspected, but to our knowledge not yet convincingly proved, in some cases of neonatal hypoglycemia (McQuarrie, Bell, Zimmerman and Wright, 1950). Vidnes and Øyasaeter (1977) reported a case of severe neonatal hypoglycemia, with impairment of gluconeogenesis, where glucagon circulating levels were low (but not zero) and where treatment with glucagon resulted in a marked clinical improvement. Bleicher, Spergel, Levy and Zarowitz (1970) reported a case where arginine infusion induced hyperinsulinemia and hypoglycemia with unmeasurable plasma glucagon. This observation supports the concept (p. 205) that the role of stimulation of glucagon secretion by amino acids is to prevent hypoglycemia from the associated insulin release. The suggestion that glucagon deficiency may play a role in the pathogenesis of certain cases of reactive hypoglycemia has been ruled out (Luyckx, 1974; Lefebvre, Luyckx and Lecomte, 1976a). In a recent investigation from our laboratory, it has been clearly demonstrated that, on the contrary, reactive hypoglycemia was always accompanied by a rise in plasma glucagon and that successful treatment of the reactive hypoglycemia was associated with the suppression of the glucagon rebound (Giugliano, Luyckx, Binder and Lefebvre, 1978).

(f) Glucagon and other endocrine diseases

(1) Acromegaly. Goldfine, Kirsteins and Lawrence (1972) demonstrated excessive plasma glucagon response to arginine in acromegalics and suggested that abnormal A-cell function exists in acromegaly, a suggestion in agreement with a previous morphologic data (Lawrence, 1972*).

(2) Cushing's disease. Excessive glucagon response to arginine has been reported in patients with Cushing's disease (Seino, Goto, Kurahachi, Sakurai, Ikeda, Kadowaki, Inoue, Mori, Taminato and Imura, 1977) as it is after glucocorticoid administration in healthy controls (Marco, Calle, Roman, Diaz-Fierros, Villanueva and Valverde, 1973a; Wise, Hendler and Felig, 1973). However, oral glucose substantially suppresses plasma glucagon in patients with Cushing's syndrome (Imura, Ikeda and Seino, 1977).

(3) Hyperthyroidism. The plasma glucagon response to arginine infusion has been reported to be slightly but not significantly reduced (Seino, Goto, Taminato, Ikeda and Imura, 1974).

(4) Hypothyroidism. Glucagon response to arginine is usually exaggerated in hypothyroidism (Seino *et al.*, 1974; Seino *et al.*, 1977).

(5) Pheochromocytoma. High fasting serum glucagon levels in five patients with pheochromocytoma have been reported by Lawrence (1966).

(6) Addison's disease. Okuno and Takenaka (1977) investigated A-cell function in a single patient with primary adrenocortical insufficiency. Basal plasma glucagon levels and the glucagon response to hypoglycemia were normal. The glucagon response to arginine, before treatment, was about half that observed in normal controls. This response became supranormal, but markedly prolonged after cortisol treatment.

(7) Multiple endocrine tumour syndrome. Hypersecretion of glucagon has been reported in multiple endocrine adenomatosis (Vance, Kitabchi, Buchanan, Stoll, Hollander and Wood, 1968; Vance, Stoll, Kitabchi, Williams and Wood, 1969).

(8) Islet-cell tumours. In two patients with metastatic pancreatic islet-cell carcinoma, Walter, Dudl and Ensinck (1972) reported extremely high basal circulating levels of plasma glucagon but attenuated response to various stimuli. In one case of organic hyperinsulinism, Luyckx (1974) reported plasma glucagon suppression by glucose, stimulation by insulin-induced hypoglycemia and inhibition by diazoxide. In another case of insulinoma, alpha-cell function has also been reported as normal (Santeusanio and Brunetti, 1976).

(g) Glucagon and obesity

For non-diabetic obese subjects, there is confusion concerning A-cell function. Paulsen and Lawrence (1968) reported high fasting glucagon levels in obese children compared with normal, non-obese controls, but the results of this study must be viewed with caution since the antibody used in the assay cross-reacted with gut GLI (p. 190). Wise, Hendler and Felig (1973) and Luyckx (1974) reported basal plasma glucagon concentrations to be similar in adult obese and in non-obese controls. In a careful recent study, plasma glucagon profiles, derived from hourly samples during a 24 hr-period, were nearly identical in 10 normal and six obese, non-diabetic subjects (Santiago, Haymond, Clarke and Pagliara, 1977). Glucagon responses of obese subjects to i.v. and oral glucose, beef meals and insulin-induced hypoglycemia have been reported as normal (Kalkhoff, Gossain and Matute, 1973; Santiago et al., 1977). The glucagon response to i.v. arginine was similar to that of normal controls (Santiago et al., 1977), but Kalkhof et al. (1973), reported an exagerated response. In contrast, the response to i.v. alanine was reduced (Wise, Hendler and Felig, 1973). The reasons for these conflicting reports have been analysed by Santiago et al. (1977). Metabolic clearance rates of glucagon and basal systemic delivery rates of the hormone in the post-absorptive state were found to be similar in obese and non-obese subjects (Fisher et al., 1976). Gel filtration profiles of plasma IRG in obese patients are similar to those reported in normal controls (cited by Jaspan and Rubenstein, 1977).

(h) Glucagon and hyperlipoproteinemia

The possible role of glucagon in lipoprotein metabolism has already been discussed p. 181. Increased plasma glucagon concentrations are usually found in hypertriglyceridaemias (Eaton, 1977*; and Tiengo et al., 1977*). Similarly, the glucagon response to arginine infusion is usually enhanced in hyperlipoproteinemia (Eaton, 1973; Tiengo, Muggeo, Assan, Fedele and Crepaldi, 1975). Clofibrate-induced reduction in plasma triglyceride levels is associated with a reduction in basal plasma glucagon concentrations but in contrast the glucagon response to arginine is enhanced (Tiengo et al., 1977). The interpretation of the hyperglucagonemia of hyperlipoproteinemia is still a matter of discussion: it is viewed by Eaton and Schade (1973) as manifestation of "glucagon resistance" while according to Tiengo et al. (1977) it is an expression of a primitive hyperactivity of the A-cell as considered by some workers to be present in diabetes (p. 205).

(i) Glucagon and renal insufficiency

The kidney plays a major role in the catabolism of endogenous glucagon (p. 186) and cessation of renal function in experimental animals induces a brisk rise in peripheral plasma glucagon levels (Bilbrey, Faloona, White

and Knochel, 1974; Lefebvre and Luyckx, 1975, 1976b) which reflects
cessation of renal catabolism of glucagon since the simultaneously measured
pancreatic secretion rates remained unchanged (Lefebvre and Luyckx,
1975). High plasma circulating levels of glucagon have been reported in
renal failure (Assan, 1972; Bilbrey et al., 1974; Daubresse, Lerson, Plomteux,
Rorive, Luyckx and Lefebvre, 1976; Kuku, Zeidler, Emmanouel, Katz,
Rubenstein, Levin and Tello, 1976; Sherwin, Bastl, Finkelstein, Fisher,
Black, Hendler and Felig, 1976). In our own investigations, all plasma IRG
values in 18 uraemic patients, but two, were above the range found in
normal subjects (Daubresse et al., 1976; Lefebvre and Luyckx, 1977). In the
study of Kuku et al. (1976), plasma IRG averaged 534 $\pm$ 32 pg/ml in 36
stable uremic subjects contrasting with a value of 113 $\pm$ 19 pg/ml found in 32
controls. The same authors demonstrated that the relative amounts of the
various plasma IRG fractions, identified by column chromatography, were
modified in renal insufficiency with 56–68% of the glucagon immunoreactivity in the 9000 dalton region (proglucagon ?, p. 200). This was later
confirmed by Valverde (1977). Sherwin et al. (1976) reported that the metabolic clearance rate of exogenous glucagon was markedly prolonged in
uremic patients, while the calculated basal systemic delivery rate remained
unchanged; in addition, the same group showed that the hyperglycemic
effect of physiological increments in glucagon was increased in undialysed
uraemic patients, suggesting that, in addition to decreased hormonal catabolism, altered tissue sensitivity might contribute to the pathophysiology
of glucagon in uraemia. The hyperglucagonemia of renal failure is abolished
by renal transplantation (Bilbrey et al., 1974).

(j) Glucagon and hepatic cirrhosis

The role of the liver in glucagon uptake has been summarised earlier (p.
185). Plasma IRG levels are elevated in many patients with compensated
cirrhosis, hepatic failure and portal-systemic shunting (Marco, Diego,
Villanueva, Diazferros, Valverde and Segovia, 1973b; Sherwin, Joshi,
Hendler, Felig and Conn, 1974; Soeters, Weir, Ebeid, James and Fischer,
1975). Recent experimental investigations of Jaspan et al. (1977) have shown
that the liver mainly extracts the 3500 dalton component of IRG (p. 185)
and Valverde (1977) has shown that, in men with cirrhosis of the liver, the
3500 dalton fraction was the only one to be elevated when compared to
normal individuals.

(k) Glucagon and stress

Plasma glucagon increases in response to exercise (p. 202) and rises in plasma
glucagon have also been described in response to trauma (Lindsey, Sante-

usanio, Braaten, Faloona and Unger, 1974b), bacterial infection (Rocha, Santeusanio, Faloona and Unger, 1973), myocardial infarction (Willerson, Hutcheson, Leshin, Faloona and Unger, 1974), burns (Wilmore, Moylan, Pruitt, Lindsey, Faloona and Unger, 1974), surgery (Russel, Walker and Bloom, 1975), pain or anxiety (Bloom, Daniel, Johnston, Ogawa and Pratt, 1973). The role of glucagon in stress-hyperglycemia has been discussed by Unger and Orci (1976) and the possible mechanisms involved have been recently analysed by Gerich and Lorenzi (1978).

(l) Glucagon and catabolic states

In 1972, Unger proposed the concept that glucagon should be viewed, not only as a hormone of glucose need, but also as a hormone of ureogenesis, functioning during accelerated protein breakdown to convert into glucose and urea the excessive quantities of amino acids entering the circulation from damaged tissues thus avoiding excessive accumulation of protein breakdown products and subsequently of ammonia. This view of one of the roles of glucagon, with its potential positive and negative aspects, has been reanalysed recently (Unger and Orci, 1976).

REFERENCES

Ahlborg, G. and Felig, P. (1976). *J. appl. physiol.* **41**, 683.

Aguilar-Parada, E., Eisentraut, A. M. and Unger, R. H. (1969). *Diabetes*, **18**, 717.

Alford, F. P., Bloom, S. R. and Nabarro, J. D. N. (1976). *J. clin. Endocr. Metab.* **42**, 830.

Alford, F. P., Bloom, S. R. and Nabarro, J. D. N. (1977). *Diabetologia*, **13**, 1.

Amatuzio, D. S., Grande, F. and Wada, S. (1962). *Metabolism*, **11**, 1240.

Andrews, S. S., Lopez, A. and Blackard, W. G. (1975). *Metabolism*, **24**, 35.

Anonymous. (1973). *Br. med. J.* **i**, 188.

Assan, R. (1972). "Glucagon. Molecular Physiology, Clinical and Therapeutic Implications" (P. Lefebvre and R. H. Unger, eds), p. 47. Pergamon Press, Oxford.

Assan, R., Hautecouverture, G., Guillemant, S., Dauchy, F., Protin, P. and Derot, M. (1969). *Pathol. Biol.* **17**, 1095.

Assan, R., Rosselin, G. and Dolais, J. (1967). *J. ann. Diabétol. Hôtel-Dieu*, **7**, 25.

Assan, R., Rosselin, G., Drouet, J., Dolais, J. and Tchobroutsky, G. (1965). *Lancet*, **ii**, 590.

Avioli, L. (1972). "Glucagon. Molecular Physiology, Clinical and Therapeutic Implications" (P. Lefebvre and R. H. Unger, eds), p. 181. Pergamon Press, Oxford.

Aydin, I., Raskin, P. and Unger, R. H. (1977). *Diabetologia*, **13**, 629.

Baetens, D., Rufener, C., Srikant, C. B., Dobbs, R., Unger, R. H. and Orci, L. (1976). *J. cell. Biol.* **69**, 455.

Barnes, A. J. and Bloom, S. R. (1976). *Lancet*, **i**, 219.

Barnes, A. J., Bloom, S. R., Alberti, K. G. M. M., Smythe, P., Alford, A. P. and Chisholm, D. J. (1977). *New Engl. J. Med.* **296**, 1250.

Baum, J., Simons, B. E., Unger, R. H. and Madison, L. L. (1962). *Diabetes*, **11**, 371.
Beck, P., Eaton, R. P., Arnett, D. M. and Alsever, R. N. (1975). *Metabolism*, **24**, 1055.
Berger, D., Crowther, R., Floyd Jr., Pek, S. and Fajans, S. S. (1977). *Diabetes*, **26** (Suppl. 1), 381.
Bilbrey, G. L., Faloona, G. R., White, M. G. and Knochel, J. P. (1974). *J. clin. Invest.* **53**, 841.
Blackard, W. G., Nelson, N. C. and Andrews, S. S. (1974). *Diabetes*, **23**, 199.
Bleicher, S. J., Spergel, G., Levy, L. and Zarowitz, H. (1970). *Clin. Res.* **18**, 355.
Bloom, S. R. (1977). "Glucagon: Its Role in Physiology and Clinical Medicine" (P. P. Foà, J. S. Bajaj and N. L. Foà, eds), p. 759. Springer Verlag, New York, Heidelberg and Berlin.
Bloom, S. R., Daniel, P. M., Johnston, D. I., Ogawa, O. and Pratt, O. E. (1972). *Psychol. Med.* **2**, 426.
Bloom, S. R., Daniel, P. M., Johnston, P. I., Ogawa, O. and Pratt, O. E. (1973). *Quat. J. exp. Physiol.* **58**, 99.
Bloom, S. R. and Johnston, D. I. (1972). *Br. med. J.* **4**, 453.
Blundell, T. L., Dockerill, S., Sasaki, K., Tickle, I. J. and Wood, S. P. (1976). *Metabolism*, **25** (Suppl. 1), 1331.
Boden, G. and Owen, O. E. (1977). *New Engl. J. Med.* **296**, 534.
Bohannon, N. V., Karam, J. H., Lorenzi, M., Gerich, J. E., Martin, S. B. and Forsham, P. H. (1977). *Diabetes*, **13**, 503.
Bomboy, J. D., Lewis, S. B., Sinclair-Smith, B. C., Lacy, W. W. and Liljenquist, J. E. (1977). *J. clin. Endocr. Metab.* **44**, 474.
Botha, J. L., Vinik, A. I., Child, P. T., Paul, M., Jackson, W. P. U. (1977). *Horm. metab. Res.* **9**, 199.
Bottger, I., Faloona, G. R., Dobbs, R. E. and Unger, R. H. (1973). *J. clin. Invest.* **52**, 2552.
Bottger, I., Schlein, E., Faloona, G. R., Knochel, J. P. and Unger, R. H. (1972). *J. clin. Endocr. Metab.* **35**, 117.
Bromer, W. W. (1961). "Measurements of Exocrine and Endocrine Function of the Pancreas" (F. W. Sunderman and F. W. Sunderman Jr., eds), p. 116. J. B. Lippincott Co., Philadelphia and Montreal.
Bromer, W. W., Boucher, M. E. and Koffenberger, J. E. (1971). *J. biol. Chem.* **246**, 2822.
Bromer, W. W., Sinn, L. G., Staub, A. and Behrens, O. K. (1957). *Diabetes*, **6**, 234.
Buchanan, K. D. and McCarroll, A. M. (1972). *Lancet*, **ii**, 1394.
Buchanan, K., Solomon, S., Vance, J., Porter, H. and Williams, R. H. (1968). *Proc. Soc. exp. biol. Med.* **128**, 620.
Carpentier, J. L., Luyckx, A. S. and Lefebvre, P. J. (1975). *Diab. Metab.* **1**, 23.
Carpentier, J. L., Malaisse-Lagae, F., Müller, W. A. and Orci, L. (1977). *J. clin. Invest.* **60**, 1174.
Cavallero, C., Capella, C., Solcia, E., Vassallo, G. and Bussolati, G. (1970). *Acta Diabetol. Lat.* **7**, 542.
Cavallero, C., Solcia, E., Vassallo, G., Capella, C. (1969). *Rend. R. R. Gastroenterology*, **1**, 51.
Chesney, T. McC. and Schofield, M. A. (1969). *Diabetes*, **18**, 627.
Cresto, J. C., Lavine, R. E., Perrino, P., Recant, L., August, G. and Hung, W. (1974). *Lancet*, **i**, 1165.
Daniel, R. R., Metzger, B. E., Freinkel, N., Faloona, G. R., Unger, R. H. and Nizan, M. (1974). *Diabetes*, **23**, 771.

Daubresse, J. C., Lerson, G., Plomteux, G., Rorive, G., Luyckx, A. S. and Lefebvre, P. J. (1976). *Eur. J. clin. Invest.* **6**, 159.

Desbuquois, B. (1975). *Eur. J. Biochem.* **53**, 569.

Desbuquois, B., Krug, F. and Cuatrecasas, P. (1974). *Biochim. biophys. Acta*, **343**, 101.

Dudl, R. J. and Ensinck, J. W. (1977). *Metabolism*, **26**, 33.

Eaton, R. P. (1973). *Metabolism*, **22**, 763.

Eaton, R. P. (1977). "Glucagon: Its Role in Physiology and Clinical Medicine" (P. P. Foà, J. S. Bajaj and N. L. Foà, eds), p. 533. Springer Verlag, New York, Heidelberg and Berlin.

Eaton, R. P. and Schade, D. S. (1973). *Lancet*, **i**, 973.

Edwards, J. C., Howell, S. L. and Taylor, K. W. (1970). *Biochim. biophys. Acta*, **215**, 297.

Edwards, J. C. and Taylor, K. W. (1970). *Biochim. biophys. Acta*, **215**, 297.

Eisentraut, A. M., Whissen, N. and Unger, R. H. (1968). *Am. J. med. Sci.* **235**, 137.

Emmanouel, D. S., Jaspan, J. B., Kuku, S. F., Rubenstein, A. H. and Katz, A. I. (1976). *J. clin. Invest.* **58**, 1266.

Ensinck, J. W. and Palmer, J. P. (1976). *Metabolism*, **25** (Suppl. 1) 1409.

Ensinck, J. W., Shepard, C., Dudl, J. and Williams, R. H. (1972). *J. clin. Endocr. Metab.* **35**, 463.

Fajans, S. S., Floyd Jr., J. C., Knopf, R. and Conn, J. W. (1967). *Rec. Prog. Horm. Res.* **23**, 617.

Falkmer, S. and Marques, M. (1972). "Glucagon. Molecular Physiology, Clinical and Therapeutic Implications" (P. J. Lefebvre and R. H. Unger, eds), p. 343. Pergamon Press, Oxford.

Fallucca, F., Iavicoli, M., Menzinger, G., Mirabella, C. and Andreani, D. (1978). *Metabolism*, **27**, 5.

Felig, P., Wharen, J. and Hendler, R. (1976). *J. clin. Invest.* **58**, 761.

Felig, P., Wahren, J., Hendler, R. and Ahlborg, G. (1972). *New Engl. J. Med.* **287**, 184.

Feliu, J. E., Hue, L., Hers, H. G. (1976). *Proc. natn. Acad. Sci. USA*, **78**, 2762.

Fisher, M., Sherwin, R. S., Hendler, R. and Felig, P. (1976). *Proc. natn. Acad. Sci. USA*, **73**, 1735.

Foà, P. P. (1976). *Metabolism*, **25** (Suppl. 1), 1489.

Foà, P. P., Bajaj, J. S. and Foà, N. L. (eds) (1977). "Glucagon: Its Role in Physiology and Clinical Medicine", 793 pp. Springer, Verlag, New York, Heidelberg and Berlin.

Galbo, H., Christensen, N. J. and Holst, J. J. (1977). *J. appl. Physiol.* **42**, 525.

Galbo, H., Holst, J. J. and Christensen, N. J. (1975). *J. appl. Physiol.* **38**, 70.

Galbo, H., Holst, J. J., Christensen, N. J. and Hilsted, J. (1976). *J. appl. Physiol.* **40**, 855.

Galloway, J. A. (1972). "Glucagon. Molecular Physiology, Clinical and Therapeutic Implications" (P. J. Lefebvre and R. H. Unger, eds), p. 299. Pergamon Press, Oxford.

Garber, A. J., Cryer, P. E., Santiago, J. V., Haymond, M. W., Pagliara, A. S. and Kipnis, D. M. (1976). *J. clin. Invest.* **58**, 7.

Gerich, J. (1977). "Glucagon: Its role in Physiology and Clinical Medicine" (P. P. Foà, J. S. Bajaj and N. L. Foà, eds) p. 617. Springer Verlag, New York, Heidelberg and Berlin.

Gerich, J. E., Charles, M. and Grodsky, G. M. (1976a). *Ann. Rev. Physiol.* **38**, 353.

Gerich, J. E., Karam, J. H. and Lorenzi, M. (1976b). *Lancet*, **i**, 855.

Gerich, J. E., Langlois, M., Schneider, V., Karam, J. H. and Noacco, C. (1974). *J. clin. Invest.* **53**, 1284.

Gerich, J. E. and Lorenzi, M. (1978). "Frontiers in Neuroendocrinology" (W. F. Ganong and L. Martini, eds), Vol. 5, p. 265. Raven Press, New York.

Gerich, J. E., Lorenzi, M., Bier, D., Schneider, V., Tsalikian, E., Karam, J. H. and Forsham, P. (1975). *New Engl. J. Med.* **292**, 985.

Gerich, J. E., Lorenzi, M., Bier, D. M., Tsalikian, E., Schneider, V., Karam, J. H. and Forsham, P. H. (1976c). *J. clin. Invest.* **57**, 875.

Gey, F., Georgi, H. and Buhler, E. (1977). "Glucagon: Its Role in Physiology and Clinical Medicine" (P. P. Foà, J. S. Bajaj and N. L. Foà, eds) p. 517. Springer Verlag, New York, Heidelberg and Berlin.

Giugliano, D., Luyckx, A. S., Binder, D. and Lefebvre, P. J. (1978). *Int. J. clin. Pharmacol.* (in press).

Glick, G. (1972). *Circulation,* **45**, 513.

Goldfine, I. D., Kirsteins, L. and Lawrence, A. M. (1972). *Horm. Metab. Res.* **4**, 97.

Goldner, M. G., Jauregui, R. M. and Weisenfled, S. (1954). *Am. J. Physiol.* **179**, 25.

Gonvers, J. J., Henchoz, L., Hofstetter, J. R. and Müller, W. A. (1977). *Schweiz. med. Wschr.* **107**, 184.

Greenwood, F. C., Hunter, W. M. and Glover, J. S. (1963). *Biochem. J.* **89**, 114.

Grey, N., McGuigan, J. E. and Kipnis, D. M. (1970). *Endocrinology,* **86**, 1383.

Gyntelberg, F., Rennie, M. J., Hickson, R. C. and Holloszy, J. O. (1977). *J. appl. Physiol.* **42**, 302.

Hanoune, J. (1976). *Biol. Gastroenterol. (Paris),* **9**, 33.

Hatfield, H. H., Banasiak, M. F., Driscoll, T., Kim, H-J. and Kalkhoff, R. K. (1977). *J. clin. Endocr. Metab.* **44**, 1080.

Hazzard, W. R., Crockford, P. M., Buchanan, K. D., Vance, J. E., Chen, R. and Williams, R. H. (1968). *Diabetes,* **17**, 179.

Heding, L. G. (1969). *Horm. Metab. Res.* **1**, 87.

Heding, L. G. (1971). *Diabetologia,* **7**, 10.

Heding, L. G. (1972). "Glucagon. Molecular Physiology, Clinical and Therapeutic Implications" (P. J. Lefebvre and R. H. Unger, eds), p. 187. Pergamon Press, Oxford.

Heding, L. G., Frandsen, E. K. and Jacobsen, H. (1976). *Metabolism,* **25** (Suppl. 1), 1327.

Hedo, J. A., Villanueva, M. L. and Marco, J. (1977). *Metabolism,* **26**, 1131.

Herbert, V., Kam-Seng, L., Gottlieb, C. W. and Bleicher, J. (1965). *J. clin. Endocr.* **25**, 1375.

Hers, H. G. (1976). *Ann. Rev. Biochem.* **45**, 167.

Hicks, D. H., Taylor, C. F., Vij, S. K., Pek, S., Knopf, R. and Fajans, S. S. (1977). *Metabolism,* **26**, 1011.

Holohan, K. N., Murphy, R. F., Buchanan, K. D. and Elmore, D. T. (1973). *Clin. chim. Acta,* **45**, 153.

Holst, J. J. (1975). *Diabetologia,* **11**, 211.

Holst, J. J. (1978). *Digestion,* **17**, 168.

Imura, H., Ikeda, M. and Seino, Y. (1977). *Jap. J. Med.* **16**, 55.

Jaspan, J. B., Huen, A. H-J., Morley, C. G., Moossa, A. R. and Rubenstein, A. H. (1977). *J. clin. Invest.* **60**, 421.

Jaspan, J. B. and Rubenstein, A. H. (1977). *Diabetes,* **26**, 887.

Jørgensen, K. H. and Larsen, U. D. (1972). *Horm. Metab. Res.* **4**, 223.

Kalkhoff, R. K., Gossain, V. V. and Matute, M. L. (1973). *New Engl. J. Med.* **289**, 465.

Kologlu, Y., Wiesell, L., Positano, V. and Anderson, G. E. (1963). *Proc. Soc. exp. Biol. Med.* **112**, 518.

Kubeš, L., Jirásek, K. and Lomský, R. (1974). *Cytologia (Tokyo)*, **39**, 179.

Kühl, C. and Holst, J. J. (1976). *Diabetes*, **25**, 16.

Kühl, C., Hornnes, P. and Klebe, J. G. (1977). *Horm. Metab. Res.* **9**, 206.

Kuku, S. F., Zeidler, A., Emmanouel, D. S., Katz, A. I., Rubenstein, A. H., Levin, N. W. and Tello, A. (1976). *J. clin. Endocr. Metab.* **42**, 173.

Langslow, D. R. and Hales, C. N. (1970). *Lancet*, **ii**, 1151.

Larsson, L-I., Holst, J. J., Håkanson, R. and Sundler, F. (1975). *Histochemistry*, **44**, 281.

Lawrence, A. M. (1966). *Proc. natn. Acad. Sci. USA*, **55**, 316.

Lawrence, A. M. (1972). "Glucagon. Molecular Physiology, Clinical and Therapeutic Implications" (P. J. Lefebvre and R. H. Unger, eds), p. 259. Pergamon Press, Oxford.

Lawrence, A. M., Tan, S., Hojvat, S., Kirsteins, L. (1976). *Science*, **195**, 70.

Leclercq-Meyer, V., Marchand, J. and Malaisse, W. J. (1974). *Diabetologia*, **10**, 215.

Leclercq-Meyer, V., Miahle, P. and Malaisse, W. J. (1970). *Diabetologia*, **6**, 121.

Leclercq-Meyer, V., Rebolledo, O., Marchand, J. and Malaisse, W. J. (1975). *Science*, **189**, 897.

Lecomte, M. J., Luyckx, A. S. and Lefebvre, P. J. (1977). *Diab. Metab.* **3**, 239.

Lefebvre, P. J. (1966). *Diabetologia*, **2**, 130.

Lefebvre, P. J. (1972). "Glucagon. Molecular Physiology, Clinical and Therapeutic Implications" (P. J. Lefebvre and R. H. Unger, eds), p. 109. Pergamon Press, Oxford.

Lefebvre, P. J. (1975). *Biochem. Pharmacol.* **24**, 1261.

Lefebvre, P. J., Fischer, U., Jutzi, E., Hommel, H. and Luyckx, A. S. (1978a). *Ann. Endocr.* **39**, 347.

Lefebvre, P. J. and Luyckx, A. (1965). *Ann. Endocr.* **26**, 369.

Lefebvre, P. J. and Luyckx, A. S. (1972). "Glucagon. Molecular Physiology, Clinical and Therapeutic Implications" (P. J. Lefebvre and R. H. Unger, eds), p. 175. Pergamon Press, Oxford.

Lefebvre, P. J. and Luyckx, A. S. (1975). *Metabolism*, **24**, 1169.

Lefebvre, P. J. and Luyckx, A. S. (1976a). *Diab. Metab.* **1**, 15.

Lefebvre, P. J. and Luyckx, A. S. (1976b). *Metabolism*, **25**, 761.

Lefebvre, P. J. and Luyckx, A. S. (1977). "Glucagon: Its Role in Physiology and Clinical Medicine" (P. P. Foà, J. S. Bajaj and N. L. Foà, eds), p. 165. Springer Verlag, New York, Heidelberg and Berlin.

Lefebvre, P. J. and Luyckx, A. S. (1978). *Diabetes*, **27**, 487.

Lefebvre, P. J. and Unger, R. H. (eds) (1972). "Glucagon. Molecular Physiology, Clinical and Therapeutic Implications", 370 pp. Pergamon Press, Oxford.

Lefebvre, P. J., Luyckx, A. S. and Nizet, A. H. (1974). *Metabolism*, **23**, 753.

Lefebvre, P. J., Luyckx, A. S. and Lecomte, M. J. (1976a). "Hypoglycemia" (D. Andreani, P. Lefebvre and V. Marks, eds), p. 91. Thieme, Stuttgart.

Lefebvre, P. J., Luyckx, A. S. and Nizet, A. H. (1978b). *Diabetologia* **12**, 359.

Lefebvre, P. J., Luyckx, A. S., Mosora, F., Lacroix, M. and Pirnay, F. (1976b). *Diabetologia*, **14**, 39.

Lesko, L., Donlon, M., Marinetti, G. V. and Hare, J. D. (1973). *Biochim. biophys. Acta*, **311**, 173.

Liljenquist, J. E., Bomboy, J. D., Lewis, S. B., Sinclair-Smith, B. C., Felts, P. W., Lacy, W. W., Crofford, O. B. and Liddle, G. W. (1974). *J. clin. Invest.* **53**, 190.

Lindsey, C. A., Faloona, G. and Unger, R. H. (1974a). *J. Am. med. Assoc.* **229**, 1771.

Lindsey, C. A., Santeusanio, F., Braaten, J., Faloona, G. R. and Unger, R. H. (1974b). *J. Am. med. Assoc.* **227**, 757.

Ljungström, O., Hjhelmquist, G. and Engström, L. (1974). *Biochim. biophys. Acta,* **358**, 289.

Loreti, L., Sugase, T. and Foà, P. P. (1974). *Horm. Res.* **5**, 278.

Luyckx, A. S. (1972). "Glucagon. Molecular Physiology, Clinical and Therapeutic Implications" (P. J. Lefebvre and R. H. Unger, eds), p. 285. Pergamon Press, Oxford.

Luyckx, A. S. (1974). "Sécrétion de l'Insuline et du Glucagon. Etude Clinique et Expérimentale", 338 p. Masson et Cie, Paris.

Luyckx, A. S. (1975). *Diab. Metab.* **1**, 201.

Luyckx, A. S., Dresse, A., Cession-Fossion, A. and Lefebvre, P. J. (1975a). *Am. J. Physiol.* **229**, 376.

Luyckx, A. S., Gaspard, U. and Lefebvre. P. J. (1978). *Metabolism,* **27**, 1033.

Luyckx, A. S., Gerard, J., Gaspard, U. and Lefebvre, P. J. (1975b). *Diabetologia,* **11**, 549.

Luyckx, A. S. and Lefebvre, P. J. (1970). *Proc. Soc. exp. Biol. Med.* **133**, 524.

Luyckx, A. S. and Lefebvre, P. J. (1974). *Diabetes,* **23**, 81.

Luyckx, A. S. and Lefebvre, P. J. (1976). "Hormones in Human Blood. Detection and Assay" (H. H. Antoniades, ed.), p. 293. Harvard University Press, Cambridge, MA.

Luyckx, A. S., Massi-Benedetti, F., Falorni, A. and Lefebvre, P. J. (1972). *Diabetologia,* **8**, 296.

Luyckx, A. S., Pirnay, F. and Lefebvre, P. J. (1978). *Eur. J. appl. Physiol.* **39**, 53.

Mallinson, C. N., Bloom, S. R., Warin, A. P., Salmon, P. R. and Cox, B. (1974). *Lancet,* **ii**, 1.

Marco, J., Calle, C., Roman, D., Diaz-Fierros, M., Villanueva, M. and Valverde, I. (1973a). *New Engl. J. Med.* **288**, 128.

Marco, J., Diego, J., Villanueva, M., Diaz-Fierros, M., Valverde, I. and Segovia, J. (1973b). *New Engl. J. Med.* **289**, 1107.

Marco, J., Hedo, J. A. and Villanueva, M. L. (1975). *Diabetes,* **24** (Suppl. 2), 411.

Marco, J., Hedo, J. A. and Villanueva, M. L. (1977). *Diabetes,* **26** (Suppl. 1), 381.

Marco, J. and Valverde, I. (1973). *Diabetologia,* **9**, 317.

Marks, V. and Samols, E. (1968). "Recent Advances in Endocrinology" (V. H. T. James, ed.), p. 111. Churchill, London.

Markussen, J., Frandsen, E. K., Heding, L. G. and Sundby, F. (1972). *Horm. Metab. Res.* **4**, 360.

Marliss, E. B., Aoki, T. T., Unger, R. H., Soeldner, J. S. and Cahill Jr., G. F. (1970). *J. clin. Invest.* **49**, 2256.

Massi-Benedetti, F., Falorni, A., Luyckx, A. S. and Lefebvre, P. J. (1974). *Horm. Metab. Res.* **6**, 392.

McEvoy, R. C., Madson, K. L. and Elde, R. P. (1977). *Horm. Metab. Res.* **9**, 272.

McGarry, J. D., Robles-Valdes, C. and Foster, D. W. (1975a). *Proc. natn. Acad. Sci. USA,* **72**, 4385.

McGarry, J. D., Wright, P. and Foster, D. (1975b). *J. clin. Invest.* **55**, 1202.

McGavran, M. H., Unger, R. H., Recant, L., Polk, H. C., Kilo, C. and Levin, M. E. (1966). *New Engl. J. Med.* **274**, 1408.

McQuarrie, I., Bell, E. T., Zimmerman, B. and Wright, W. S. (1950). *Fed. Proc.* **9**, 337.

Miller, R. E., Chernish, S. M., Brunelle, R. L. and Rosenak, B. D. (1978). *Radiology,* **127**, 55.

Mirsky, A., Perisutti, G. and Davis, N. C. (1959). *Endocrinology*, **64**, 992.

Miyata, M., Yamamoyo, T., Yamaguchi, M., Nakao, K. and Yoshida, T. (1976). *Proc. Soc. exp. Biol. Med.* **152**, 540.

Mortimore, G. E. (1973). *Am. J. Physiol.* **204**, 699.

Müller, W. A., Aoki, T. T., Egdahl, R. H. and Cahill Jr., G. F. (1977). *Diabetologia*, **13**, 55.

Müller, W. A., Brennan, M. F., Tan, M. H. and Aoki, T. T. (1974). *Diabetes*, **23**, 512.

Müller, W. A., Faloona, G. R. and Unger, R. H. (1971). *New Engl. J. Med.* **285**, 1450.

Müller, W. A., Faloona, G. R., Aguilar-Parada, E. and Unger, R. H. (1970). *New Engl. J. Med.* **283**, 109.

Munger, B. L. (1972). "Glucagon. Molecular Physiology, Clinical and Therapeutic Implications" (P. J. Lefebvre and R. H. Unger, eds), p. 7. Pergamon Press, Oxford.

Muñoz-Barragan, L., Rufener, C., Srikant, C. B., Dobbs, R. E., Shannon Jr., W. A., Baetens, D. and Unger, R. H. (1977). *Horm. Metab. Res.* **9**, 37.

Narahara, H. T., Everett, N. B., Simons, B. S. and Williams, R. H. (1958). *Am. J. Physiol.* **192**, 227.

Noe, B. D. (1976). *Metabolism*, **25** (Suppl. 1), 1339.

Noe, B. D. and Bauer, G. E. (1971). *Endocrinology*, **89**, 642.

Noe, B. D. and Bauer, G. E. (1975). *Endocrinology*, **97**, 868.

Nonaka, K. and Foà, P. P. (1969). *Proc. Soc. exp. Biol. Med.*, **130**, 330.

Ohneda, A., Ishii, S., Horigome, K. and Yamagata, S. (1975). *Diabetes*, **24**, 811.

Okuno, G. and Takenaka, H. (1977). "Glucagon: Its Role in Physiology and Clinical Medicine" (P. P. Foà, J. S. Bajaj and N. L. Foà, eds), p. 777. Springer Verlag, New York, Heidelberg and Berlin.

Orci, L. (1976a). "Polypeptide Hormones: Molecular and Cellular Aspects", p. 344. Ciba Foundation Symposium (New series) Elsevier, North-Holland, Amsterdam.

Orci, L. (1976b). Metabolism, **25** (Suppl. 1), 1303.

Orci, L. (1977). "Insulin and Metabolism" (J. S. Bajaj, ed.), p. 1. Excerpta Medica, Amsterdam, London, New York.

Orci, L., Forssman, W. G., Forssman, W. and Roullier, C. (1968). "Electron Microscopy", 4th European Regional Conference. (S. D. Bocchiarelli, ed.), p. 369. Tikografia Poliglotto Vaticana, Rome.

Orci, L., Malaisse-Lagae, F., Amherdt, M., Ravazzola, M., Weisswange, A., Dobbs, R. E., Perrelet, A. and Unger, R. H. (1975a). *J. clin. Endocr. Metab.* **41**, 841.

Orci, L., Malaisse-Lagae, F., Ravazzola, M., Rouiller, C., Renold, A. E., Perrelet, A. and Unger, R. H. (1975b). *J. clin. Invest.* **56**, 1066.

Orci, L. and Unger, R. H. (1975). *Lancet*, **ii**, 1243.

Östenson, C. G., Andersson, A., Brolin, S. E., Petersson, B. and Hellerström, C. (1977). "Glucagon: Its Role in Physiology and Clinical Medicine" (P. P. Foà, J. S. Bajaj and N. L. Foà, eds), p. 243. Springer Verlag, New York, Heidelberg and Berlin.

Palmer, J. P., Werner, P. L., Benson, J. W. and Ensinck, J. W. (1976). *Metabolism*, **25** (Suppl. 1), 1483.

Park, C. R. and Exton, J. H. (1972). "Glucagon. Molecular Physiology, Clinical and Therapeutic Implications" (P. J. Lefebvre and R. H. Unger, eds), p. 77. Pergamon Press, Oxford.

Parmley, W. W. and Sonnenblick, E. H. (1971). *Am. J. Cardiol.* **27**, 298.

Parving, H. H., Noer, J., Kehlet, H., Mogensen, C. E., Svendsen, P. A. and Heding, L. (1977). *Diabetologia*, **13**, 323.

Passa, P., Luyckx, A. S., Carpentier, J. L., Lefebvre, P. J. and Canivet, J. (1977). *Diabetologia*, **13**, 509.

Paulsen, E. P. and Lawrence, A. M. (1968). *Lancet*, **ii**, 110.

Pek, S., Fajans, S. S., Floyd Jr., J. C., Knopf, R. F. and Conn, J. W. (1972). *Diabetes*, **21**, 216.

Podolsky, S. and Lawrence, A. M. (1977). "Glucagon: Its Role in Physiology and Clinical Medicine" (P. P. Foà, J. S. Bajaj and N. L. Foà, eds), p. 711. Springer Verlag, New York, Heidelberg and Berlin.

Pollock, H. G. and Kimmel, J. R. (1975). *J. biol. Chem.* **250**, 9377.

Quabbe, H. J., Ramek, W. and Luyckx, A. S. (1977). *J. clin. Endocr. Metab.* **44**, 383.

Raskin, P., Aydin, I. and Unger, R. H. (1976). *Diabetes*, **25**, 227.

Rocha, D. M., Santeusanio, F., Faloona, G. R. and Unger, R. H. (1973). *New Engl. J. Med.* **288**, 700.

Röjdmark, S., Bloom, G., Chou, M. C. Y. and Field, J. B. (1978). *Endocrinology*, **102**, 806.

Rosselin, G., Freychet, P., Bataille, D. and Kitabgi, P. (1974). *Israel J. med. Sci.* **10**, 1314.

Rowlinson, H. R. and Lesford, J. H. (1951). *J. Pharm. Pharmacol.* **3**, 887.

Russel, R. C. G., Walker, W. J. and Bloom, S. R. (1975). *Br. med. J.* **i**, 10.

Samols, E., Marri, G. and Marks, V. (1965). *Lancet*, **ii**, 417.

Samols, E., Tyler, J. M., Marks, V. (1972). "Glucagon. Molecular Physiology, Clinical and Therapeutic Implications" (P. J. Lefebvre and R. H. Unger, eds), p. 151. Pergamon Press, Oxford.

Santeusanio, F. and Brunetti, P. (1976). "Hypoglycemia" (D. Andreani, P. Lefebvre and V. Marks, eds), p. 69. Thieme, Stuttgart.

Santeusanio, F., Massi-Benedetti, M., Angeletti, G. and Brunetti, P. (1977). *Horm. Metab. Res.* **9**, 337.

Santiago, J. V., Haymond, M. W., Clarke, W. L. and Pagliara, A. S. (1977). *Metabolism*, **26**, 1115.

Sasagawa, T., Kobayashi, S. and Fujita, T. (1974). "Gastroentero–Pancreatic Endocrine System. A Cell Biological approach" (T. Fujita, ed), p. 17. Igahu Shoin, Tokyo.

Sasaki, K., Dockerill, S., Adamiak, D., Tickle, I. J. and Blundell, T. (1975a). *Nature, Lond.* **257**, 751.

Sasaki, H., Rubalcalva, B., Baetens, D., Blazquez, E., Srikant, C. B., Orci, L. and Unger, R. H. (1975b). *J. clin. Invest.* **56**, 135.

Schade, D. S. and Eaton, R. P. (1975). *Diabetes*, **24**, 502.

Schopman, W., Hacking, W. H. L. and Steendijck, C. (1967). *Acta endocr.* **54**, 527.

Sebel, E. F., Hull, R. D., Kleerekoper, M. and Stokes, G. S. (1974). *Am. J. Med. Sci.* **267**, 337.

Seino, Y., Goto, Y., Kurahachi, H., Sakurai, H., Ikeda, M., Kadowaki, S., Inoue, Y., Mori, K., Taminato, T. and Imura, H. (1977). *Horm. Metab. Res.* **9**, 28.

Seino, Y., Goto, Y., Taminato, T., Ikeda, M. and Imura, H. (1974). *J. clin. Endocr. Metab.* **38**, 1136.

Senyk, G., Nitecki, D. E. and Goodman, J. W. (1971). *Science*, **171**, 407.

Senyk, G., Nitecki, D. E., Spitler, L. and Goodman, J. W. (1972). *Immunochemistry*, **9**, 97.

Sherwin, R. S., Bastl, C., Finkelstein, F. O., Fisher, M., Black, B., Hendler, R. and Felig, P. (1976). *J. clin. Invest.* **57**, 722.

Sherwin, R., Joshi, P., Hendler, R., Felig, P. and Conn, H. (1974). *N. Engl. J. Med.* **290**, 239.

Shima, K. and Foà, P. P. (1968). *Clin. chim. Acta*, **22**, 511.

Soeters, P., Weir, G., Ebeid, A. M., James, J. H. and Fischer, J. E. (1975). *Gastroenterology*, **69**, 867 (abstract).

Sokal, J. E. (1970). *Endocrinology*, **87**, 1338.

Sokal, J. E. (1972). "Glucagon". Molecular Physiology, Clinical and Therapeutic Implications" (P. J. Lefebvre and R. H. Unger, eds), p. 275. Pergamon Press, Oxford.

Sokal, J. E. and Ezdinli, E. Z. (1967). *J. clin. Invest.* **46**, 778.

Sokal, J. E. and Weintraub, B. (1966). *Am. J. Physiol.* **210**, 63.

Solcia, E., Vassallo, G. and Capella, C. (1970). "Origin, Physiology and Pathophysiology of the Gastrointestinal Hormones" (W. Creutzfeldt, ed.), p. 3. F. K. Schattauer Verlag, Stuttgart:

Solomon, Y., Londos, C. and Rodbell, M. (1974). *Ann. Biochem.* **58**, 541.

Sperling, M. A., Delamater, P. V., Phelps, D., Fisher, R. H., Oh, W. and Fisher, D. A. (1974). *J. clin. Invest.* **53**, 1159.

Srikant, C. B., McCorckle, K. and Unger, R. H. (1977). *J. clin. Invest.* **252**, 1847.

Stahl, M., Nars, P. W., Herz, G., Baumann, J. B. and Girard, J. (1972). *Horm. metab. Res.* **4**, 224.

Stalmans, W., De Wulf, H. and Hers, H. G. (1971). *Eur. J. Biochem.* **18**, 582.

Staub, A. and Behrens, O. K. (1954). *J. clin. Invest.* **33**, 1629.

Staub, A., Sinn, L. and Behrens, O. K. (1953). *Science*, **117**, 628.

Staub, A., Sinn, L. and Behrens, O. K. (1955). *J. biol. Chem.* **214**, 619.

Steinberg, D. and Huttunen, J. K. (1972). "Advances in Cyclic Nucleotide Research" (P. Greengard and A. Robison, eds), Vol. 1, p. 47. Raven Press, New York.

Sundby, F. (1970). 7th Cong. Int. Diabetes Fed., Buenos-Aires.

Sundby, F. (1976). *Metabolism*, **25** (Suppl. 1), 1319.

Sundby, F., Frandsen, E. K., Thomsen, J., Kristiansen, K. and Brunfeldt, K. (1972). *FEBS Letts*, **26**, 289.

Sundby, F., Jacobsen, H. and Moody, A. J. (1976). *Horn. Metab. Res.* **8**, 366.

Sutherland, E. W. and De Duve, C. (1948). *J. biol. Chem.* **175**, 663.

Tager, H. S., Hohenboken, M. and Markese, J. (1977). *Endocrinology*, **100**, 367.

Tager, H. S. and Steiner, D. F. (1973). *Proc. natn. Acad. Sci. USA*, **70**, 2321.

Tamborlane, W. V., Sherwin, R. S., Hendler, R. and Felig, P. (1977). *New Engl. J. Med.* **297**, 181.

Telner, A. H., Taylor, C. I., Pek, S., Crowther, R. L., Floyd, Jr, J. D. and Fajans, S. S. (1977). "Glucagon: Its Role in Physiology and Clinical Medicine" (P. P. Foà, J. S. Bajaj and N. L. Foà, eds), p. 723. Springer Verlag, New York, Heidelberg and Berlin.

Thomsen, J., Kristiansen, K., Brunfeldt, K. and Sundby, F. (1972). *FEBS Letts*, **21**, 315.

Tiengo, A., Muggeo, M., Assan, R., Fedele, D. and Crepaldi, G. (1975). *Metabolism*, **24**, 901.

Tiengo, A., Nosadini, R., Garotti, M. C., Fedele, D., Muggeo, M. and Crepaldi, G. (1977). "Glucagon: Its Role in Physiology and Clinical Medicine" (P. P. Foà, J. S. Bajaj and N. L. Foà, eds), p. 735. Springer Verlag, New York, Heidelberg and Berlin.

Trakatellis, A. C., Tada, K., Yamati, K. and Gardini-Kouidou, P. (1975). *Biochemistry*, **14**, 1508.

Tsalikian, E., Dunphy, T., Bohannon, N., Lorenzi, M., Gerich, J., Matin, S. B. and Forsham, P. H. (1976). *Diabetes*, **25** (Suppl. 1), 387.

Unger, R. H. (1972). "Glucagon. Molecular Physiology, Clinical and Therapeutic implications" (P. J. Lefebvre and R. H. Unger, eds), p. 245. Pergamon Press, Oxford.

Unger, R. H. (1976). *Metabolism*, **25** (Suppl. 1), IX.

Unger, R. H., Aguilar-Parada, E., Müller, W. A. and Eisentraut, A. M. (1970). *J. clin. Invest.* **49**, 837.

Unger, R. H., Dobbs, R. E. and Orci, L. (1978). *Ann. Rev. Physiol.* **40**, 307.

Unger, R. H. and Eisentraut, A. M. (1967). *J. ann. Diabétol. Hôtel-Dieu*, **7**, 7.

Unger, R. H., Eisentraut, A. M., Keller, S., Lang, H. C. and Madison, L. L. (1959). *Proc. Soc. exp. Biol. Med.* **102**, 621.

Unger, R. H., Eisentraut, A. M., McGall, M. S. and Madison, L. L. (1961). *J. clin. Invest.* **40**, 1280.

Unger, R. H. and Lefebvre, P. J. (1972). "Glucagon. Molecular Physiology, Clinical and Therapeutic Implications" (P. J. Lefebvre and R. H. Unger, eds), p. 213. Pergamon Press, Oxford.

Unger, R. H., Ohneda, A., Aguilar-Parada, E. and Eisentraut, A. M. (1969). *J. clin. Invest.* **48**, 810.

Unger, R. H. and Orci, L. (1975). *Lancet*, **i**, 14.

Unger, R. H. and Orci, L. (1976). *Physiol. Rev.* **56**, 778.

Unger, R. H., Srere, P., Bromer, W. W. and Felig, P. (Eds). (1976). *Metabolism*, **25**, (Suppl. 1), 1303.

Valverde, I. (1977). "Glucagon: Its Role in Physiology and Clinical Medicine" (P. P. Foà, J. S. Bajaj and N. L. Foà, eds), p. 77. Springer Verlag, New York, Heidelberg, Berlin.

Valverde, I., Villanueva, M. L., Lozano, I. and Marco, J. (1974). *J. clin. Endocr. Metab.* **39**, 1090.

Vance, J. E., Kitabchi, A. E., Buchanan, K. D., Stoll, R. W., Hollander, D. and Wood Jr., F. C. (1968). *Diabetes*, **17**, (Suppl.1) 299.

Vance, J. E., Stoll, R. W., Kitabchi, A. E., Williams, R. H. and Wood Jr., F. C. (1969). *J. Am. med. Assoc.* **207**, 1679.

Vidnes, J. and Øyasaeter, S. (1977). *Pediat. Res.* **11**, 943.

Villalpando, S. and Drash, A. (1976). *Diabetes*, **25** (Suppl. 1), 334.

Von Schenk, H., Larsson, I. and Thorell, J. I. (1976). *Clin. chim. Acta*, **69**, 225.

Vranic, M. (1976). *Metabolism*, **25** (Suppl. 1), 1490.

Vuylsteke, C. A. and De Duve, C. (1957). *Arch. Int. Pharmacodyn. Ther.* **3**, 437.

Walter, R. M., Dudl, R. J. and Ensinck, J. W. (1972). *Diabetes*, **21** (Suppl. 1), 333.

Weinges, K. F. (1968). "Labeled Proteins in Tracer Studies", p. 271. European Atomic Energy Community Euratom, Brussels.

Weir, G. (1977). "Glucagon: Its Role in Physiology and Clinical Medicine" (P. P. Foà, J. S. Bajaj and N. L. Foà, eds), p. 65. Springer Verlag, New York, Heidelberg and Berlin.

Weir, G., Horton, E. S., Aoki, T. T., Slovik, D., Jaspan, J. and Rubenstein, A. H. (1977). *J. clin. Invest.* **59**, 325.

Weir, G., Knowlton, S. D. and Martin, D. B. (1975a). *Endocrinology*, **97**, 932.

Weir, G. C., Knowlton, S. D. and Martin, D. B. (1975b). *J. clin. Endocr. Metab.* **40**, 296.

Weir, G. C., Turner, R. C. and Martin, D. B. (1973), *Horm. Metab. Res.* **5**, 241.

Whalen, G. E. (1974). *Gastroenterology*, **67**, 1284.

Wilmore, D. W., Moylan, J. A., Pruitt, B. A., Lindsey, C. A., Faloona, C. R. and Unger, R. H. (1974). *Lancet*, **i**, 73.

Willerson, J. T., Hutcheson, D., Leshin, S. J., Faloona, G. R. and Unger, R. H. (1974). (1974). *Am. J. Med.* **27**, 747.

Wise, J. K., Hendler, R. and Felig, P. (1973). *J. clin. Invest.* **52**, 2774.

Wollheim, C. B., Blondel, B., Renold, A. E. and Sharp, G. W. G. (1976). *Diabetologia*, **12**, 269.

Wünsch, E. and Weinges, K. F. (1972). "Glucagon. Molecular Physiology, Clinical and Therapeutic Implications" (P. J. Lefebvre and R. H. Unger, eds), p. 31. Pergamon Press, Oxford.

IV. Growth Hormone

P. H. SÖNKSEN and T. E. T. WEST

INTRODUCTION

Greenwood (1967) summarised the work on human and animal growth hormone including many of the advances that had followed rapidly and directly from the introduction of the radioimmunoassay for human growth hormone. There were still many methodological pitfalls and growth hormone assays were available at only a few specialist centres. Since then, most of these problems have been overcome and radioimmunoassays for human and animal growth hormones are readily available. In clinical practice, the measurement of plasma growth hormone concentrations have not only proven themselves reliable in the diagnosis of disorders of growth, but have been shown to be a most helpful index of pituitary function. The availability of sensitive and specific assays for rat, dog and other animal growth hormones has greatly encouraged more fundamental research. The last ten years has also seen the isolation and characterisation of human prolactin (see Chapter VI). Human growth hormone had always been found to contain intrinsic lactogenic activity and until very recently there had been considerable doubt about the existence of a separate lactogenic hormone in man. Widespread interest in hormone-receptors has advanced our understanding of the complex and intricate interrelationships (both evolutionary as well as functionally) between growth hormones, prolactins and chorionic somatomammotrophic hormones (see Chapter VII). The relationship between growth hormone and tissue growth factors has become a little clearer (see Chapter V).

There have been two further international symposia on growth hormone since the last edition, the most recent in September 1975 (Pecile and Müller, 1976). There have been several excellent books (Franchimont and Burger, 1975, Martini and Besser, 1977; Martin, Reichlin and Brown, 1977) and review articles which cover the subject and the reader will often be referred to these as a source of further reading and references.

A. ISOLATION, PROPERTIES AND STRUCTURE

1. Isolation

Growth hormone is the most readily isolated pituitary hormone with yields in the range of 1–6 mg of hormone per gram of pituitary. Since, unlike insulin, growth hormone for clinical use has to be extracted from human tissues, it is imperative that pituitary glands are harvested and extracted with maximum efficiency. Just as was the case with insulin, it seems that the clinical grades of hGH contain related peptides of various molecular weights. Although some of these may be physiologically occurring peptides, many of them appear to be aggregates that are produced during the extraction procedure. Since these aggregates have lower avidity for receptors (Gordon, Lesniak, Hendricks, Roth, McGuffin and Gavin, 1974; Soman and Goodman, 1977; Moore and Jin, 1978) it is likely that they are biologically less active. This is in keeping with reduced growth-promoting action in clinical trials in man (Moore, 1978) and indicates the need for improvements in the techniques for growth hormone extraction and preparation for clinical use.

Some of these problems can be improved upon by avoiding ethanol as a precipitating agent during extraction (Brown, Catt and Martin, 1967; Parlow and Shorne, 1976) with consequent increased yield and higher proportion of monomeric hGH in the resulting preparation. There is however, remarkably little information on the stability (in terms of aggregation/dimerisation, etc.) of clinical preparations. From what is known about the tendency of radioactively labelled hGH to change from monomeric to aggregated forms, it might be anticipated that clinical grades of hCG are much less stable than clinical preparations of insulin, and indeed preliminary data suggest that this is true (Moore, 1978). It might be anticipated that, just as was the case with insulin, the high mw hGH aggregates are more immunogenic than the monomeric species. Further information is needed on the importance of the use of monomer hGH in clinical practice and on ways of preventing the progressive aggregation of hGH that seems inevitably to accompany storage.

2. Physico-chemical Properties and Structure

The tendency of hGH in solution to change its apparent molecular weight and perhaps also its biological activity, is at variance with the resistance that the molecule appears to have to denaturation by solvents. Growth hormone possesses a remarkable ability to regain its native secondary and tertiary structures after exposure to extremely severe solvent conditions, such as 50% acetic acid or 5M guanidine-hydrochloride, even in the absence of the disulphide bonds (Bewley and Li, 1975). Although these solvents are known to cause denaturation of hCG, the reversibility of all conformational changes is paralleled by restoration of complete biological potency. The molecular weight of human growth hormone determined from amino acid sequence is 22, 125 daltons, which is in excellent agreement with values calculated from physical measurement. The isoelectric point measured directly in phosphate buffer (ionic strength 0·1) was 4·9 which differs from that measured by minimal solubility in salt-free solutions (5·5) or that calculated from the amino acid composition (5·98). The reasons for these differences are not clear (Bewley and Li, 1975). Sequence analyses indicate that hGH is a single polypeptide chain containing two disulphide bonds with no carbohydrate or prosthetic groups. Figure 1 shows the primary structure of hGH, containing a total of 191 amino acids. Studies on secondary and tertiary structure indicate that hCG is a globular molecule that undergoes reversible conformational changes in powerful denaturing agents.

Comparison of the amino acid sequence of hGH with other mammalian pituitary growth hormones, prolactins and chorionic somatomammotrophins (placental lactogens) reveals homologies that indicate origin from a

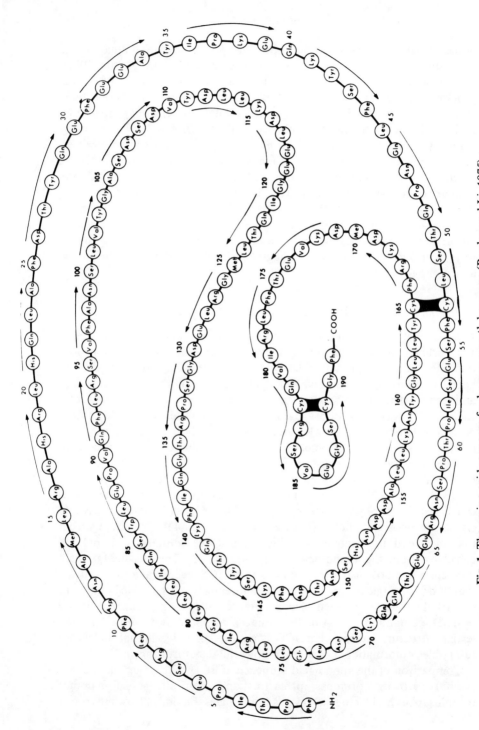

Fig. 1. The amino acid sequence for human growth hormone (Bewley and Li, 1975).

common ancestral molecule (Bewley and Li, 1975; Wallis and Davies, 1976). Human growth hormone and chorionic somatomammotrophin (hCS) have more than 85 % of their primary structure in common and both possess lactogenic and growth promoting activity (although the latter activity of hCS is only 0·03 % that of hGH). There is a high degree of sequence homology between hGH, hCS and ovine prolactin with sufficient evidence to suggest they were derived from a common ancestor. Of interest in this respect is the observation of Carr and Friesen (1976), that ovine chorionic

Table 1

Classification of hormones and receptors (activity shown as a percentage). From Lesnick, Gordon and Roth (1977).

Group	Hormones	Receptors for primate GH	Receptors for non-primate GH	Receptors for lactogenic hormones
I	primate UH	100	100	100
	oCS	100	100	100
II	non-primate	0·03	100	0
III	hCS	0·03	0	100
	oPRL	0·03	0	100
	hPRL	0	0	100

somatomammotrophin (oCS) is equipotent with hGH in competing for ^{125}I-hGH binding sites on human liver. Somewhat surprisingly it was found that primate chorionic somatomammotrophins (placental lactogens) exhibited a potency of only 0·5–1·0 % that of hGH. These unexpected findings were later confirmed by Lesniak, Gordon and Roth (1977), this time using hGH receptors on cultured human lymphocytes. They extended their study to show that bovine and ovine growth hormones reacted with similar potencies to that of hCS (0·03 %). As a result of their own work and from previously published data they proposed a classification of hormones and receptors shown in Table 1. These hormones not only competed with ^{125}I-hGH for binding to the hGH receptors on the lymphocytes but were also able to induce receptor-loss when incubated with the cells for 18–24 hr at 37°, although their activity in this respect did not tally exactly with their activity in competing with [125]I hGH for the hGH receptor. This induced receptor-loss was interpreted as an indication of biological activity of the various preparations and the relative potencies thus derived were shown to be of a similar order of magnitude to those previously found from minimal effective doses in man. No data are yet available on the biological activity of oCS in man but from its receptor activity one must anticipate that it may be considerable and thus of potential clinical interest. Thus the active sites in oCS and hGH are sterically more similar than those in the non-primate growth hormones. Comparative studies on growth hormone sequences have thrown much light on the structural relationships within this family of protein hormones and receptor-binding studies are beginning to give more details of the three-dimensional conformation than has previously been possible. There are, however, many questions that still remain unanswered— thus we still do not understand why hCS has more lactogenic than growth-promoting activity when its primary structure is more like hGH than hPRL. The lactogenic activity of hGH has been known for a long time and this activity is in keeping with recent estimates of its potency for competing with ^{125}I hPRL for lactogenic receptors but it is not clear why non-primate growth hormones are devoid of lactogenic activity. No doubt answers to these and other related questions will be available before the next edition of this book.

It is already clear that the surface topology of the molecule dictates its biological activity and in the case of hGH and its related hormones, this is formed around and supported by a rigid underlying framework. This remarkably stable framework is determined mainly by the primary amino acid sequence which in its turn, is derived from the genome that has, over countless generations, been modified to produce a family of related peptides. It is hardly surprising that attempts to find an "active-core" to the hGH molecule have been largely without success. As is the case with insulin, it seems that the globular nature of the molecule is fairly rigid and in contrast to linear peptides such as ACTH, disturbances of this structure rapidly lead to loss of biological activity.

Unlike insulin however, is the remarkable degree of species-specificity that has evolved. This specificity is only partly accounted for by changes in the structure of the hormone. Evolution has affected the conformation of the receptor in such a way that the primates share a receptor that is highly specific for primate growth hormone, while lower-mammals have receptors that, like the insulin receptor, react equally well with primate and native growth hormones.

3. Immunochemistry

Human growth hormone is highly immunogenic in rabbits, guinea-pigs and rats and the high-titre, high-avidity antibodies that are produced have hGH-neutralising as well as binding activity. With most antisera to hGH, there appears to be cross-reactivity between hGH and monkey growth hormone, although the extent of this varies between antisera. When compared with the monomers, high molecular weight aggregates of hGH have much reduced immunoreactivity with most antisera to hGH although in some receptor assays the aggregates may be fully active (Moore and Jin, 1978).

Comparisons between radioreceptor assays and radioimmunoassays for hGH in plasma have generally shown a high degree of concordance (Jacobs, Sneid, Garland, Laron and Daughaday, 1976; Garnier and Job, 1977) although there is evidence to suggest that this is not always the case (Gordon, Lesniak, Eastman, Hendricks and Roth, 1976). It would hardly be surprising to find that antibodies raised against hGH differed in their specificity and cross-reactivity with monomeric, dimeric and aggregated hGH, occasionally leading to discrepancies between radioreceptor and radioimmunoassays.

Antibodies raised against hGH are usually highly specific—perhaps even more so than the hGH receptor, generally sharing no cross-reactivity with non-primate growth hormones or primate and non-primate prolactins but usually some cross-reactivity with hCS. Although the cross-reactivity with hCS is usually low it is sufficient to interfere with the assay of plasma hGH in pregnancy since hCS concentrations are so high in the maternal plasma. It is often possible to saturate the hCS binding sites with excess hCS and still leave sufficient sites specific for hGH to allow a valid, sensitive and specific assay (Varma, Sönksen, Varma, Soeldner, Selenkow and Emerson, 1971).

B. ORGANS OF ORIGIN, METABOLISM AND EXCRETION

1. Pituitary

The anterior pituitary in man contains between 1 and 6 mg of hGH per gram of tissue. The hGH content remains approximately constant throughout life. Growth hormone is secreted by the acidophil cells that tend to occupy the posterolateral part of the anterior pituitary (Doniach, 1977). Classical staining techniques have not been very helpful in pituitary histology but the introduction of immunofluorescence and immunocytochemistry has allowed for the first time, unequivocal demonstration of the cells of origin of the anterior pituitary hormones. Separate cells of origin have been demonstrated for growth hormone and prolactin—both of which appear as acidophils with conventional stains (Zimmerman, Defendini and Frantz, 1974).

Ultrastructural examination demonstrates secretory granules in virtually all the cells, irrespective of their staining characteristics. Cells can be readily classified according to granule size, with prolactin (average diameter 550 nm) and growth hormone (average diameter 450 nm) secreting cells containing the largest granules, while thyrotrophin-secreting cells contain the smallest (average diameter 135 nm). The combination of immunocyto-chemistry with electron microscopy has greatly facilitated the study of pituitary cytology and with more widespread availability, should lead to a long-overdue improvement in our understanding of pituitary pathology.

2. Placenta

Although hCS is phylogenetically related to hGH and is likely to have physiological growth promoting, as well as lactogenic action, there is no evidence that the placenta produces another peptide more closely related to growth hormone.

3. Other Tissues

Although ectopic hGH production from lung cancer was reported as long ago as 1972 (Beck and Burger, 1972; Greenberg, Beck, Martin and Burger, 1972) it has been generally accepted that the prognosis is so poor that death supervenes before there has been time for a clinical syndrome to appear (Rees, 1976). The association of acromegaly with bronchial carcinoid adenomas has long been recognised and usually accepted as an example of the pluriglandular syndrome (Sönksen, Ayres, Braimbridge, Corrin, Davies, Jeremiah, Oaten, Lowy and West, 1976a). Dabek *et al.* (1974) recently reported the biochemical cure of two patients with acromegaly and bronchial carcinoid tumours after removal of the bronchial adenoma. Only one of the two tumours removed contained significant amounts of growth hormone. Just before publication of Dabek's cases, we also had a patient with an identical syndrome who was biochemically cured of acromegaly by removal of a bronchial adenoma. The tumour contained no extractable hGH, neither did it produce hGH in tissue culture. Since the patient had an en-larged pituitary fossa we presumed that the carcinoid tumour was producing a substance that stimulated the somatotroph cells either directly or via the hypothalamus. Although the tumour contained catecholamines we were not able to demonstrate the production of a "releasing-substance" by the tumour in tissue culture (Sönksen *et al.*, 1976a). Several points emerge from this:

(i) ectopic hGH production undoubtedly occurs—either from carcinoid tumours or the closely related (perhaps even identical) and more malignant oat cell tumours of the lung;

(ii) just as with ACTH, the tumours may not secrete the hormone itself (in this case hGH) but rather a releasing substance;

(iii) that cases of the pluriglandular syndrome may not indicate spon-taneous tumour development simultaneously in several different glands but rather that one gland may produce a substance (endocrine growth factor?) that leads to growth and eventual tumour development in one or more endocrine glands (Skrabanek and Powell, 1978);

(iv) that this is not all that uncommon—two cases of acromegaly cured by removal of a bronchial carcinoid (one of whom we managed to identify from microfilmed records) in whom the surgeon's recollection was confirmed by clinical photographs taken before and five years after surgery at a time when hGH radioimmunoassays had not yet been introduced (Sönksen et al., 1976a).

4. Distribution and Metabolism

After secretion from the anterior pituitary, hGH appears to reach equilibrium in a "space" slightly larger than plasma volume. Since it is known that hGH is carried as a simple solution in plasma, without significant binding to other plasma proteins, this indicates that diffusion from the vascular pool is limited and that a concentration gradient is likely to exist between the plasma and tissue fluid hGH concentrations. Under some pathological conditions—such as hepatic failure, renal failure and possibly also uncontrolled diabetes mellitus—capillary permeability increases and the apparent distribution space increases to values approaching that of extracellular fluid (Owens, Srivastava, Tompkins, Nabarro and Sönksen, 1973).

Normally hGH is metabolised by the liver and kidneys each accounting for approximately half of the total disposal of hGH (McCormick, Sönksen, Soeldner and Egdahl, 1969). The overall clearance of hGH from the blood stream (metabolic clearance rate—MCR) averages 3 ml kg/min (1751 $day^{-1} M^{-2}$) and is constant at all plasma hGH concentrations (Owens et al., 1973). It is of importance to note that with hGH, MCR values are similar when determined with ^{125}I, ^{131}I or unlabelled hormone (Franchimont and Burger, 1975); this indicates that radiolabelled hGH is a valid tracer for the hormone and is in contrast to insulin where the rate of metabolism of labelled hormone is much reduced depending on the degree and site of iodine incorporation (Ellis, Jones, Thomas, Geiger, Teetz and Sönksen, 1977). The MCR of hGH is low compared with insulin and this is reflected in a longer half life of approximately 20 min compared with that of 4 min for insulin (Owens et al., 1973, Sönksen, Srivastava, Tompkins and Nabarro, 1972). Growth hormone metabolism is reduced in renal failure and in myxoedema but surprisingly little impaired in patients with liver disease. This seems to be due to increased capillary permeability associated with severe liver failure and a resultant increase in extravascular hGH metabolism in tissues other than the liver (Owens et al., 1973). In thyrotoxicosis hGH metabolism is slightly increased but thyroid hormone status does not seem to have a very important effect on hGH metabolism. Although changing from the horizontal to upright posture reduces hGH metabolism (probably as a result of a reduction in hepatic blood flow), most of the fluctuation in hGH concentration in plasma reflects hGH secretion rather than changes in degradation.

Although the kidneys are an important site of hGH metabolism, urinary excretion of hGH is normally very small. Urinary hGH concentrations are so low that considerable skill is required to operate valid assays. This includes dialysis (to remove low molecular weight substances such as urea and salt that interfere with the radioimmunoassay) and subsequent concentration by lyophilisation. Much effort has been expended in attempts to set up valid assays for urinary hGH which have considerable diagnostic potential. The overwhelming conclusion has been that the difficulties far outweigh the benefits and this accounts for the paucity of data on urinary hGH excretion.

Although hGH concentrations in the plasma fluctuate widely throughout the day and night, there is agreement that the average hGH concentrations in the plasma is around 3 ng/ml (6 mu/l). Knowing the MCR of hGH to be approximately 3 ml/kg/min, this implies a daily production rate of around 1 mg in a 70 kg adult. This is in keeping with the levels of hGH in plasma after treatment with different doses of hGH (Sönksen et al., 1976b) and suggests that hGH therapy might be more rationally given as a daily injection on a body weight basis (e.g. 15 µg/kg/day); this would represent a significant reduction in dosage according to most treatment schedules and hence a considerable saving of a scarce commodity. Although the growth rate on higher-dosage regimes is bound to be greater (Preece, Tanner, Whitehouse and Cameron, 1976) this does not itself seem a logical argument against a more economic and rational approach to the use of an expensive substance, when low-doses tailored to body weight lead to the attainment of normal growth rates (Frasier, Aceto, Hayles and Mikity, 1977).

C. MECHANISMS CONTROLLING SECRETION

1. Neuroendocrine

Research into neuroendocrine control of anterior pituitary function has provided a wealth of information on the regulation of hGH release and has provided a rational explanation for many of the abnormalities in secretion of this hormone. This section summarises briefly the current knowledge in this field (for excellent reviews see Müller, 1973; Martin, 1976; Smythe, 1977).

It has long been recognised that hypothalamic and other brain lesions are associated with disorders of growth and pituitary function. Since the important early work of Harris (1948) neuroendocrinology has become a major branch of endocrinology. The current state of knowledge is based upon pharmacological and electrophysiological studies as well as upon the effects of destructive lesions of the hypothalamus.

The importance of particular areas of the hypothalamus in GH regulation have been identified by destructive lesions of the hypothalamus and pituitary stalk and pituitary transplantation studies which result in lowered plasma levels and blunting or loss of the GH response to insulin-induced hypoglycaemia and sleep (Krieger and Glick, 1974). In experimental animals small lesions of the median eminence and midline basal hypothalamus block GH release following insulin (Abrams, Parker, Blanco, Reichlin and Daughaday, 1966) and stress (Brown, Schalch and Reichlin, 1971). Lesions of the ventromedial nucleus in young rats produce lowered plasma and pituitary GH concentrations associated with growth retardation (Frohman and Bernardis, 1968). Lesions of the hypothalamus which do not involve the ventromedial-arcuate nucleus area are not associated with GH deficiency, suggesting that this area is a specific stimulatory area in the control of GH secretion.

This hypothesis is supported by the results of electrical stimulation of the hypothalamus. Stimulation of the medial basal hypothalamus causes GH secretion (Martin, 1972) whether the stimulus is unilatral or bilateral. Stimulation outside the ventromedial-arcuate nucleus complex is without effect. If the stimulus is applied to the preoptic area significant inhibition of GH secretion is seen confirming earlier speculation of a GH inhibitory area in the anterior hypothalamus and parachiasmatic region. This area is now known to contain high concentrations of somatostatin (growth hormone release inhibiting hormone, GHRIH) (Elde, Hökfelt, Johansson, Efendic and Luft, 1976.

Hypothalamic stimulation probably influences GH secretion by excitation of tuberoinfundibular peptidergic neurones which are distributed widely throughout the medial basal hypothalamus (Martin and Renaud, 1974). Sites for TSH and LH release are more extensive than those for GH release.

The final common path for the control of GH secretion probably involves the release from the ventromedial-arcuate nucleus region of GH-releasing hormone (GHRH). Although GHRH activity has been found in hypophyseal portal blood (Wilber and Porter, 1970), Schally and his colleagues (1973) isolated a decapeptide from porcine hypothalamic extracts which was biologically active in releasing GH *in vivo* and *in vitro*. Disappointingly, subsequent synthesis yielded an inactive substance which turned out to be identifiable as a portion of the β chain of pork haemoglobin. However, further studies have confirmed that hypothalamic extracts will cause the release of GH. Earlier reports of hypothalamic extracts which were inactive in releasing GH may have been due to contamination with hypothalamic GHRIH. GHRH activity can be demonstrated to be an entity which is distinct from vasopressin and thyroid releasing hormone (TRH) both of which have GH releasing properties.

GHRIH, a tetradecapeptide, first discovered in the hypothalamus (Brazeau, Vale, Burgus, Ling, Butcher, Rivier and Guillemin, 1973) is now known (by immunohistochemical and radioimmunoassay studies) to be distributed widely in other parts of the nervous system as well as in peripheral endocrine cells (for review article see Luft, Efendic and Hökfelt, 1978). In the hypothalamus GHRIH has been found in both cell bodies and neuronal fibres. GHRIH positive cells are also distributed throughout the brain particularly in the cortex and GHRIH positive fibres originating from cell bodies in the anterior hypothalamus have been found in the median eminence extending down into the pituitary stalk. The dense plexuses of GHRIH positive fibres in the ventromedial and arcuate nuclei are compatible with the hypothesis that GHRIH has a transmitter or modulator role which is important in the control of GH secretion as well as that of other anterior pituitary hormones.

GHRIH inhibits GH secretion whatever stimulus is applied suggesting that the action of this hormone is to inhibit the final common path of GH release. When infused intravenously the inhibition of GH secretion is rapid and after cessation of infusion plasma GH concentrations tend to rebound to levels higher than those prior to infusion. This action has been shown in both humans and in experimental animals. Lesions of the ventromedial nucleus, in the rat, prevent the postinhibitory GH rebound after GHRIH administration suggesting the possibility that a short-loop negative feedback mechanism may operate for GH secretion (i.e. that increased GH levels may inhibit further GH secretion). On the other hand the postinhibitory GH surge after GHRIH is also seen in isolated rat pituitaries *in vitro*.

The observations that stress and sleep stimulate GH secretion indicate that extrahypothalamic areas of the brain may influence GH secretion, although the isolated hypothalamus can maintain reasonably normal basal GH secretion (Halasz, Schalch and Gorski, 1971) including pulsatile release. Extensive anatomical studies in the rat have shown that the hippocampus, amygdala and reticular formation have connections with the medial basal hypothalamus (ventromedial-arcuate nucleus region). It is probably an over-simplification to attribute specific roles for GH secretion control to complex neuronal structures such as these but electrical stimulation studies suggest that activation of hippocampus and basolateral amygdala stimulate GH release while stimulation of the corticomedial amygdala inhibits GH release. Stimulation of other parts of the brain also stimulate GH secretion; one such site is the region surrounding the interpeduncular nucleus which has dopaminergic inputs to higher centres. Stimulation of the raphe nucleus of the brain stem (which contains serotinergic neurones) inhibits GH release during stimulation followed by a postinhibitory rebound (similar to the results of ventromedial nucleus stimulation).

The existence of such pathways explain the GH release following stress and sleep since the hippocampus is involved in the alerting response, the amygdala in emotional responses (including aggression) and the raphe nuclei in the induction of slow wave sleep. The high concentrations of mono-amines (dopamine, noradrenaline and serotonin) in the hypothalamus, particularly in the region of the median eminence, suggest the possibility that these may be important in the regulation of the hypothalamic-hypo-physiotrophic hormones. There is a considerable body of evidence for the stimulatory roles of monoamines in GH secretion in man and primates although there is discussion as to whether serotonin or dopamine is the more important in causing stimulation of GH release (Smythe, 1977).

L-dopa, given by mouth, crosses the blood brain barrier and evokes GH secretion (Boyd, Lebovitz and Pfeiffer, 1970). L-dopa is a precursor of both dopamine and noradrenaline and its effects are blocked by phentolamine, an α-adrenergic blocking agent (Kansal, Buse, Talbert and Base, 1972) as is GH secretion stimulated by insulin hypoglycaemia, vasopressin and exercise, but not sleep-related GH secretion. This suggests that the effects of L-dopa on GH secretion are mediated by noradrenaline (α-adrenergic agents enhance GH release and β-stimulation inhibits GH release while appropriate adrenergic blockade produce the converse effects).

However, specific central dopaminergic agents such as apomorphine and bromocriptine can stimulate GH secretion, although pretreatment with glucose diminishes the GH response, showing that glucoreceptor activity may partially overide monoaminergic stimuli.

Serotonin and its analogues can also provoke GH release in man and primates although the response is not great (Imura, Nakai and Hoshimi, 1973). The serotonin antagonists methysergide and cyproheptadine will also block the GH release after insulin hypoglycaemia indicating some inter-play between the various mono-aminergic mechanisms rather than specific, exclusive physiological roles.

There are important species differences in the GH response to different pharmacological stimuli and there is probably no animal model that precisely duplicates GH control in man. Changes in monoaminergic control mechanisms have been suggested as a possible explanation for abnormal GH secretion in disease. Acromegalic patients usually show a paradoxical fall in elevated plasma GH levels in response to L-dopa (Liuzzi, Chiodini, Botalla, Cremascoli and Silvestrini, 1972) or bromocriptine (Liuzzi, Chiodini, Botalla, Cremascoli, Müller and Silvestrini, 1974). In some

I

cases the abnormality may be a secondary disorder. Hoyte and Martin
(1975) have reported return of the normal hGH response to L-dopa, apomorphine and TRH after removal of an adenoma secreting hGH. Smythe
(1977), on the other hand has suggested as an alternative explanation that the
"paradoxical" effects of dopaminergic drugs on hGH secretion in acromegaly
may be due to dopamine acting on serotonin receptors. In support of this
hypothesis Smythe cites evidence that L-dopa can, in normal subjects,
inhibit as well as stimulate hGH release and that L-dopa stimulated hGH
secretion can be inhibited by serotoninergic blockade. These "cross-effects"
may be explained by certain structural similarities between dopamine and
serotonin (as well as ergoline) ring systems. This apparent lack of specificity
is supported by the finding in the same neurone of both noradrenaline and
GHRIH (Hökfelt, Elfvin, Elde, Schultzberg, Goldstein and Luft, 1977)
for which there is corroborative evidence in the invertebrates. Another
possible explanation for the "paradoxical effects" of dopaminergic agents
in acromegaly is the existence of dopaminergic receptors in the pituitary as
well as in the hypothalamus. Martin, Renaud and Brazeau (1975) have
suggested that the hypothalamic peptidergic-neurones (secreting GHRH
and GHRIH) like the monoaminergic neurones are involved in a diffuse
neural network with a widespread distribution in the central nervous
system. Release of peptides into the hypophyseal portal system may be
only one aspect of their biological roles and this may account for the complexity of the control mechanisms and the apparent paradoxes found in
disease states. Finally there is evidence of a short-loop feedback control of
GH secretion (see above) as well as evidence that levels of somatomedin or
other growth factors may be important in controlling GH secretion
(Daughaday, Herington and Phillips, 1975).

2. Metabolic

Metabolic factors governing GH secretion have been extensively reviewed
by Reichlin (1975) and will be briefly summarised here. GH is an important
regulator of energy homeostasis by its lipolytic action and its effects as an
anabolic hormone and an insulin antagonist. It is, therefore, not surprising
that alterations in the concentrations of circulating energy substrates influence
GH secretion.

Hypoglycaemia is a well known potent stimulus for hGH secretion in man
(Roth, Glick, Yalow and Berson, 1963) and most other mammalian species.
There is good evidence for a hypoglycaemic threshold for hGH release (Luft,
Cerasi, Madison, von Euler, Della Casa and Roovete, 1966; West and
Sönksen, 1977).

Hyperglycaemia will inhibit basal GH secretion and rises in plasma GH associated with exercise and arginine infusion but will not block sleep or stress-related release of hGH. Some adaptation of glucoreceptors occurs in relation to chronic blood glucose changes and GH release is observed during recovery from hyperglycaemia even though absolute blood glucose levels are elevated (Irie, Sakuma, Tsushima, Shizume and Nakao, 1967b).

Experimental studies in animals have shown that the hypothalamus contains areas which act as glucoreceptors and are important in relation to GH secretion. Blanco, Schalch and Reichlin (1966) were able to block the GH response to insulin hypoglycaemia in the squirrel monkey by glucose perfusion of the median eminence region. Induction of intracellular gluco-penia in the hypothalamus using injection of 2-deoxy-D-glucose in the rhesus monkey (Himsworth, Carmel and Frantz, 1972) released GH when the injections were given into the lateral hypothalamus alongside the mid part of the ventromedial nucleus. It has been suggested that the results of these two studies can be interpreted by the explanation that the lateral hypothala-mus is sensitive to a fall in blood glucose and the ventromedial nucleus to a rise in blood glucose. This theory is compatible with views that the lateral hypothalamus controls food drive while the ventromedial nucleus contains "satiety centre". Prolonged fasting in man is characterised by rises in plasma concentrations of free fatty acids (FFA) and ketone bodies as well as hGH. Concrete evidence that either of these two substrates can themselves regulate hGH secretion is lacking. Enormous elevations of FFA induced by fat intake and heparin injection have no effect on hGH levels in man (Schalch and Kipnis, 1965) and elevation of plasma β-hydroxybutyrate concentrations in the monkey do not stimulate GH release. Although increases in FFA levels block the GH secretion in response to insulin hypoglycaemia (Blackard, Boylen, Hinson and Nelson, 1969) and sleep (Lipman, Taylor, Schenk and Mintz, 1972), the concentrations of FFA achieved are highly unphysiological and therefore the relevance of these findings to day to day regulation of GH secretion is uncertain. It seems more likely that the metabolic adaptations to starvation are mainly produced by inhibition of insulin secretion and that the rise in GH levels is due to food deprivation (see below). The increase in FFA levels may therefore result from the dual effects of the lipolytic effect of raised GH levels and loss of the antilipolytic action of insulin.

It has been suggested that a lowering of FFA concentration can stimulate GH secretion (Irie, Sakuma, Tsushima, Matsuyaki, Shizume and Nakao, 1967a; Quabbe, Ramek and Luyckx, 1977). However, FFA depression is unlikely to be as important as hypoglycaemia in hGH regulation since a fall in FFA levels occurs after insulin administration irrespective of whether glucose is given as well but hGH levels only rise when blood glucose levels have also fallen (West and Sönksen, 1977).

Certain amino acids, particularly arginine, which stimulate insulin secretion have also been found to cause GH release. The physiological relevance of these findings has been questioned (Reichlin, 1975) because of the large doses required to stimulate GH secretion and the age and sex differences in the response. Cyclic AMP and calcium ions are effective *in vitro* as well as *in vivo* in causing GH release and probably act directly on pituitary somatotrophs. It appeared initially that cAMP was the second messenger involved in GH release but Peake (1973) showed that highly purified GHRH did not increase cAMP within the pituitary but increased cGMP levels which in turn promoted calcium uptake into the pituitary and released GH. Cyclic nucleotides influence hormone release without affecting their synthesis. Parsons (1970) has summarised the stimulus secretion coupling hypothesis of Douglas as it applies to GH secretion.

Metabolic factors now appear to be less important in the day to day regulation of GH secretion than the more complex and subtle neuroendocrine mechanisms although metabolic factors may act in concert with neuroendocrine and other endocrine secretions in emergency.

D. METHODS OF DETERMINATION IN BLOOD AND TISSUE FLUIDS

1. Biological Assays

Remarkably little has been added to this field since the chapter by Korner (1961) in the first edition of this book. The assay of growth hormone has recently been reviewed by Wilhelmi (1973) and Friesen and Carr (1976).

Although bioassay remains fundamental to the measurement of activity of purified growth hormone and provides the basis for comparison of reference standards throughout the world, the assays are too insensitive and non-specific for valid measurement of hGH in blood and tissue fluids. The tibial width assay is most commonly used and is also the most sensitive (Greenspan, Li, Simpson and Evans, 1949). Over a limited range of GH doses, the growth of the epiphyseal cartilage in the hypophysectomised rat is linearly related to the logarithm of the dose of growth hormone administered to the rats. Female rats are hypophysectomised at 26–28 days of age and after a recovery period of two weeks, injected daily with GH for four days. Following this the animals are killed, the tibias divided and the width of the tibial plate measured microscopically. The minimal effective dose is in the region of 5 μg per animal per day and a maximum response occurs with about 400 μg/day. Attempts to assay hGH in plasma have either found undetectably low values or values in the range of 2–200 μg hGH per ml plasma; greatly in excess of hGH concentration measured by radioimmuno-assay. The most likely explanation for this discrepancy is the lack of sensitivity and specificity of the bioassays rather than the presence of GH with biological but not immunological reactivity, since more recent data with the more sensitive and specific radioreceptor assays agree well with the radioimmuno-assay. It is known that plasma contains some substances other than hGH, which are active in the tibial assay (Thorngren and Hansson, 1977; Ching, Trakulrungsi, Somana, Evans and Evans, 1977) and these will all tend to lead to an elevated ratio of bioassayable to immunoassayable hGH concentration.

2. Radioreceptor Assays

Although experience with radioreceptor assays (RRA) is still rather limited, results suggest that they may well combine the specificity of the radio-immunoassay with the biological importance of the bioassay. If data for growth hormone eventually proves to be similar to those for insulin, then there will be a close relationship between biological potency of various growth hormones, chemical analogues and related peptides and their ability to compete with radiolabelled hGH for hGH receptors (Roth, Kahn, Lesniak, Gorden, De Meyts, Megyesi, Neville, Gavin, Sol, Freychet, Goldfine, Bar and Archer, 1975). While an antibody may bind to any part of the growth hormone molecule, the GH-receptor only reacts with the biologically active site. The measurement of hormone concentration by RRA is thus a more accurate reflection of its biological potency. Different patterns of cross-reactivity are seen between hGH and related peptides depending on the particular receptor that is chosen for RRA and the radioligand selected. The number of variables is immense and the potential degree of cross-reactivity between growth hormones, prolactins and chorionic somato-mammotrophins from different species is considerable.

Since hGH has both somatotrophic as well as lactotrophic activity, it might be expected to react with both types of receptor—this is indeed the case with lactogenic receptors from rat liver; with ^{125}I-hGH as ligand, hGH and hPRL have equal activity in inhibiting radioligand binding. Rabbit liver contains receptors that show high-specificity for hGH and other non-primate growth hormones but little activity with prolactin (Etzrodt, Musch, Schleyer and Pfeiffer, 1976). Human liver and cultured monocytes contain receptors that are specific for hGH, showing little or no cross-reactivity with non-primate growth hormones and primate or non-primate prolactins (Carr and Friesen, 1976; Lesniak, Gorden and Roth, 1977), and this is in keeping with the failure of non-primate GH to promote growth in hGH-deficient patients.

The principle and practical details of radioreceptor assays for hGH have been recently reviewed in detail by Friesen and Carr (1976). Sensitivity is generally lower than that of RIA although assays have been reported with sensitivities as low as 2 ng hGH per ml of plasma (Garnier and Job, 1977) allowing detection of hGH in basal samples taken from normal subjects.

In contrast to the wide discrepancies between bioassay and RIA, the results of RRA are in close agreement with those of the RIA. Garnier and Job (1977) found remarkably close correlation between RRA and RIA in the assay of hGH in plasma from normal and hypopituitary children treated with exogenous hGH (RRA/RIA ratios 1·03 and 1·05 respectively). Not all studies have found such concordance and it seems that the choice of receptor and radioligand can influence the results as can the proportion of aggregated to monomeric GH in the samples (Soman and Goodman, 1977; Gordon et al., 1976; Moore and Jin, 1978).

Despite these occasional differences between RRA and RIA, the general pattern of results has shown good agreement between the two types of assay both in terms of the absolute concentration of hGH in plasma in different diseases as well as the pattern of hGH responses to stimulation and suppression tests. The RRA has been helpful in elucidating at least one clinical problem: Jacobs et al. (1976) have shown that the high circulating hGH concentrations in Laron dwarfs (Laron, Pertzelan and Karp, 1968) previously documented by RIA, is also detectable by RRA, suggesting that the defect lies not with the circulating hGH but with the tissue receptors. This is in keeping with the failure of hGH therapy to cause growth, metabolic responses or generation of somatomedin in these patients (Daughaday, 1977).

3. Radioimmunoassays

Since the last edition, the radioimmunoassay (RIA) of hGH has moved from the experimental field to one of prominence in clinical practice. Although initially one of the more difficult RIAs in terms of development, radioiodination of ligand, interference and lack of consistency of results (Greenwood, 1967), it is now perhaps, the most widely available and frequently used hormone RIA and we are indebted to Greenwood (1967) for much of this pioneering work.

The practical details of the RIA for hGH have recently been reviewed in considerable detail (Friesen and Carr, 1976; Sönksen, 1976a) and will only be touched on here. Although any form of separation of "free" from "bound" radioligand may be used, the authors prefer and strongly recommend the double-antibody procedure (Sönksen, 1976b), which has in their hands been working consistently for more than ten years. The major advantage is its specificity, due to the immunological nature of the reaction. This ensures that the precipitate at the bottom of the test tube after centrifugation is immunologically intact, thus confering a degree of specificity lacking in most separation procedures.

Radioiodination of hGH is best performed using ^{125}I, because of its higher isotopic abundance and purity. The technique for introducing ^{125}I into the hGH molecule does not seem of critical importance and the Chloramine-T method originally introduced by Greenwood, Hunter and Glover (1963), still remains the simplest and most satisfactory. Good incorporation of radioactivity into hGH does not always occur but is facilitated by minimising the reaction volume. Purification of the radioligand is essential before use. This is conveniently carried out on small columns (30 × 2 cm) of Sephadex G-50 fine, developed in an albumin-containing buffer. Monomeric ^{125}I-hGH must be separated from the aggregated ^{125}I-hGH that elutes in the void volume and from free ^{125}Iodide. The radioligand (like the parent molecule) is rather unstable and tends to aggregate on storage. For this reason we routinely repurify ^{125}I hGH before each assay.

There seems to be general agreement on current international standards for hGH. There is an international reference preparation (IRP 66/217) issued by the National Institute for Biological Standards and Control (Holly Hill, Hampstead, London NW3 6RB, UK) for use in radioimmunoassays both as a standard and for radioiodination. The introduction of a national hGH quality control scheme in the UK revealed some alarming discrepancies between centres, and was helpful in determining the causes for this and re-solving many of the differences.

Human growth hormone is highly immunogenic and specific antibodies of high titre and avidity are readily available. There is remarkable little difference between plasma hGH values determined with different antisera. When comparing insulin concentrations in plasma using ten separate insulin antibodies, we found wide discrepancies in apparent insulin content, particularly in fasting samples (Sönksen, 1976a). Similar studies with ten separate antisera produced against hGH showed no significant variation.

Antisera to hGH commonly cross-react with hCS and for this reason "routine" hGH assays will not give valid results from plasma from pregnant patients. It is possible in most instances, to saturate the hCS-reactive sites with excess hCS added to the assay tube and still leave sufficient hGH-specific sites for a sensitive and specific assay of hGH in pregnancy-plasma (Varma et al., 1971). Because of the lack of cross-reactivity of hGH with other peptide and glycoprotein hormones, it is possible to assay more than one hormone simultaneously in plasma using ^{125}I and ^{131}I radioligands. This has considerable advantages, particularly in terms of economy. We have been assaying insulin and hGH simultaneously (using ^{131}I-insulin and ^{125}I-hGH) for more than ten years and have found it most convenient and to work extremely well (Sönksen, 1976a).

The within-assay variability of most RIAs has been very small, averaging in good hands less than 2 % (coefficient of variation). Between-assay variability on the other hand has never been so good usually averaging 10%. This means a very considerable between-assay imprecision, the causes of which have not yet been identified. Whenever possible, experimental design should take notice of this and samples from a given patient before and after treatment should be included in the same assay.

The periods of incubation of the assay can be varied widely without serious effect on sensitivity. It is easily possible to modify the hGH assay to be sufficiently sensitive for clinical use and provide an answer within 24 hr. If this is important (and it seldom is sufficiently important to justify the extra effort and cost involved) an instantaneous separation technique such as dextran-charcoal is advantageous.

There are several variations on the standard RIA, such as the immuno-radiometric assay (Miles and Hales, 1968) and the two-site assay (Addison and Hales, 1971) which although offering advantages for other hormones, seem to have little to recommend them over the standard RIA, in the case of hGH.

The likely development of RIA for hGH will be away from the use of radio-ligands towards other forms of labelling that will facilitate the handling of large batches of samples and reduce the counting time and costs. The remarkable thing about the current RIAs of hGH is their general availability and freedom from the technical problems which troubled earlier investigators.

E. PLASMA LEVELS OF HUMAN GROWTH HORMONE

The widespread availability of reliable radioimmunological techniques for the measurement of hGH has provided extensive information on the effects of physiological and disease states on the secretion of hGH.

1. Normal Subjects

hGH is secreted episodically by the pituitary (Glick and Goldsmith, 1968) and cleared rapidly from the plasma (Owens et al., 1973). A "normal" plasma level can, therefore, only be defined in terms of the conditions under which the blood sample was obtained. Plasma hGH is usually undetectable after an overnight fast in normal adult humans. In the normal human foetus (from

70 days to midgestation) plasma hGH levels are comparable with those found in acromegalic patients (Kaplan, Grumbach and Shephard, 1972) but fall progressively towards full term. The levels at birth are still markedly elevated compared with the normal adult and continue to fall, rapidly during the first two weeks of life and then more slowly to the end of the first year of life. The elevated plasma hGH levels persist longer in premature infants (Cornblath, Parker, Reisner, Forbes and Daughaday, 1965). Secretion of hGH in older adults is diminished as compared with younger adults (Finkelstein, Roffward, Boyar, Kream and Hellman, 1972) or children and adolescents (Thompson, Rodriquez, Kowarski, Migeon and Blizzard, 1972). That these changes are due to differences in secretion rather than metabolism of hGH is confirmed by the absence of a change in the metabolic clearance rate of hGH with increasing age (Taylor, Zinster and Mintz, 1969). The responsiveness of the pituitary, as judged by rises in hGH, ACTH and possibly the gonadotrophins following provocative stimuli, also shows some decline with increasing age (Bazarre, Johanson, Huseman, Varma and Blizzard, 1976).

Basal fasting concentrations of hGH are indistinguishable in men and women but the spontaneous fluctuations and the responses to exercise, stress and arginine infusion are greater in women. These differences are probably due to the effects of oestrogens since (i) the hGH response to arginine in women is maximal at midcycle—corresponding to the oestrogen peak (Merimee, Fineberg and Tyson, 1969) and (ii) hGH response to arginine in men can be augmented by oestrogen treatment. The increased hGH responsiveness in women is due partly to increased pituitary responsiveness and partly to decreased end organ response to hGH induced by oestrogens (Josimovich, Mintz and Finster, 1967). hGH responses to insulin hypoglycaemia do not differ between men and women.

The secretion pattern of hGH during the day is characterised by bursts of secretion following exericse (Hunter and Greenwood, 1964), stress (Glick, Roth, Yalow and Berson, 1965) and following carbohydrate-rich meals. In addition unexplained episodes of secretion are also seen during the day (Glick and Goldsmith, 1968). The most striking increases in plasma hGH levels are seen during sleep. Quabbe, Schilling and Helge (1966) in normal adults found intermittent peaks of hGH secretion during the night—usually related to deep sleep although they made no objective measurements of the depth of sleep. This work was confirmed and extended by Takahashi, Kipnis, Daughaday (1968) who found peaks of hGH appearing with the onset of deep sleep (slow wave sleep), stages III and IV as assessed by EEG recordings. These changes in plasma hGH were unrelated to changes in blood glucose, cortisol or insulin concentrations.

2. Pathological States

(a) Hypothalamic and pituitary disease

Active acromegaly is characterised by hypersecretion of hGH as a consequence of an acidophil adenoma although in·some cases the responses of plasma hGH to dynamic tests suggest a primary hypothalamic disorder. Because plasma hGH concentrations can vary widely even in fasting normal individuals random hGH measurements are unreliable as a means of establishing or refuting the diagnosis of acromegaly (Sönksen, 1974). The diagnosis can best be made by showing failure of suppression of plasma hGH after an oral glucose load. In normal subjects plasma hGH falls below 2 mu/l (often to less than 0·4 mu/l) at some point during an oral glucose tolerance test, usually between 90 and 120 min after glucose ingestion. In acromegaly the most common finding is a high fasting plasma hGH concentration which shows little or no suppression after oral glucose although paradoxical rises in hGH after oral glucose are seen and may be coincident with increases in plasma insulin. "Burnt-out" acromegaly is a dubious clinical entity and most cases of spontaneous regression of acromegaly are due to a pituitary apoplexy.

The problem caused by the variability of plasma hGH has been resolved by continuous sampling of blood to yield an integrated plasma level of hGH (Frantz and Holub, 1968; Daggett and Nabarro, 1977); this is more reliable than basal hGH for assessment of the response to treatment in acromegaly but not as convenient as blood sampling after oral glucose.

Successful treatment of acromegaly is usually associated with a fall in basal plasma hGH to below 10 mu/l and/or normal suppression after oral glucose. Trans-sphenoidal hypophysectomy has been shown to be an effective form of treatment in acromegaly. Williams and his colleagues found successful lowering of plasma hGH in 39 out of 59 patients treated by this operation alone and in seven other patients treated with radiotherapy and surgery (Williams, Jacobs, Kurtz, Millar, Oakley, Spathis, Sulway and Nabarro, 1974). Cryohypophysectomy has been reported to be successful in lowering the raised hGH levels in acromegaly by Cross, Glynne, Grossart, Jennett, Kellett, Lazarus, Thomson and Webster, (1972), although the actual concentrations of hGH were not reported (Cross et al., 1972). The effects of conventional pituitary irradiation are less spectacular and are usually slow in onset (Roth, Gordon and Brace, 1970; Hunter, McGurk, McLelland, Hibbert, Strong, Gillingham and Harris, 1971) as is the response to yttrium implantation (Wright, Hartog, Palter, Tevaarwerk, Doyle, Arnot, Joplin and Fraser, 1970). Early reports of proton beam irradiation suggested that this might have little more to offer than conventional radiotherapy but more recently Kjellberg and Kliman (1975) have claimed results as good as with trans-sphenoidal hypophysectomy using the stereotatic Bragg peak proton beam. The most controversial aspect of current treatment for acromegaly concerns the efficacy of the dopaminergic agent bromocriptine. Marked clinical and hormonal improvements have been reported by one group (Wass, Thorner, Morris, Rees, Mason, Jones and Besser, 1977), although in only 15 of their 73 patients did mean daily hGH fall to 10 mu/l or less. Other centres, however, have reported less satisfactory results (Summers, Hipkin, Diver and Davis, 1975; Dunn, Donald and Espiner, 1977). Bromocriptine may be a useful adjunct to other forms of therapy in acromegaly (Holdaway, Frengley, Scott and Ibbertson, 1978). Reports of good clinical response to treatment of acromegaly despite an inadequate fall in plasma hGH may be due to changes in somatomedin synthesis but this is speculative. The converse of acromegaly and gigantism associated with elevated plasma somatomedin A levels but normal hGH has been described (Hoffenberg, Howella, Epstein, Pimstone, Fryklund, Hall, Schwalbe and Rudd, 1977).

The measurement of plasma hGH response to dynamic tests (see below) is a useful means of assessing pituitary function in known or suspected pituitary or hypothalamic disease, the failure of hGH release being an early feature of pituitary disease. In addition it is a means of identifying those children and adolescents with short stature who may benefit from hGH therapy (Tanner, Whitehouse, Hughes and Vince, 1971). Deficiency of hGH may occur in association with other anterior pituitary hormone deficiencies or in isolation. Isolated hGH deficiency has been reported as a recessively inherited defect (Rimoin, Merimee and McKusick, 1966).

(b) Other endocrine disorders

In hyperthyroidism hGH secretion is normal but is impaired in myxoedema. The secretion of hGH in response to provocative stimuli returns to normal after correction of hypothyroidism (Tunbridge, Marshall and Burke, 1973). Whether thyroxine directly stimulates protein synthesis in the anterior pituitary as it does in other tissues (e.g. liver and kidney) or whether it acts by altering hypothalamic function is unknown.

Cushing's syndrome (either spontaneous or iatrogenic) is usually associated with impairment of the hGH response to insulin hypoglycaemia. However, some workers have shown no inhibition of hGH release following corticosteroid administration (Morris, Jorgensen and Jenkins, 1968) and high doses of exogenous corticosteroids do not inhibit hGH secretion during sleep in normal men (Krieger, Albin, Paget and Glick, 1972). It is possible that dose, duration of therapy and closeness in time between administration and study may be important factors in explaining these seemingly irreconcilable differences. ACTH therapy does not inhibit hGH secretion and this may account for the lack of growth inhibition in children treated with ACTH for long periods. It is not clear from the findings outlined above whether prolonged corticosteroid therapy inhibits growth in children by suppressing hGH secretion or by a peripheral antagonism of hGH action. The persistence of abnormal hGH secretion during sleep after successful treatment of Cushing's disease lends support to the hypothesis of an underlying hypothalamic cause of this disorder. (Krieger and Glick, 1972).

Excessive and erratic hGH secretion is found in patients with poorly controlled diabetes mellitus and the responses to stimuli such as exercise are exaggerated (Hansen, 1970). Strict control of blood glucose abolishes the hypersecretion of hGH (Hansen, 1971). Since hGH is implicated as a factor in the pathogenesis of diabetic retinopathy control of hyperglycemia would be expected to protect against the development of this complication. Paradoxical rises in plasma hGH have been found in prediabetic males (Sönksen, Soeldner, Gleason and Boden, 1973a) as well as in a miscellany of other conditions. Rises in plasma hGH are seen during treatment of diabetic ketoacidosis and appear to be in response to insulin administration rather than to the fall in blood glucose (Sönksen, Srivastava, Tompkins and Nabarro, 1972).

Patients with hypoglycaemia due to endogenous hyperinsulinism (insulinoma or nesidioblastosis) may show normal or elevated plasma hGH concentrations. The secretion of hGH appears to be related to the presence of symptoms rather than the absolute level of plasma glucose.

(c) Non-endocrine disease

Plasma hGH concentrations may be altered by non-endocrine disease. If this occurs in childhood growth is impaired. A number of reports have documented impairment of hGH secretion in children with severe emotional deprivation (Brown and Reichlin, 1972). James Barrie (author of Peter Pan) is said to be the archetype of this condition. Such children show impaired hGH release after insulin hypoglycaemia or arginine infusion and to a lesser extent may have impairment of ACTH and gonadotrophin secretion. Growth and normal neuroendocrine response return when the child is placed in a more suitable environment (usually hospital). It has, in one case, been shown that β-adrenergic blockade with propranolol released hGH (Imura, Yoshimi and Ikekubo, 1971) suggesting that the underlying cause of this syndrome involved excessive β-adrenergic inhibition of hGH secretion. Resistance of hepatic receptors to hGH has been proposed to explain dwarfism associated with high plasma hGH concentrations (Laron, Pertzelan and Karp, 1968). Recently it has been shown that somatomedin levels are low in Laron

dwarfism suggesting that feedback regulation of hGH may involve somatomedin. End-organ resistance in Laron dwarfism has been demonstrated
by failure of exogenous hGH therapy to cause nitrogen retention or an
increase in growth velocity (Najjar, Khachadurian, Ilbani and Blizzard,
1971). The mechanism of the stunted growth of the African pygmy is also
probably due to end-organ resistance (Merimee, Rimolin, Cavalli-Sforza,
Rabinonitz and McKusick, 1968), although by analogy with Laron dwarfism
it is difficult to understand why plasma hGH responses to provocative
stimuli are similar to those found in normal adult controls (Rimoin, Merimee,
Rabinonitz, McKusick and Cavalli-Sforza, 1967).

During starvation, hGH secretion rises (Kipnis, Hertelendy and Machlin,
1969) and is probably an important homeostatic adaptation to malnutrition.
In most patients with anorexia nervosa plasma hGH levels are elevated,
often above 100 mu/l. Garfinkel (1975) has shown that the hGH elevation
in anorexia nervosa is directly related to the lowered energy intake.

Acute and chronic stress (both physical and psychological) are well known
to cause increased secretion of hGH (Reichlin, 1966). Abnormalities in
hGH secretion found in patients receiving drugs with effects on the hypothalamus are now well documented (see above) and biochemical abnormalities
in hypothalamic function probably explain the abnormal hGH release in
depression.

Obese subjects are usually reported to show sluggish hGH responses to
most stimuli, although if the stimulus given to an obese patient is adequate,
normal release of hGH is eventually observed (West, Owens, Sönksen,
Srivastava, Tompkins and Nabarro, 1975).

Bronchial tumours can secrete hGH ectopically (Steiner, Dahlbäck and
Waldenström, 1968; Rees and Ratcliffe, 1974). Acromegaly has been reported
in patients with bronchial carcinoid tumours (Dabek, 1974; Sönksen et al.,
1976a) but in the majority of such cases the hypersecretion is probably due
to the production of hGH releasing substances (possibly monoamines)
from the tumour rather than true ectopic secretion of hGH.

3. Tests for Human Growth Hormone Secretory Reserve

Of the many provocative tests which are available for investigation of the
ability to secrete hGH, insulin hypoglycaemia is the most reliable and
reproducible. It is usually the yardstick by which other tests have been
judged or used as an arbiter where other tests have given dubious answers.
It is essential however, that adequate hypoglycaemia is achieved (unequivocal
hypoglycaemic symptoms and/or blood glucose $< 1·5$ mmol/l). Intravenous
arginine can be used in adults but men require 48 hr pretreatment with
stilboestrol (Merimee, Rabinowitz, Riggs, Burgess, Rimoin and McKusick,

1967). Injection of glucagon has been used as a test of hGH and ACTH reserve but the side effects are unpleasant and normal subjects may fail to show a hGH response. Oral administration of "Bovril" has been used as an alternative to insulin hypoglycaemia in children (Jackson, Grant and Clayton, 1968). Oral L-dopa given to normal subjects has been found to be a reliable provocative test of hGH release comparing favourably with insulin hypoglycaemia and being more reliable than arginine, vasopressin and glucagon (Eddy, Gilliland, Ibarra, McMurry and Thompson, 1974).

In cases where the insulin test yields an ambiguous result the test should be repeated. If the result of the repeat test is still doubtful one of the alternative stimuli may be used. Under these circumstances a sleep study may be the most helpful alternative (Mace, Gotlin and Beck, 1972; Sönksen, 1974).

REFERENCES

Abrams, R. I., Parker, M. L., Blanco, S., Reichlin, S. and Daughaday, W. (1966). *Endocrinology*, **78**, 605.
Addison, G. M. and Hales, C. N. (1971). *Horm. Metab. Res.* **3**, 59.
Bazarre, T. L., Johanson, A. J., Huseman, C. A., Varma, M. M. and Blizzard, R. M. (1976). *In* "Growth Hormone and Related Peptides" (A. Pecile and E. E. Müller, eds), p. 261. Excerpta Medica, Amsterdam.
Beck, C. and Burger, H. G. (1972). *Cancer*, **30**, 75.
Bewley, T. A. and Li, C. L. (1975). *Adv. Enzymol.* **42**, 73.
Blackard, W. G., Boylen, C. T., Hinson, T. C. and Nelson, N. C. (1969). *Endocrinology*, **85**, 1180.
Blanco, S., Schalch, D. S. and Reichlin, S. (1966). *Fed. Proc.* **25**, 191.
Boyd, A. E., Lebovitz, H. E. and Pfeiffer, J. B. (1970). *New Engl. J. Med.* **283**, 1425.
Brazeau, P., Vale, W., Burgus, R., Ling, N., Butcher, M., Rivier, J. and Guillemin, R. (1973). *Science*, **179**, 77.
Brown, G. M. and Reichlin, S. (1972). *Psychosom. Med.* **34**, 45.
Brown, G. M., Schalch, D. S. and Reichlin, S. (1971). *Endocrinology*, **89**, 694.
Brown, J. B., Catt, K. J. and Martin, F. I. R. (1967). *J. Endocr.* **38**, 451.
Carr, D. and Friesen, H. G. (1976). *J. clin. Endocr.* **42**, 484.
Chung, M., Trakulrungsi, C., Somano, R., Evans, A. B. and Evans, E. S. (1977). *Acta endocr., Copenh.* **85**, 25.
Cornblath, M., Parker, M. L., Reisner, S. H., Forbes, A. E. and Daughaday, W. H. (1965). *J. clin. Endocr. Metab.* **25**, 209.
Cross, J. N., Glynne, A., Grossart, K. W. M., Jennett, W. B., Kellett, R. J., Lazarus, J. H., Thomson, J. A. and Webster, M. H. C. (1972). *Lancet*, **i**, 215.
Dabek, J. T. (1974). *J. clin. Endocr.* **28**, 329.
Daggett, P. R. and Nabarro, J. D. N. (1977). *Clin. Endocr.* **7**, 437.
Daughaday, W. H. (1977). *Clin. Endocr. Metab.* **6**, 117.
Daughaday, W. H., Herington, A. C. and Phillips, L. S. (1975). *A. Rev. Physiol.* **37**, 211.
Doniach, I. (1977). *Clin. Endocr. Metab.* **6**, 21.

Dunn, P. J., Donald, R. A. and Espiner, E. A. (1977). *Clin. Endocr.* 7, 273.

Eddy, R. L., Gilliland, P. F., Ibarra, J. D., McMurry, J. F. and Thompson, J. Q. (1974). *Am. J. Med.* **56**, 179.

Elde, R., Hökfelt, T., Johansson, O., Efendic, S. and Luft, R. (1976). *Neuroscience*, **2**, 759.

Ellis, M. J., Jones, R. H., Thomas, J. H., Geiger, R., Teetz, V. and Sönksen, P. H. (1977). *Diabetologia*, **13**, 257.

Etzrodt, H., Musch, K. A., Schleyer, M. and Pfeiffer, E. P. (1976). *J. clin. Endocr.* **42**, 1184.

Finkelstein, J., Roffwarg, H., Boyar, R., Kream, J. and Hellman, C. (1972). *J. clin. Endocr. Metab.* **35**, 665.

Franchimont, P. and Burger, H. (1975). "Human Growth Hormone and Gonadotrophins in Health and Disease." North-Holland/American Elsevier.

Frantz, A. G. and Holub, D. A. (1968). *Excerpta Med. Found. Int. Cong. Ser.* **157**, 18 (C. Gual, ed.).

Frasier, S. D., Aceto, Jr., T., Hayles, A. B. and Mikity, V. G. (1977). *J. clin. Endocr. Metab.* **44**, 22.

Friesen, H. and Carr, D. (1976). *In* "Hormones in Human Blood" (H. Antoniades, ed.), p. 349. Harvard University Press.

Friesen, H., Guyda, H. and Hardy, J. (1970). *J. clin. Endocr.* **31**, 611.

Frohman, L. A. and Bernardis, L. L. (1968). *Endocrinology*, **82**, 1125.

Garfinkel, P. E. (1975). *Arch. gen. Psychiat.* **32**, 739.

Garnier, P. E. and Job, J. C. (1977). *Acta endocr., Copenh.* **86**, 50.

Glick, S. M. and Goldsmith, S. (1968). *In* "Growth Hormone", p. 84. Excerpta Medica, Amsterdam.

Glick, S. M., Roth, J., Yalow, R. S. and Barson, S. A. (1965). *Rec. Prog. Horm. Res.* **21**, 241.

Gorden, P., Lesniak, M. A., Eastman, R., Hendricks, C. M. and Roth, J. (1976). *J. clin. Endocr. Metab.* **43**, 364.

Gorden, P., Lesniak, M. A., Hendricks, C. M., Roth, J., McGuffin, W. and Gavin, J. R. (1974). *Isr. J. med. Sci.* **10**, 1239.

Greenberg, P. B., Beck, C., Martin, T. J. and Burger, H. G. (1972). *Lancet*, **i**, 350.

Greenspan, F. S., Li, C. H., Simpson, M. E. and Evans, H. M. (1949). *Endocrinology*, **45**, 455.

Greenwood, F. C. (1967). *In* "Hormones in Blood" (C. H. Gray and A. L. Bacharach, eds), Vol. 1, p. 195. Academic Press, London and New York.

Greenwood, F. C., Hunter, W. M. and Glover, J. S. (1963). *Biochem. J.* **89**, 114.

Halasz, B., Schalch, D. S. and Gorski, R. A. (1971). *Endocrinology*, **89**, 198.

Hansen, Aa. P. (1970). *J. clin. Invest.* **47**, 1467.

Hansen, Aa. P. (1971). *J. clin. Invest.* **50**, 1806.

Harris, G. W. (1948). *J. Physiol.* **107**, 418.

Himsworth, R. L., Carmel, P. W. and Frantz, A. G. (1972). *Endocrinology*, **91**, 217.

Hoffenberg, R., Howell, A., Epstein, S., Pimstone, B. L., Fryklund, L., Hall, K., Schwalbe, S. and Rudd, B. T. (1977). *Clin. Endocr.* **6**, 443.

Holdaway, I. M., Frengley, P. A., Scott, D. J. and Ibbertson, H. K. (1978). *Clin. Endocr.* **8**, 45.

Hökfelt, T., Elfin, L. G., Elde, R., Schultzberg, M., Goldstein, M. and Luft, R. (1977). *Proc. natn. Acad. Sci., USA*, **74**, 3587.

Hoyte, K. and Martin, J. B. (1975). *J. clin. Endocr. Metab.* **41**, 656.

Hunter, W. M. and Greenwood, F. C. (1964). *Br. Med. J.* **1**, 804.

252 P. H. SÖNKSEN AND T. E. T. WEST

Hunter, W. M., McGurk, F. M., McLelland, J., Hibbert, D. J., Strong, J. A., Gillingham, F. J. and Harris, P. (1971). *Excerpta Med. Found. Int. Cong. Ser.* **236**, 168.
Imura, H., Nakai, Y. and Hoshimi, T. (1973). *J. clin. Endocr. Metab.* **36**, 204.
Imura, H., Yoshimi, T. and Ikekubo, K. (1971). *Endocr. jap.* **18**, 301.
Irie, M., Sakuma, M., Tsushima, T., Matsuyaki, F., Shizume, K. and Nakao, K. (1967a). *Proc. Soc. exp. Biol. Med.* **125**, 1314.
Irie, M., Sakuma, M., Tsushima, T., Shizume, C. and Nakao, K. (1967b). *Proc. Soc. exp. Biol. Med.* **126**, 708.
Jacobs, L., Sneid, D. S., Garland, J. T., Laron, L. and Daughaday, W. H. (1976). *J. clin. Endocr. Metab.* **42**, 403.
Jackson, D., Grant, D. B. and Clayton, B. E. (1968). *Lancet,* **ii**, 373.
Josimovich, J. B., Mintz, D. H. and Finster, J. L. (1967). *Endocrinology,* **81**, 1428.
Kansal, P. C., Buse, J., Talbert, O. R. and Base, M. G. (1972). *J. clin. Endocr. Metab.* **34**, 99.
Kaplan, S. L., Grumbach, M. M. and Shephard, T. H. (1972). *J. clin. Invest.* **51**, 3080.
Kipnis, D. M., Hertelendy, F. and Machlin, L. J. (1969). "Progress in Endocrinology", p. 601. Excerpta Medica, Amsterdam.
Kjellberg, R. N. and Kliman, B. (1975). "International Symposium on Growth Hormone and Related Peptides", p. 95. Ricorca Scientifica ed Educazione Permanente, University of Milan.
Korner, A. (1961). *In* "Hormones in Blood" (C. H. Gray and A. L. Bacharach, eds), 1st edition, p. 210. Academic Press, London and New York.
Krieger, D. T., Albin, J., Paget, S. and Glick, S. (1972). *Horm. Metab. Res.* **4**, 463.
Krieger, D. T. and Glick, S. M. (1972). *Am. J. Med.* **52**, 25.
Krieger, D. T. and Glick, S. (1974). *J. clin. Endocr. Metab.* **39**, 986.
Laron, Z., Pertzelan, A. and Karp, M. (1968). *Isr. J. med. Sci.* **4**, 883.
Lesniak, M. A., Gorden, P. and Roth, J. (1977). *J. clin. Endocr. Metab.* **44**, 838.
Lipman, R. L., Taylor, A. L., Schenk, S. and Mintz, D. H. (1972). *J. clin. Endocr. Metab.* **35**, 592.
Liuzzi, A., Chiodini, P. G., Botalla, L., Cremascoli, G. and Silvestrine, F. (1972). *J. clin. Endocr. Metab.* **35**, 941.
Liuzzi, A., Chiodini, P. G., Botalla, L., Cremascoli, G., Müller, E. E. and Silvestrini, F. (1974). *J. clin. Endocr. Metab.* **38**, 910.
Luft, R., Cerasi, E., Madison, L. L., von Euler, U.S., Della Casa, L. and Roovete, A. (1966). *Lancet,* **ii**, 254.
Luft, R., Efendic, S. and Hökfelt, T. (1978). *Diabetologia,* **14**, 1.
Mace, J., Gotlin, R. N. and Beck, P. (1972). *J. clin. Endocr. Metab.* **34**, 339.
Martin, J. B. (1972). *Endocrinology,* **91**, 107.
Martin, J. B. (1976). *In* "Frontiers in Neuroendocrinology", Vol. 4, p. 129. Raven Press, New York.
Martin, J. B., Reichlin, S. and Brown, G. M. (1977). "Clinical Neuroendocrinology" F. A. Davis, Philadelphia.
Martin, J. B. and Renaud, L. P. (1974). "Neuroendocrine Integration: Basic and Applied Aspects". Raven Press, New York.
Martin, J. B., Renaud, L. P. and Brazeau, P. (1975). *Lancet,* **ii**, 393.
Martini, L. and Besser, G. M. (1977). "Clinical Neuroendocrinology." Academic Press, London and New York.
McCormick, J. R., Sönksen, P. H., Soeldner, J. S. and Egdahl, R. (1969). *Surgery,* **66**, 175.
Merimee, T. J., Fineberg, S. E. and Tyson, J. E. (1969). *Metabolism,* **18**, 606.

Merimee, T. J., Rabinonitz, D., Riggs, L., Burgess, J. A., Rimoin, D. L. and McKusick, V. A. (1967). *New Engl. J. Med.*, **276**, 434.

Merimee, T. J., Rimon, D. L., Cavalli-Sforza, L. C., Rabinonitz, D. and McKusick, V. A. (1968). *Lancet*, **ii**, 194.

Miles, L. E. M. and Hales, C. N. (1968). *Lancet*, **ii**, 492.

Moore, W. V. (1978). *J. clin. Endocr. Metab.* **46**, 20.

Moore, W. V. and Jin, D. (1978). *J. clin. Endocr.* **46**, 374.

Morris, H. G., Jorgensen, J. R. and Jenkinson, S. A. (1968). *J. clin. Invest.* **47**, 427.

Müller, E. E. (1973). *Neuroendocrinology*, **11**, 338.

Najjar, S. S., Khachadurian, A. K., Ilbani, M. N. and Blizzard, R. M. (1971). *New Engl. J. Med.* **284**, 809.

Owens, D., Srivastava, M. C., Tompkins, C. V., Nabarro, J. D. N. and Sönksen, P. H. (1973). *Eur. J. clin. Invest.* **3**, 284.

Parlow, A. F. and Shome, B. (1976). *J. clin. Endocr. Metab.* **43**, 229.

Parsons, J. A. (1970). *J. Physiol., Lond.* **210**, 973.

Peake, G. T. (1973). "Frontiers in Neuroendocrinology", p. 173. Academic Press, New York and London.

Pecile, A. and Müller, E. E. (1976). "Growth Hormone and Related Peptides". Excepta Medica, Amsterdam.

Preece, M. A., Tanner, J. M., Whitehouse, R. H. and Cameron, N. (1976). *J. clin. Endocr. Metab.* **42**, 477.

Quabbe, H. J., Ramer, W. and Luyckx, A. S. (1977). *J. clin. Endocr. Metab.* **44**, 383.

Quabbe, H. J., Schilling, E. and Helge, H. (1966). *J. clin. Endocr.* **26**, 1173.

Rees, L. H. (1976). *Clin. Endocr.* **5**, 3635.

Rees, L. H. and Ratcliffe, J. G. (1974). *Clin. Endocr.* **3**, 263.

Reichlin, S. (1966). *New Engl. J. Med.* **275**, 600.

Reichlin, S. (1975). "Handbook of Physiology", Section 7: Endocrinology, Vol. 4, Part 2, p. 405. Williams and Wilkins, Baltimore.

Rimoin, D. L., Merimee, T. J. and McKusick, V. A. (1966). *Science*, **152**, 1635.

Rimoin, D. L., Merimee, T. J., Rabinonitz, D., McKusick, V. A. and Cavalli-Sforza, L. L. (1967). *Lancet*, **ii**, 523.

Roth, J. S., Glick, M., Yalow, R. S. and Berson, S. A. (1963). *Science*, **140**, 987.

Roth, J., Gorden, P. and Brace, K. (1970). *New Engl. J. Med.* **282**, 1385.

Roth, J., Kahn, R., Lesniak, M. A., Gorden, P., De Meyts, P., Megyesi, K., Neville Jr., D. M., Gavin III, J. R., Sol, A. H., Freychet, P., Goldfine, I. D., Bar, R. S. and Archer, J. A. (1975). *Rec. Prog. Horm. Res.* **31**, 95.

Schalch, D. S. and Kipnis, D. M. (1965). *J. clin. Invest.* **44**, 2010.

Schally, A. V., Arimura, A. and Kastin, A. J. (1973). *Science*, **179**, 341.

Skrabanek and Powell (1978). *Clin. Endocr.* **9**, 141.

Smythe, G. A. (1977). *Clin. Endocr.* **7**, 325.

Soman, V. and Goodman, A. D. (1977). *J. clin. Endocr.* **44**, 569.

Sönksen, P. H. (1974). *J. R. Coll. Physcns, Lond.* **8**, 220.

Sönksen, P. H. (1976a). *In* "Hormones in Human Blood" (H. Antioniades, ed.), p. 176. Harvard University Press.

Sönksen, P. H. (1976b). *In* "Hormones in Human Blood" (H. Antoniades, ed.), p. 121. Harvard University Press.

Sönksen, P. H., Ayres, A. B., Braimbridge, M., Corrin, B., Davies, D. R., Jeremiah, G. M., Oaten, S. W., Lowy, C. and West, T. E. T. (1976a). *Clin. Endocr.* **5**, 503.

Sönksen, P. H., Soeldner, J. S., Gleason, L. E. and Boden, G. (1973a). *Diabetologia*, **9**, 426.

Sönksen, P. H., Srivastava, M. C., Tompkins, C. V. and Nabarro, J. D. N. (1972). *Lancet*, **ii**, 155.

Sönksen, P. H., Tompkins, C. V., Srivastava, M. C. and Nabarro, J. D. N. (1973b). *Clin. Sci. mol. Med.* **45**, 633.

Sönksen, P. H., West, T. E. T., Lowy, C., Prunty, F. T. G., Scopes, J. V., Wilson, B. D. R. and Jeremiah, G. M. (1976b). *Br. Med. J.* **1**, 709.

Steiner, H., Dahlbäck, O. and Waldenström, J. (1968). *Lancet*, **i**, 783.

Summers, V. K., Hipkin, L. J., Diver, M. J. and Davis, J. C. (1975). *J. clin. Endocr. Metab.* **40**, 904.

Takahashi, Y., Kipnis, D. M. and Daughaday, W. H. (1968). *J. clin. Invest.* **47**, 2079.

Tanner, J. M., Whitehouse, R. H., Hughes, P. C. R. and Vince, F. P. (1971). *Arch. Dis. Child.* **46**, 745.

Taylor, A., Zinster, J. and Mintz, D. (1969). *J. clin. Invest.* **48**, 2349.

Thompson, R., Rodriquez, A., Kowarski, A., Migeon, C. J. and Blizzard, R. M. (1972). *J. clin. Endocr. Metab.* **35**, 334.

Thorngren, K. G. and Hansson, L. I. (1977). *Acta endocr.* **48**, 485.

Tunbridge, W. M. G., Marshall, J. C. and Burke, C. W. (1973). *Br. Med. J.* **1**, 153.

Varma, S. K., Sönksen, P. H., Varma, K., Soeldner, J. S., Selenkow, H. A. and Emerson Jr., K. (1971). *J. clin. Endocr.* **32**, 328.

Wallis, M. and Davies, R. V. (1976). *In* "Growth Hormone and Related Peptides" (A. Pecile and E. E. Müller, eds), p. 1. Excerpta Medica, Amsterdam.

Wass, J. A. H., Thorner, M. O., Morris, D. V., Rees, L. H., Mason, A. S., Jones, A. E. Besser, G. M. (1977). *Br. Med. J.* **1**, 875.

West, T. E. T., Owens, D., Sönksen, P. H., Srivastava, M. C., Tompkins, C. V. and Nabarro, J. D. N. (1975). *Clin. Endocr.* **4**, 573.

West, T. E. T. and Sönksen, P. H. (1977). *Clin. Endocr.* **7**, 283.

Wilber, J. F. and Porter, J. C. (1970). *Endocrinology*, **87**, 807.

Wilhelmi, A. E. (1973). *In* "Methods in Investigative and Diagnostic Endocrinology" (S. A. Berson and R. S. Yalow, eds), Part 2, p. 297. North Holland Publishing Company, Amsterdam.

Williams, R. A., Jacobs, H. S., Kurtz, A. B., Millar, J. G. B., Oakley, N. W., Spathis, G. S., Sulway, M. J. and Nabarro, J. D. N. (1974). *Quart. J. Med.* **XLIV**, 79.

Wright, A. D., Hartog, M., Palter, H., Tevaarwerk, G., Doyle, F. H., Arnot, R., Joplin, G. F. and Fraser, T. R. (1970). *Proc. R. Soc. Med.* **63**, 221.

Zimmerman, E. A., Defendini, R. and Frantz, A. G. (1974). *J. clin. Endocr. Metab.* **38**, 577.

V. Somatomedins

KERSTEN HALL and LINDA FRYKLUND

INTRODUCTION

The pituitary hormone somatotrophin (GH) *in vivo* promotes skeletal growth, both in mammals and man. GH in physiological doses has, on the contrary, scarcely any effect on cartilage *in vitro*. In 1957, Salmon and Daughaday, as a result of their *in vitro* studies on cartilage sulphation postulated that the growth promoting action of GH could be mediated by secondary factors found in serum. This GH-dependent sulphation factor activity was subsequently found to have a more widespread anabolic action and the term somatomedin (SM) was introduced (Daughaday, Hall, Raben, Salmon, Van den Brande and Van Wyk, 1972). This term was selected since "somato" implies a hormonal relationship to somatotrophin but "soma" can also indicate the target tissue. "Medin" indicates the mediatory role. The anabolic hormone insulin, is also to some extent GH-regulated but was not included in the definition since it has scarcely any *in vitro* effect on cartilage.

With different isolation procedures two somatomedins active on cartilage have been isolated. Somatomedin A (SM-A) is a neutral polypeptide, mw 7000, whereas somatomedin C (SM-C) is basic (Hall, 1972; Fryklund, Uthne and Sievertsson, 1974a; Van Wyk, Underwood, Baseman, Hintz, Clemmons and Marshall, 1975; Fryklund, Skottner and Hall, 1978).

An anabolic hormone, in the same way as insulin, would be expected to stimulate glucose uptake in the target tissue, and SM-A was also shown to enhance the uptake and conversion of ^{14}C-glucose into ^{14}CO$_2$ in rat adipose tissue (Hall and Uthne, 1971). This discovery, with the knowledge that human serum contains more insulin-like activity (ILA) than can be attributed to its insulin content, suggests a relationship between somatomedins and ILA. The major part of ILA, immunologically different from insulin, was called non-suppressible insulin-like activity (NSILA) (Froesch, Bürgi, Ramseier, Bally and Labhart, 1963). NSILA purified from acidified Cohn fraction III of human serum was also shown to stimulate sulphate uptake in rat and chick cartilage (Humbel, Bünzli, Mülly, Oelz, Froesch and Ritschard, 1971; Zingg and Froesch, 1973; Froesch, Schlumpf, Heimann, Zapf, Humbel and Ritschard, 1975a). In addition, NSILA has been shown to be least partly GH-dependent (Schlumpf, Heimann, Zapf and Froesch, 1976) and therefore fulfills the criteria for a SM. However, Rinderknecht and Humbel (1976a, b) who isolated two homologous NSILA polypeptides termed them insulin-like growth factors 1 and 2 (IGF-1 and IGF-2).*

Purified SM and NSILA stimulate the incorporation of thymidine into DNA and the multiplication of chick fibroblasts (Froesch, Zapf, Meuli, Mäder, Waldvogel, Kaufmann and Morell, 1975b). This biological activity thereby associates these substances with another polypeptide, called multiplication-stimulating activity (MSA). MSA was partially purified from calf plasma and rat liver conditioned (see below) medium (Dulak and Temin, 1973a, b) and when isolated has been shown to have an insulin-like effect *in vitro* (Rechler, Podskalny and Nissley, 1976; Moses, Rechler and Nissley, 1977).

SM-A, SM-C, IGF-1, and IGF-2 purified from human serum and MSA purified from rat liver conditioned medium have many target organs in common. All have insulin-like action in rat adipose tissue and rat muscle, stimulate the synthesis of proteoglycans in cartilage and stimulate multiplication and DNA synthesis in human skin fibroblasts, and embryonic chick fibroblasts (Hall and Uthne, 1971; Werner, Hall and Löw, 1974; Underwood,

---

* NSILA in the text refers to an impure preparation, IGF to the pure characterised peptides.

Hintz, Voina and Van Wyk, 1972; Van Wyk *et al.*, 1975; Rechler, Fryklund, Nissley, Hall, Podskalny, Skottner and Moses, 1978) (Table 1). This family of insulin-like polypeptides appears to have a more widespread and potent action on tissues other than those classically associated with insulin.

Table 1

Somatomedin-like peptides.

Peptide	Bioassay	Source
Somatomedin A	$^{35}SO_4$ uptake into embryonic chick cartilage	human plasma
Somatomedin C	$^{35}SO_4$ and ^3H-thymidine uptake into rat cartilage	human plasma
IGF I (insulin-like growth factor)	^{14}C-glucose uptake into rat epididymal fat tissue	human plasma
IGF II	^{14}C-glucose uptake into rat epididymal fat tissue	human plasma
MSA (multiplication stimulating activity)	^3H-thymidine uptake into DNA of embryonic chick fibroblasts	calf plasma, rat liver, cell conditioned media
NSILP (non-suppressible insulin-like protein)	^{14}C-glucose uptake into rat epididymal fat tissue	human plasma

Somatomedin B (SM-B) purified from human plasma is also a GH-dependent factor, but it has no insulin action in adipose tissue and does not stimulate sulphate uptake. This polypeptide will be discussed separately (Fryklund, Uthne, Sievertsson and Westermark, 1974b; Westermark, Wasteson and Uthne, 1975; Fryklund and Sievertsson, 1978).

A. ISOLATION AND CHEMICAL PROPERTIES

With the exception of MSA, the somatomedin-like peptides have been isolated from human plasma. The large-scale method has involved a Cohn fraction as starting material with subsequent acid-ethanol extraction before a separation procedure involving gel filtration, ion exchange and electrophoresis. Although the original Cohn fraction has large amounts of somatomedin-like activity, the unmanageable nature of this material results in large losses which have to date only been partly avoided. The starting material for SM-A and SM-C was Cohn Fraction IV from Kabi (Fryklund, Skottner, Sievertsson and Hall, 1975; Van Wyk *et al.*, 1975). This fraction is first homogenised with water, acidified and then the pH raised before acetone precipitation. Recently the procedure for SM-A has been revised, since the acetone precipitation was found to be very inefficient. This acetone step is now omitted, and an ion-exchange step substituted.

Rinderknecht and Humbel (1976a, b) started from an acetone powder derived from Cohn Fraction III and instead extracted with 0·5 M acetic acid before gel filtration in the same medium. Subsequent steps were preparative polyacrylamide electrophoresis and SE-Sephadex C-25 gel filtration at 55°. Two almost identical and homologous peptides IGF-1 and IGF-2 have been isolated and structurally identified; the mw is 7600 and isoelectric point 8·2 (for IGF-1) (Rinderknecht and Humbel, 1976a, b; Humbel and Rinderknecht, 1978). There is a close sequence homology with insulin but certain invariable amino acids of insulin are not present in the N-terminal region of IGF (Fig. 1). The two regions homologous to the A and B-chains of insulin are linked by a connecting peptide, which is not however homologous in sequence to the C-peptide of proinsulin. The A-chain counterpart also has additional amino acids at the C terminus. The 3-dimensional structure has been proposed to be similar but not identical to insulin and also proinsulin (Blundell, Bedarker, Rinderknecht and Humbel, 1978). IGF-1 and -2, unlike insulin, are single chain peptides. These authors suggest a reason why IGF does not cross-react with insulin antibodies although close structural homology is found to the antibody binding region of insulin which is composed of the C-terminal part of the B-chain. The IGF "C" peptide can lie on the surface and thereby partly cover this region. The extra sequence on the A-chain also appears to mask this area. A protein, non-suppressible insulin-like protein (NSILP) with NSILA activity mw 100,000, has been isolated by Poffenbarger (1975). This is apparently not convertable into IGF-1 or -2 (Poffenbarger, 1978).

SM-A has been isolated by gel filtration on Sephadex G-50 after formic acid extraction of the acid-ethanol extract (Hall, 1972; Uthne, 1973). Subsequent steps involve electrophoresis on cellulose at 2 or 3 different pH values and finally by Sephadex G-50 gel filtration (Fryklund et al., 1974a, 1975, 1978). The amino acid composition is shown for SM-A and IGF-1 (Table 2). This indicates that the substances are not fragments of GH, nor are they apparently closely related, since there are several differences in the amino acid composition, notably the cysteine and histidine content. SM-C is purified after the first Sephadex G-50 by isoelectric focusing, SP-Sephadex and preparative gel electrophoresis (Van Wyk et al., 1975). SM-C is more basic than SM-A, perhaps more like IGF-1 or -2 but no chemical data for SM-C are yet available, so no comparison can be made (Van Wyk, Furlanetto, Underwood, d'Ercole and Decedie, 1976).

MSA has been purified from medium conditioned by a cloned line of Buffalo rat liver cells, BRL 3a2, by chromatography on Dowex 50, gel filtration on Sephadex G-50 followed by preparative polyacrylamide

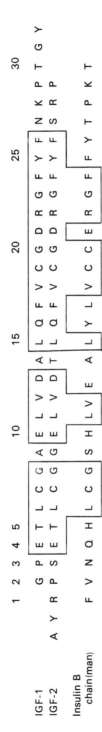

Fig. 1. Sequence comparison between insulin and IGF (Rinderknecht and Humbel, 1976a, b). The amino acid residues are represented by the letters recommended by the IUPAC–IUB Commission on Biochemical Nomenclature (1968) *J. biol. Chem.* **243**, 3557–3559.

Table 2

Amino acid compositions of somatomedin A and IGF-I (Humbel *et al.*, 1978).

	SM-A	IGF
Asp	5	5
Thr	3	3
Ser	4	5
Glu	10	6
Pro	4	5
Gly	4	7
Ala	5	6
Cys	1	6
Val	3	3
Met	1	1
Ile	1	1
Leu	5	6
Tyr	1	3
Phe	1	4
His	2	—
Lys	5	3
Arg	4	6
TOTAL	59	70

electrophoresis (Nissley, Passamani and Short, 1976). The mw is approximately 7500 and the peptide is somewhat basic. The amino acid composition (Moses, unpublished data) indicates that it is different from IGF and SM-A.

B. BIOLOGICAL ACTIVITY *IN VITRO*

Originally the somatomedin-like peptides were identified by different bioassays (Table 1), sulphate uptake into chick and rat cartilage (SM-A and SM-C, respectively) (Hall, 1970; Van Wyk, Hall, Van den Brande, Weaver, Uthne, Hintz, Harrison and Mathewson, 1972), conversion of ^{14}C-glucose to ^{14}C-CO_2 (NSILA) (Froesch *et al.*, 1963) and thymidine incorporation into embryonic chick fibroblasts (Rechler *et al.*, 1976) for MSA. However, it has been shown subsequently that all of these substances are active in all of the respective bioassays which were at first presumed specific, although potency differences occur.

The biological effects which have been studied *in vitro* are either related to effects on fat and carbohydrate metabolism or growth-promoting effects including protein synthesis. The effects on rat adipose tissue, which is one of the target organs for insulin, have been extensively studied by Froesch *et al.* (1975b). An insulin-like spectrum of activity was observed, both with respect to the conversion of ^{14}C-glucose to CO_2 and its incorporation into fat as well as the inhibitory effect on glycerol release. The potency on a molar basis, however, in comparison with insulin is approximately 50 fold less. IGF-2 is more potent than both IGF-1 and SM-A (Zapf, Schoenle and Froesch, 1978). In diaphragm muscle both IGF and SM-A, like insulin, stimulate amino acid uptake (Salmon and DuVall, 1970; Uthne, Reagan, Gimpel and Kostyo, 1974) but the potency difference is reduced, and in heart muscle even reversed where IGF is even more potent than insulin (Meuli and Froesch, 1975). So far no results are available from liver of effects on glycolysis and glycogenesis, but SM-A has an inhibitory effect on glucagon-stimulated cAMP production (Hall, Fryklund, Löw, Skottner and Zederman, 1978).

Multiplication-stimulating effects have been studied in growing tissues and cells, such as embryonic chick fibroblasts, human skin fibroblasts, and rat myoblasts (Morell and Froesch, 1973; Rechler, Nissley, Podskalny, Moses and Fryklund, 1977; Florini, Nicholson and Dulak, 1977; Rechler *et al.*, 1978). In both fibroblast systems, the SM-peptides are equipotent (Rechler *et al.*, 1978, unpublished) with insulin. However, the active concentration range for insulin in these systems is many times greater than the normal physiological levels, whereas the somatomedin-like peptides are active within the physiological range.

The effects on thymidine incorporation into DNA have been studied in rat cartilage (Daughaday and Reeder, 1966; Van Wyk *et al.*, 1972, 1976), in fibroblasts (Rechler *et al.*, 1976, 1977), and embryonic brain cells (Sara, Hall, Wetterberg, Fryklund, Wahlund, Sjögren and Skottner, 1978). While insulin is not active on cartilage or brain cells, the SM peptides have a stimulatory effect.

Gibson, Ben-Porath, Doller and Segen (1978) have examined protein synthesis in embryonic chick cartilage and found that SM-A and IGF were equipotent whereas MSA was considerably less active, the relative potency effects were the same for sulphation; insulin was again without effect. According to Zapf *et al.* (1978) IGF-1 and IGF-2 can be distinguished in rat cartilage, IGF-1 like SM-A is considerably more effective at lower doses.

C. METHODS OF DETERMINATION

The somatomedins have been determined by bioassay and more recently by radioligandassay.

1. Bioassay

Most bioassays for somatomedins are based on the incorporation of labelled sulphate into cartilage. Sulphation is the last step in the synthesis of proteoglycans and can be used as an index of protein synthesis in cartilage in a fully supplemented system. The optimal concentrations of glucose and amino acids, especially glutamine and serine, have been thoroughly investigated (Salmon and Daughaday, 1958; Salmon, 1960; Koumans and Daughaday, 1963; Hall, 1970). In order to evaluate the stimulatory effects of biological fluids on the uptake of labelled sulphate it is also necessary to correct for the sulphate in the medium. Although "sulphation activity" assays are used widely for SM activity in serum samples, the need for sulphate determination has not always been recognised (Phillips, Pennisi, Belosky, Uittenbogaart, Ettenger, Malekzadeh and Fine, 1978).

The original "sulphation factor" assay utilised costal cartilage from hypophysectomised rats (Salmon et al., 1957). A linear dose-response curve was found between the uptake of sulphate and the logarithm of the concentrations of serum. The precision was improved by a 4-point design of the assay (Almqvist, 1961; Van den Brande, Van Wyk, Weaver and Mayberry, 1971). In order either to improve the precision of the assay or to simplify the procedure a variety of cartilage assays have been developed using costal cartilage from fasted rats, embryonic chick pelves, costal cartilage from pigs and rabbits (Yde, 1968; Hall, 1970; Van den Brande and Du Caju, 1974; Bala, Hankins and Smith, 1975). In general, cartilage from younger or hypophysectomised animals is more sensitive than from older intact animals (Heins, Garland and Daughaday, 1970; Beaton, 1976).

Cartilage from different mammals and chick responds to the GH-dependent activity present in human serum. However, a species difference is observed with respect to the sensitivity to thyroid and steroid hormones. Cortisol and its analogues in high concentrations have a direct inhibitory effect on sulphate uptake, but it is only in pig cartilage that physiological amounts of cortisol influence the results of somatomedin activity in serum samples (Keret, Schimpff and Girard, 1976; Van den Brande and van Buul, 1978). In general, oestrogens inhibit sulphate uptake but the effect of androgens has not been fully elucidated. Embryonic chick cartilage responds to both thyroxine and triiodothyronine (Audhya and Gibson, 1975; Gibson et al., 1978).

NSILA activity on rat epididymal adipose tissue and isolated fat cells (Froesch et al., 1963; Froesch, Bürgi, Müller, Humbel, Jakob and Labhart, 1967) has been determined in the presence of an excess of insulin antibodies, where insulin is used for the standard curve. Quantitative determinations in serum are of limited value because of interference from plasma proteins.

NSILA therefore is usually determined in serum after acidification and gel filtration (Schlumpf et al., 1976). Although it has not been investigated completely it seems that IGF-2 is more effective than SM-A and IGF-1 on adipose tissue, while the converse is true for cartilage (Zapf et al., 1978).

2. Radioreceptor Assay

Once the purified peptides were available radioreceptor assays (RRA) were developed. A variety of tissues from humans, monkeys and rats have specific binding sites for SM and IGF and can be used as matrix in the RRA (Hintz, Clemmons, Underwood and Van Wyk, 1972; Takano, Hall, Fryklund and Sievertsson, 1976a; Thorsson and Hintz, 1977). Until eventual species differences are excluded for the SM binding sites, it is preferable to use a human tissue for measuring SM levels in human serum. Placental tissue is readily available and is rich in binding sites for SM-C as well as SM-A and particulate placental membranes have been used in the RRA for these peptides (Marshall, Underwood, Voina, Foushee and Van Wyk, 1974; Hall, Takano and Fryklund, 1974). As expected, NSILA can also be used as the labelled peptide in the placental RRA (Posner, Guydal and Omori, 1977). For the RRA of IGF, Zapf and co-workers used chick embryo fibroblasts whereas Megyesi utilised rat liver membranes, with either MSA or NSILA as the labelled peptide (Megyesi, Kahn, Roth, Froesch, Humbel, Zapf and Neville, 1974a; Megyesi, Kahn, Roth, Neville, Nissley, Humbel and Froesch, 1975; Zapf, Mäder, Waldvogel, Schalch and Froesch, 1975a).

The RRA based on placental membranes allows determinations of SM levels directly in serum samples, whereas it is necessary to dissociate the SM from their carrier proteins before determination in rat liver membrane assays. The latter method entails dissociation and purification by gel chromatography before the samples can be assayed. This difference is probably due to a difference in affinity between the peptides and the binding sites in the two tissues. The high affinity constant between placental membranes and SM-A was calculated to be 2.5×10^8 l/mol.

The procedure for the SM-A RRA is as follows (Takano, Hall, Ritzén, Iselius, and Sievertsson, 1976b). Fresh or frozen human placenta is homogenized in sucrose and purified by stepwise ultracentrifugations. About 5–10 μg of membrane protein are obtained from each gram of tissue. The assays are carried out in siliconised glass tubes or albuminised plastic tubes and the incubation buffer is 0·05 M Tris-HCl, pH 7·4, containing 1% of human albumin. Serum or standard, labelled hormone, and human placental membrane (100–150 μg protein) are incubated for 16 hr at $+4°$, followed by centrifugation at 6000 g for 15 min. Different techniques have been used for iodination such as the lactoperoxidase method for SM-A and chloramine T method for the other peptides. Attempts to achieve high specific activity result in peptide destruction and it is necessary to purify the labelled peptide. SM-A was purified on CMC cellulose on a pH gradient and SM-C by ion exchange resin, or on a SM-C antibody column (Hall, Luft, Takano and Fryklund, 1976; Van Wyk et al., 1976). The affinity of a peptide

Table 3

Specificity studies of the placental somatomedin A binding sites.

Hormone	Concentration (ng/ml)	% of initial binding
Competitive		
Somatomedin A, 1200 u/mg	30	50
Somatomedin C	90	50
IGF-1	35	50
Rat MSA	35	50
Porcine insulin	10×10^3	50
Porcine proinsulin	25×10^3	50
Nerve growth factor	100×10^3	50
Porcine calcitonin	250×10^3	50
Non-competitive		
Somatostatin	3×10^3	100
Somatomedin B	10×10^3	100
Fibroblast growth factor	11×10^3	100
hGH	14×10^3	100
Bovine ACTH	700×10^3	100

for a receptor can also be used for purifying labelled preparations. With a good labelled peptide the specific and unspecific binding are 30% and 3% respectively, of total radioactivity.

Neither the RRA for SM-A nor that for SM-C is specific for the respective peptide. In the SM-A RRA, both IGF-1 and MSA are equipotent with SM-A, and SM-C cross-reacts (Takano, 1975; Rechler et al., 1977, 1978). SM-A cross-reacts in the SM-C RRA and it is probable that all of these peptides bind to the same receptor. Insulin and calcitonin in high doses can compete with SM-A for the placental membrane binding sites but the potency is 1000–20,000 times lower respectively. This cross-reaction is therefore of no importance when determining SM levels in serum samples. Structurally unrelated polypeptides such as GH, SM-B, epidermal growth factor (EGF), and nerve growth factor (NGF) do not cross-react (Table 3).

Serum in increasing doses between 0·5 μl and 40 μl gives a dose-response curve which is superimposable on that for the pure polypeptide (Fig. 2). 100% recovery of pure polypeptide is found after addition to the serum samples. However, parallelism does not ensure that SM in serum is quantitatively measured. After dissociation of SM by acidification from the binding proteins in acromegalic serum more than 100% activity is found in the

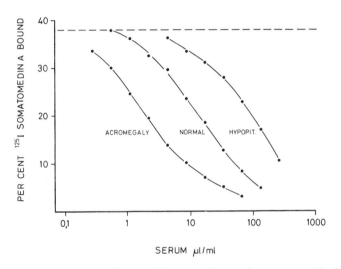

Fig. 2. Radioreceptor assay for SM-A with human placental membrane. Displacement curves with different sera are shown.

low molecular weight fraction. The results, the precision and the reproducibility obtained with the RRA for SM-A and SM-C are similar. One difference has been observed, however; both serum and plasma samples can be used for SM-C determination whereas only serum samples can be used for SM-A determination. For some unexplained reason plasma or heparin addition to serum causes a spurious increase in the measured levels of SM-A.

In the liver membrane RRA for NSILA, either labelled NSILA and MSA were used (Megyesi *et al.*, 1974a, 1975). These authors assume that NSILA and MSA bind to the same receptor. Rechler *et al.* (1978) who also used the Neveille rat liver membrane preparation, found that of the SM peptides only labelled IGF-2 and MSA will bind, so presumably Megyesi and co-workers are measuring preferentially IGF-2 rather than the other SM-like peptides in human serum. In the fibroblast RRA, Zapf *et al.* (1975a) used cultured chick embryo fibroblasts. The apparent intrinsic association constant for binding of IGF to intact cells is 10^9 mol/l. IGF-1 and IGF-2 were equipotent in displacing the label in this system, and insulin 100 fold less effective. Rechler *et al.* (1978) using a different assay system for chick embryo fibroblasts found no difference between insulin and the SM-peptides.

3. Protein Binding Assay

A protein binding assay has been developed for NSILA (Zapf, Kaufmann, Eigenmann and Froesch, 1977). The binding protein was obtained after gel filtration in acetic acid of an acetone powder of human serum. The fraction which elutes as albumin is pooled, and dialysed against phosphate buffer. An aliquot of this acidified protein fraction is incubated together with labelled NSILA and the sample or standard. After 2 hr of incubation at room temperature the free and bound forms are separated with charcoal. IGF-2 is in fact twice as effective in displacing the labelled peptide. NSILA levels in serum are measured after acidification and gel chromatography to isolate the low molecular weight fraction.

4. Radioimmunoassay

Radioimmunoassays (RIA) have recently been developed for the insulin-like somatomedins, SM-A, SM-C, MSA, NSILA, and NSILP (Reber and Liske, 1976; Poffenbarger and Boully, 1976; Furlanetto, Underwood, Van Wyk and D'Ercole, 1977; Hall, Brant, Enberg and Fryklund, 1979; Moses, Nissley, Rechler and Short, 1978). Antibodies were raised in rabbits against all of these peptides, with the exception of SM-A, where Leghorn hens were used. MSA, SM-A and NSILA antibodies were of low titre, and were used in a final dilution of less than 1:2000. SM-C antibodies were used in a dilution of 1:10,000. The calculated affinity constants between SM-A and its antibodies was 1×10^9 l/mol and for SM-C, $4·6 \times 10^{10}$ l/mol. Different techniques were used for separating bound and free polypeptides. The double antibody technique has been used, except for SM-A RIA where Sepharose-bound antibodies were used. The assays for SM-A and SM-C were modified to allow direct determination on serum samples. Cross-reaction has so far only been studied with SM-A RIA. IGF-1 and SM-C cross-reacted in this assay but IGF-2 was considerably less potent and MSA showed no cross-reaction at all. The calculated amount of immunoreactive SM-A in normal serum is 1 µg SM-like peptides/ml. The SM-C RIA was apparently more specific, since SM-A, the only peptide tested, showed very low activity. The calculated level of SM-C was about 200 ng/ml. Reber *et al.*

(1976) used an antigen which was about 90% pure and found only 4 ng NSILA/mg in normal sera. Since acidification leads to a considerable increase in the values, it is doubtful whether they are measuring total amounts. The RIA for MSA is also apparently very specific since IGF-1, -2 and SM-A hardly cross-react; this could however reflect a species variation. The calculated level in normal rat serum is approximately 100 ng/ml; rat serum is considerably more potent than human serum in both SM-A and SM-C RIA.

D. CIRCULATING FORMS

When plasma or serum is fractioned by gel chromatography or ultrafiltration, the somatomedin activity has an apparent molecular weight above 50,000 (Koumans and Daughaday, 1963; Van Wyk, Hall and Weaver, 1969; Hall, 1972; Bala, Blakeley and Smith, 1976). In dissociating conditions, however, such as low pH, most of the biological activity appears in the low molecular weight range (Hall, 1972), suggesting that some form of non-covalent complex is present in serum.

The existence of a specific carrier-protein became more apparent when the iodinated peptides could be used (Kaufmann, Zapf, Toretti and Froesch, 1977; Hintz and Liu, 1977). The gel chromatography pattern of a mixture containing human serum and labelled NSILA or SM-A indicates that at least two forms are present, one eluting just after globulins (Form I), the other as albumin (Form II) (Zapf, Waldvogel and Froesch 1975b). The same pattern was confirmed by the measurements of biological activity of the respective fractions. Moreover, when comparing serum from hypopituitary patients with normal and acromegalic subjects it was obvious that Form I is not present in serum from untreated patients with GH deficiency (Fryklund et al., 1978). A GH-dependence of Form I carrier is observed also in rat serum when labelled MSA is used (Moses, Nissley, Cohen and Rechler, 1976). Nothing is known about the affinity of the different SM-like peptides to these two different forms. Zapf et al. (1978), using the acidified high molecular weight serum fraction in a specific binding assay have shown that there are affinity differences between IGF-1, -2, SM-A and MSA; IGF-2 being most potent. The issue is further confused since Fryklund et al. (1978) found when isolating carrier protein Form I that an apparent molecular weight decrease to that of Form II occurred after acidification. The two forms, however, differ by charge so presumably a simple dissociation of a dimer to monomer is not involved. Another variant of the high molecular weight forms which has recently been confirmed is NSILP.

NSILP is a protein, mw 80,000, consisting of two dissimilar chains cross-linked by disulphide bonds (Poffenbarger, 1978). This was originally assumed to be undissociated carrier protein but recently two other groups have confirmed that there is a non-acid or -urea dissociable form present in plasma corresponding to about 10% (Zapf and Froesch, 1978; Enberg, Fryklund and Hall, 1978; Hall et al., 1978a, b). Whether NSILP represents a precursor which also has insulin-like activity or some other form is not yet clear. Sulphation activity has not been found.

Less than 1% of the SM in serum is present in the free form. Whether this represents the biologically active fraction or whether variations in affinity to the binding protein or to tissue receptors determine the biological effect is not known for different tissues.

E. BLOOD LEVELS

1. Normal Levels

Comparison between absolute values from different laboratories is difficult since there is no universal reference serum. The activity in 1 ml pooled serum is arbitrarily defined as 1 unit. For example the mean level of SM-A in healthy adult subjects was 1·07 according to Hall et al. (1975a, b, 1976) whereas Van Wyk et al. (1975), found it to be 1·5–2·0 u/ml. Insulin has been used as a reference material in the bioassay for NSILA.

Besides being subjected to hormonal influences and changes in pathological conditions SM activity varies with the age of the individual. The change is gradual with age; it is low at birth and increases progressively until adult levels are reached at age six (Van den Brande, van Buul, Heinrich, van Roon, Zurcher and van Steirtegen, 1975; Van den Brande et al., 1978). Since it has been demonstrated in both rats and rabbits, that cartilage sensitivity is much greater in the young organism, it is conceivable that the low levels in small children are sufficient for supporting their high growth rate.

The age dependency of SM levels is confirmed by the radioligand assays. SM levels are found by both SM-A and SM-C RRA to be 50% of adult values at birth with a rise until puberty (Hall et al., 1976; D'Ercole, Underwood and Van Wyk, 1977). In adults a decline is observed after the age of 40 (Takano, Hall, Kastrup, Hizuka, Shizume, Kawai, Akimoto, Takuma and Sugina, 1978a). No significant diurnal variation was observed using the RRA for SM-A although there was a tendency to increase slightly in the morning. This is in contrast to the pig cartilage assay, where higher levels were observed in the afternoon than in the morning. Because their assay is sensitive to cortisol it probably reflects the diurnal variation of cortisol (Van den Brande *et al.*, 1978).

Since RIA is a recent development, insufficient data are available. However, preliminary data indicate that immunoreactive SM-A and SM-C follow the same age dependent pattern as found with RRA (Furlanetto *et al.*, 1977; Hall *et al.*, 1978a).

Nutrition is obviously involved in the maintenance of normal levels since a decrease is seen after a three day fast (Takano, Hizuka, Kawai and Shizume, 1978b). This change is faster and more severe in rats. The rate of disappearance is the same as that observed after hypophysectomy (Takano *et al.*, 1978a). Presumably the carrier proteins are involved in the maintenance of serum/plasma levels.

2. Growth Hormone Dependence

The different bioassays clearly show the GH dependency of SM. An invariable elevation is seen in acromegaly, and a depression in patients with growth hormone deficiency (Daughaday, 1971; Hall, Takano, Fryklund and Sievertsson, 1975b; Van Wyk and Underwood, 1975). After administration of GH to children with GH deficiency a lapse of 2–3 hr occurs before any increase in levels of SM is detectable (Daughaday, Laron, Pertzelan and Heins, 1969; Hall, 1971). During long-term treatment with GH, a correlation was found between the SM level and the growth rate (Hall and Olin, 1972).

When NSILA in extracted serum is measured by the fat pad bioassay a similar significant difference was also found between levels in acromegaly and GH deficiency (Schlumpf *et al.*, 1976; Franklin, Rennie, Burger and Cameron, 1976). A good correlation is observed between the values determined in the bioassay and the protein-binding assays, although the latter values are 2-fold higher (Zapf, *et al.*, 1977).

Both the RRA for SM-A and SM-C show that the mean levels of SM are significantly higher in patients with acromegaly than in healthy controls; and significantly lower patients with GH deficiency (Marshall *et al.*, 1974; Hall *et al.*, 1974, 1976; Takano *et al.*, 1976b). The half life after successful hypophysectomy in acromegalic patients was about 24 hr (Takano, 1975). After a single intramuscular injection of GH to children with GH deficiency a maximum level of SM-A is obtained after 24 hr, declining to the basal level after 48 hr (Takano, Hizuku, Shizume and Hall, 1977a). The magnitude of the increase was correlated to the GH dose. A discrepancy has been reported using the rat liver membrane RRA (Megyesi, Gorden and Kahn, 1977). No difference was observed between healthy individuals and patients with acromegaly. It is not however completely clear whether MSA or a partially pure NSILA was in fact used as label.

K

Both immunoreactive SM-A and SM-C show a GH-dependency in the respective RIA. A potency ratio of 30 between levels in acromegaly and GH-deficiency was found with both methods, indicating that SM-A and SM-C are GH-dependent (Furlanetto et al., 1977; Hall et al., 1979). The difference is however more pronounced than that found earlier by RRA. A possible explanation for this finding is the fact that the SM-A RIA is relatively insensitive to IGF-2 and SM-C RIA is considered specific. This would seem to indicate that SM-A and IGF-1 as well as SM-C are GH-dependent.

3. Other Disorders

The lowest levels of SM-like peptides, by SM-A RRA, cartilage bioassay and protein binding assay for NSILA are found in Laron dwarfs (Daughaday et al., 1969; Takano et al., 1976b; Zapf et al., 1977). These patients have the same phenotype as GH-deficient patients, but plasma GH levels are high, and these patients do not respond to exogenous GH therapy (Laron, Pertzelan, Karp and Daughaday, 1971). The basic failure in this disease is assumed to be a defective generation of SM. A defective SM generation has also been suggested in liver diseases, because decreased levels of SM activity as well as SM-A has been found in patients with liver cirrhosis (Marek, Schullerová, and Schreiberová, 1976; Schimpff, Donnadieu, Glasinoiv, Warnet and Girard, 1976; Takano, Hizuka, Shizume, Hayashi, Motoika and Obata, 1977b).

Normal levels of SM activity have been demonstrated in serum from African pygmies (Daughaday et al., 1969). In Turner's syndrome the growth retardation is accompanied by normal levels of SM activity and this finding has been confirmed with the RRA (Daughaday and Parker, 1963; Almqvist, Lindsten and Lindell, 1963; Takano et al., 1976b). Therefore, the most likely explanation of the retarded skeletal growth in Turner's syndrome is resistance to SM in the epiphyseal growth plate. Normal levels of SM-A RRA were also found in short children with age-related skeletal age and normal GH production (Takano, Shizume, Hizuka, Kawai, Fryklund and Hall, 1978b). In tall girls with a body height above + 3 s.d.m. we have observed a tendency for elevated levels of SM-A by RRA. During oestrogen therapy these levels decreased significantly which is in accordance with earlier results, indicating a decrease of SM activity (Wiedemann and Schwartz, 1972). Cortisol, which depresses the levels of SM activity does not affect the SM-A levels determined by RRA.

The levels of SM are not changed in human diabetes mellitus which is in contrast to the decreased levels of NSILA found in dogs after induced diabetes

(Eigenmann, Becker, Kammermann, Leemann, Heimann, Zapf and Froesch, 1977).

In general there is a good agreement between the levels of SM activity by bioassay and the levels obtained by RRA. However, discrepancies exist. In uremia, low levels are reported (Saenger, Wiedemann, Schwartz, Korth-Schutz, Lewy, Riggo, Rurin, Stenzel and New, 1974; Schwalbe, Betts, Rayner and Rudd, 1977) but high levels are found with the SM-A RRA (Watson, Spencer, Uthne, Piel and Holliday, 1977; Takano et al., 1976b, 1979).

The apparently low levels of SM activity found in uremic plasma can partly be ascribed to an increased sulphate concentration in this condition. Phillips et al (1978) found normal values after correcting for this. However, since RRA in fact indicates values above normal it is probable that some type of inhibitor is present. Inhibitors also appear to be formed in malnutrition, although it is not yet clear whether there is an absolute change in SM levels. It is important to remember that biological systems measure the net effect of both stimulators and inhibitors. A decrease can therefore be a result of either a decrease in SM or an increase in inhibitors.

A few groups of tumour patients have been investigated. Increased levels of SM-A by RRA were found in a few patients with osteosarcoma (Hall et al., 1976). Tumour patients with hypoglycemia have been investigated and found to have high levels of NSILA-like peptides when measured by RRA on rat liver membrane (Megyesi, Kahn, Roth and Gorden, 1974b) which has not been confirmed by others. This assay apparently measures preferentially IGF-2 which is more active on fat and liver tissue than the other SM (Moses et al., 1977; Rechler et al., 1978).

4. Somatomedins and Foetal Growth

The factors involved in foetal growth are not yet characterised (Hall and Sara, 1978). Whether the SM have any significance for foetal growth is not proved, but can be assumed for the following reasons. Firstly, they have a mitogenic action on foetal cells in vitro (Sara et al., 1978). Secondly, a variety of foetal tissues have specific binding sites for SM (D'Ercole, Foushee and Underwood, 1976). Thirdly, immunoreactive SM-A is present in human foetal serum (Hall et al., 1978). Fourthly, foetal serum from various species contains polypeptides which cross-react with SM-A and SM-C for their binding sites. Finally, a correlation between SM levels and birth weight in human new-borns has been found (D'Ercole et al., 1976; Svan, Hall, Ritzén, Takano and Skottner, 1977). The supply of pure SM and their antibodies does not yet allow their use in animal foetuses. Consequently, it has not yet been possible to prove directly the importance of SM for foetal growth.

F. SOMATOMEDIN B

Somatomedin B activity, stimulating DNA synthesis in glial cells was apparently also GH-dependent (Westermark *et al.*, 1975). After acid-ethanol extraction of Cohn Fraction IV as in the isolation procedure for SM-B the peptide was further purified by gel filtration and cellulose column electro-phoresis (Fryklund *et al.*, 1974b). It was found to be an acidic single chain polypeptide, mw 5000. Several forms, differing in charge but not composition suggested that perhaps deamidation had occurred during isolation. A unique sequence (Fig. 3) (Fryklund *et al.*, 1978) was obtained, which showed no obvious relationship to insulin or any of the other known growth factors.

```
1    2    3    4    5    6    7    8    9    10  11
Asp–Gln–Glu–Ser–Cys–Lys–Gly–Arg–Cys–Thr–Glu–

12  13  14  15  16  17  18  19  20  21  22  23
Gly–Phe–Asn–Val–Asp–Lys–Lys–Cys–Gln–Cys–Asp–Glu–

24  25  26  27  28  29  30  31  32  33
Leu–Cys–Ser–Tyr–Tyr–Gln–Ser–Asn–Cys–Thr–

34  35  36  37  38  39  40  41  42  43  44
Cys–Tyr–Thr–Ala–Glu–Cys–Lys–Pro–Gln–Val–Thr–OH
```

Fig. 3. Somatomedin B, primary structure.

This is in accordance with the known biological effects, since SM-B lacks insulin-like activity, and is in fact a poor growth factor in *in vitro* systems. A closer examination of the structure indicated a possible relationship to protease inhibitors and in fact a region, residues 5–8, shows a close homology with the trypsin binding site of the bovine pancreatic trypsin inhibitor. Weak antitrypsin activity but not anti-thrombin or anti-plasmin has been found. A radioimmunoassay developed from rabbit serum by both Yalow, Hall and Luft (1975) and Hall *et al.* (1976) showed that immunogenic SM-B was species-specific, and that plasma levels were greatly elevated in acro-megaly. Hypopituitary children were in general at the lower limit of the normal range (Hall *et al.*, 1976). SM-B antibodies were used in a dilution of 1:4000 and charcoal adsorption was used to separate bound from free peptide. Immunoreactive SM-B indicates that a slight age dependence is seen. There is no apparent diurnal variation (Hall *et al.*, 1976).

SM-B, while found in urine as a low molecular weight form, appears in plasma as a complex with a mw 100,000. The carrier appears also to be cold-labile since aggregation to a higher molecular weight readily occurs on cooling and freezing. Only about 10% of SM-B can be dissociated on acid treatment, suggesting that perhaps a covalent bond is involved. The carrier protein is definitely different from that for the insulin-like somatomedins.

GH is not the only hormone affecting SM-B levels; oestrogens also can cause an increase. SM-B is not a classical growth factor like the other SM, but it is easy to suggest a role for a protease inhibitor in growth. Controlled proteolysis is for example involved in tissue growth and the conversion of prohormones to active hormones and perhaps even in the unmasking of hormone receptors on the cell surface. These questions must today be left unanswered.

CONCLUSIONS AND PERSPECTIVES

It is clear that the polypeptides with insulin-like and sulphation-stimulating activity form a family. Two of the peptides, IGF-1 and -2, although close structural homologues, exhibit considerable differences in immunogeneity, bioactivity and binding affinity. It is not known at present which part of the molecule is involved in the expression of these differences. The stretch of peptide chain, corresponding to the C peptide of proinsulin, which is on the surface of the molecule (Blundell et al., 1978) can perhaps be the specificity-determining region. The close correspondence in bioactivity between IGF-1 and SM-A cannot yet be explained due to lack of structural information on SM-A. We do not know at present whether the high molecular weight forms are biologically active at the target.

The biological effect of the somatomedins has to be the result of an equilibrium in the system where the binding proteins and the receptor on the target organ compete for SM. The different affinity constants will then determine the biological effect. Differences in chemical nature can affect affinity to both binding protein and receptor. The whole carrier protein situation is considerably more complex and surely also of more clinical importance than was realised earlier. The nature, requirements and localisation of SM receptors need investigating, likewise the situation in normal growth conditions.

Although it is obvious that GH is intimately involved in the regulation of SM-A, SM-C and IGF-1, the situation as regards IGF-2 is not so certain. It is probable that GH also is involved in the regulation of at least one of the carrier proteins, which is absent in untreated hypopituitary patients. NSILP, the non-acid-dissociable form is a third form with high molecular weight; the clinical significance of this has not yet been resolved. The serum levels of insulin-like peptides reflect GH status and can also be used to follow therapy. Ectopic production has been found in some tumour cases. The lack of diurnal variation simplifies measurement problems normally encountered with GH.

Results obtained with animal experiments indicate that nutrition and hormones other than GH are involved in the regulation of SM (Phillips and Young, 1976; Eigenmann et al., 1977; Takano et al., 1978b). In analogy with insulin, where glucose acts as the primary stimulator, we could expect that some nutrient would have the same function for somatomedins. The liver has been postulated as the site of synthesis but as yet the evidence is not complete.

The role of SM-B in the GH-dependent peptide family is not at all clear. It is neither an insulin-like SM or even a growth factor but perhaps some type of enzyme inhibitor or modulator, which can be of prime importance in the regulation of tissue growth.

The in vitro growth promoting activity of the somatomedin-like peptides has been well documented, but whether they can replace GH in postnatal life and are foetal growth factors are problems which will perhaps be solved in the next decade. The function of these insulin-like peptides in carbohydrate metabolism and the pathogenesis of diabetes is another field of exploration.

Although considerable progress has been made during the last ten years, we have only just begun to discern the contours of this new and exciting area of endocrinology.

REFERENCES

Almqvist, S. (1961). Acta endocr., Copenh. **36**, 31.

Almqvist, S., Lindsten, J. and Lindvall, N. (1963). Acta endocr., Copenh. **42**, 168.

Audhya, T. K. and Gibson, K. D. (1975). Proc. natn. Acad. Sci. USA, **72**, 604.

Bala, R. M., Blakeley, E. D. and Smith, G. R. (1976). J. clin. Endocr. Metab. **43**, 1110.

Bala, R. M., Hankins, C. and Smith, G. R. (1975). Can. J. Physiol. Pharmac. **53**, 403.

Beaton, G. R. (1976). Thesis. Faculty of Science, University of Witwatersrand, Johannesburg.

Blundell, T. L., Bedarkar, S., Rinderknecht, E. and Humbel, R. E. (1978). Proc. natn. Acad. Sci. USA, **75**, 180.

Daughaday, W. H. (1971). Adv. int. Med. **17**, 237.

Daughaday, W. H., Hall, K., Raben, M. S., Salmon Jr., W. D., Van den Brande, J. L. and Van Wyk, J. J. (1972). Nature, Lond. **236**, 107.

Daughaday, W. H., Laron, Z., Pertzelan, A. and Heins, J. N. (1969). Trans. Assoc. Am. Phycns, **82**, 129.

Daughaday, W. H. and Parker, M. L. (1963). J. clin. Endocr. Metab. **23**, 638.

Daughaday, W. H. and Reeder, C. (1966). J. Lab. clin. Med. **68**, 357.

D'Ercole, A. J., Foushee, D. B. and Underwood, L. E. (1976). *J. clin. Endocr. Metab.* **43**, 1069.

D'Ercole, A. J., Underwood, L. E. and Van Wyk, J. J. (1977). *J. Pediat.* **90**, 375.

Dulak, N. C. and Temin, H. M. (1973a). *J. cell. Physiol.* **81**, 153.

Dulak, N. C. and Temin, H. M. (1973b). *J. cell. Physiol.* **81**, 161.

Eigenmann, J. E., Becker, M., Kammermann, B., Leemann, W., Heimann, R., Zapf, J. and Froesch, E. R. (1977). *Acta endocr., Copenh.* **85**, 818.

Enberg, G., Fryklund, L. and Hall, K. (1978). Int. Symp. Somatomedins and Growth, Genoa, Italy, p. 36 (abstract).

Florini, J. R., Nicholson, M. L. and Dulak, N. C. (1977). *Endocrinology,* **101**, 32.

Franklin, R. C., Rennie, G. C., Burger, H. G. and Cameron, D. P. (1976). *J. clin. Endocr. Metab.* **43**, 1164.

Froesch, E. R., Bürgi, H., Müller, W. A., Humbel, R. E., Jakob, A. and Labhart, A. (1967). *Rec. Prog. Horm. Res.* **23**, 565.

Froesch, E. R., Bürgi, H., Ramseier, E. B., Bally, P. and Labhart, A. (1963). *J. clin. Invest.* **42**, 1816.

Froesch, E. R., Schlumpf, U., Heimann, R., Zapf, J., Humbel, R. E. and Ritschard, W. J. (1975a). *Adv. metab. Disord.* **8**, 203.

Froesch, E. R., Zapf, J., Meuli, C., Mäder, M., Waldvogel, M., Kaufmann, U. and Morell, B. (1975b). *Adv. metab. Disord.* **8**, 211.

Fryklund, L. and Sievertsson, H. (1978). *Fedn. Eur. biochem. Soc. Lett.* **87**, 55.

Fryklund, L., Skottner, A. and Hall, K. (1978). Proc. 11th FEBS Meeting: Growth Factors (K. W. Kastrup and J. H. Nielsen, eds), Vol. 48, p. 65. Pergamon Press, Oxford.

Fryklund, L., Skottner, A., Sievertsson, H. and Hall, K. (1975). Excerpta Medica International Congress Series, No. 381 "Growth Hormone and Related Peptides", p. 156. Excerpta Medica, Amsterdam.

Fryklund, L., Uthne, K. and Sievertsson, H. (1974a). *Biochem. biophys. Res. Commun.* **61**, 957.

Fryklund, L., Uthne, K., Sievertsson, H. and Westermark, B. (1974b). *Biochem. biophys. Res. Commun.* **61**, 950.

Furlanetto, R. W., Underwood, L. E., Van Wyk, J. J. and D'Ercole, J. (1977). *J. clin. Invest.* **60**, 648.

Gibson, K. D., Ben-Porath, E., Doller, H. J. and Segen, B. J. (1978). *In* Proc. 11th FEBS Meeting: Growth Factors (K. W. Kastrup and J. H. Nielsen, eds), Vol. 48, p. 101. Pergamon Press, Oxford.

Hall, K. (1970) *Acta endocr., Copenh.* **63**, 338.

Hall, K. (1971). *Acta endocr., Copenh.* **66**, 491.

Hall, K. (1972). *Acta endocr., Copenh.* (Suppl. 16), 1.

Hall, K., Brant, J., Enberg, G. and Fryklund, L. (1979). *J. clin. Endocr. Metab.* **48**, 271–278.

Hall, K., Fryklund, L., Löw, H., Skottner, A. and Zederman, R. (1978). *In* Proc. 11th FEBS Meeting: Growth Factors (K. W. Kastrup and J. H. Nielsen, eds), Vol. 48, p. 59. Pergamon Press, Oxford.

Hall, K., Luft, R., Takano, K. and Fryklund, L. (1976). Excerpta Medica International Congress Series, No. 403. Proc. 5th Int. Cong. Endocr., Hamburg, Vol. 2, p. 162. (V. H. T. James, ed.). Excerpta Medica, Amsterdam.

Hall, K. and Olin, P. (1972). *Acta endocr., Copenh.* **69**, 417.

Hall, K. and Sara, V. (1978). Proc. Dahlem Conf. Abnormal Foetal Growth, Biological Bases and Consequences (F. Naffolin, ed.), p. 121.

Hall, K., Takano, K. and Fryklund, L. (1974). *J. clin. Endocr. Metab.* **39**, 973.

Hall, K., Takano, K., Fryklund, L. and Sievertsson, H. (1975a). *Adv. metab. Disord.* **8**, 19.

Hall, K., Takano, K., Fryklund, L. and Sievertsson, H. (1975b). Convegno Int. Endocr. Ped., Bologna, p. 209. Pacini, Pisa.

Hall, K. and Uthne, K. (1971). *Acta med. scand.* **190**, 137.

Heins, J. N., Garland, J. T. and Daughaday, W. H. (1970). *Endocrinology,* **87**, 688.

Hintz, R. L. and Liu, F. (1977). *J. clin. Endocr. Metab.* **45**, 988.

Hintz, R. L., Clemmons, D. R., Underwood, L. E. and Van Wyk, J. J. (1972). *Proc. natn. Acad. Sci. USA,* **69**, 2351.

Humbel, R. E., Bünzli, H., Mülly, K., Oelz, O., Froesch, E. R. and Ritschard, W. J. (1971). *In* "Diabetes" (R. R. Rodrigues and J. Vallance-Owen, eds), p. 306. Excerpta Medica, Amsterdam.

Humbel, R. E. and Rinderknecht, E. (1978). *In* Proc. 11th FEBS Meeting: Growth Factors (K. W. Kastrup and J. H. Nielsen, eds), Vol. 48, p. 55. Pergamon Press, Oxford.

Kaufmann, U., Zapf, J., Torretti, B. and Froesch, E. R. (1977). *J. clin. Endocr. Metab.* **44**, 160.

Keret, R., Schimpff, R. M. and Girard. F. (1976). *Hormone Res.* **7**, 254.

Koumans, J. and Daughaday, W. H. (1963). *Trans. Ass. Am. Phycns,* **76**, 152.

Laron, Z., Pertzelan, A., Karp, M. and Daughaday, W. H. (1971). *J. clin. Endocr. Metab.* **33**, 332.

Marek, J., Schullerová, M. and Schreiberová, O. (1976). *Rev. Czech. Med.* **22**, 194.

Marshall, R. N., Underwood, L. E., Voina, S. J., Foushee, D. B. and Van Wyk, J. J. (1974). *J. clin. Endocr. Metab.* **39**, 283.

Megyesi, K., Gorden, P. and Kahn, C. R. (1977), *J. clin. Endocr. Metab.* **45**, 330.

Megyesi, K., Kahn, C. R., Roth, J., Froesch, E. R., Humbel, R. E., Zapf, J. and Neville, D. M. (1974a). *Biochem. biophys. Res. Commun.* **57**, 307.

Megyesi, K., Kahn, C. R., Roth, J. and Gorden, P. (1974b). *J. clin. Endocr. Metab.* **38**, 931.

Megyesi, K., Kahn, C. R., Roth, J., Neville, D. M., Nissley, S. P., Humbel, R. E. and Froesch. E. R. (1975). *J. biol. Chem.* **250**, 8990.

Meuli, C. and Froesch, E. R. (1975). *Eur. J. clin. Invest.* **5**, 93.

Morell, B. and Froesch, E. R. (1973). *Eur. J. clin. Invest.* **3**, 119.

Moses, A. C., Nissley, S., Cohen, K. L. and Rechler, M. M. (1976). *Nature, Lond.* **263**, 137.

Moses, A. C., Nissley, S. P., Rechler, M. M. and Short, P. A. (1978). The Endocrine Society (abstract).

Moses, A. C., Rechler, M. M. and Nissley, S. P. (1977). The Endocrine Society (abstract).

Nissley, S. P., Passamani, J. and Short, P. (1976). *J. cell. Physiol.* **89**, 393.

Phillips, L. S., Pennisi, A. J., Belosky, D. C., Uittenbogaart, C., Ettenger, R. B., Malekzadeh, M. H. and Fine, R. N. (1978). *J. clin. Endocr. Metab.* **46**, 165.

Phillips, L. S. and Young, H. S. (1976). *Diabetes,* **25**, 516.

Poffenbarger, P. L. (1975). *J. clin. Invest.* **56**, 1455.

Poffenbarger, P. L. (1978). Int. Symp. Somatomedins and Growth, Genoa, Italy, p. 19 (abstract).

Poffenbarger, P. L. and Boully, L. A. (1976). 5th Int. Congr. Endocr., Hamburg, p. 163. Brühlsche Universitätsdruckerei, Giessen.

Posner, B. I., Guydal, H. J. and Omori, Y. (1977). *J. Steroid Biochem.* **8**, 387.

Reber, K. and Liske, R. (1976). *Horm. metab. Res.* **7**, 201.

Rechler, M. M., Fryklund, L., Nissley, S. P., Hall, K., Podskalny, J. M., Skottner, A. and Moses, A. C. (1978). *Eur. J. Biochem.* **82**, 5.

Rechler, M. M., Nissley, S. P., Podskalny, J. M., Moses, A. C. and Fryklund, L. (1977). *J. clin. Endocr. Metab.* **44**, 820.

Rechler, M. M., Podskalny, J. M. and Nissley, S. P. (1976). *Nature, Lond.* **259**, 134.

Rinderknecht, E. and Humbel, R. E. (1976a). *Proc. natn. Acad. Sci. USA*, **73**, 2365.

Rinderknecht, E. and Humbel, R. E. (1976b). *Proc. natn. Acad. Sci. USA*, **73**, 4379.

Saenger, P., Wiedermann, E., Schwartz, E., Korth-Schutz, S., Lewy, J. E., Riggo, R. R., Rubin, A. L., Stenzel, K. H. and New, M. I. (1974). *Pediat. Res.* **8**, 163.

Salmon Jr., W. D. (1960). *J. Lab. clin. Med.* **56**, 673.

Salmon Jr., W. D. and Daughaday, W. H. (1957). *J. Lab. clin. Med.* **49**, 825.

Salmon Jr., W. D. and Daughaday, W. H. (1958). *J. Lab. clin. Med.* **51**, 167.

Salmon Jr., W. D. and DuVall, M. R. (1970). *Endocrinology*, **87**, 1168.

Sara, V. R., Hall, K., Wetterberg, L., Fryklund, L., Wahlund, L. O., Sjögren, B. and Skottner, A. (1978). Int. Symp. Somatomedins and Growth, Genoa, Italy, p. 45 (abstract).

Schimpff, R. M., Donhadieu, M., Glasinovic, J. G., Warnet, J. M. and Girard, F. (1976). *Acta endocr., Copenh.* **83**, 365.

Schlumpf, U., Heimann, R., Zapf, J. and Froesch, E. R. (1976). *Acta endocr., Copenh.* **81**, 28.

Schwalbe, S. L., Betts, P. R., Rayner, P. H. W. and Rudd, B. T. (1977). *Br. med. J.* **1**, 679.

Svan, H., Hall, K., Ritzén, M., Takano, K. and Skottner, A. (1977). *Acta endocr., Copenh.* **85**, 636.

Takano, K. (1975). Thesis, Karolinska Institute, Stockholm.

Takano, K., Hall, K., Fryklund, L. and Sievertsson, H. (1976a). *Horm. metab. Res.* **8**, 16.

Takano, K., Hall, K., Kastrup, K. W., Hizuka, N., Shizume, K., Kawai, K., Akimoto, M., Takuma, T. and Sugino, N. (1979). *J. clin. Endocr. Metab.* **48**, 371–376.

Takano, K., Hall, K., Ritzén, M., Iselius, L. and Sievertsson, H. (1976b). *Acta endocr., Copenh.* **82**, 449.

Takano, K., Hizuka, N., Kawai, K. and Shizume, K. (1978a). *Acta endocr., Copenh.* **87**, 485.

Takano, K., Hizuka, N., Shizume, K. and Hall, K. (1977a). *Endocr. jap.* **24**, 359.

Takano, K., Hizuka, N., Shizume, K., Hayashi, N., Motoike, Y. and Obata, H. (1977b). *J. clin. Endocr. Metab.* **45**, 828.

Takano, K., Shizume, K., Hizuka, N., Kawai, K., Fryklund, L. and Hall, K. (1978b). Int. Symp. Somatomedins and Growth. Genoa. Italy, p. 58.

Thorsson, A. V. and Hintz, R. L. (1977). *Biochem. biophys. Res. Commun.*, **74**, 1566.

Underwood, L. E., Hintz, R. L., Voina, S. J. and Van Wyk, J. J. (1972). *J. clin. Endocr. Metab.* **35**, 194.

Uthne, K. (1973). *Acta endocr., Copenh.* (*Suppl.* 175), 1.

Uthne, K., Reagan, C. R., Gimpel, L. P. and Kostyo, J. L. (1974). *J. clin. Endocr. Metab.* **39**, 548.

Van den Brande, J. L. and Du Caju, M. V. L. (1974). *Acta endocr., Copenh.* **75**, 233.

Van den Brande, J. L. and van Buul, S. (1978). *Annls Biol. anim. Biochim. Biophys.* **18**, 11.

Van den Brande, J. L., van Buul, S., Heinrich, U., van Roon, F., Zurcher, T. and van Steirtegem, A. C. (1975). *Adv. metab. Disord.* **8**, 171.

Van den Brande, J. L., Van Wyk, J. J., Weaver, R. P. and Mayberry, H. E. (1971). *Acta endocr., Copenh.* **66**, 65.

Van Wyk, J. J., Furlanetto, R. W., Underwood, L. E., D'Ercole, A. J. and Decedie, C. J. (1976). 5th Int. Congress Endocr., Hamburg.

Van Wyk, J. J., Hall, K., Van den Brande, J. L., Weaver, R. P., Uthne, K., Hintz, R. L., Harrison, J. H. and Mathewson, P. (1972). In Proc. 2nd Int. Symp. Growth Hormone (A. Pecile and E. Müeller, eds), p. 155. Excerpta Medica, Amsterdam.

Van Wyk, J. J., Hall, K. and Weaver, R. P. (1969). Biochim. biophys. Acta, 192, 560.

Van Wyk, J. J. and Underwood, L. E. (1975). A. Rev. Med. 26, 427.

Van Wyk, J. J., Underwood, L. E., Baseman, J. B., Hintz, R. L., Clemmons, D. R. and Marshall, R. N. (1975). Adv. metab. Disorder. 8, 127.

Watson, A. C., Spencer, E. M., Uthne, K. O., Piel, C. F. and Holliday, M. A. (1977) Pediat. Res. 11, 546.

Werner, S., Hall, K. and Löw, H. (1974). Horm. metab. Res. 6, 319.

Westermark, B., Wasteson, Å. and Uthne, K. (1975). Exp. cell. Res. 96, 58.

Wiedemann, E. and Schwartz, E. (1972). J. clin. Endocr. Metab. 34, 51.

Yalow, R. S., Hall, K. and Luft, R. (1975). J. clin. Invest. 55, 127.

Yde, H. (1968). Acta endocr., Copenh. 57, 557.

Zapf, J. and Froesch, E. R. (1978). Int. Symp. Somatomedins and Growth, Genoa, Italy, p. 26 (abstract).

Zapf, J., Kaufmann, U., Eigenmann, E. J. and Froesch, E. R. (1977). Clin. Chem. 23, 677.

Zapf, J., Mäder, M., Waldvogel, M., Schalch, S. and Froesch, E. R. (1975a). Archs Biochem. Biophys. 168, 630.

Zapf, J., Schoenle, E. and Froesch, E. R. (1978). In Proc. 11th FEBS Meeting: "Growth Factors" (K. W. Kastrup and J. H. Nielsen, eds), Vol. 48, p. 45. Pergamon Press, Oxford.

Zapf, J., Waldvogel, M. and Froesch, E. R. (1975b). Archs Biochem. Biophys. 168, 638.

Zingg, A. E. and Froesch, E. R. (1973). Diabetologia, 9, 472.

VI. Prolactin

S. FRANKS

INTRODUCTION

Prolactin was identified half a century ago as a lactogenic hormone secreted by the pituitary (Striker and Grueter, 1928). Although knowledge of its structure and physiological role in mammals steadily advanced, the nature of prolactin in the human has remained elusive until the last decade. In the last edition of "Hormones in Blood", Isabel Forsyth (Forsyth, 1967) drew attention to the recent progress in the understanding of the structure, biological effects and control of secretion of prolactin in non-primate species, but stressed the necessity to identify prolactin in man and to develop a sensitive assay for the hormone in human blood. Dr. Forsyth herself was one of the scientists, who, in the late 1960's and early 1970's, contributed evidence for the identity of human prolactin as a hormone separate from growth hormone (HGH) (Frantz and Kleinberg, 1970; Forsyth, Besser, Edwards, Francis and Myres, 1971). At the same time, prolactin was finally isolated from both monkey and human pituitary glands (Guyda and Friesen, 1971; Lewis, Singh and Seavey, 1971a; Hwang, Guyda and Friesen, 1972). This evidence, together with the development of bioassay techniques (Forsyth and Myres, 1971; Frantz, Kleinberg and Noel, 1972) and subsequently, sensitive and specific radioimmunoassay methods (Hwang, Guyda and Friesen, 1971; Frantz *et al.*, 1972; Greenwood, Lino and Bryant, 1973; Sinha, Selby, Vanderlaan and Lewis, 1973) have led to the remarkable wealth of knowledge of the physiology and pathophysiology of prolactin secretion which has been acquired in the last ten years.

The aim in this chapter is to review the important recent developments in research on human prolactin and to raise some questions as to direction of future investigation into its nature and physiology.

A. CHEMICAL CONSTITUTION AND MAIN PHYSICAL PROPERTIES

1. Isolation and Purification

(a) Pituitary glands

Prolactin was not isolated from human pituitary tissues until 1971, but the attempts to separate prolactin from growth hormone by biochemical means were encouraged by considerable evidence, from clinical and immunological studies, for the existence of a lactogenic hormone discrete from HGH (reviewed by Sherwood, 1971). Indeed, from early clinical reports of disorders characterised by abnormal lactation, it was obvious that inappropriate lactation could occur in the absence of features suggesting acromegaly (Haenel, 1928; Krestin, 1932; Argonz and del Castillo, 1953; Forbes, Henneman, Griswold and Albright, 1954). Guyda and Friesen (1971) were able to separate monkey prolactin from growth hormone by affinity chromatography; using a human placental lactogen (HPL) antibody, coupled to a solid phase (sepharose), they were able to remove 99% of monkey growth hormone (MGH) from pituitary preparations. After immunoabsorption of the MGH, the unabsorbed fractions from the tissue homogenates or incubation media of monkey pituitary glands were found to contain prolactin bioactivity (as estimated by pigeon crop sac assay); the dose curves of these fractions paralleled that of ovine prolactin standard. This crude preparation of monkey prolactin was subsequently used successfully in a radioimmunoassay for human prolactin (see Introduction and Section E.2).

Shortly after Guyda and Friesen's work was published, Lewis *et al.* (1971a) reported the isolation and purification of human prolactin. An alkaline extract of freshly frozen human pituitary glands (60 gm or about 120 glands) was first chromatographed on Sephadex G-150 and the fraction containing HGH and prolactin was then rechromatographed on a DEAE-cellulose column. The protein was eluted by a gradient of 0·1 M and 0·1 M ammonium bicarbonate and prolactin appeared in the fractions just before HGH. The pattern on disc electrophoresis of the "prolactin fractions" showed a slow-moving component which was distinct from growth hormone and which, as had previously been shown by these workers (Lewis, Singh, Sinha and Vanderlaan, 1971b), possessed potent lactogenic activity. The molecular weight of this component was estimated to be similar to that of HGH at about 21,000. The growth hormone activity of the prolactin was assessed at about 10% of that of HGH in both bioassay and radioimmunoassay systems. Hwang and colleagues (1972) then described a method for the extraction and purification of prolactin from acetone-dried human pituitary powder from which HGH had been removed according to Raben's method (Raben, 1959). After gel filtration and DEAE-cellulose chromatography, the prolactin-rich fractions were pooled and repurified on a carboxy-methyl cellulose (CMC) ion exchange column. The overall yield was estimated to be about 40% (although other workers reported a recovery of less than 10% by this method). The HGH contamination at the end of the third step was less than 1%. Later Hwang and colleagues (Hwang, Robertson, Guyda and Friesen, 1973) applied this method successfully to the purification of prolactin from stored frozen pituitary glands and obtained a yield of 40–50 μg of prolactin/gland, i.e. up to 50% of the total pituitary content. A major problem in these methods was the significant amount of prolactin which appeared in aggregated form and was unavailable for further purification. A modification of the above methods, avoiding the necessity for an alkaline extraction and resulting in a higher recovery of prolactin, was suggested by Scott and Lowry (1973).

Hummel and colleagues (Hummel, Brown, Hwang and Friesen (1975) reported that monkey or human GH and prolactin could be separated by isoelectric focusing (the major prolactin component having an i.p. of pH 5·93–6·04) and Rathnam and Saxena (1977) incorporated this technique in a method for purification of prolactin from acetone-dried pituitary powder. These workers argued that the acetone-dried preparation was available in relatively plentiful supply; their yield of prolactin was 23 mg/kg pituitary powder. Skyler and colleagues (Skyler, Rogol, Lovenberg and Knazek (1977) raised the question of human pituitary tissue in culture as a potentially rich source of prolactin, particularly since long term viability of lactotrophs seemed feasible (Knazek and Skyler, 1976). The value of this method remains to be established, but it seems unlikely that it will replace the previously described techniques.

(b) Amniotic fluid

Early radioimmunoassay studies indicated that prolactin was present in high concentrations in human amniotic fluid (Hwang et al., 1971) (see Sections C.2 and F.1), and it was soon realised that this was a possible source of large amounts of prolactin. In early 1974, two groups published a preliminary method for the isolation and purification of prolactin from human amniotic fluid (Ben David and Chrambach, 1974; Hwang, Murray, Jacobs, Niall and Friesen, 1974). Hwang et al. (1974) were able to determine the amino-terminal sequence of prolactin in material purified by affinity chromatography (see Section A.3). Recent refinements of the methods for extraction and purification of prolactin from amniotic fluid have enabled yields of highly purified hormone to be obtained in milligram quantities (Rathnam, Cederqvist and Saxena, 1977; Ben-David and Chrambach, 1977).

2. Heterogeneity of Human Prolactin

(a) Pituitary and amniotic fluid

Heterogeneity of human prolactin isolated from pituitary and amniotic fluid was described by several workers whose studies have been discussed in the previous section. Lewis and Singh (1973) noted that during chromatography of the alkaline–ethanol pituitary extract on Sephadex G-150, a significant amount of prolactin (as measured by a radioimmunoassay) appeared in higher molecular weight forms. A similar finding was recorded by Hwang et al. (1973). The origin of these larger molecules was not clear but Lewis and Singh suggested that these might represent aggregation of prolactin after extraction (Pensky, Murray, Mozaffarrien and Pearson, 1972). These larger molecular weight forms were removed during subsequent purification of the hormone. Isoelectric focusing of both pituitary (Hummel et al., 1975; Rathnam et al., 1975) and amniotic fluid prolactin (Ben-David and Chrambach, 1977) has also revealed heterogeneity of prolactin, but this does not necessarily represent differences in molecular size (Ben-David and Chrambach, 1977).

(b) Peripheral plasma

The initial reports of heterogeneity of prolactin in pituitary extracts were soon confirmed and, furthermore, prolactin components of differing molecular size were demonstrated in peripheral plasma (Suh and Frantz, 1974; Rogol and Rosen, 1974; Guyda, 1975). Two main components of prolactin were identified (in both pituitary extracts and plasma) by chromatography on Sephadex G-100; one (K_{av} 0·4) which was eluted with the monomeric prolactin marker (mw 21,000) and the other (K_{av} 0·2) which was assumed to be a larger form (termed "little" and "big" prolactin by Suh and Frantz). The proportion of "little" to "big" forms varied with different clinical states (Fig. 1) with the monomeric form predominating in serum from thyrotrophin-releasing hormone (TRH) treated normal subjects, patients during pregnancy and the puerperium and some but not all patients with prolactin-secreting pituitary tumours. A recent report has shown that such heterogeneity may also be seen in plasma from non-TRH stimulated normal subjects. In addition, this study provided further evidence for the presence of a third, very large prolactin component—"big, big" prolactin (accounting for up to 30% of the total radioimmunoactivity in baseline plasma samples) which appeared close to the void volume of the G-100 Sephadex column. It is of interest that the relative amount of this very large form was noted to decrease after TRH-stimulation (Farkouh, Packer and Frantz, 1977). Other workers however, have been unable to identify this component in either pituitary or plasma extracts (Guyda, 1975). It should be noted that although differences in the elution pattern on Sephadex chromatography probably represent variations in molecular size, they could also be due to differences in molecular configuration. Additional evidence for changes in size of the prolactin molecule (e.g. gel electrophoresis) was not given in the above studies.

The origin, nature and significance of large molecular weight forms of prolactin, all of which seem to have similar receptor binding and immunological properties, are not fully understood. It has been suggested that the presence of "big" prolactin in pituitary culture media is supportive evidence that prolactin may be secreted as a prohormone (Guyda, 1975) and indeed,

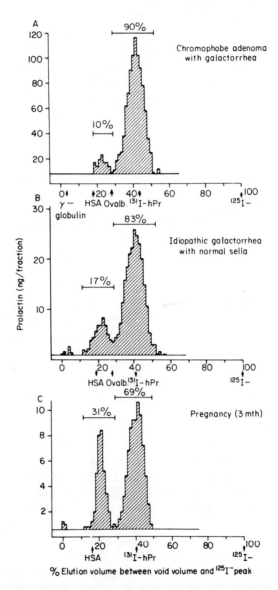

Fig. 1. Elution pattern of ^{125}I-prolactin of plasma samples from three different subjects. The mobility is expressed as a percentage of the effluent volume emerging between the void volume, determined with blue dextran, and the ^{125}I peak. Other markers used were human serum albumin (HSA) and ovalbumin (ovalb. mw 45,000). From Suh and Frantz (1974) with permission.

in vitro biosynthesis of prolactin may result in a product of larger molecular weight than the monomeric marker (Seo, Refetoff, Vassart and Scherberg, 1977) (see Section B). However, big prolactin may simply be a dimer in which the two prolactin molecules are linked by a disulphide bond in a similar manner to the larger molecular weight forms of HGH and human placental lactogen (HPL) (Benveniste and Frohman, 1978).

Heterogeneity of prolactin appears to be present also in the *cerebrospinal fluid* of hyperprolactinaemic patients (Kiefer and Malarkey, 1978).

3. Structure of Human Prolactin

The structure of a number of primate prolactins has been known for more than a decade and comparisons of the structures of ovine prolactin with HPL and HGH have proved a useful basis for the understanding of the nature of human prolactin (Li, Dixon and Chung, 1971). Analysis of the amino-terminal of the human pituitary prolactin isolated by Hwang *et al.* (1972) was performed by Niall and a single residue (leucine) was identified. Subsequently, Niall and co-workers (Niall, Hogan, Tregear, Segre, Hwang and Friesen, 1973) established the sequence of 40 amino acid residues from the amino-terminal of the molecule, and noted the similarity in ovine and human prolactins. However, the complete amino acid sequence of human prolactin remained undetermined until very recently. In 1977, Shome and Parlow reported for the first time the entire linear amino acid sequence comprising 198 residues. The similarity of human and ovine prolactin was again apparent, as was the large number of differences from HGH and HPL. The structure showed a 73% identity with ovine prolactin in terms of amino acid sequence (77% with porcine and 60% with rat prolactin) but only 32 of the 198 residues corresponded to those of HGH. The sequence of the 40 amino-terminal residues was in agreement with that previously shown by Niall, save for a serine residue compared with asparagine at position 38. The complete amino acid sequence of prolactin, as defined by Shome and Parlow is shown in Fig. 2.

B. CELLS OF ORIGIN AND BIOSYNTHESIS

1. Pituitary Lactotrophs

(a) *Morphology of prolactin-secreting cells*

The presence of specific prolactin-secreting cells in the anterior pituitary of the human had been clearly established by morphological studies even before isolation of prolactin from the gland provided the final proof of the

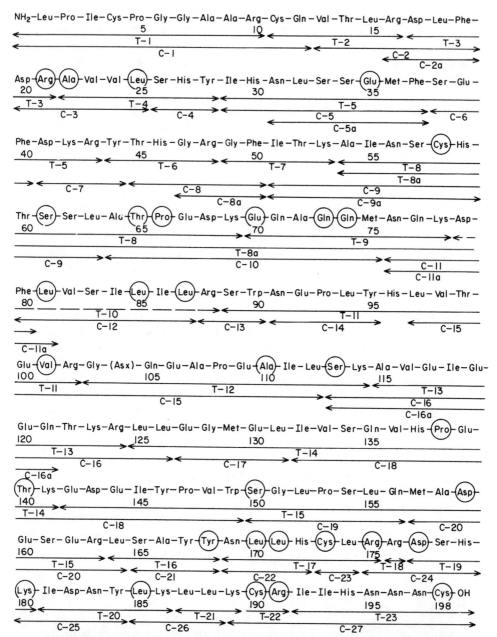

Fig. 2. The complete linear aminoacid sequence of human prolactin. The encircled residues indicate the only points of identity with HGH (C = Chymotrypsin split residues, T = Trypsin fragments). From Shome and Parlow (1977) with permission.

separate identities of prolactin and HGH. A number of staining techniques were used to identify pituitary lactotrophs among the acidophilic cells of the anterior hypophysis (reviewed by Forsyth, 1967; Baker and Yu, 1977) and it became clear from immunohistochemical studies that prolactin-secreting cells were present in both sexes in adult humans; these cells underwent hypertrophy during the last two trimesters of pregnancy and could be found in tumours of the pituitary in patients who had galactorrhoea but no evidence of excessive HGH secretion. Electron microscope studies of the lactotroph (reviewed by Guyda, Robert, Collu and Hardy, 1973) show a characteristic appearance which is common to both normal cells and those from prolactin-secreting tumours. These features include irregular, densely staining nuclei, and larger, more evenly distributed secreting granules compared with somatotrophs. The lactotrophs appear to be localised mainly in the postero-lateral wings of the pars distalis but recent work has suggested that the cells show morphological and topographical heterogeneity (Baker and Yu, 1977). Baker and Yu have observed that mammotrophs first appear in the foetal hypophysis at 14 weeks of gestation, that there is little difference in the cell numbers seen in adult men and non-pregnant or non-puerperal women, and that the numbers regress in both sexes in old age.

(b) Biosynthesis by pituitary gland

Biosynthesis of prolactin by human pituitary cells was first clearly demonstrated by Friesen, Guyda and Hwang (1970); after incubation of human pituitary glands with ^{3}H-leucine, a protein with a similar molecular weight to HGH (which was not precipitated by an antibody to HGH) was eluted by gel filtration. The total amount of protein identified as prolactin which was produced by the glands was calculated to be much less than that of HGH but was more rapidly synthesised and released into the medium than was HGH. Recent studies using rat pituitary cell cultures from the GH_3 tumour cell line have proved a useful model for examination of the biosynthesis of prolactin. Biswas and Tashjian (1974) presented evidence indicating that prolactin synthesis is largely confined to the membrane-bound polysome fractions. Cytoplasmic mRNA from GH_3 cells, translated in a cell free system by a wheat germ embryo extract, is able to direct the synthesis of prolactin; this synthesis is influenced by the addition of factors such as TRH and oestrogens to the culture medium (Evans and Rosenfield, 1976; Dannies and Tashjian, 1976). Seo et al. (1977) have since demonstrated cell free translation of human prolactin by mRNA (derived from a prolactin-secreting tumour) and noted that the translated product was larger (though only by some 500 daltons) than I^{125} prolactin used as a marker. This was thought to be a precursor molecule.

2. Other Sources of Prolactin

(a) Amniotic fluid

The origin of the very high concentrations of prolactin in amniotic fluid is not known. The maternal plasma may make some contribution in the rhesus monkey (Josimovich, 1977) but this probably does not apply to the human, (Friesen, Hwang, Guyda, Tolis, Tyson and Myres, 1972). Some studies indicate that the source may be foetal urine (Badawi, Perez-Lopez and Robyn, 1973) but others favour the placental membranes (Friesen et al., 1972). Healy, Muller and Burger (1977) have localised prolactin (by immunofluorescence) to the cytoplasm of human amniotic epithelial cells and have postulated that these cells are capable of prolactin secretion. However, biosynthesis by the placental membranes has not yet been proven by direct studies.

(b) Non-pituitary tumours

Ectopic prolactin secretion by tumour tissue is rare, but has been reported to occur in neoplasms of the lung and kidney (Turkington, 1972a; Rees, Bloomfield, Rees, Corrin, Franks and Ratcliffe, 1974). However, Turkington's data must be interpreted with caution since bioassay measurements were used in this study and cross-reaction of other lactogenic hormones cannot be ruled out.

C. BIOLOGICAL EFFECTS AND MECHANISMS OF ACTION

1. Comparative Physiology

More than 100 physiological actions have been reported for prolactin in vertebrates (Nicoll and Bern, 1972; Nicoll, Buntin, Clemons, Schreibman and Russell, 1977). Nicoll and Bern (1972) have suggested that these actions can be divided into five main categories:

  (i) effects related to reproduction,
 (ii) effects on water and electrolyte balance,
(iii) effects on somatic growth or metabolism,
(iv) effects on integumentary structures or ectodermal derivatives,
 (v) actions involving synergism with adrenal or gonadal steroids.

The understanding of the biological function of prolactin in man has lagged considerably behind that of lower vertebrate physiology, mainly due to the doubt, until recently, about the existence of a separate human prolactin.

In the last few years, many physiological actions have been proposed for human prolactin. It is probably reasonable to state, however, that as yet, only its role in lactation and reproduction has been established with any certainty. The physiological actions of prolactin, proven or postulated, will be reviewed in the following section.

2. Biological Effects in Man

(a) Lactation and reproduction

It is not certain whether prolactin affects normal pubertal breast development in the human (Frantz, 1978) but its importance in lactation has now been firmly established (Tyson, Hwang, Guyda and Friesen, 1972; Tyson, Khojandi, Huth and Andreassen, 1975). Prolactin, interacting with gonadal steroids (and probably also adrenal steroids, insulin and thyroid hormones) is required for the initiation of lactation and probably is also necessary for its maintenance. Whilst it is true that at 2–3 months post-partum lactation continues even when serum prolactin levels have fallen to 30 ng/ml or below, further suppression of prolactin secretion by hypophysectomy or by dopamine-agonist drugs leads to cessation of milk production (reviewed by Frantz, 1978). The relationship of prolactin secretion to inappropriate lactation will be discussed below (Section F.2).

Lactation is classically associated with amenorrhoea and there is considerable evidence that the anovulation is caused by hyperprolactinaemia (Del Pozo and Fluckiger, 1973; Rolland and Schellekens, 1973; Robyn, Delvoye, Van Exter, Vekemens, Caufriez, de Nayer, Delogne-Desnoeck and L'Hermite, 1977). Similarly, pathological hyperprolactinaemia may impair gonadal function in both women and men (Section F. 2), but it is not certain whether prolactin has a more general role in the control of normal gonadal function in the human. The luteotrophic and luteolytic actions of prolactin in the rat are well known and it has been shown that there are specific binding sites for prolactin in the ovarian tissue of many mammalian species, including man (Saito and Saxena, 1975). Working with human ovarian follicles in vitro, McNatty, Sawyers and McNeilly (1974) reported that prolactin appeared to be important in normal follicular steroidogenesis. These workers showed that the addition of prolactin to the culture medium was necessary for progesterone synthesis, but that excessive amounts of prolactin inhibited progesterone output. Patients on prolactin-lowering drugs, who may have subnormal plasma levels of prolactin, may ovulate normally and this has been put forward as an argument against a role of prolactin in normal ovarian steroidogenesis. However, McNatty et al. (1974) have shown that the follicle may concentrate prolactin from the blood so that very low plasma levels may still be adequate for progesterone synthesis. Verification of this action of prolactin awaits further studies.

Although little is known of the physiological significance of prolactin in human male reproduction, the finding of specific binding sites in rat testis suggests that this may be a target organ for prolactin (Aragona and Friesen, 1975; Charreau, Attramadal, Torjesen, Purvis, Calandra and Hansson, 1977). It has been shown that prolactin may have either stimulatory or inhibitory effects on testicular steroidogenesis both in the rat and in man, although in the latter, high circulating concentrations of prolactin are usually associated with low plasma testosterone levels (Section F. 3), (Hafiez, Lloyd and Bartke, 1972; Negro-Vilar, Krulich and McCann, 1973; Fang, Refetoff, Rosenfield, 1974; Rubin, Poland and Tower, 1976). Some recent studies in the rat have drawn attention to the possible supportive role of prolactin to gonadotrophin-stimulated testosterone serum levels (Bartke, 1977; Swerdloff and Odell, 1977) but it remains to be determined whether this action is physiologically important in man.

(b) Water and electrolyte balance

Prolactin serves an important osmoregulatory function in lower vertebrates and there are some indications that it influences kidney function in mammals (for review see Nicoll, 1973). On the basis of experiments performed in the rat and cat (Lockett, 1965) the possibility that prolactin is involved in the regulation of salt and water balance in man has been explored by a number of workers. Horrobin, Lloyd, Lipton, Burtsyn, Durkin and Muiriri (1971) found that exogenous ovine prolactin administered to healthy volunteers reduced renal excretion of sodium and potassium and increased plasma sodium and osmolarity. Buckman and Peake (1973) measured endogenous prolactin levels in response to a salt or water load and produced results suggesting that prolactin was important in the regulation of osmolar balance. Subsequent studies, however, have failed to support these findings (Adler, Noel, Wartofsky and Frantz, 1975; Keeler and Wilson, 1976; Carey, Johansen and Seif, 1977).

Although the physiological importance of plasma prolactin as a regulator of salt and water balance in man must be seriously questioned, (e.g. there is no evidence of osmolar imbalance in patients who have prolactin-secreting tumours and plasma levels of more than 1000 ng/ml), there are data in the monkey to suggest that prolactin in amniotic fluid may contribute to the maintenance of normal water balance in the amniotic sac (Josimovitch, 1977); this may be one of the reasons for the presence in primates of such large amounts of prolactin in this compartment. The relevance of this finding to the physiology of human pregnancy, however, remains in question.

(c) Metabolic effects—vitamin D metabolism

One of the most fascinating recent developments in the field of prolactin physiology is the finding that prolactin may be involved in the regulation of vitamin D metabolism in the kidney (Lancet, 1977). MacIntyre and colleagues (Spanos, Colston, Evans, Galante, MacAuley and MacIntyre, 1976a) found that prolactin stimulated the enzyme in chick kidney which produces 1,25 dihydroxycholecalciferol (1,25 $(OH)_2D_3$)—the active metabolite of vitamin D. A subsequent study confirmed that the prolactin-induced enzyme effects were followed by a rise in plasma levels of 1,25 $(OH)_2D_3$ (Spanos, Pike, Haussler, Colston, Evans, Goldner, McCain and MacIntyre, 1976b). Furthermore, lactation is associated with a 4-fold rise in 1,25 $(OH)_2D_3$ levels in experimental animals. That prolactin may be important in the major changes in calcium absorption observed during pregnancy is therefore an attractive hypothesis but its application to human prolactin physiology awaits further, more direct evidence.

(d) Interaction with adrenal steroid hormones

Abnormalities of adrenal steroid metabolism have been reported in patients with pathological hyperprolactinaemia (Forbes et al., 1954; Giusti, Bassi, Borsi, Cattaneo, Giannotti, Lanza, Pazzagli, Vigiani and Serio, 1977; Carter, Tyson, Warner, McNeilly, Faiman and Friesen, 1977), but the physiological significance of an interaction of prolactin with ACTH and adrenal steroids in man remains to be established. Of particular interest is the recent observation that human prolactin is able to stimulate cortisol release from human foetal adrenal cells in culture (Glickman, Carson, Naftolin and Challis, 1978) suggesting an adrenocorticotrophic role for prolactin in the foetus (Winters, Colston, MacDonald and Porter, 1975); but these data require support from further in vitro and from in vivo studies.

(e) Foetal lung maturation

Further evidence that prolactin is an important hormone to the developing human foetus comes from a report by Hauth, Parker, MacDonald, Porter and Johnston (1978). In an analysis of data from 191 neonates, these workers noted that the incidence of respiratory distress syndrome (RDS) was much higher in babies whose cord prolactin levels were less than 200 ng/ml. Furthermore, there was a significant correlation of prolactin levels (but not cortisol levels) with foetal weight and gestational age. Because prolactin has been reported to stimulate surfactant production in the rabbit foetus (Hamosh and Hamosh 1977), Hauth et al. (1978) have suggested that foetal prolactin has a similar role in human foetal lung maturation. However, subsequent studies in the rabbit and sheep, using a highly purified ovine prolactin, have failed to demonstrate a direct effect on surfactant production (Gluckman, Ballard, Kitterman, Kaplan and Grumbach, 1978). Gluckman *et al.* (1978) were able to confirm the correlation of RDS with low foetal prolactin levels but suggested that this association may be a reflection of the independent effects of oestrogen on both body weight and lung maturation.

In conclusion it may be asked what, if any, is the feature common to these apparently widely diverse actions of prolactin? Nicoll and Bern (1972) view prolactin as a hormone which may "condition" the responses of the target organ to the trophic effects of other hormones. This mechanism might still operate by means of a common effect at cellular level—perhaps by influencing ion permeability and thereby the intracellular ion concentrations (Nicoll and Bern, 1972).

3. Hormone–Receptor Interaction and Mechanism of Action

Specific binding sites for prolactin have been demonstrated in a wide variety of animal tissues including mammary gland, liver, ovary, testis and adrenal (Posner, Kelly, Shiu and Friesen, 1974). The relation of prolactin receptors to biological function has, in part, been discussed above. In this section, the characteristics and regulation of specific prolactin-binding sites will be discussed in relation to data acquired from the finding of high affinity, limited capacity binding sites in tissues from a variety of species, including man, (reviewed by Posner, 1977). Evidence that the prolactin receptor, as defined from binding studies, is important in modulating the action of prolactin is provided by the studies of Shiu and Friesen (1974, 1976). These workers showed that an antibody to the prolactin receptor blocked prolactin binding and at the same time inhibited the prolactin-mediated incorporation of ^{3}H-leucine into mammary gland casein.

Prolactin-binding sites in rat liver can be induced by oestrogens (and possibly other gonadal steroids), and by prolactin itself (Posner, Kelly and Friesen, 1975). This ability of prolactin to induce and maintain its own receptor in rat liver probably also applies to other tissues (for example, breast) and other species (including man) and may, for example, explain the maintenance of lactation in women despite low circulating levels of prolactin late in the puerperium (Franks, Kiwi and Nabarro, 1977b). The possible mechanisms by which prolactin can regulate its own receptor have been summarised by Posner (1977).

Although it appears that the biological actions of prolactin (at least in the mammary gland) are mediated by binding to a specific plasma membrane receptor (Shiu and Friesen, 1974, 1976), the prolactin molecule itself may participate in the cellular response of the target organ (Nolin and Witorsch,

1976; Nolin, 1978). These data (which are based on immunohistochemical studies) are, however, open to question and although the nature and role of the second messenger for prolactin action remains uncertain there is evidence that the effects of prolactin on the cell membrane may alone be sufficient to trigger RNA synthesis in milk-secreting cells (Rillema and Wild, 1977).

D. CONTROL OF PROLACTIN SECRETION

In 1938, Westman and Jacobsohn observed that pituitary stalk section resulted in pseudopregnancy in the rat. This response, however, was attributed to concurrent cervical stimulation and the significance of this finding was not realised until 1954 when Everett demonstrated that disassociation of the pituitary from the hypothalamus was, alone, capable of resulting in prolonged hypersecretion of prolactin, as judged by mammary growth and luteotrophic activity. Since then much has been learned of the nature of hypothalamic control of prolactin and the physiological and pharmacological factors which influence its secretion in the human, as well as in the rat (Fig. 3).

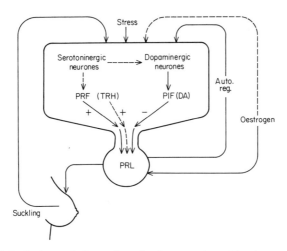

Fig. 3. Physiological regulation of prolactin secretion. The interrupted arrows indicate pathways whose existence are inferred from experimental data in animals and man but whose physiological importance have not yet been established (PRL = prolactin, DA = dopamine, PRF = prolactin releasing factor, TRH = TSH-releasing hormone, PIF = prolactin-inhibiting factor) Auto. reg. = autoregulation by "short-loop" feedback.

1. Prolactin Inhibiting Factor (PIF) and Biogenic Amines

(a) PIF and catecholamines

The presence of a PIF in the rat hypothalamus was first clearly demonstrated in the elegant studies of Pasteels (1962) and Meites, Nicoll and Talwalker (1963). These studies showed that pituitary glands removed from intimate contact with the hypothalamus secreted increasingly large amounts of prolactin. Further evidence for the presence of PIF has been provided by several workers (reviewed by Meites, 1973). The chemical nature of PIF has been the subject of much research in recent years. From both *in vivo* and *in vitro* studies it has been shown that prolactin secretion may be influenced by monoamines. Van Maanen and Smelik (1968) showed that depletion of the catecholamine content of the hypothalamus by reserpine implants increased prolactin secretion in the rat. A direct inhibitory effect of catecholamines (of which the most active was dopamine) on rat pituitary explants was reported by MacLeod (1969), Koch, Lu and Meites (1970), Birge, Jacobs, Hammer and Daughaday (1970) and MacLeod and Lehmeyer (1972). Kamberi, Mical and Porter (1971a) observed that prolactin secretion in the intact animal was suppressed by the intraventricular infusion of dopamine. MacLeod (1969) suggested that PIF was dopamine itself and subsequently Takahara, Arimura and Schally (1974) showed that a purified preparation of porcine hypothalami with high PIF activity contained large concentrations of catecholamines. They demonstrated that the *in vivo* activity of PIF infused in the hypophyseal portal system of the rat was closely related to dopamine content, thus providing strong support for the concept that dopamine itself is an important PIF. This finding has since been confirmed by a number of groups. That dopamine may not be the only PIF is suggested by recent studies which have shown that hypothalamic extracts which are free of catecholamines may still have PIF activity (Schally, Dupont, Arimura, Takahara, Redding, Clemens and Shaar, 1976; Enjalbert, Moos, Carbonell, Priam and Kordon, 1977); but the physiological importance of this dopamine-free prolactin inhibitory activity remains to be determined.

(b) Serotonin and melatonin

While dopamine has been shown to inhibit prolactin release, serotonin appears to stimulate its secretion. Kamberi, Mical and Porter (1971b) reported a rise in serum prolactin concentrations after injection of serotonin into the third ventricle of the rat. Serotonin is not thought to cross the blood–brain barrier, and not surprisingly, a systemic injection in the rat was ineffective; but i.v. injection of the serotonin precursor, 5 hydroxy-tryptophan (5 HTP) has been shown to increase prolactin levels (Meites, 1973). Studies in the rat suggest that serotoninergic neurones in the hypothalamus have the capacity to stimulate prolactin secretion, either by a direct effect on pro-lactin-releasing factor or by interacting with the dopaminergic system (Talwalker, Ratner and Meites, 1963; Neill, 1974; Kordon, Blake, Terkel and Sawyer, 1973; Advis, Simpkins, Bennett and Meites, 1977). Although the serotonergic control of prolactin secretion may be important, it appears from pharmacological experiments in the rat that the dopaminergic pathway is dominant (MacLeod, 1977). There is, at present, little direct evidence that serotonin affects prolactin secretion in man, but 5-HTP has been shown to stimulate prolactin secretion in normal subjects, (Kato, Nakai, Imura, Chihara and Ohgo, 1974). The serotonin antagonist, methysergide, lowers prolactin levels but these data must be interpreted with caution since this drug has been shown also to possess dopamine-agonist properties (Login and MacLeod, 1977).

There is some evidence that the pineal gland has prolactin-regulatory activity (Blask, Vaughan, Reiter, Johnson and Vaughan, 1976) and in this context, melatonin (a product of serotonin) has been shown to stimulate prolactin secretion (Meites, 1973).

2. Prolactin Releasing Factor (PRF) and TRH

The presence of a physiologically important hypothalamic PRF was postu-lated by Valverde, Chieffo and Reichlin (1972) who prepared an extract from porcine hypothalami which could stimulate prolactin secretion in oestrogen- and progesterone-primed rats. Following reports that native TRH stimulated prolactin release from rat pituitary cells in culture (Tashjian, Barowsky and Jensen, 1971), there have been a number of *in vivo* studies which indicate that exogenous TRH is a potent stimulator of prolactin secretion. The prolactin response to TRH is modified by the sex and thyroid status of the subject tested (Bowers, Friesen, Hwang, Guyda and Folkers, 1971; Bowers, Friesen and Folkers, 1973; Jacobs, Snyder, Utiger and Daughaday, 1973) (see also Section F.2). The finding that a detectable rise in prolactin levels may be seen after a very small dose of TRH (a dose which is too small to stimulate a measurable increase of TSH) (Jacobs *et al.*, 1973) has led to speculation that TRH is the physiological releasing factor for both TSH and prolactin. This seems unlikely since, in many respects (e.g. during nursing) the control of TSH and prolactin are clearly independent (Reichlin, Martin, Mitnick, Boshans, Grimm, Bollinger, Gordon and Malacara, 1972). Furthermore, it has been demonstrated that PRF activity is present in hypothalamic extracts which are free from TRH (Valverde *et al.*, 1972).

3. Autoregulation of Prolactin Secretion

Several workers have provided evidence that prolactin may regulate its own secretion by a "short-loop" feedback from the pituitary to the hypothalamic regulatory centres (reviewed by Neill, 1974). In the rat, transplants beneath the renal capsule of either a normal pituitary or of a prolactin-secreting pituitary adenoma will reduce the prolactin content of the *in situ* pituitary; cultured *in vitro*, the *in situ* gland incorporates less amino acid. A pituitary transplant will reduce the rise in prolactin content of the *in situ* gland which is normally induced by suckling. Implants of prolactin to the rat median eminence reduce both serum prolactin levels and pituitary content. These hypothalamic implants have profound physiological effects in that they have been shown to block pseudopregnancy and to block milk secretion in the lactating rat. Iontophoretic application of prolactin to hypothalamic neurones in the rat suggest that the hypothalamic areas involved in the control of prolactin secretion are within the dorsomedial, ventromedial and habenular nuclei (Yamada, 1975). The results of experiments using iontophoretic techniques must always be viewed with care but if the data hold true it seems that the feedback control of prolactin is mediated through hypothalamic areas which are at the brain side of the blood–brain barrier. The route by which circulating prolactin reaches them is not known, but it has been postulated that CSF mediates this transport (MacLeod and Login, 1977). The intriguing finding that there are specific binding sites for prolactin in the choroid plexus of many mammalian species (Walsh, Posner, Kopriwa and Brawer, 1978) raises the question of the presence of a specific transport mechanism for prolactin in this organ.

4. Suckling Stress and Sleep

Physiological stimuli of prolactin secretion include suckling, stress and sleep, all of which appear to be mediated by neuro-regulatory pathways terminating in dopaminergic or serotoninergic neurones in the hypothalamus. A description of the neural pathways involved in the control of prolactin secretion in the rat and human is beyond the scope of this chapter, but these have been well reviewed by Neill (1974) and Martin, Reichlin and Brown (1977).

The rise in prolactin induced by suckling (Hwang *et al.*, 1971; Tyson *et al.*, 1972; Frantz *et al.*, 1972; Noel, Suh and Frantz, 1974) is clearly important in the maintenance of puerperal lactation and is thought to be effected by a neuro-endocrine reflex triggered by nipple stimulation. A rise in prolactin has also been observed in response to nipple stimulation in a small proportion of normal non-lactating women and occasionally in men (Kolodny, Jacobs and Daughaday, 1972; Noel *et al.*, 1974). These and other studies suggest that the suckling reflex may be altered by psychological factors.

Both physical and psychological stress may lead to a significant increase in prolactin secretion (Neill, 1970; 1974; Frantz *et al.*, 1972) and it is therefore important to consider this factor in interpretation of results of all studies of prolactin secretion. The stress associated with the induction of anaesthesia and with surgical procedures has been reported to be an important stimulant of prolactin release (Frantz *et al.*, 1972; Frantz, 1973). The "stress" of hypoglycaemia also raises prolactin levels and insulin-induced hypoglycaemia has been used as a dynamic test of prolactin secretion (Frantz *et al.*, 1972 and see Section F.2).

The sleep related rise in prolactin levels in normal subjects will be discussed in Section F.1.

5. Oestrogens

Oestrogens have been shown to stimulate prolactin secretion in both experimental animals and in the human (for reviews see Meites, 1973; Frantz *et al.*, 1972; Neill, 1974; MacLeod, 1976). Indeed, in the rat, prolonged oestrogen stimulation has been shown to induce chronic hypersecretion of prolactin and proliferation of pituitary lactotrophs (Lloyd, Meares and Jacobi, 1973). Endogenous oestrogen secretion is thought to account for the sex difference in both basal and stimulated prolactin levels and for the rise in prolactin levels observed during pregnancy (see Section F.1). There is some controversy as to whether there is any significant variation of prolactin levels during the menstrual cycle (Section F.1). Oral contraceptives containing as little as 30 µg ethinyl oestradiol have been shown to increase prolactin levels, although these concentrations are rarely outside the normal range (Abu-Fadil, Devane, Siler and Yen, 1976; Deriks-Tan and Taubert, 1976; Franks, 1977). However, there is no evidence that the oral contraceptive is an important factor in the aetiology of prolactin-secreting pituitary tumours in women with hyperprolactinaemic amenorrhoea (Jacobs, Knuth, Hull and Franks, 1977; G. Tolis, personal communication, 1978). The site of action of oestrogens appears to be both at hypothalamic level and directly on the pituitary (Neill, 1974; Labrie, Ferland, DeLean, Legacé, Drouin, Beaulieu, Vincent and Massicotte, 1978).

6. Peptide Hormones

A most interesting development in the last year has been the observation that a number of naturally occurring small peptides are able to stimulate the secretion of prolactin. These include beta-endorphin, neurotensin, substance P and bombesin (Rivier, Brown and Vale, 1977; Rivier, Vale, Ling, Brown and Guillemin, 1977; Rivier, Rivier and Vale, 1978). It should be stressed that many of these studies are preliminary and have been performed in experimental animals; thus the role of these peptides in human prolactin physiology remains to be ascertained.

7. Drugs Which Affect Prolactin Secretion

A large number of pharmacological agents has been shown to influence prolactin secretion (Fluckiger, 1972; Daughaday, 1974; Besser and Thorner, 1976) (Table 1). Drugs which deplete the hypothalamic content of dopamine

Table 1
Drugs which influence serum prolactin concentrations.

Drugs which raise prolactin concentrations	Drugs which lower prolactin concentrations
Dopamine depleting drugs	Dopamine agonists
α-methyl dopa	L-dopa
reserpine	apomorphine
Dopamine receptor blocking agents	ergot derivatives
phenothiazines (chlorpromazine)	(bromocriptine, lergotrile,
pimozide	lisuride, metergoline)
benzamides (sulpiride, metoclopramide)	Serotonin antagonists
butyrophenones (haloperidol)	methysergide[b]
opiates[a] (morphine)	
TRH	
Oestrogens	

[a] The mechanism of action of these compounds is not certainly known but opiates are probably dopamine receptor blocking drugs.
[b] Methysergide may also possess a dopamine receptor blocking action.

(such as alpha-methyl-dopa and reserpine) or antagonise the action of dopamine at the receptor level (e.g. phenothiazines, sulpiride, metoclopramide) all tend to raise prolactin levels (Calaf, 1973; Thorner, Besser, Hagen, and McNeilly, 1974a). The stimulatory actions of TRH and oestrogens have been discussed above (Sections D.2, 5).

Dopamine agonists and drugs which increase the hypothalamic (or pituitary) content of dopamine suppress prolactin secretion. Recent studies suggest that a direct action of dopamine agonists or antagonists may be of considerable, and in many cases, primary importance in the control of prolactin secretion by these agents (MacLeod, 1976). The finding that L-dopa was effective in reducing serum prolactin levels in both normoprolactinaemic and hyperprolactinaemic subjects (Malarkey, Jacobs and Daughaday, 1971; Frantz *et al.*, 1972) led to trials of L-dopa in the suppression of both puerperal and inappropriate lactation. However, the action of L-dopa is both short-lived and unpredictable and in therapeutic use it has been superseded by bromocriptine (2-brom-α-ergocryptine, CB154—a Sandoz product). Both drugs appear to act, principally, by activation of dopamine receptors on the lactotrophs but bromocriptine, a semi-synthetic ergot alkaloid, is a long-acting dopamine agonist which is effective in suppressing prolactin levels for up to 12 hr after a single dose. Its use has greatly facilitated the treatment of hyperprolactinaemic conditions (Section F.3).

E. METHODS OF MEASUREMENT

The last seven to eight years have seen significant development in the techniques of prolactin assay. Since Forsyth's review in 1967, bioassay methods have become more sensitive and the widespread availability of radio-immunoassay has inevitably resulted in rapid advancement of our understanding of normal and disordered prolactin secretion.

1. Bioassay

(a) *The pigeon crop sac assay*

The classical method of measurement of prolactin was the pigeon crop sac assay developed by Riddle, Bates and Dykshorn (1933). Although this proved to be a useful marker for lactogenic activity in human serum (Canfield and Bates, 1965) modifications of this method (reviewed by Forsyth, 1967; Forsyth and Parke, 1973) have failed to increase the specificity or sensitivity of the assay sufficiently to allow confident quantitation of circulating prolactin levels in man.

(b) In vitro *mammary gland stimulation assays*

A few years ago *in vitro* bioassay systems using isolated mammary gland tissue were developed for the measurement of human serum prolactin levels. These assays relied on the secretory activity, in response to prolactin, of breast tissue from the pregnant mouse (Loewenstein, Mariz, Peake and Daughaday, 1971; Turkington, 1971; Frantz *et al.*, 1972) or mammary tissue from the pseudopregnant rabbit (Forsyth and Myres, 1971). Forsyth and Myres (1971) and Frantz *et al.*, (1972) used an histological end point to assess the tissue response. The precision and sensitivity of these assays showed considerable improvement over the previous bioassays, but even so, it was not possible to detect, with any reliability, basal prolactin levels in non-lactating women and in normal men. The mouse assay appeared the more sensitive, but the coefficient of variation of measurements of serum samples was about 30% (Frantz *et al.*, 1972). The rabbit assay was even less precise and was considered by Forsyth and Parke (1973) to be only semi-quantitative.

The ability of prolactin to stimulate the production of milk proteins, fats, and sugars prompted a number of groups to use biochemical markers to determine the end point of the mammary gland bioassay. Loewenstein *et al.* (1971) for example, estimated the *n*-acetyl-lactosamine synthetic activity in pregnant mouse glands and Turkington (1971) measured the incorporation of ^{32}P into casein. These and other workers reported good precision but no great improvement of sensitivity compared with histological methods (Forsyth and Parke, 1973). Furthermore, the complexity of these methods limited their use as routine assays. Both HGH and HPL cross-reacted in all bioassay systems but this problem could be overcome by neutralisation of these hormones by the addition of specific antisera. The use of bioassay for the routine measurement of prolactin has been largely superseded by radioimmunoassay which offers the advantages of greater simplicity, sensitivity, precision and the ability to process large numbers of samples. However, bioassay still has a place in comparative physiology and in the assessment of biological activity of reference preparations or plasma samples.

2. Radioimmunoassay (RIA)

The successful isolation of prolactin from primate pituitary tissue (Guyda and Friesen, 1971; Lewis *et al.*, 1971b; Hwang *et al.*, 1972; 1973) has led to the development of specific RIA methods for human prolactin. The ideal requirements of an RIA for prolactin are that it should be specific enough to distinguish prolactin from growth hormone or placental lactogen and that it should be sensitive enough to measure circulating levels in normal men and in non-puerperal women as well as detecting levels during lactation and in pathological states such as galactorrhoea.

(a) Heterologous and homologous radioimmunoassay

Early RIA's for human prolactin were of two types:

(i) Homologous systems utilising the same prolactin (sheep, monkey or baboon) for preparation of radioactive label and antibody, with reference preparations obtained from human pituitary or plasma (Hwang et al., 1971; Frantz et al., 1972; L'Hermite, Delvoye, Nokin, Vekemans and Robyn, 1972).

(ii) Heterologous assays in which the materials used for iodination and for raising antisera were obtained from animals of different species (Josimovich, Bocella and Levitt, 1971; Jacobs, Mariz and Daughaday, 1972; Aubert, Grumbach and Kaplan, 1974b). These assays appeared to be specific for prolactin, showed parallelism between standards and plasma samples and were sensitive enough to measure levels in normal subjects; but the main disadvantage of these systems was the lack of precision in plasma measurements (Robyn, 1973; Jacobs, 1973; Greenwood, et al., 1973).

When purified preparations of human pituitary prolactin became more widely available, homologous radioimmunoassay utilising human prolactin ^{125}I or ^{131}I label and anti-human-prolactin antiserum became the method of choice in most circumstances. In the published methods (most of which employ a double antibody method for separating bound from free radioactivity) specificity, sensitivity and precision seem highly satisfactory. Specificity of RIA depends in part on the characteristics of the labelled antigen and the antibody. In most assays in current use, parallelism of pituitary and plasma standards has been noted and HGH or HPL do not cross-react at all with prolactin. This specificity is important since prolactin levels are often measured during pregnancy or in patients with acromegaly. Radioimmunoassay does not appear to distinguish between monomeric prolactin or higher molecular weight forms in the serum (Lequin and Rolland, 1977); however these heterogeneous forms also appear to possess similar receptor binding properties as judged from other methods of assay. The detection limit of homologous radioimmunoassays using human materials is in the region of 0·5–1 ng/ml (Franks, 1977), i.e. at the lower limit or below the physiological range of plasma levels in normal subjects (Section F.1).

There have been few problems associated with the RIA of prolactin. Intermittent difficulties have been encountered in the iodination of prolactin using the chloramine-T method (reviewed by Franks, 1977), but this process has generally not presented any difficulties. The one major problem is that of standardisation of results between laboratories; this will be discussed in detail below.

(b) *Comparison of radioimmunoassay and bioassay results*

Since RIA measures immunological activity of the hormone and not biological activity, correlative studies of results obtained in the same serum samples by the two methods of assay are clearly of importance (Bangham and Borth, 1972). Early reports showed a rank order correlation of bioassay and RIA values (Greenwood *et al.*, 1973); these findings were confirmed by Frantz *et al.*, (1972) and Besser, Parke, Edwards, Forsyth and McNeilly (1972) who were able to show good agreement in the absolute values in samples measured by the two methods (Fig. 4).

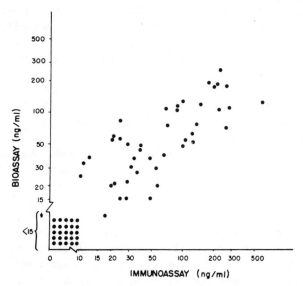

Fig. 4. Correlation of results of plasma prolactin concentrations measured by bioassay (mouse mammary gland) and radioimmunoassay. Bioassay results are expressed in terms of NIH-P-S8 ovine standard and radioimmunoassay levels in terms of a Friesen human pituitary standard. From Frantz *et al.* (1972) with permission.

(c) Pituitary prolactin standards and problems in standardisation of RIA

The original RIA's for human prolactin were developed before purified human prolactin was available and, not surprisingly, used a wide range of reference preparations, most of which were human serum samples which had high prolactin activity, calibrated against sub-primate pituitary prolactin standards. The subsequent widespread use of purified human prolactin and specific antisera supplied by laboratories of Dr. Friesen and Dr. Lewis* resulted in some continuity between laboratories in the choice of refe ence preparation. A collaborative study was conducted by the National Pituitary Agency (NPA) (Aubert, Becker, Saxena and Raiti, 1974a)

* These preparations have been generously made available to interested research workers by the National Pituitary Agency (NIAMDD, USA).

using the RIA "kits" supplied by Lewis and by Friesen. Analysis of serum samples by seven RIA methods using these kits in three laboratories generally showed good agreement in serum prolactin levels measured against either the Lewis or Friesen standard, but values in the range of 1–10 ng/ml were much more variable. Iodination of the pituitary preparations yielded satisfactory results using the chloramine-T method. The choice of antiserum did not affect the absolute serum concentrations measured, although at equivalent titres the Friesen antiserum produced a steeper standard curve; these results were encouraging but the need for an international reference preparation for prolactin was clear (Cotes, 1972, 1973). Cotes (1972) distributed a human prolactin standard prepared by Dr. Friesen (Hwang *et al.*, 1972) which was termed MRC research standard A, preparation 71/222. This was designated as containing a 10 mu/ampoule. The purity of this standard was estimated at between 30 and 50% and its potency defined in both bioassay and radioimmunoassay systems. However, for a number of reasons, this standard has proved unsatisfactory. In particular, the contents of the ampoule estimated against widely used NPA standards has varied considerably between laboratories and in some cases, lack of parallelism between the dose response curve of 71/222 and pituitary or plasma preparations has been noted (Cotes, 1973; Franks, 1977). The result is that 71/222 has not been widely adopted as a reference preparation and a new standard has been prepared and tested on behalf of the WHO (20th Expert Committee on Biological Standardisation).

The report of the new International Reference Preparation (IRP) for Human Prolactin describes the results of a collaborative study involving 15 laboratories across the world (Cotes and Das, 1978). IRP is a purified pituitary prolactin preparation (supplied by the NPA) which is stable and which gives a dose-response curve which is parallel to other purified prolactin standards and (in most cases) to serum standards. Estimations of plasma and serum samples measured against IRP showed good rank order correlation between assay systems. There was, however, considerable variability in absolute values in the different laboratories and there was also poor agreement in consecutive measurements made in the same laboratory. This latter observation was thought to indicate problems inherent in calibrating any new laboratory standard. Nevertheless, IRP showed important improvements over 71/222 particularly in stability and identity with pituitary and plasma standards.

Overall, IRP was considered to meet the requirements of an international research standard for prolactin and this preparation is now available on request from the National Institute of Biological Standards and Control, Hampstead, London. To provide continuity with the old standard, 71/222, it has been proposed that, based on figures from comparative studies in the

WHO report, the IRP should, by definition, contain 650 mu (equivalent to 20 µg) per ampoule.

3. Radioreceptor Assay

The uptake and binding of ^{125}I prolactin to rabbit mammary tissue was detected by Falconer (1972) and, subsequently, specific binding sites for prolactin were identified in a number of tissues (Turkington and Frantz, 1972; Shiu, Kelly and Friesen, 1973). Turkington, Frantz and Majumder (1973) and Shiu et al. (1973) took advantage of this phenomenon to develop a radioreceptor assay for prolactin. Friesen and colleagues (Shiu et al., 1973) used an assay based on the binding of ^{125}I-prolactin to mammary tissue from the mid-pregnant rabbit pretreated with cortisol and HPL. This assay had the advantage of simplicity over regular bioassays and could be considered to reflect biological activity (although apart from in the breast, it may not always be correct to assume that the presence of specific binding sites for prolactin in a tissue necessarily implies biological activity in that tissue). There was a good correlation of results obtained by radioreceptor assay and RIA, but Friesen and colleagues found that the sensitivity of the radioreceptor assay was insufficient to allow quantitation of basal serum prolactin levels in normal subjects. Like the mammary gland bioassays described above, the radioreceptor assay is not specific for human prolactin; ^{125}I-prolactin could be displaced by prolactins from a number of species as well as by HPL and HGH. However, as Friesen pointed out, radioreceptor assay is not intended to replace RIA but rather to act as a complement to it; radioreceptor assay produces a quick and simple means for the assessment of lactogenic hormones in general and is an ideal tool for comparative studies for prolactin from any number of avian or mammalian species (Friesen, Tolis, Shiu and Hwang, 1973).

F. PLASMA LEVELS

1. Normal Subjects

(a) Age and sex differences in adults

Basal prolactin levels in adult males and females, as measured by radio-immunoassay, were reported in early studies to range from 0–30 ng/ml, with a mean of 10–15 ng/ml (Hwang et al., 1971; Friesen et al., 1972; Frantz et al., 1972; Sinha et al., 1973). Later studies from Friesen's laboratory indicated that the mean levels in terms of Friesen's standard were rather lower than had been previously reported (7·9 ± 0·4, (s.e.m.) ng/ml in women and

5·2 ± 0·55 in men) and that there was a statistically significant difference in prolactin concentrations between adult men and women. Postmenopausal levels were not significantly different from those obtained in women of reproductive age (Guyda and Friesen, 1973). Data from our own laboratory (Franks, Murray, Jequier, Steele, Nabarro and Jacobs, 1975; Franks, 1977) are in agreement with these figures. The mean prolactin concentrations in 50 premenopausal women was 7·2 ± 0·4 (s.e.m.) ng/ml, in 40 postmenopausal women was 6·8 ± 0·3 and in 30 men was 6·2 ± 0·3. There was no significant difference between levels in the three groups.

(b) Twenty-four hour pattern of secretion

The 24 hr pattern of secretion has been well defined. Prolactin appears to be released in a pulsatile fashion, but these pulses are not large except during sleep when marked rises in prolactin concentrations have been noted (Nokin, Vekemens, L'Hermite and Robyn, 1972; Sassin, Frantz, Kapen and Weitzman, 1973; Parker and Rossman, 1973). Nevertheless, it is advisable to assess basal prolactin levels on the basis of at least two plasma samples since pulsatility together with the stress of venepuncture may occasionally give misleadingly high levels (Parker and Rossman, 1973; Frantz et al., 1972). Nokin et al. (1972) suggested that, like ACTH, prolactin showed a true circadian rhythm independent of sleep, but a more recent study (Sassin et al., 1973) showed that the nocturnal rise of prolactin was dependent on sleep (Fig. 5). Although Sassin et al. (1973) were unable to correlate the surge in prolactin secretion to a particular stage of sleep, Parker, Rossman and Vanderlaan (1974) have suggested that peak levels correspond to periods of non-REM (rapid eye movement) sleep. The sleep-related rise in prolactin is usually absent in patients with prolactin-secreting tumours (Section F. 3) (Jacobs and Daughaday, 1973; Franks, Jacobs, Hull, Steele and Nabarro, 1977a) and in patients with anorexia nervosa (G. Tolis, 1978, personal communication). The nocturnal rise in prolactin can be inhibited by dopamine-agonist drugs and by methysergide (Mendelson, Jacobs, Reichman, Othmer, Cryer, Trivedi and Daughaday, 1975).

(c) Menstrual cycle

There is still some controversy regarding the variability in prolactin levels throughout the menstrual cycle. L'Hermite, Vekemens, Delvoye, Nokin and Robyn (1973) reported that there was a significant increase of prolactin in the luteal phase of the cycle but McNeilly and Chard (1974), whilst noting that levels in the luteal phase were higher in some cases, showed that in eight women the mean basal concentrations were not significantly different in the two phases of the cycle. In addition, McNeilly and Chard were unable

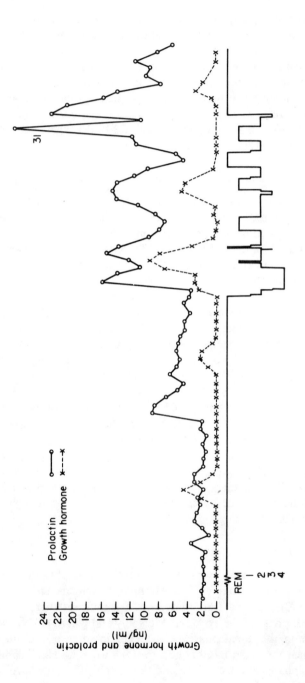

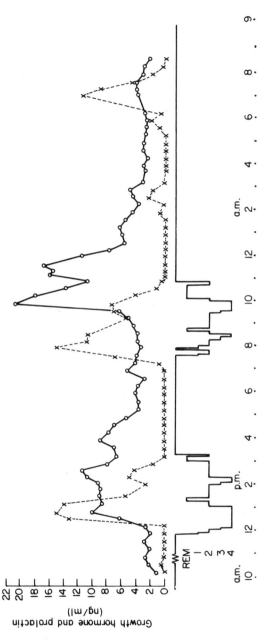

Fig. 5. 24 hr pattern of prolactin secretion in a normal male subject. The upper panel shows prolactin and HGH concentrations during a normal day in a single subject and the lower panel shows the hormone levels, in the same subject, after reversal of the normal sleep pattern. Note the episodic nature of prolactin secretion particularly during sleep (REM = rapid eye movement). From Sassin *et al.* (1973) with permission.

to show a correlation of prolactin concentrations with oestradiol-17β as had been reported by L'Hermite and colleagues. In both these studies the day-to-day fluctuation of prolactin levels throughout the cycle was confirmed. However, a more recent study from Robyn's laboratory (Robyn *et al.*, 1977) showed that in an analysis of a total of 51 normal menstrual cycles there was a consistent and significant mid-cycle peak of prolactin and levels during the luteal phase were clearly higher than those obtained in the follicular phase of the cycle. Any change in prolactin levels during the cycle is likely to be secondary to changes in oestradiol secretion (Robyn *et al.*, 1977) and not functionally important in normal ovulation since patients whose prolactin secretion is suppressed by bromocriptine may still have ovulatory cycles (see Section C.2).

(d) Pregnancy and lactation

Prolactin levels rise steadily during pregnancy reaching a maximum in the third trimester (Hwang *et al.*, 1971; Tyson *et al.*, 1972; Friesen, 1973; Tyson

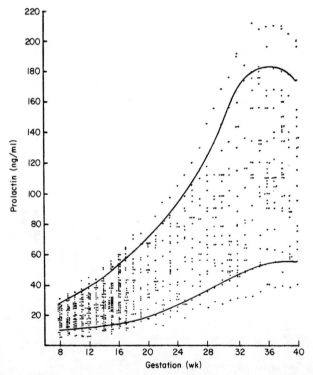

Fig. 6. Plasma prolactin concentrations in normal pregnancy. The solid lines indicate the 90th and 10th centiles. From Biswas and Rodeck (1976) with permission.

et al., 1975, Biswas and Rodeck, 1976) (Fig. 6). In the puerperium, basal prolactin concentrations return to pre-partum levels, often within a week, but for up to three months after delivery, prolactin secretion increases in response to suckling. Thereafter, lactation continues even though suckling induces only a small or no rise in prolactin (Fig. 7). However, lactating mothers in Central Africa who nurse on demand, for up to 24 months post-partum, have persistently elevated prolactin levels during lactation (Robyn *et al.*, 1977). The role of prolactin secretion in the maintenance of lactation has been discussed above (Section C.2).

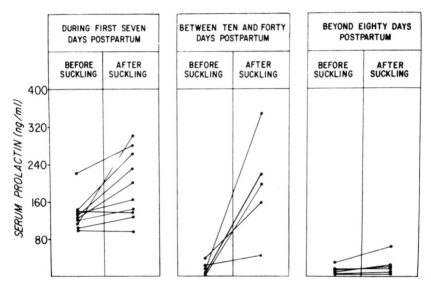

Fig. 7. Serum prolactin concentrations in response to suckling in normal post-partum women. From Tyson *et al.* (1972) with permission.

(e) *Amniotic fluid and foetal pituitary and plasma levels*

As previously described, amniotic fluid contains very large amounts of prolactin. The concentration increases rapidly from the 12th to the 24th week of pregnancy to reach about 4 µg/ml (Tyson *et al.*, 1972; McNeilly, Gilmore, Jeffery, Dobbie and Chard, 1977) and although levels decrease during the last six weeks of pregnancy, the mean concentration at term is still in the region of 10 times the maternal plasma level (Schenker, Ben David and Polishuk, 1975). Few data are available on prolactin levels in the human foetus. Kaplan, Grumbach and Aubert (1976) in a study of 55 human foetuses reported a rise in pituitary prolactin concentrations from about 100 days of gestation. Prolactin is detectable in the serum at about 90 days, but levels remain low until 180 days. There is then a steady increase so that at term the mean umbilical vein plasma level is about 200 ng/ml.

(f) Infancy, childhood and puberty

Serum prolactin levels are between 200–300 ng/ml in the first three days of life and then decline to reach a plateau of about 100 ng/ml until four weeks of age. Thereafter, there is a progressive fall towards prepubertal levels so that the mean concentration between three and 12 months of age is approximately 10 ng/ml (Guyda and Friesen, 1973; Aubert, Grumbach and Kaplan, 1975). In the premature infant, plasma prolactin levels during the first three days of life are significantly lower than in a healthy infant, but at six weeks of age levels in premature babies are higher than in normal infants. Between the ages of two and 12 years prolactin levels are not significantly different from those in adults (Guyda and Friesen, 1973; Ehara, Yen and Siler, 1975; 1975; Lee, Jaffe and Midgley, 1974; Franks and Brook, 1976). In a longitudinal study through puberty, Ehara and colleagues noted an increase in prolactin levels in girls between the ages of 14 and 15 (i.e. late puberty) and these data have since been confirmed by Aubert et al. (1975) and Thorner, Round, Jones, Fahmy, Groom, Butcher and Thompson (1977). This rise in prolactin in late puberty appears to be secondary to an increase in serum oestradiol levels. Although changes in prolactin secretion have been implicated in timing the onset of puberty in the rat (Wuttke and Gelato, 1976) it is not known whether prolactin has a similar role in man.

2. Dynamic Tests of Prolactin Secretion

(a) TRH

The administration of exogenous TRH is a safe, practical and informative test of the pituitary prolactin reserve. 100 µg of TRH will produce a maximal prolactin response (Jacobs et al., 1973) but, as the optimal dose for the stimulation of TSH is 200 µg, this dose is usually chosen for the test. As with TSH, the prolactin response to TRH is greater in men than in women, is impaired in hyperthyroidism and increased in hypothyroidism (Fig. 8). The TRH-stimulated prolactin levels in prepubertal children of either sex are not significantly different from those found in men (Foley, Jacobs, Hoffman, Daughaday and Blizzard, 1972; Guyda and Friesen, 1973; Franks and Brook, 1976). The TRH test is a useful indication of pituitary prolactin reserve in patients with hypopituitarism. Basal prolactin levels are rarely unmeasurable, even after hypophysectomy, but the response to TRH denotes the functional capacity of the remaining lactotrophs. The diagnostic role of the TRH test in hyperprolactinaemic conditions is discussed below (Section F.3).

(b) Chlorpromazine, sulpiride and metoclopramide

The knowledge that phenothiazines and related drugs stimulate prolactin release has been utilised in the development of chlorpromazine or sulpiride stimulation tests. Consistency of results has been reported when the drug is given by intramuscular injection (Turkington, 1972a; Frantz *et al.*, 1972;

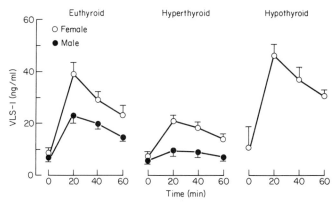

Fig. 8. Prolactin response to TRH. M ± S.E.M. prolactin concentration before and after 200 μg TRH are shown in normal subjects and in those with thyroid disease.

Thorner *et al.*, 1974a). The anti-emetic metoclopromide is also a potent stimulant of prolactin secretion and evaluation of the prolactin response to an intramuscular injection of 10 mg of metoclopramide has been advocated as a simple and reliable test of pituitary prolactin reserve (Judd, Lazarus and Smythe, 1976). The site of action of these drugs is not entirely clear; they may have a direct effect on the pituitary as well as a hypothalamic action (MacLeod, 1976). In general, these tests have no practical advantages over the TRH test.

(c) Intravenous insulin

The fact that insulin-induced hypoglycemia will induce a rise in serum prolactin has led to its use as a test for prolactin secretion. Frantz *et al.* (1972) have shown that with adequate hypoglycemia all subjects tested showed a prolactin response of i.v. insulin, but the peak level varied from

2–19 times the basal level. More recent studies have shown more reliable responses and suggested that a fall in blood glucose to 1·7 mmol/l (35 mg/dl) or below is sufficient to evoke a response (Copinschi, L'Hermite, Vanhaelst, Leclercq, Bruno, Golstein, Ooms and Robyn, 1973). There appears to be no significant difference in the mean prolactin response to hypolglycaemia in men compared with women or in adults compared with children (Franks, 1977). Because of the problems associated with hypoglycaemia, the insulin test is rarely used as a primary test of prolactin reserve but it is convenient to measure prolactin levels in patients with pituitary disease who are undergoing the test for assessment of HGH or ACTH secretion.

(d) L-*Dopa and bromocriptine*

Dopamine agonist drugs such as L-dopa and bromocriptine lower prolactin concentrations and at one time it was thought that they might provide a useful way to discriminate between hypothalamic and pituitary hyperprolactinaemia. However, it is clear that both these drugs may act directly at the pituitary level and have the ability to suppress prolactin secretion, even when hyperprolactinaemia is due to the presence of a pituitary tumour.

3. Disorders of Prolactin Secretion

Once reliable methods of measurement of human prolactin became widely available, it became clear that elevated plasma levels of prolactin in patients with or without galactorrhea could be found in a variety of diseases of the pituitary and hypothalamus (Frantz *et al.*, 1972; Jacobs and Daughaday, 1973) and the potential importance of prolactin measurements in the investigation and management of patients with pituitary and hypothalamic diseases was recognised. Disorders of prolactin secretion probably represent the most prevalent form of hypothalamic or pituitary disease seen in clinical practice today.

(a) *Causes of hyperprolactinaemia*

As has been previously discussed, a number of drugs may result in excessive secretion of prolactin and this is an important consideration in evaluating the patient with hyperprolactinaemia. The phenothiazines are perhaps responsible for most cases of drug-induced hyperprolactinaemia and management of these patients presents a problem since it is not always possible to withdraw the psychotrophic drugs. If it is necessary to lower prolactin levels, preliminary evidence suggests that bromocriptine does not interfere with the psychotrophic action of the phenothiazines (Beumont, Breuwer.

Pimstone, Vinik and Utian, 1975), but further studies are required to substantiate this claim.

Primary hypothyroidism may be associated with hyperprolactinaemia and galactorrhoea (Van Wyk and Grumbach, 1960; Kinch, Plunkett and Delvin, 1969; Edwards, Forsyth and Besser, 1971). Treatment with thyroxine, in most cases, results in a fall of prolactin levels to normal (Edwards et al., 1971; Franks et al., 1977a). In such cases, if pituitary enlargement is present, the radiological changes regress during treatment, but occasionally a concurrent autonomous prolactin-secreting tumour is present. The TRH test is a useful discriminating index—patients without a tumour have an exaggerated prolactin response to TRH, whilst those with tumours have a blunted response (Tolis and MacKenzie, 1976; Franks, 1977).

Patients with pituitary tumours frequently have hyperprolactinaemia. The tumour itself may secrete prolactin but in some cases hyperprolactinaemia is secondary to upward extension of a non-prolactin-secreting tumour interfering with the production or transport of PIF. Similarly, primary hypothalamic disease may result in hypersecretion of prolactin as does pituitary stalk section.

There are a number of other, rarer causes of hyperprolactinaemia. These include post-encephalitic parkinsonism and injuries to the chest wall (for review see Besser and Edwards, 1972).

(b) Diseases of the pituitary and hypothalamus

Raised serum prolactin concentrations were first demonstrated (by pigeon crop sac bioassay) in patients with pituitary enlargement and galactorrhoea by Canfield and Bates (1965). These findings were subsequently supported by data from other bioassay measurements (Forsyth et al., 1971; Frantz et al., 1972) and later confirmed by specific radioimmunoassay measurements (Frantz et al., 1972; Hwang et al., 1971). In an analysis of 18 patients with chromophobe adenoma of the pituitary, Frantz et al. (1972) reported elevated prolactin levels in more than half of the patients, but noted that galactorrhoea occurred in a minority of hyperprolactinaemic patients. Jacobs and Daughaday (1973) found that raised prolactin levels occurred in 30% of the 13 patients with "functionless" tumours and in a more recent series, Nader, Mashiter, Doyle and Joplin (1976) showed that prolactin levels were elevated in 27 of 34 women with a radiologically abnormal pituitary fossa. Franks, Nabarro and Jacobs (1977c) studied prolactin levels in 111 patients with so-called "functionless" tumours of the pituitary, i.e. with radiological enlargement of the pituitary fossa but with no evidence of acromegaly or Cushing's syndrome. Elevated prolactin concentrations were found in 45 of 64 (70%) patients studied before treatment and in 15 of 47 patients after pituitary surgery (Fig. 9). This figure possibly overestimates the incidence of a prolactinoma as a cause of an enlarged sella turcica; 12 of 45 patients had only slightly elevated prolactin levels which (from the evidence of air encephalographic studies) may have been related to suprasellar extension of a non-functioning pituitary tumour. The tumour may still have been a

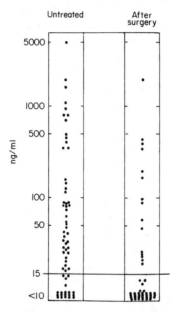

Fig. 9. Serum prolactin concentrations in 111 patients with "functionless" tumours of the pituitary; the horizontal line indicates the upper limit of normal. From Franks *et al.* (1977c) with permission.

prolactinoma, but in the absence of information about specific staining or electron microscopy this remains uncertain. Nevertheless, the significance of the finding of even slightly elevated prolactin levels is illustrated by the fact that suppression of prolactin secretion may lead to return of menstruation in patients in this group (Franks *et al.*, 1977a). In other ways, this study may under-estimate the incidence of prolactinomas; in 14 of the patients with normal prolactin levels and large pituitary fossa, air encephalography was not performed and the possibility of an enlarged but "empty" sella (Kaufman, Pearson and Chamberlin, 1973) could not be ruled out. The majority of hyperprolactinaemic patients presented with amenorrhoea or impotence but galactorrhoea was the exception rather than the rule (Fig. 10). By contrast, reproductive symptoms were uncommon in the group with normal prolactin levels, the diagnosis frequently being made on a skull

X-ray taken for other reasons. An important finding was the delay in recognition of the pituitary tumour as the cause of the reproductive symptoms. Although eight of the men of this series had consulted their physicians on account of impotence, in only one was the pituitary tumour recognised at an early stage. Similarly, in about one-third of women who presented with

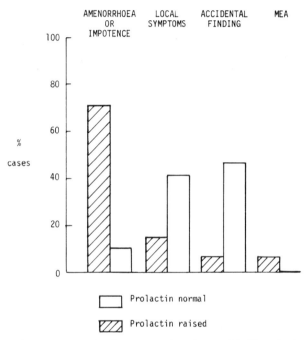

Fig. 10. Presenting symptoms in 64 untreated patients with "functionless" tumours of the pituitary. The mode of presentation in the group of 45 hyperprolactinaemic patients is compared with that in the group of 19 with normal prolactin levels (MEA = multiple endocrine adenomata). The difference between the groups is significant ($\chi^2 = 23; p = <0.001$).

amenorrhoea, the presence of a tumour was not detected until pressure symptoms had occurred. For these reasons, measurement of serum prolactin levels is important in assessment of any patient who presents with amenorrhoea or impotence.

Since growth hormone was known to possess lactogenic properties in many bioassay systems, the occasional finding of galactorrhoea in patients with acromegaly (Davidoff, 1926) had been attributed to high HGH levels. Since RIA measurements have been utilised, raised prolactin levels have been reported to occur in between 8 and 40 % of patients with acromegaly (Hwang *et al.*, 1971; Turkington, 1972b; Sinha *et al.*, 1973; Frantz *et al.*, 1972; Jacobs and Daughaday, 1973). In a recent study of 82 patients with acromegaly, hyperprolactinaemia was found in 26 % of 50 untreated patients but only one of these patients had galactorrhoea (Franks, Jacobs and Nabarro, 1976; Franks, 1977). There was no correlation between prolactin and HGH concentrations. Hypersecretion of prolactin in acromegaly may result from one of two mechanisms:

(i) interference with the synthesis or transport of PIF by suprasellar extension of the growth hormone-secreting tumour (Turkington, 1972b).

(ii) direct hypersecretion of both prolactin and HGH by a single tumour cell type, by two cell types in the same tumour or even by two discrete adenomas (Guyda *et al.*, 1973; Zimmerman, Defendi and Frantz, 1974; Corenblum, Sirek, Horvath, Kovacs and Ezrin, 1976; Tolis, Bertrand, Carpenter and McKenzie, 1978). In the series reported by Franks *et al.* (1976) the second explanation was appropriate in five of 13 cases, but in the majority of patients hypersecretion of prolactin was thought to be secondary to suprasellar extension of the growth hormone secreting tumour. For this reason, the finding of a raised serum prolactin concentration in a patient with acromegaly should be considered an indication for air encephalography, even in the absence of clinical evidence of upward extension of the tumour and even when acromegaly itself is not considered serious enough to warrant surgical treatment. Extrasellar enlargement of the pituitary tumour is usually the explanation for the occasional finding of elevated prolactin levels in patients with Nelson's syndrome.

Hyperprolactinaemia is common in patients with destructive lesions of the hypothalamus. These include tumours such as craniopharyngiomas and granulomatous lesions (Turkington, 1972b; Frantz *et al.*, 1972; Friesen *et al.*, 1973; Jacobs and Daughaday, 1973). Elevated prolactin levels may be the only evidence of endocrine dysfunction in some patients with hypothalamic lesions (Turkington, 1972b; Franks, 1977). Hyperprolactinaemia in patients with hypothalamic disease is associated with prolactin levels which tend to be lower than those seen in patients with prolactin-secreting tumours; prolactin levels of a similar magnitude may be observed in patients following pituitary stalk section (Frantz *et al.*, 1972).

(c) Hyperprolactinaemia and female reproductive function

Both normal and inappropriate lactation may be associated with amenorrhoea. The mechanism causing anovulation and amenorrhoea, in both cases, is thought to involve hypersecretion of prolactin since treatment which reduces serum prolactin concentrations arrests milk formation and restores fertility. These observations have been made both in women lactating after childbirth (Del Pozo and Fluckiger, 1973; Rolland and Schellekens, 1973) and in those with galactorrhoea (Lutterbeck, Pryor, Varga and Wenner, 1971; Besser *et al.*, 1972; Del Pozo, Varga, Wyss, Tolis, Friesen, Wenner, Welter and Uettwiler, 1974; Thorner, McNeilly, Hagen and Besser, 1974b). Since elevated serum prolactin levels may occur without accompanying galactorrhoea, a number of recent studies have attempted to assess the prevalence of hyperprolactinaemia in women presenting with amenorrhoea regardless of presence of galactorrhoea. The results of these studies indicate that hyperprolactinaemia is common and may be found in between 13 and 20% of women with amenorrhoea (Franks *et al.*, 1975; Bohnet, Dahlen, Wuttke and Schneider, 1976; Glass, Williams, Butt, Logan-Edwards and London, 1976; Van Look, McNeilly, Hunter and Baird, 1977). The minority of hyperprolactinaemic patients have radiological evidence of a pituitary tumour and galactorrhoea has been shown to occur in only about 30% of such patients (Franks *et al.*, 1975). In a subsequent prospective study of 100 unselected patients with amenorrhoea (Jacobs, Hull, Murray and Franks, 1975; Franks, 1977) hyperprolactinaemia was found in 19 patients, none of whom was hypothyroid or was taking any drug known to raise prolactin levels. Galactorrhoea occurred in six women, and seven of the 19 patients had abnormalities of the pituitary fossa (i.e. pituitary tumours occurred in 7% of patients with amenorrhoea in this series). Plain radiographs of the skull are not sufficient to exclude the presence of a pituitary tumour. Pro-lactin-secreting tumours are often less than 1 cm in diameter ("micro-tumours"—Hardy, 1973) and may cause asymmetrical enlargement of the fossa. Anterior–posterior and lateral tomography may be needed to make or exclude the diagnosis of a prolactinoma (Hardy, 1973; Vezina and Sutton, 1974; Besser, 1976; Franks and Jacobs, 1977; Vezina, 1978), antunes, Housepian and Frantz (1977) reported that nine of 45 patients with hyper-prolactinaemia had sellar volumes that were within the normal range but that tomography of the fossa revealed abnormalities in eight of the nine. The cause of elevated prolactin levels in patients with normal tomograms remains uncertain; prolactin levels in such patients tend to be below 100 ng/ml (Jacobs, Franks, Murray, Hull, Steele and Nabarro, 1976) and there is evidence to support the hypothesis that these patients too have small pituitary tumours (Jacobs and Franks, 1975).

The endocrine characteristics of hyperprolactinaemic amenorrhoea have been well documented. The episodic release of prolactin in such patients is preserved, but the sleep-related rise in prolactin secretion is absent, even in patients with marginally elevated prolactin levels (Franks *et al.*, 1977a; Fig. 11). The prolactin response to TRH is impaired in patients with hyper-prolactinaemia regardless of the appearance of the pituitary X-rays (Jacobs *et al.*, 1976; Van Look *et al.*, 1977; Corbey, Lequin and Rolland, 1977). In general, stimulation or suppression tests have not been found useful in evaluation of hyperprolactinaemic conditions (Frantz, 1978) but measurements of the prolactin response to TRH may provide a means to assess the functional significance of borderline raised prolactin levels (Franks and Jacobs, 1977; Corby *et al.*, 1977). Patients with hyperprolactinaemia and

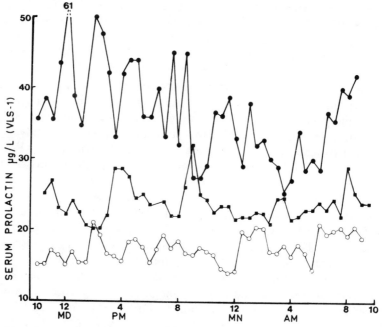

Fig. 11. 24 hr pattern of secretion of prolactin in three women with hyperprolactinaemic amenorrhoea but without enlargement of the pituitary fossa. Note the marked pulsatile secretion but the absence of a sleep-related rise in prolactin even in the patient with marginally elevated prolactin concentrations. From Franks *et al.* (1977a) with permission.

amenorrhoea have clinical, biological and biochemical evidence of oestrogen deficiency. Plasma oestradiol concentrations are low and are frequently below the range of levels seen in normal women during the early follicular phase of the cycle. However, both basal and stimulated gonadotrophin concentrations, even in patients with radiologically apparent pituitary tumours, are comparable to values obtained in normal women during the follicular phase of the cycle (Jacobs *et al.*, 1976). Furthermore, these patients rarely ovulate in response to clomiphene (Jacobs *et al.*, 1976; Bohnet *et al.*, 1976) suggesting a disturbance in the normal hypothalamic-pituitary control of gonadotrophin secretion. Loss of the normal pulsatile pattern of LH secretion (Bohnet *et al.*, 1976) and absence of the oestrogen-mediated positive feedback mechanism (Glass, Shaw, Butt, Logan Edwards and London, 1975; Aono, Miyake, Shioji, Kiwigasa, Oshini and Kurachi, 1976) are additional features which indicate that the primary reproductive disorder in hyper-prolactinaemic amenorrhoea resides at the hypothalamic–pituitary level. Nevertheless, a direct, deleterious action of prolactin on the ovary cannot be discounted (reviewed by Thorner and Besser, 1977).

Amenorrhoea is not the only manifestation of an adverse effect of prolactin on female reproductive function. Although very high prolactin levels are usually associated with complete absence of menses, patients with moderate elevation of prolactin concentrations may present with oligomenorrhoea and infertility or occasionally with regular cycles but a short luteal phase (Del Pozo, Wyss and Varga, 1976). As in patients with amenorrhoea, lowering prolactin levels with bromocriptine or by surgery restores fertility. Hirsutism is recognised to be a feature of hyperprolactinaemic amenorrhoea and recent studies suggest that excessive androgen production may be related to stimulation of the $\Delta 5$ steroid biosynthetic pathway of the adrenal by prolactin (Giusti *et al.*, 1977, Carter *et al.*, 1977).

From the view-point of assessing the patient who presents with galactor-rhoea a few points should be borne in mind. The most common form of galactorrhoea is that associated with normal menses; the majority of such patients have normal basal and stimulated prolactin levels (Kleinberg, Noel and Frantz, 1977). The mechanism of inappropriate milk secretion in these patients is not fully understood but it seems to be prolactin-dependent, since bromocriptine is effective in abolishing the galactorrhoea. Conversely when galactorrhoea is accompanied by amenorrhoea, prolactin levels are almost always elevated.

(d) *Hyperprolactinaemia and male reproductive function*

Friesen *et al.* (1973), in a study of men with prolactin-secreting pituitary tumours, reported low testosterone but normal gonadotrophin levels in patients complaining of impotence. These findings were later confirmed by Faglia and colleagues (Beck-Peccoz, Travaglini, Ambrosi, Rondenna, Paracchi, Spada, Weber, Bara and Rouzin 1977) and by Thorner and Besser (1977) but the latter reported a more variable picture with low or normal testosterone concentrations and impaired, normal or even exaggerated gonadotrophin responses to the gonadotrophin-releasing hormone. In a more recent study, Franks, Jacobs, Martin and Nabarro (1978) analysed the clinical and endocrine features in 29 men with pituitary tumours and hyper-secretion of prolactin. Twenty-one patients had "functionless" pituitary tumours and the remaining eight had acromegaly. None of the patients in this series had galactorrhoea, which emphasises the rarity of this sign in men with

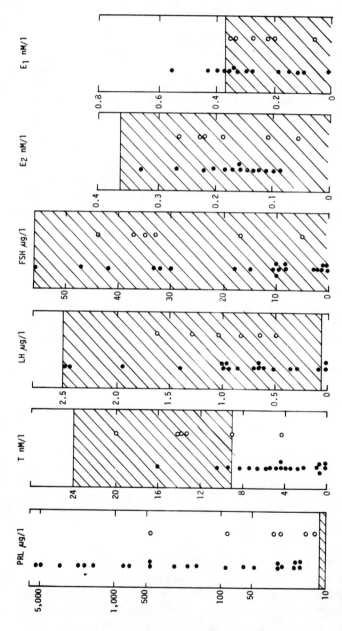

Fig. 12. Concentrations of serum prolactin (PRL) testosterone (T), LH, FSH, oestradiol-17β, (E₂) and oestrone (E₁) in men with hyper-prolactinaemia who have impaired (solid circles) or normal (open circles) sexual function. The hatched areas indicate the normal ranges. From Franks *et al.* (1978) with permission.

hyperprolactinaemia (Kleinberg *et al.*, 1977). Of the 29 men, 23 complained of impotence or loss of libido and the remaining six claimed normal sexual function. Prolactin concentrations were significantly higher and testosterone levels lower in the impotent men than in those with normal sexual function; 18 of 21 impotent patients had sub-normal testosterone levels (Fig. 12) but the testosterone response to HCG was within normal limits. Gonado-trophin concentrations were within the normal range in both groups of hyperprolactinaemic men and the responses of LH and FSH to LH-RH were also normal apart from in two patients who had panhypopituitarism after pituitary surgery. Treatment which lowered prolactin levels resulted in a rise of testosterone and return of potency, without significant changes in gonadotrophin levels. Tolis and Van Vliet (1976) have described loss of normal pulsatile pattern of LH secretion in hyperprolactinaemic men; the pulsatile secretion is restored by reduction of prolactin levels. Thus, the available data suggest that impaired testicular function in hyperprolac-tinaemia is caused by a prolactin-mediated disturbance of hypothalamic-pituitary function. Further studies of the effects of excessive prolactin levels on testicular function is required; little is known about its effect on spermato-genesis (the few semen analyses that have been performed have shown oligospermia) or on Leydig cell morphology. As in patients with amenor-rhoea, hyperprolactinaemia may also have a direct action on the testis in addition to its effects on gonadotrophin secretion.

(e) *Management of hyperprolactinaemic conditions**

The management of a patient with hyperprolactinaemia is the subject of considerable controversy at present (Jacobs, 1976). Clearly, pituitary ablative therapy (usually in the form of surgical removal of the tumour) is mandatory in the presence of a prolactin-secreting tumour which is large enough to cause local symptoms. However, the majority of patients with hyperprolactinaemia do not require pituitary surgery on purely neurological grounds and the approach to management depends on the endocrine manifestations of hyperprolactinaemia. In the patient with hyperprolac-tinaemic amenorrhoea, the major indications for treatment are infertility, galactorrhoea, and symptoms of oestrogen deficiency (dyspareunia, flushes) (Franks *et al.*, 1977a). If, after tomography of the pituitary fossa, there is no radiological evidence of a pituitary tumour, it is the policy of most centres to treat the patient with bromocriptine (Thorner *et al.*, 1974b; Franks *et al.*, 1977a). Bromocriptine has been used with considerable success in the treat-ment of hyperprolactinaemic hypogonadism with or without galactorrhoea. In the series reported from our own laboratory (Franks *et al.*, 1977a) ovula-

*Recent reviews of this subject are by Jacobs, H. S. and Wright, C. (1978). *Br. J. Hosp. Med.* **20**, 652; Reichlin, S. (1979). *New Engl. J. Med.* **300**, 313; Franks, S. (1979). *Drugs* (in press).

tion resumed in all 32 patients who received bromocriptine as primary therapy. Bromocriptine is equally effective in restoring reproductive function in hyperprolactinaemic impotence (Thorner *et al.*, 1974b; Franks *et al.*, 1978).

The most contentious issue in the management of hyperprolactinaemic hypogonadism is the choice of therapy for the patient who has radiological evidence of a pituitary tumour and who wishes to become pregnant. There is a risk of dangerous enlargement of the pituitary tumour during pregnancy (Gemzell, 1975; Lancet, 1976) and although bromocriptine is effective in restoring fertility, even in patients with overt pituitary tumours, the evidence that this drug can reduce tumour growth in man is, at present somewhat anecdotal (reviewed by Franks *et al.*, 1977a). Thus, most endocrinologists advise primary treatment of the tumour by either pituitary surgery or radiotherapy. Irradiation may not result in a significant fall in plasma prolactin levels for several months (Reyes, Gomez and Faiman, 1977) but when supplemented by bromocriptine therapy, it is successful in restoring ovulation and appears to prevent pituitary enlargement during subsequent pregnancy (Child, Gordon, Mashiter and Joplin, 1975; Thorner, Besser, Jones, Dacie and Jones, 1975). However, in centres where the expertise is available, the treatment of choice is surgical removal of the tumour. If a "microtumour" is present, selective transsphenoidal adenomectomy gives highly successful results (Hardy, 1973, 1978). With larger tumours, provided the adenoma is confined to the pituitary fossa, the prognosis after treatment, in terms of return of fertility and preservation of normal pituitary function, is excellent (Franks *et al.*, 1977a; Bertrand and Tolis, 1978). Secondary treatment with bromocriptine may be instituted if necessary. If the aim is not pregnancy but simply restoration of normal menses (and normal oestrogen production), then bromocriptine alone may be given, provided contraceptive measures are taken (Franks *et al.*, 1977a). In men, treatment with bromocriptine alone may be appropriate except in cases where signs of local spread of a pituitary tumour make pituitary ablative therapy necessary.

(f) Prolactin and breast cancer

Whilst there is little doubt that prolactin is capable of stimulating breast tumour growth in rats (for review see McGuire, 1977), the role of prolactin secretion in the development of human mammary tumours remains uncertain. A number of studies have shown that serum prolactin levels are not significantly higher in patients with breast cancer than in normal women or those with benign tumours of the breast (Wilson, Buchan, Roberts, Forrest, Boynes, Cole and Griffiths, 1974; Kwa, De Jong-Bakker, Engelsman and Cléton, 1974; Franks, Ralphs, Seagroatt and Jacobs, 1974), but *in vitro* studies have shown that the growth of some breast cancers is dependent on prolactin (Salih, Flax, Brander and Hobbs, 1972). In patients with hormone-dependent breast cancers, the complex interaction of prolactin and ovarian or adrenal hormone steroids, at the level of the steroid receptor, remains to be clarified (McGuire, 1977).

ACKNOWLEDGEMENTS

During the preparation of this chapter, I was in receipt of an MRC Travelling Research Fellowship. I am indebted to Doctors Harvey Guyda and Bernard Robaire for reviewing the manuscript and for their helpful comments thereon.

REFERENCES

Abu-fadil, S., Devane, G., Siler, T. M. and Yen, S. S. C. (1976). *Contraception*, **13**, 79.

Adler, R. A., Noel, G. L., Wartofsky, L. and Frantz, A. G. (1975). *J. clin. Endocr. Metab.* **41**, 383.

Advis, T. P., Simpkins, J. W., Bennett, J. and Meites, J. (1977). Prog. 59th Meet. Endocr. Soc., Chicago, Illinois. Abst. No. 396.

Antunes, J. L., Housepian, E. M. and Frantz, A. G. (1977). *Ann. Neurol.* **2**, 148.

Aono, T., Migake, A., Shioji, T., Kinugasa, T., Oshini, T. and Kurachi, K. (1976). *J. clin. Endocr. Metab.* **42**, 696.

Aragona, C. and Friesen, H. (1975). *Endocrinology* **97**, 677.

Argonz, J. and del Castillo, E. B. (1953). *J. clin. Endocr.* **13**, 79.

Aubert, M. L., Bedar, R. L., Saxena, B. B. and Raiti, S. (1974a). *J. clin. Endocr. Metab.* **38**, 1115.

Aubert, M. L., Grumbach, M. M. and Kaplan, S. L. (1974b). *Acta endocr., Copnh.* **77**, 460.

Aubert, M. L., Grumbach, M. M. and Kaplan, S. L. (1975). *J. clin Invest.* **56**, 155.

Badawi, M., Perez-Lopez, F. P. and Robyn, C. (1973), *Acta endocr., Copnh.* (Suppl. **177**), 237.

Baker, B. L. and Yu, Y. Y. (1977). *Am. J. Anat.* **148**, 217.

Bangham, D. R. and Borth, R. (1972). *Acta endocr., Copenh.* **71**, 625.

Bartke, A. A. (1977). *In* "The Testis in Normal and Infertile Men" (P. Troen and H. R. Nankin, ed.) p. 367. Raven Press, New York.

Ben-David, M. and Chrambach, A. (1974). *Endocr. Res. Commun.* **1**, 193.

Ben-David, M. and Chrambach, A. (1977). *Endocrinology*, **101**, 250.

Benveniste, R. and Frohman, L. A. (1978). *Endocrinology*, **102**, 198.

Bertrand, G. and Tolis, G. (1979). *In* "Clinical Neuroendocrinology—A Pathophysiologic Approach" (G. Tolis, ed.). Raven Press, New York.

Besser, G. M. (1976). *Br. J. Radiol.* **49**, 652.

Besser, G. M. and Edwards, C. R. W. (1972). *Br. med. J.* **2**, 280.

Besser, G. M., Parke, L., Edwards, C. R. W., Forsyth, L. A. and McNeilly, A. S. (1972). *Br. med. J.* **3**, 669.

Besser, G. M. and Thorner, M. O. (1976). *Postgrad. med. J.* **52** (Suppl. 1), 64.

Beumont, P., Bruwer, J., Pimstone, B., Vinik, A. and Utian, W. (1975). *Br. J. Psychiat.* **126**, 285.

Birge, C. A., Jacobs, L. S., Hammer, C. T. and Daughaday, W. H. (1970). *Endocrinology,* **86**, 120.

Biswas, D. K. and Tashjian, A. H. (1974). *Biochem. biophys. Res. Commun.* **60**, 241.

Biswas, S. and Rodeck, C. H. (1976). *Br. J. Obstet. Gynaec.* **83**, 683.

Blask, D., Vaughan, M., Reiter, R., Johnson, L. and Vaughan, G. (1976). *Endocrinology,* **99**, 152.

Bohnet, H. G., Dahlen, H. G., Wuttke, W. and Schneider, H. P. G. (1976). *J. clin. Endocr. Metab.* **42**, 132.

Bowers, C. Y., Friesen, H. G. and Folkers, K. (1973). *Biochem. biophys. Res. Commun.* **51**, 512.

Bowers, C. Y., Friesen, H. G., Hwang, P., Guyda, H. J. and Folkers, K. (1971). *Biochem. biophys. Res. Commun.* **45**, 1033.

Buckman, M. T. and Peake, G. T. (1973). *Science,* **181**, 755.

Calaf, P. (1973). *In* "Human Prolactin" (J. C. Pasteels and C. Robyn, eds), p. 217. Excerpta Medica, Amsterdam.

Canfield, C. J. and Bates, R. W. (1965). *New Engl. J. Med.* **273**, 897.

Carey, R. M., Johanson, A. J. and Seif, S. M. (1977). *J. clin. Endocr. Metab.* **44**, 850.

Carter, J., Tyson, J., Warne, G., McNeilly, A., Faiman, C. and Friesen, H. (1977). *J. clin. Endocr. Metab.* **45**, 973.

Charreau, F. H., Attramadal, A., Torjeson, P. A., Purvis, K., Calandra, R. and Hansson, V. (1977). *In* "The Testis in Normal and Infertile Men" (P. Troen and H. R. Nankin, eds), p. 387. Raven Press, New York.

Child, D. F., Gordon, H., Mashiter, K. and Joplin, G. F. (1975). *Br. med. J.* **4**, 87.

Copinschi, G., L'Hermite, M., Vanhaelst, L., Leclercq, R., Bruno, O. D., Golstein, J., Ooms, H. A. and Robyn, C. (1973). *Lancet,* **i**, 945.

Corbey, R. S., Lequin, R. M. and Rolland, R. (1977). *In* "Prolactin and Human Reproduction" (P. G. Crosignani and C. Robyn, eds), p. 203. Academic Press, London and New York.

Corenblum, B., Sirek, A. M. T., Horvath, E., Kovacs, K. and Ezrin, C. (1976). *J. clin. Endocr. Metab.* **42**, 857.

Cotes, P. M. (1972). *In* "Prolactin and Carcinogenesis" (A. P. Boyns and K. Griffiths, eds), p. 111. Alpha Omega Alpha Publishing, Cardiff.

Cotes, P. M. (1973). *In* "Human Prolactin" (J. L. Pasteels and C. Robyn, eds), p. 97. Excerpta Medica, Amsterdam.

Cotes, P. M. and Das, R. E. G. (1978). *Br. J. Obstet. Gynaec.* **85**, 451.

Dannies, P. S. and Tashjian, A. H. (1976) *Biochem. biophys. Res. Commun.* **70**, 1180.

Daughaday, W. H. (1974). *In* "Textbook of Endocrinology" (R. H. Williams, ed.), p. 31. W. B. Saunders, London, Philadelphia and Toronto.

Davidoff, L. M. (1926). *Endocrinology,* **10**, 461.

Del Pozo, E. and Fluckiger, E. (1973). *In* "Human Prolactin" (J. L. Pasteels and C. Robyn, eds), p. 291. Excerpta Medica, Amsterdam.

Del Pozo, E., Varga, L., Wyss, H., Tolis, G., Friesen, H., Wenner, R., Vetter, L. and Uettwiler, A. (1974). *J. clin. Endocr. Metab.* **39**, 18.

Del Pozo, E., Wyss, H. and Varga, L. (1976). *In* "Ovulation in the Human" (P. G. Crosignani, ed.), p. 297. Academic Press, London and New York.

Deriks-Tan, J. S. A. and Taubert, H. D. (1976). *Contraception,* **14**, 1.

Edwards, C. R. W., Forsyth, I. A. and Besser, G. M. (1971). *Br. med. J.* **3**, 462.

Ehara, Y., Yen, S. S. C. and Siler, T. M. (1975). *Am. J. Obstet. Gynecol.* **121**, 995.

Enjalbert, A., Moos, F., Carbonell, L., Priam, M. and Kordon, C. (1977). *Neuroendocrinology*, **24**, 147.

Evans, G. A. and Rosenfeld, M. G. (1976). *J. biol. Chem.* **251**, 2842.

Everett, J. W. (1954). *Endocrinology*, **54**, 685.

Faglia, G., Beck-Peccoz, P., Travaglini, P., Ambrosi, B., Rondenna, M., Paracchi, A., Spada, A., Weber, G., Bara, R. and Rouzin, A. (1977). *In* "Prolactin and Human Reproduction" (P. G. Crosignani and C. Robyn, eds), p. 225. Academic Press, London and New York.

Falconer, I. R. (1972). *Biochem. J.* **126**, 8p.

Fang, V. S., Refetoff, S. and Rosenfield, R. L. (1974). *Endocrinology*, **95**, 991.

Farkouh, N. H., Packer, M. G. and Frantz, A. G. (1977). Prog. 59th Ann. Meet. Endocr. Soc., Chicago, Illinois. Abst. No. 135.

Foley, T., Jacobs, L., Hoffman, W., Daughaday, W. and Blizzard, R. (1972). *J. clin. Invest.* **51**, 2143.

Forbes, A. P., Henneman, P. H., Griswold, G. C. and Albright, F. (1954). *J. clin. Endocr.* **14**, 265.

Forsyth, I. A. (1967). *In* "Hormones in Blood" (C. H. Gray and A. L. Bacharach, eds), 2nd edition, p. 234. Academic Press, London and New York.

Forsyth, I. A., Besser, G. M., Edwards, C. W., Francis, L. and Myres, R. P. (1971). *Br. med. J.* **3**, 225.

Forsyth, I. A. and Myres, R. P. (1971). *J. Endocr.* **51**, 157.

Forsyth, I. A. and Parke, L. (1973). *In* "Human Prolactin" (J. L. Pasteels and C. Robyn, eds), p. 71. Excerpta Medica, Amsterdam.

Franks, S. (1977). "Disorders of Human Prolactin Secretion", M.D. Thesis, University of London.

Franks, S. and Brook, C. G. D. (1976). *Horm. Res.* **7**, 65.

Franks, S. and Jacobs, H. S. (1977). *In* "Prolactin and Human Reproduction" (P. G. Crosignani and C. Robyn, eds), p. 245. Academic Press, London and New York.

Franks, S., Jacobs, H. S., Hull, M. G. R., Steele, S. J. and Nabarro, J. D. N. (1977a). *Br. J. Obstet. Gynaec.* **84**, 241.

Franks, S., Jacobs, H. S., Martin, N. and Nabarro, J. D. N. (1978). *Clin. Endocr.* **8**, 277.

Franks, S., Jacobs, H. S. and Nabarro, J. D. N. (1976). *Clin. Endocr.* **5**, 63.

Franks, S., Kiwi, R. and Nabarro, J. D. N. (1977b). *Br. med. J.* **1**, 882.

Franks, S., Murray, M. A. F., Jequier, A. M., Steele, S. J., Nabarro, J. D. N. and Jacobs, H. S. (1975). *Clin. Endocr.* **4**, 597.

Franks, S., Nabarro, J. D. N. and Jacobs, H. S. (1977c). *Lancet*, **i**, 778.

Franks, S., Ralphs, D. N. L., Seagroatt, V. and Jacobs, H. S. (1974). *Br. med. J.* **4**, 320.

Frantz, A. G. (1973). *Prog. Brain Res.* **39**, 311.

Frantz, A. G. (1978). *New Engl. J. Med.* **298**, 201.

Frantz, A. G. and Kleinberg, D. L. (1970). *Science*, **170**, 745.

Frantz, A. G., Kleinberg, D. L. and Noel, G. L. (1972). *Rec. Prog. Hormone Res.* **28**, 527.

Friesen, H., Guyda, H. and Hardy, J. (1970). *J. clin. Endocr. Metab.* **31**, 611.

Friesen, H. G., Hwang, P., Guyda, H. J., Tolis, G., Tyson, J. E. and Myers, R. (1972). *In* "Prolactin and Carcinogenesis" (A. R. Boyns and K. Griffiths, eds), p. 64. Alpha Omega Alpha Publishing, Cardiff.

Friesen, H., Tolis, G., Shiu, R. and Hwang, P. (1973). *In* "Human Prolactin" (J. L. Pasteels and C. Robyn, eds). Excerpta Medica, Amsterdam.

Gemzell, C. (1975). *Am. J. Obstet. Gynec.* **121**, 311.

Giusti, G., Bassi, F., Borsi, L., Cattaneo, S., Giannotti, P., Lanza, L., Pazzagli, P., Vigiani, G. and Serio, M. (1977). *In* "Human Prolactin" (P. G. Crosignani and C. Robyn, eds), p. 239. Academic Press, London and New York.

Glass, M. R., Shaw, R. W., Butt, W. R., Logan Edwards, R. and London, D. R. (1975). *Br. med. J.* 3, 274.

Glass, M. R., Williams, J. W., Butt, W. R., Logan Edwards, R. and London, D. R. (1976). *Br. J. Obstet. Gynaec.* 83, 495.

Glickman, J. A., Carson, G., Naftolin, F. and Challis, J. R. G. (1978). Prog. 60th Ann. Meet. Endocr. Soc., Miami, Florida.

Gluckman, P. W., Ballard, P. L., Kitterman, J. A., Kaplan, S. L. and Grumbach, M. M. (1978). *Pediatr. Res.* 12, 524.

Greenwood, F. C., Lino, C. G. and Bryant, G. D. (1973). *In* "Human Prolactin" (J. L. Pasteels and C. Robyn, eds), p. 82. Excerpta Medica, Amsterdam.

Guyda, H. J. (1975). *J. clin. Endocr. Metab.* 41, 953.

Guyda, H. J. and Friesen, H. (1971). *Biochem. biophys. Res. Commun.* 42, 1068.

Guyda, H. J. and Friesen, H. G. (1973). *Pediatr. Res.* 7, 534.

Guyda, H., Robert, F., Collu, R. and Hardy, J. (1973). *J. Clin. Endocr. Metab.* 36, 531.

Haenel, H. (1928). *Munch. med. Wschr.* 75, 261.

Hafiez, A. A., Lloyd, C. W. and Bartke, A. (1972). *J. Endocr.* 52, 327.

Hamosh, M. and Hamosh, P. (1977). *J. clin. Invest.* 59, 1002.

Hardy, J. (1973). *In* "Diagnosis and Treatment of Pituitary Tumours" (P. O. Kohler and G. T. Ross, eds), p. 179. Excerpta Medica, Amsterdam.

Hardy, J., Beauregard, H. and Robert, F. (1978). *In* "Progress in Prolactin Physiology and Pathology" (C. Robyn and M. Harter, eds), p. 361. Elsevier, Amsterdam.

Hauth, J. C., Parker, C. R., MacDonald, P. C., Porter, J. C. and Johnston, J. M. (1978). *Obstet. Gynec.* 51, 81.

Healy, D. L., Muller, H. K. and Burger, H. G. (1977). *Nature, Lond.* 265, 642.

Horrobin, D., Lloyd, I., Lipton, A., Burtsyn, P., Durkin, N. and Miuriri, K. L. (1971). *Lancet*, ii, 352.

Hummel, B. C., Brown, G. M., Hwang, P. and Friesen, H. (1975). *Endocrinology*, 97, 855.

Hwang, P., Guyda, H. and Friesen, H. (1971). *Proc. natn. Acad. Sci., USA*, 68, 1902.

Hwang, P., Guyda, H. and Friesen, H. (1972). *J. biol. Chem.* 247, 1955.

Hwang, P., Murray, J. B., Jacobs, J. W., Niall, H. D. and Friesen, H. (1974). *Biochemistry*, 13, 2354.

Hwang, P., Robertson, M., Guyda, H. and Friesen, H. (1973). *J. clin. Endocr. Metab.* 36, 1110.

Jacobs, H. S. (1976). *New Engl. J. Med.* 295, 954.

Jacobs, H. S. and Franks, S. (1975). *Br. med. J.* ii, 141.

Jacobs, H. S., Franks, S., Murray, M. A. F., Hull, M. G. R., Steele, S. J. and Nabarro, J. D. N. (1976). *Clin. Endocr.* 5, 439.

Jacobs, H. S., Hull, M. G. R., Murray, M. A. F. and Franks, S. (1975). *Horm. Res.* 6, 268.

Jacobs, H. S., Knuth, U., Hull, M. G. R. and Franks, S. (1977). *Br. med. J.*, 2, 940.

Jacobs, L. S. (1973). *In* "Human Prolactin" (J. L. Pasteels and C. Robyn, eds), p. 94. Excerpta Medica, Amsterdam.

Jacobs, L. S. and Daughaday, W. H. (1973). *In* "Human Prolactin (J. L. Pasteels and C. Robyn, eds), p. 189. Excerpta Medica, Amsterdam.

PROLACTIN 327

Jacobs, L. S., Mariz, I. K. and Daughaday, W. H. (1972). *J. clin. Endocr. Metab.* **34**, 484.
Jacobs, L. S., Snyder, P. G., Utiger, R. D. and Daughaday, W. H. (1973). *J. clin. Endocr. Metab.* **36**, 1069.
Josimovich, J. B. (1977). *In* "Prolactin and Human Reproduction" (P. G. Crosignani and C. Robyn, eds), p. 27. Academic Press, London and New York.
Josimovich, J. B., Bocella, L. and Levitt, M. J. (1971). *J. clin. Endocr. Metab.* **33**, 77.
Judd, S. J., Lazarus, L. and Smythe, G. (1976). *J. clin. Endocr. Metab.* **43**, 313.
Kamberi, I. A., Mical, R. S. and Porter, J. C. (1971a). *Endocrinology*, **88**, 1012.
Kamberi, I. A., Mical, R. S. and Porter, J. C. (1971b). *Endocrinology*, **88**, 1288.
Kaplan, S. L., Grumbach, M. M. and Aubert, M. L. (1976). *Rec. Prog. Hormone Res.* **32**, 161.
Kato, Y., Nakai, Y., Imura, H., Chihara, K. and Ohgo, S. (1974). *J. clin. Endocr. Metab.* **38**, 695.
Kaufman, B., Pearson, O. H. and Chamberlin, W. B. (1973). *In* "Diagnosis and Treatment of Pituitary Tumours" (P. O. Kohler and G. T. Ross, eds), p. 100. Excerpta Medica, Amsterdam.
Keeler, R. and Wilson, N. (1976). *Can. J. Physiol. Pharmacol.* **54**, 887.
Kiefer, K. A. and Malarky, W. B. (1978). *J. clin. Endocr. Metab.* **46**, 119.
Kinch, R. A. H., Plunkitt, E. R. and Devlin, M. C. (1969). *Am. J. Obstet Gynecol.* **105**, 766.
Kleinberg, D. L., Noel, G. L. and Frantz, A. G. (1977). *New Engl. J. Med.* **296**, 589.
Koch, Y., Lu, K. H. and Meites, J. (1970). *Endocrinology*, **87**, 673.
Kolodny, R. C., Jacobs, L. S. and Daughaday, W. H. (1972). *Nature, Lond.* **238**, 284.
Kordon, C., Blake, C. A., Terkel, J. and Sawyer, C. H. (1973). *Neuroendocrinology*, **13**, 213.
Knazek, R. A. and Skyler, J. S. (1976). *Proc. Soc. exp. biol. Med.* **151**, 561.
Krestin, D. (1932). *Lancet*, **i**, 928.
Kwa, H. G., De Jong-Bakker, M., Engelsman, E. and Cleton, F. J. (1974). *Lancet*, **i**, 433.
Labrie, F., Ferland, L., De Léan, L., Légace, L., Drouin, J., Beaulieu, M., Vincent, R. and Massicotte, J. (1979). *In* "Clinical Neuroendocrinology—A Pathophysiologic Approach" (G. Tolis, ed.). Raven Press, New York.
Lancet (1976). **i**, 401.
Lancet (1977). **i**, 840.
Lee, P. A., Jaffe, R. B. and Midgley, A. R. (1974). *J. clin. Endocr. Metab.* **39**, 664.
Lequin, R. M. and Rolland, R. (1977). *In* "Prolactin and Human Reproduction" (P. G. Crosignani and C. Robyn, eds), p. 1. Academic Press, London and New York.
Lewis, U. J. and Singh, R. N. P. (1973). *In* "Human Prolactin" (J. L. Pasteels and C. Robyn, eds), p. 1. Excerpta Medica, Amsterdam.
Lewis, U. J., Singh, R. N. P. and Seavey, B. K. (1971a). *Biochem. biophys. Res. Commun.* **44**, 1169.
Lewis, U. J., Singh, R. N. P., Sinha, Y. N. and Vanderlaan, W. P. (1971b). *J. clin. Endocr. Metab.* **33**, 153.
L'Hermite, M., Delvoye, P., Nokin, J., Vekemans, M. and Robyn, C. (1972). *In* "Prolactin and Carcinogenesis" (A. R. Boyns and K. Griffiths, eds). Alpha Omega Alpha Publishing, Cardiff.
L'Hermite, M., Vekemans, M., Delvoye, P., Nokin, J. and Robyn, C. (1973). *Proc. R. Soc. Med.* **66**, 864.
Lloyd, H. M., Meares, J. D. and Jacobi, J. (1973). *Int. J. Cancer*, **2**, 90.

Lockett, M. F. (1965). *J. Physiol. (Lond).* **181**, 192.

Loewenstein, J. E., Mariz, I. K., Peake, G. T. and Daughaday, W. H. (1971). *J. clin. Endocr. Metab.* **33**, 217.

Lutterbeck, P. M., Pryor, J. S., Varga, L. and Wenner, R. (1971). *Br. med. J.* **3**, 228.

MacLeod, R. M. (1969). *Endocrinology,* **85**, 916.

MacLeod, R. M. (1976). *In* "Frontiers in Neuroendocrinology" (L. Martini and W. F. Ganong, eds), Vol. 4, p. 169. Raven Press, New York.

MacLeod, R. M. (1977). Prog. 59th Meet. Endocr. Soc., Chicago, Illinois. Abstr. No. 339.

MacLeod, R. M. and Lehmeyer, J. E. (1972). *In* "Lactogenic Hormones" (G. E. W. Wolstenholme and J. Knight, eds), p. 53. Churchill Livingstone, London.

MacLeod, R. M. and Login, I. S. (1977). *Adv. biochem. Psychopharmacol.* **16**, 147.

Malarkey, W. B., Jacobs, L. S. and Daughaday, W. H. (1971). *New Engl. J. Med.* **285**, 1160.

Martin, J. B., Reichlin, S. and Brown, G. M. (1977). "Clinical Neuroendocrinology", p. 135. F. A. Davis, Philadelphia.

McGuire, W. L. (1977). *In* "Prolactin and Human Reproduction" (P. G. Crosignani and C. Robyn, eds), p. 143. Academic Press, London and New York.

McNatty, K. P., Sawyers, R. S. and MacNeilly, A. S. (1974). *Nature, Lond.* **250**, 653.

McNeilly, A. S. and Chard, T. (1974). *Clin. Endocr.* **3**, 105.

McNeilly, A. S., Gilmore, D., Jeffery, D., Dobbie, E. and Chard, T. (1977). *In* "Prolactin and Human Reproduction" (P. G. Crosignani and C. Robyn, eds), p. 21. Academic Press, London and New York.

Meites, J. (1973). *In* "Human Prolactin" (J. L. Pasteels and C. Robyn, eds), p. 105. Excerpta Medica, Amsterdam.

Meites, J., Nicoll, C. S. and Talwalker, P. K. (1963). *In* "Advances in Neuroendocrinology" (A. V. Nalbandov, ed.), p. 238. University of Illinois Press.

Mendelson, W. B., Jacobs, L. S., Reichman, J. D., Othmer, E., Cryer, P. E., Trivedi, B. and Daughaday, W. H. (1975). *J. clin. Invest.* **56**, 690.

Nader, S., Mashiter, K., Doyle, F. H. and Joplin, G. F. (1976). *Clin. Endocr.* **5**, 245.

Negro-Vilar, A., Krulich, L. and McCann, S. M. (1973). *Endocrinology,* **93**, 660.

Neill, J. D. (1970). *Endocrinology,* **87**, 1192.

Neill, J. D. (1974). *In* "Handbook of Physiology", Section 7: Endocrinology (E. Knobil and W. H. Sawyer, eds), Vol. IV, p. 2. Am. Physiol. Soc., Washington, DC.

Niall, H. D., Hogan, M. L., Tregear, G. W., Segre, G. V., Hwang, P. and Friesen, H. (1973). *Rec. Prog. Hormone Res.* **29**, 387.

Nicoll, C. S. (1973). *In* "Human Prolactin" (J. L. Pasteels and C. Robyn, eds), p. 119. Excerpta Medica, Amsterdam.

Nicoll, C. S. and Bern, H. A. (1972). *In* "Lactogenic Hormones" (G. E. W. Wolstenholme and J. Knight, eds), p. 299. Churchill Livingstone, London.

Nicoll, C., Buntin, J., Clemons, G., Schreibman, M. and Russell, S. (1977). *In* "Endocrinology" (V. H. T. James, ed.), Vol. 2, p. 293. Excerpta Medica, Amsterdam.

Noel, G. L., Suh, H. K. and Frantz, A. G. (1974). *J. Clin. Endocr. Metab.* **38**, 413.

Nokin, J., Vekemans, M., L'Hermite, M. and Robyn, C. (1972). *Br. med. J.* **3**, 561.

Nolin, J. M. (1978). *Endocrinology,* **102**, 402.

Nolin, J. M. and Witorsch, R. J. (1976). *Endocrinology,* **99**, 949.

Parker, D. C. and Rossman, L. G. (1973). *Clin. Res.* **21**, 213.

Parker, D. C., Rossman, L. G. and Vanderlaan, E. F. (1974). *J. clin. Endocr.* **38**, 646.

Pasteels, J. L. (1962). *C.R. Soc. Biol. (Paris),* **254**, 2664.

Pensky, J., Murray, R. M. J., Mozaffarian, G. and Pearson, O. H. (1972). *In* "Prolactin and Carcinogenesis" (A. R. Boyns and K. Griffiths, eds), p. 24. Alpha Omega Alpha Publishing, Cardiff.

Posner, B. I. (1977). *In* "Endocrinology" (V. H. T. James, ed.), Vol. 2, p. 178. Excerpta Medica, Amsterdam.

Posner, B. I., Kelly, P. A. and Friesen, H. G. (1975). *Science*, **187**, 57.

Posner, B. I., Kelly, P. A., Shiu, R. P. C. and Friesen, H. G. (1974). *Endocrinology*, **95**, 521.

Raben, M. S. (1959). *Rec. Prog. Hormone Res.* **15**, 71.

Rathnam, P., Cederqvist, L. and Saxena, B. B. (1977). *Biochim. biophys, Acta*, **492**, 186.

Rathnam, P. and Saxena, B. B. (1977). *Endocrinology*, **100**, 1403.

Rees, L. H., Bloomfield, G. A., Rees, G. M., Corrin, B., Franks, L. M. and Ratcliffe, J. G. (1974). *J. clin. Endocr. Metab.* **38**, 1090.

Reichlin, S., Martin, J., Mitnick, M., Boshans, R., Grimm, Y., Bollinger, J., Gordon, J. and Malacara, J. (1972). *Rec. Prog. Hormone Res.* **28**, 229.

Reyes, F. I., Gomez, F. and Faiman, C. (1977). *In* "Prolactin and Human Reproduction" (P. G. Crosignani and C. Robyn, eds), p. 259. Academic Press, London and New York.

Riddle, O., Bates, R. W. and Dykshorn, S. (1933). *Am. J. Physiol.* **105**, 191.

Rillema, J. A. and Wild, E. A. (1977). *Endocrinology*, **100**, 1219.

Rivier, C., Brown, M. and Vale, W. (1977). *Endocrinology*, **100**, 751.

Rivier, C., Rivier, J. and Vale, W. (1978). *Endocrinology*, **102**, 519.

Rivier, C., Vale, W., Ling, N., Brown, M. and Guillemin, R. (1977). *Endocrinology*, **100**, 238.

Robyn, C. (1973), *In* "Human Prolactin" (J. L. Pasteels and C. Robyn, eds), p. 94. Excerpta Medica, Amsterdam.

Robyn, C., Delvoye, P., Vam Exter, C., Vekemans, M., Caufriez, A., deNayer, A., Delogne-Desnoeck, J. and L'Hermite, M. (1977). *In* "Prolactin and Human Reproduction" (P. G. Crosignani and C. Robyn, eds), p. 71. Academic Press, London and New York.

Rogal, A. D. and Rosen, S. W. (1974). *J. clin. Endocr. Metab.* **38**, 714.

Rolland, R. and Schellekens, L. (1973). *J. Obstet. Gynaec. Br. Commonw.* **80**, 945.

Rubin, R. T., Poland, R. E. and Tower, B. B. (1976). *J. clin. Endocr. Metab.* **42**, 112.

Saito, T. and Saxena, B. B. (1975). *Acta endocr., Copenh.* **80**, 126.

Salih, H., Flax, H., Brander, W. and Hobbs, J. R. (1972). *Lancet*, **ii**, 1103.

Sassin, J. F., Frantz, A. G., Kapen, S. and Weitzman, E. D. (1973). *J. Clin. Endocr. Metab.* **37**, 436.

Schally, A. V., Dupont, A., Arimura, A., Takahara, J., Redding, T. W., Clemens, J. and Shaar, C. (1976). *Acta endocr., Copenh.* **82**, 1.

Schenker, J. G., Ben-David, M. and Polishuk (1975). *Am. J. Obstet. Gynec.* **123**, 834.

Scott, A. M. and Lowry, P. J. (1973). *J. Endocr.* **63**, 43p.

Seo, H., Refetoff, S., Vassart, G. and Scherberg, N. (1977). Prog. 59th Ann. Meet. Endocr. Soc., Chicago, Illinois. Abst. No. 134.

Sherwood, L. (1971). *New Engl. J. Med.* **284**, 774.

Shiu, R. P. C. and Friesen, H. G. (1974). *J. biol. Chem.* **249**, 7902.

Shiu, R. P. C. and Friesen, H. G. (1976). *Science*, **192**, 259.

Shiu, R. P. C., Kelly, P. A. and Friesen, H. G. (1973). *Science*, **180**, 968.

Shome, B. and Parlow, A. F. (1977). *J. clin. Endocr. Metab.* **45**, 1112.

Sinha, Y. N., Selby, F. W., Lewis, U. J. and Vanderlaan, W. P. (1973). *J. clin. Endocr. Metab.* **56**, 509.

Skyler, J. S., Rogol, A. D., Lovenberg, W. and Knazek, R. A. (1977). *Endocrinology,* **100**, 283.

Spanos, E., Colston, K. W., Evans, I. M. A., Galante, L. S., MacAuley, S. J. and MacIntyre, I. (1976a). *Mol. cell. Endocr.* **5**, 163.

Spanos, E., Pike, J. W., Haussler, M. R., Colston, K. W., Evans, I. M. A., Goldner, A. M., McCain, T. A. and MacIntyre, I. (1976b). *Life, Sci.* **19**, 1751.

Striker, P. and Grueter, F. (1928). *C.r. Soc. Biol. (Paris),* **99**, 1978.

Suh, H. K. and Frantz, A. G. (1974). *J. clin. Endocr. Metab.* **39**, 928.

Swerdoff, R. S. and Odell, W. D. (1977). *In* "The Testis in Normal and Infertile Men" (P. Troen and H. R. Nakkin, eds), p. 395. Raven Press, New York.

Takahara, J., Arimura, A. and Schally, A. V. (1974). *Endocrinology,* **95**, 462.

Talwalker, P. K., Ratner, A. and Meites, J. (1963). *Am. J. Physiol.* **205**, 213.

Tashjian, A. H., Barowsky, N. J. and Jensen, D. K. (1971). *Biochem. biophys. Res. Commun.* **43**, 516.

Thorner, M. O. and Besser, G. M. (1977). *In* "Prolactin and Human Reproduction" (P. G. Crosignani and C. Robyn, eds), p. 285. Academic Press, London and New York.

Thorner, M. O., Besser, G. M., Hagen, C. and McNeilly, A. S. (1974a). *J. Endocr.* **61**, XXXII.

Thorner, M. O., Besser, G. M., Jones, A., Dacie, J. and Jones, A. E. (1975). *Br. med. J.* **4**, 694.

Thorner, M. O., McNeilly, A. S., Hagen, C. and Besser, G. M. (1974b). *Br. med. J.* **2**, 419.

Thorner, M. O., Round, J., Jones, A., Fahmy, D., Groom, G., Butcher, S. and Thompson, K. (1977). *Clin. Endocr.* **7**, 463.

Tolis, G., Bertrand, G., Carpenter, S. and McKenzie, J. M. (1978). *Ann. int. Med.* **89**, 345.

Tolis, G. and McKenzie, T. M. (1976). Prog. 7th Ann. Meet. Eur. Thyroid Assoc., Helsinki. Abst. No. 57.

Tolis, G. and VanVliet, S. (1976). *Clin. Res.* **24**, 279A.

Turkington, R. W. (1971). *New Engl. J. Med.* **285**, 1455.

Turkington, R. W. (1976). *J. clin. Endocr. Metab.* **33**, 210.

Turkington, R. W. (1972a). *J. clin. Endocr. Metab.* **34**, 247.

Turkington, R. W. (1972b). *J. clin. Endocr. Metab.* **34**, 159.

Turkington, R. W. and Frantz, W. L. (1972). *In* "Prolactin and Carcinogenesis" (A. R. Boyns and K. Griffiths, eds), p. 39. Alpha Omega Alpha Publishing, Cardiff.

Turkington, R. W., Frantz, W. L. and Majunder, G. C. (1973). *In* "Human Prolactin" (J. L. Pasteels and C. Robyn, eds), p. 24. Excerpta Medica, Amsterdam.

Tyson, J. E., Hwang, P., Gudya, H. and Friesen, H. (1972). *Am. J. Obstet. Gynec.* **113**, 14.

Tyson, J. E., Kohjandi, M., Huth, J. and Andreassen, B. (1975). *J. clin. Endocr. Metab.* **40**, 764.

Valverde, R. C., Chieffo, V. and Reichlin, S. (1972). *Endocrinology,* **91**, 982.

Van Look, P., McNeilly, A., Hunter, W. and Baird, D. (1977). *In* "Prolactin and Human Reproduction" (P. G. Crosignani and C. Robyn, eds), p. 217. Academic Press, London and New York.

Van Maanen, J. H. and Smelik, P. G. (1968). *Neuroendocrinology,* **3**, 177.

Van Wyk, J. J. and Grumbach, M. M. (1960). *J. Pediat.* **57**, 416.

Vezina, J. L. and Sutton, T. J. (1974). *Am. J. Roentgen.* **120**, 46.

Walsh, R., Posner, B. I., Kopriwa, B. and Brawer, J. (1978). *Science,* **201,** 1041.

Westman, A. and Jacobsohn, D. (1938). *Acta Pathol. Microbiol. Scand.* **15,** 445.

Wilson, R. G., Buchan, R., Roberts, M. M., Forrest, A. P. M., Boynes, A. R., Cole, E. N. and Griffiths, K. (1976). *Cancer,* **33,** 1325.

Winters, A. J., Colston, C., MacDonald, P. C. and Porter, J. C. (1975). *J. clin. Endocr. Metab.* **41,** 626.

Wuttke, W. and Gelato, M. (1976). *Ann. biol. Anim. Biochem. biophys.* **16,** 349.

Yamada, Y. (1975). *Neuroendocrinology,* **18,** 263.

Zimmerman, E. A., Defendi, R. and Frantz, A. G. (1974). *J. clin. Endocr. Metab.* **38,** 577.

VII. Human Placental Lactogen

T. CHARD

INTRODUCTION

The presence in the human placenta of a substance having mammotrophic activity was first clearly demonstrated by Ito and Higashi (1961). Josimovich

M

and MacLaren (1962) demonstrated that the material was similar immunochemically to human pituitary growth hormone (hGH), and that it occurred
in maternal peripheral serum, retroplacental serum and placental extracts.
These pioneering studies have now been widely confirmed and extended,
and detailed investigations have yielded a very full picture of the physiology
and pathophysiology of the hormone. Furthermore, the measurement of
placental lactogen in maternal blood during pregnancy has become what is
probably the most universally accepted biochemical test of placental function
per se, and is a common clinical adjunct to the use of oestrogens (see Vol. 3
Chapter VI) as a means for studying the well-being of the foetus and placenta
in current obstetric practice. The literature on both the physiology and the
clinical applications of placental lactogen has been the subject of several
comprehensive reviews (Hartog, 1972; Chard, 1972; Letchworth, 1976).

A. NOMENCLATURE

There has been considerable confusion over the nomenclature of the protein
which, for the purposes of this chapter, will be referred to as human placental
lactogen or hPL. However, several other designations have been put forward,
including human chorionic growth hormone-prolactin (hCGP) (Grumbach
and Kaplan, 1964), purified placental protein (PPP) (Florini, Tonelli, Brewer,
Coppola, Ringler and Bell, 1966), and human chorionic somato-mammo-
trophin (hCS) (Li, Grumbach, Kaplan, Josimovich, Friesen and Catt, 1968).
The last term is widely used and has been strongly defended by Bewley
and Li (1974) on the grounds that it provides a clear-cut description of the
relationship of this protein to other "irrevocably" named hormones. Furthermore, the use of the term "chorionic" is more specific than "placental" and
is in common use for other placental hormones such as chorionic gonadotrophin and chorionic corticotrophin. However, many workers consider
the term chorionic somatomammotrophin to be inelegant and cumbersome
and therefore prefer the original name of placental lactogen. This must
probably be accepted in the absence of any clear-cut rules for the nomenclature of hormonal proteins comparable to those which exist for enzymes.

B. PLACENTAL LACTOGENIC HORMONES IN OTHER SPECIES

Similar placental lactogenic hormones have been found in other species,
such as the goat (Buttle, Forsyth and Knaggs, 1972), the Rhesus monkey
(Walsh, Wolf, Meyer, Aubert and Friesen, 1977), and the sheep (Handwerger,

Crenshaw, Maurer, Barrett, Hurley, Colander and Fellows, 1977). Since the existence of such hormones seems to be a function of the experimental ability to find them in a given species it seems likely that they occur in all species forming a placenta.

C. PLACENTAL LACTOGEN AND OTHER PLACENTAL PROTEINS

Placental lactogen is only one of a large number of placental specific proteins (see Table 1) some of which appear to be unique in the sense of having no

Table 1

Proteins produced by the human placenta.

Protein	Abbreviation
Human chorionic gonadotrophin	hCG
Human placental lactogen	hPL
Human chorionic somatomammotrophin	hCS
Human chorionic thyrotrophin	hCT
Human chorionic corticotrophin	hCCT
Human chorionic gonadotrophin releasing hormone	hC-LRH
Schwangerschafts-spezifiches glykoprotein 1	SP, 1
Pregnancy associated plasma protein A	PAPP-A
Pregnancy associated plasma protein B	PAPP-B
Heat stable alkaline phosphatase	HSAP
Cystine aminopeptidase (oxytocinase)	CAP
Diamine oxidase (histaminase)	DO
Placental protein 5	PP5

obvious counterpart in the adult while others, including hPL, are closely related but not necessarily identical with adult products. The synthesis of this wide range of materials, many of which have no obvious physiological function but may recur in association with tumours in adult life, is a major biological enigma (Gordon and Chard, 1979).

D. SYNTHESIS

In common with other specific placental proteins and hormones, hPL appears to be a product of the syncytiotrophoblast. However, the only experimental evidence for this arises from immunohistochemical studies (e.g. Currie, Beck, Ellis and Reed, 1966; Ikonicoff and Cedard, 1973). The technical basis of these investigations has been criticised on the grounds of lack of appropriate controls, and because a theoretical analysis has indicated that the actual concentrations of the hormone in the cytoplasm of the trophoblast cell would be inaccessible to present techniques (Gau and Chard, 1976). The most

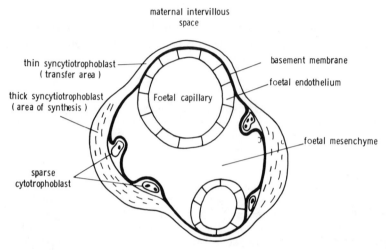

Fig. 1. Diagram of a section across the chorionic villus, showing the principle structures involved in placental synthesis and transfer.

definitive evidence, which would be demonstration of *de novo* synthesis of hPL in tissue culture, is not available because it is impossible to be certain of the homogeneity of placental material *in vitro*. Nevertheless, the vast bulk of indirect evidence would support the hypothesis of a trophoblastic origin.

There have been a number of studies on the localisation of the protein synthesising machinery within the trophoblast. These include the observations by Burgos and Rodrigues (1966) of a clear differentiation between thick areas of the trophoblast cytoplasm which are rich in endoplasmic reticulum and microvilli and therefore appear to be specialised for protein synthesis, together with thin areas without microvilli which lie in proximity to foetal capillaries and appear to be specialised for the transport of nutrients and waste products (Fig. 1). The differentiation between these areas is of considerable clinical significance because it is possible to envisage a process which could damage the critically important transfer areas while leaving the synthetic areas intact. However, since trophoblast pathology is usually secondary to factors such as occlusion of maternal decidual arterioles or foetal capillaries in the chorionic villus it is likely in practice that all areas will be equally affected.

E. IMMUNOCHEMICAL NATURE

Several groups have described the isolation and purification of hPL (Cohen, Grumbach and Kaplan, 1964; Friesen, 1965; Turtle, Beck and Daughaday, 1966; Florini et al., 1966). After initial extraction from placental tissue, followed by chemical precipitation, final purification is achieved by combinations of gel filtration, ion-exchange chromatography, and electrophoresis. Human placental tissue is easily obtained, large scale extraction is feasible, and for this reason highly purified hPL is readily available. Large amounts have been prepared commercially, arising from a programme in which it was proposed to use hPL as a substitute for growth hormone in the treatment of dwarfed children.

Human placental lactogen is a polypeptide of mw 21,000 with a single chain of 190 amino acids and two intrachain disulphide bonds (Sherwood, Handwerger, McLaurin and Lanner, 1971; Handwerger and Sherwood, 1974). However, Niall, Hogan, Sauer, Rosenblum, Tregear, Segre, Hwang and Friesen (1973) have reported that the total number of amino acid residues in HPL is 191 with an additional glutamine residue at position 68 from the amino-terminus (Fig. 2). The amino acid composition is very similar to that of hGH, the only differences being in the number of methionine, histidine and proline residues. The amino acid sequence of the two hormones is identical at 163 of the 190 residues (86% sequence homology), and the disulphide bonds are located in homologous portions of each molecule. Most of the differences lie at or near the NH_2-terminus, and of the observed substitutions only one requires more than a single base change in the triplet codon. The sequences of hPL and hGH are also somewhat similar to that of prolactin (13% sequence homology with hPL, 16% with hGH). However, prolactin has 198 amino acids and three intrachain disulphide bonds (Shome and Parlow, 1977). Because there are several regions of internal homology, all three hormones may have originated from a shorter primordial peptide of 25–30 amino acids. At an early stage there was a structural divergence which produced two major evolutionary lines: one with primarily lactogenic activity; the other with somatotrophic activity. At a later stage individual species showed further divergence within these lines, yielding the observed differences between, for example, the structures of sheep and human pituitary growth hormone and prolactin. Finally, there occurred divergences within an individual species leading to the existence of separate pituitary and

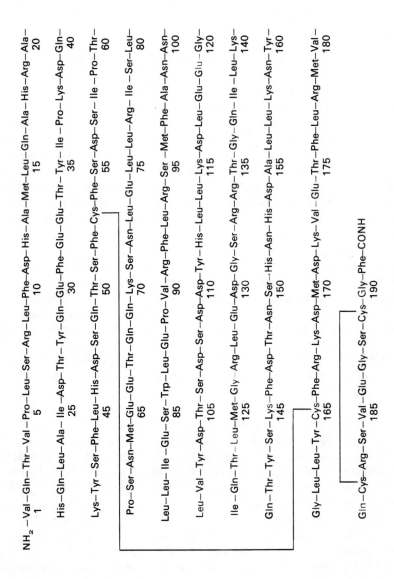

Fig. 2. The amino acid sequence of hPL (modified from Li, Dixon and Chung, 1971).

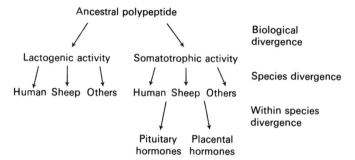

Ancestral polypeptide

Lactogenic activity   Somatotrophic activity

Human Sheep Others   Human Sheep Others

Biological
divergence

Species divergence

Within species
divergence

Pituitary   Placental
hormones   hormones

Fig. 3. Diagrammatic representation of the evolutionary divergence of the lactogenic and somatotrophic hormones (modified from Bewley and Li, 1974). It should be noted that the divergence between pituitary and placental forms seems to be universal, since it has been found in all species so far examined.

placental proteins within the general lines of somatotrophic hormones. These concepts are illustrated diagrammatically in Fig. 3.

F. BIOLOGICAL NATURE

A number of biological activities have been proposed for hPL including lactogenesis, growth promotion, stimulation of the corpus luteum, an effect on carbohydrate and lipid metabolism, erythropoiesis, inhibition of fibrinolysis, and immunosuppression. Although very similar to hGH, hPL has very weak somatotrophic activity equivalent to only 0·1–1 % of that of the pituitary peptide. The extent of the lactogenic activity of hPL has been the subject of dispute. The first reports suggested that its potency was some 75 % that of a reference preparation of sheep prolactin (Josimovich and Brande, 1964). However, later studies suggested considerably lower activity (Friesen, 1965; Florini *et al.*, 1966) of the order of 1–4 u/mg in the pigeon crop-sac assay. Forsyth (1967) noted that the potency in the rabbit intraductal assay was substantially greater than that in the pigeon crop-sac assay, a discrepancy similar to that which has been observed for human growth hormone. Investigations using intact animals have given estimates ranging from 20–100% of that of prolactin (Handwerger and Sherwood, 1974). It would appear that the apparent lactogenic potency of hPL is highly dependent on the purity of the material examined, on the type of assay, and even on the animal species used for the assay. For all these reasons it is difficult and perhaps impossible to assign an exact potency.

In rodents hPL has luteotrophic activity; it is also possible that it might influence placental progesterone secretion, in particular the interconversion of progesterone and the biologically inactive 20α-dihydroprogesterone (Josimovich and Archer, 1977). In animals administration of hPL leads to a rise in blood sugar and impairment of carbohydrate tolerance (Burt, Leake and Pruitt, 1966; Handwerger, Fellows, Crenshaw, Hurley, Barrett and Maurer, 1976); this is probably due to increased peripheral resistance to the action of insulin, though it has been shown in hypophysectomised rats that hPL can cause an increase in insulin release *in vitro* from islet cells (Martin and Friesen, 1969).

In mice hPL can stimulate erythropoietin and thus the incorporation of iron into red blood cells (Jepson and Friesen, 1968). Both hPL and hCG can suppress the lymphocyte transformation induced by phytohemagglutinin and may thus play a role in the immune survival of a pregnancy (Contractor and Davies, 1973).

G. BIOLOGICAL FUNCTIONS

It is very important to differentiate between activity and function. A naturally occurring molecule may have a specific effect in an experimental system but this does not guarantee that it is responsible for that effect in a physiological system. The differentiation is particularly striking with all of the biologically active placental proteins: none can be clearly identified as being entirely and exclusively essential for any physiological event, and it has even been suggested that the placental proteins have no biological function but instead are waste products of the general activities of the placenta as an independent organism (Gordon and Chard, 1979).

An important function of hPL during normal pregnancy could be the preparation of the breast for lactation. There are several other candidates for this, including placental oestrogens and progesterone and maternal pituitary prolactin all of which are elevated at the same time. Administration of hPL to non-pregnant subjects in amounts sufficient to yield blood levels comparable to those in mid-gestation does not appear to induce lactation (Josimovich, Stock and Tobon, 1974). Furthermore, full lactation can be induced by appropriate breast stimulation in subjects not only who are not pregnant but who have never been pregnant.

Similar remarks can be addressed to the possible role of hPL in carbohydrate and lipid metabolism in normal pregnancy. It is well known that pregnancy constitues a diabetogenic stress: impairment of carbohydrate tolerance and elevated levels of circulating insulin and free fatty acids are normal findings. An attractive teleological hypothesis can be put forward for these observations: that the pregnant woman will tend to retain glucose within her circulation where it is available for transport across the placenta to the developing foetus, and particularly to the foetal brain for which glucose is the essential and only energy source. Many experimental observations would tend to support the possible role of hPL in this process. Administration of hPL to non-pregnant subjects leads to impaired carbohydrate tolerance and increased levels of insulin (Beck and Daughaday, 1967; Kalkhoff, Richardson and Beck, 1969), and plasma free fatty acids (Riggi, Boshart, Bell and Ringler, 1966). The circulating levels of hPL decrease following administration of i.v. glucose (Burt, Leake and Rhyne, 1970;

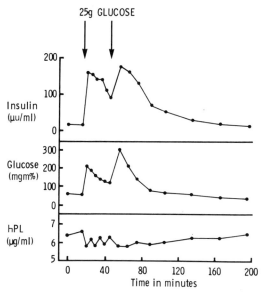

Fig. 4. Plasma levels of insulin, glucose, and hPL in 10 subjects following i.v. injection of glucose (from Pavlou *et al.*, 1973).

Spellacy, Buhi, Schram, Birk and McCreary, 1971; Pavlou, Chard, Landon and Letchworth, 1973) (Fig. 4), though Pavlou and his colleagues pointed out that the change is small and inconsistent, and might easily be explained by trivial mechanisms such as the osmotic expansion of plasma volume which results from injection of a hypertonic solution; no response has been claimed after oral administration of glucose (Pavlou *et al.*, 1973). Other workers have shown apparent increases during insulin-induced hypoglycemia (Spellacy *et al.*, 1971) and prolonged starvation (Tyson, Austin and Farinholt, 1971; Kim and Felig, 1971); but again, the changes are small by comparison with those of pituitary growth hormone under similar experimental circumstances. The case that hPL might have effects on carbohydrate metabolism is clearcut. The case that it is solely responsible for the changes seen in pregnancy is much less so; an equally good candidate would be the steroid hormones of the placenta (oestrogens and progesterone) which at levels considerably lower than those found in late gestation (for example in subjects on oral contraceptive agents) can readily produce all the changes characteristic of a prediabetic state.

Finally, it would be attractive to speculate that hPL, through its somatotrophic effect, is an important growth promoting factor for the foetus. However, this possibility is virtually ruled out by two observations: first, that the somatotrophic activity of hPL is extremely low (1 % or less) compared with that of pituitary growth hormone; second, the levels of hPL in the foetal circulation are 1000 fold less than those in the mother.

H. CONTROL MECHANISMS

In common with other placental proteins there is little indication for the existence of control mechanisms in the sense that they occur for comparable products of the normal adult. No releasing or inhibiting factors have been identified and where mechanisms have been suggested (e.g. the changes in hPL during experimental manipulation of carbohydrate metabolism) the evidence is often disputed and subject to alternative explanations (p. 341).

A hypothesis has been put forward (Chard, 1976; and Fig. 5) which proposes that the potential for placental protein production is a function of the total mass of the trophoblast; that the rate of release depends on the concentration of the protein in the maternal blood in the intervillous space; and that this concentration, in turn, depends on the rate of blood-flow in the intervillous space. In other words, hPL will diffuse from the trophoblast cell down a concentration gradient: the faster the rate of blood-flow the more rapid is the removal of hPL and hence the steeper the gradient. This hypothesis is not at variance with any accepted facts, and has the important

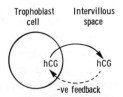

Fig. 5. The rate of hormone release by the trophoblast and intervillous blood flow. A low concentration in the intervillous space leads to an increased rate of release on the basis of a simple "mass-action" feedback. If intervillous blood flow increases the hormone is removed more rapidly and the rate of release also increases.

implication that the rate of hPL production and its circulating levels in the mother will be closely related to utero–placental blood flow. It may also explain why products of the foetus and placenta, such as oestriol, and products of the placenta, such as hPL, often show a simultaneous decrease in abnormal states.

I. METABOLISM AND CLEARANCE

The half life of hPL in the maternal circulation, estimated by its rate of disappearance after delivery of the placenta, is 10–20 min (Spellacy, Carlson and Birk, 1966; Pavlou, Chard and Letchworth, 1972). As with virtually all biological molecules, the disappearance is biphasic with an initial rapid fall (yielding the half life stated above) followed by a period when the decrease is much less rapid. Pavlou *et al.* (1972) noted that the differences in half lives between individual subjects could not be explained by observational error alone, and concluded that each subject had her own characteristic half life of hPL. This can be attributed to differences in the mode of delivery and the physiological state of the patient.

The rate of synthesis of hPL has been estimated at 1–12 g/day (Beck, Parker and Daughaday, 1965; Kaplan, Gurpide, Sciarra and Grumbach, 1968). This is considerably greater than that of any other known protein hormone from any site, an interesting observation in the light of the dispute as to whether it has any function (see above).

All investigators have agreed that maternal levels of hPL show no nycto-hemeral rhythm (Beck, Parker and Daughaday, 1965; Samaan, Yen, Friesen and Pearson, 1966; Keller, Gerber, Greub and Schreiner, 1970; Pavlou, Chard and Letchworth, 1972; Lindberg and Nilsson, 1973a). However, Pavlou *et al.* (1972) in studies on 10 subjects showed that the variation over a 24 hr period was rather greater than that which could be attributed to the assay itself. Thus a single sample taken from an individual will not necessarily be representative of all samples taken from the individual, and the diagnostic significance of hPL levels is increased if serial levels are available. It is not clear what factors might be responsible for the observed variation. Posture has no effect (Ylikorkala, Haapalahti and Jarvinen, 1973), nor does strenuous physical exercise (Lindberg and Nilsson, 1973a; Pavlou *et al.*, 1973). There is no change in levels following the infusion of amino acids or ingestion of a protein meal (Tyson, Austin and Farinholt, 1971), nor following i.v. infusion of prostaglandins or oxytocin (Spellacy, 1972). A number of workers have claimed that there are wide fluctuations in levels during normal labour (e.g. Cramer, Beck and Makowski, 1971) but this has not been confirmed in other studies (Gillard, Letchworth and Chard, 1973).

J. LEVELS IN DIFFERENT BIOLOGICAL FLUIDS

The levels of hPL in foetal blood are 100 fold less than those in maternal blood (Kaplan and Grumbach, 1965; Crosignani, Nencioni and Brambati, 1972). This differential appears to be universal to all the specific proteins of the human placenta, with the possible exception of placental protein 5 (Grudzinskas, personal communication). It is probably due to the fact that the trophoblast is in direct contact with the maternal circulation, whereas it is separated from the foetal circulation by a basement membrane and the foetal capillary endothelium.

The levels of hPL in amniotic fluid are 10 fold less than those in maternal blood (Niven, Ward and Chard, 1974). These authors also showed that there was a direct relation between the concentration in amniotic fluid and that in maternal blood, but no relation between the total amount of hPL in the two compartments. Only small amounts of hPL are excreted in maternal urine (0·5 mg/day) against a production rate of 1 g/day, a finding which is not unexpected for a protein of this molecular weight.

K. ASSAY IN BLOOD

1. Biological Assay

In principle it would be possible to measure hPL in any of a variety of presently available assays for lactogenic activity. However, the reservations already expressed about estimation of the lactogenic potency of the hPL molecule, together with the technical problems of the methods themselves, render this approach impractical. The only value of bioassays would be in defining the properties of a placental lactogenic protein in a species not hitherto examined.

2. Radioreceptor Assay

A radioligand receptor assay for lactogenic hormones has been described (Shiu and Friesen, 1973). Cell membrane fractions produced by ultracentrifugation of homogenates of lactating mammary glands from pseudopregnant rabbits are used as receptor. The maximum sensitivity of this procedure (1 ng/ml) is rather less than that of radioimmunoassay (0·1 ng/ml). Furthermore, the system is liable to non-specific interference from serum proteins and requires substantial dilution of samples.

3. Radioimmunoassay

The vast majority of studies on hPL have been carried out using radio-immunoassay, though other types of immunological assay have been developed including haemagglutination inhibition (Gusdon, 1969), complement fixation (Zuckerman, Fallow, Tashjian, Levine and Friesen, 1970; Varma, Varma, Selenkow and Emerson, 1970) and radial immunodiffusion (Seppala and Ruoslahti, 1970). An enzymoimmunoassay based on the ELISA technique is commercially available (Organon).

(a) Purified hPL, International Reference Preparation and standards

As already noted, purified hPL suitable for iodination is commercially available. Very recently, an International Reference Preparation has been established (Cotes and Das, 1978) consisting of a batch of 3500 ampoules code labelled 73/545; each contains 1 mg of a preparation of purified hPL freeze-dried in mannitol. As a result of a collaborative study the content of each ampoule has been defined as 850 μu.

Table 2

Preparation of standards for hPL assay.

Tube No.	Volume exchanged (ml)	Standard concentration (μg/ml)
1	1·2	12
2	0·8	8
3	0·6	6
4	0·4	4
5	0·2	2
6	0·1	1

A procedure for preparing hPL standard for use in a routine assay is given below:

(i) Weigh out 10 mg highly purified hPL.

(ii) Dissolve in 10 ml hPL-free serum (from a non-pregnant human or an animal species).

(iii) Aliquot as lots of 0·5 ml and store deep frozen.

(iv) Dilute an aliquot 1:10 (0·4 ml + 3·6 ml hPL-free serum) to give a solution of 100 μg/ml.

(v) Set out six tubes (see Table 2), each containing 10 ml of hPL-free serum.

(vi) Remove an appropriate volume from each tube and replace it with the solution from (iv) above.

(vii) Deep-freeze as aliquots each sufficient for 1 week of assays (0·2–0·4 ml).

(b) Iodination of pPL

Purified preparations of hPL are readily iodinated by the chloramine T technique, though other procedures such as enzymatic iodination using lactoperoxidase are probably equally suitable (Edwards, personal communication). The following are details of a method using chloramine T (diluent buffer is phosphate 0·05 M, pH 7·4 with no added protein):

(i) Dissolve purified hPL (50 μg) in 0·02 ml buffer in a conical vial (for convenience a number of aliquots of this type may be prepared by freeze-drying the appropriate volume of a solution of hPL in a series of vials).

(ii) Add 2 mCi carrier-free sodium ^{125}I (volume approx 0·02 ml).

(iii) Add chloramine T (10 μg) in 0·02 ml buffer. The solution should be prepared immediately before the iodination.

(iv) Mix thoroughly but briefly (10–15 sec).

(v) Add and mix sodium metabisulphite (20 μg) in 0·02 ml buffer.

(vi) Add 0·5 ml diluent buffer containing 2 mg/ml bovine serum albumin,

(vii) Transfer carefully to a 1 × 15 cm (approx) column of Sephadex G75, previously eluted with diluent buffer containing albumin

(viii) Elute with diluent buffer containing 2 mg/ml bovine serum albumin, collect fractions of approx 0·5 ml.

(ix) Assess total counts in each fraction and binding in the presence and absence of anti-hPL.

(x) Collect fractions yielding highest binding in presence of antibody, and store as deep frozen aliquots.

The yield is usually 80% or greater, and the binding of tracer 90% or greater in the presence of an excess of antibody. Stored in aliquots at $-20°$ the tracer is stable for 4–6 weeks.

(c) Antiserum to hPL

Purified hPL is highly immunogenic. Serial injections into any of a variety of animal species yields a vigorous antibody response within 2–4 months and most of the resulting antisera are suitable for use in a radioimmunoassay. Because of the relatively high concentrations in which it is used, substantial stocks of antiserum are necessary for the conduct of a routine assay.

A method for immunisation with hPL is shown below:

(i) Dissolve 0·6 mg of purified hPL in 2 ml phosphate buffer containing no protein (use a glass tube).

(ii) Add 4·5 ml of complete Freund's adjuvant (Difco).

(iii) Homogenise thoroughly: a convenient method for this is repeated aspiration and expulsion from an all-glass syringe fitted with an all-metal needle. Plastic should be avoided as some types are attacked by components of the adjuvant. An alternative method is the use of a Potter–Elvehjem homogeniser.

(iv) Inject 1 ml of the homogenate into each of six adult female New Zealand White rabbits. The injection should be subcutaneous and divided among six or more sites around the neck and shoulders. There is no need to shave the animal for this procedure.

(v) Wait 6 weeks and repeat the procedure, but using 25 µg immunogen per animal rather than 92 µg.

(vi) After a further 2 weeks take a test bleed (2 ml) and repeat the booster immunisation when this has been examined.

(vii) Repeat for four booster injections in total, and then repeat at 1–3 month intervals according to the results and the requirements for antiserum.

(viii) If the test bleeds reveal a useful antiserum, a larger bleed (50 ml) should be collected prior to the next booster injection.

(ix) For a larger animal (sheep, goat) a similar schedule may be followed but the amount of immunogen should be increased 2–3 times.

(d) Separation of bound and free hormone

The main differences in the many radioimmunoassays which have been described reside in the preparation of hormone used, and the technique of separation of antibody-bound and free peptide. The methods include chromatoelectrophoresis (Grumbach and Kaplan, 1964; Frantz, Rabkin and Friesen, 1965), double antibody (Beck, Parker and Daughaday, 1965; Samaan, Yen, Friesen and Pearson, 1966; Spellacy, Carlson and Birk, 1966; Gaspard, Goulart and Franchimont, 1971; El Tomi, Crystle and Stevens, 1970), dextran charcoal (Sciarra, Sherwood, Varma and Lundberg, 1968; Saxena, Refetoff, Emerson and Selenkow, 1968b; Josimovich, Kosor, Bocella, Mintz and Hutchinson, 1970; Haour, Cohen and Bertrand, 1970; Kim and Felig, 1971), solid-phase antibody (Leake and Burt, 1969; Spona and Janisch, 1971; Teoh, Spellacy and Buhi, 1971; Spenser, 1971; Gardner, Bailey and Chard, 1974), and dioxan (Haour, 1971), or ethanol precipitation (Letchworth, Boardman, Bristow, Landon and Chard, 1971a). The last of these is the most simple, cheap and reliable; it is the basis of a semi-automated procedure with a throughput of many hundreds of samples in a working day (Letchworth, Boardman, Bristow, Landon and Chard, 1971b), and of several commercial kits.

(e) Assay protocol for hPL

A typical assay protocol, using ethanol precipitation of the bound fraction, is shown below. It should be noted that the hPL assay is "robust", and that substantial variations on the procedure are possible without significantly affecting the results. Diluent buffer is phosphate 0·05 M, pH 7·4, with 2 mg/ml bovine serum albumin.

(i) Dispense 0·05 ml of standard (see Table 1) or sample into duplicate tubes; include two pairs containing hPL-free serum alone to act as assay blank and "O" standard.

(ii) To each tube add 0·2 ml of solution of ^{125}I hPL, diluted such that the total counts per tube are approx 10,000–15,000 in 10 sec. Include one pair of tubes containing tracer alone for measurement of total counts.

(iii) To each tube add 0·25 ml of a 1:500 dilution of antiserum to hPL; in the case of the assay blank tubes add 0·25 ml diluent buffer in place of this.

(iv) Incubate for 1 hr at room temperature.

(v) Add 1 ml of absolute ethanol and mix.

(vi) Centrifuge for 30 min at 2000 g at room temperature.

(vii) Decant or aspirate the supernatant.

(viii) Count each precipitate.

(ix) Plot the results as per cent tracer bound on the vertical axis against the concentration of standard on a log scale on the horizontal axis.

(f) Specificity of the hPL assay

The only biological materials which have the potential for interference in the hPL assay are pituitary growth hormone and prolactin: with both molecules the cross-reaction is less than 1% (i.e. sufficient purified GH and prolactin is not available to test lower levels). Since the levels of hPL in normal pregnancy are several orders of magnitude greater than those of GH or prolactin, specificity is not a problem.

(g) Sensitivity of the hPL assay

When fully optimised for sensitivity (Chard, 1978) the hPL assay has a minimum detection limit of 0·1 ng/ml. However, for clinical application great sensitivity is not a requirement since from an early stage of gestation levels are in excess of 1 µg/ml, and in the third trimester the assay should be designed in such a way that 4 µg/ml (the cut-off point between normality and abnormality) should lie in the middle of the standard curve (Letchworth et al., 1971a). This is achieved by the use of high concentrations of reagents, particularly of antibody, which typically is used at final dilutions of 1 in 500–1000. In this way the assay shows a number of advantages. First, it enables a sample to be introduced into the assay without prior dilution and the errors to which this can give rise. Second, the system reaches equilibrium in minutes rather than hours and results can be made available within a few hours of the sample being drawn. Third, the use of a high concentration of antibody permits an increase in the amount of tracer with a concomitant reduction in both counting times and the requirement for high specific activity.

L. MATERNAL LEVELS IN NORMAL PREGNANCY

Placental lactogen is detectable in maternal blood soon after implantation, and the levels rise progressively to reach a plateau after the 35th week (Fig. 6). The increase follows the type of sigmoid curve which seems to be characteristic of all the specific placental proteins and which parallels closely the growth of the placenta both in weight and in DNA content. There is no change

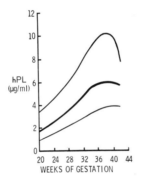

Fig. 6. The normal range of circulating hPL levels in the mother from the 20th–42nd week of gestation. The mean ± two standard deviations are shown. The distribution is skewed, the variation above the mean being greater than that below it.

in levels associated with the onset of labour, and the absolute levels are not related to the time of onset of labour (Gillard, Letchworth and Chard, 1973). The exact values for hPL in late pregnancy have differed widely between different authors, with estimates for the mean at term ranging from 3·3–25 μg/ml (Letchworth, 1976). Most of these differences can be explained by variation among standard preparations, and this should be substantially eliminated by the introduction of the International Reference Preparation.

The normal range of hPL levels in the later part of pregnancy, derived from serial samples on 200 well-defined subjects, is shown in Fig. 6. In common with most other biochemical parameters the variation around the mean shows a skewed distribution (Chard, 1976). The range of variation is greater above the mean than below it. For this reason the best approximation to the true mean and standard deviations is obtained after logarithmic transformation of the data. An alternative approach is the use of non-parametric statistics in which the results are expressed as a median and centiles. Correct analysis of the normal range is the key to the adequate definition of cut-off points between normality and abnormality.

The overall spread of hPL values in normal pregnancies (coefficient of variation 36%) is less than that of circulating oestrogens, but slightly greater than that of the placental protein SP_1 (Klopper, Masson and Wilson, 1977). All other things being equal, the material showing the lowest coefficient of variation should be the best clinical test (Chard, 1976).

M. INTERPRETATION OF BIOCHEMICAL TESTS OF PLACENTAL FUNCTION

The literature on the clinical application of biochemical tests of placental function is frequently confusing and contradictory. One group of workers will demonstrate that a test is of great value, another will disparage the procedure. Furthermore, it is not infrequently asked whether any such test is of any value at all when set against the strict criterion of whether it contributes to a decrease in perinatal mortality and morbidity. However, certain generalisations can be made about the interpretation of these tests and, possibly more important, on the interpretation of the literature about them (see also Chard, 1976):

(i) A test is of no value unless a carefully analysed normal range is available. A normal range should usually be based on results from at least 50 subjects at each week of gestation, and a clear definition of "normality" should be stated.

(ii) The normal range should be submitted to appropriate statistical evaluation. As already noted, a Gaussian distribution is unusual and results should usually be analysed after transformation or in non-parametric form.

(iii) It is essential for any individual laboratory or group of laboratories to establish its own normal range. Because of differences in methodology the use of a published normal range is frequently misleading.

(iv) Ranges should be established for clinically-defined abnormalities according to whether or not they are associated with foetal risk. For example, it is of little value to know that the levels of a given material are generally low in pre-eclampsia: the clinician requires to know which case of pre-eclampsia is at greatest risk.

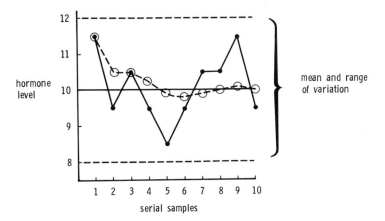

Fig. 7. Diagram to show the value of serial as opposed to single samples. The hormone has an overall day-to-day variation of $\pm 20\%$, and serial samples (●—●) fluctuate within these limits. Calculation of the cumulative mean (O—O) shows that this becomes stable when five or more serial results are available, thus providing a very accurate estimate of the true situation in an individual patient.

(v) It must be appreciated that there is no such thing as a perfect test. All will show a degree of overlap between normality and abnormality, with a "grey-zone" between. It is much better to interpret a result as a risk and not a certainty.

(vi) Serial levels are invariably of greater value than a single level. It is often thought that this is because a trend may be apparent, i.e. a fall in a high-risk case. But far more important is the fact that serial levels give much greater confidence to the observed relation between an individual subject and the population of which that subject is part (Fig 7).

N. MATERNAL LEVELS IN COMPLICATIONS OF PREGNANCY

1. Trophoblastic Tumours

Trophoblastic tumours produce hPL but in amounts smaller than those in normal pregnancy (Samaan *et al.*, 1966; Saxena, Goldstein, Emerson and Selenkow, 1968a; Goldstein, 1971). It has been suggested that low levels of hPL in the presence of an enlarged uterus might alert the clinician to the presence of trophoblastic disease. The maternal levels appear to be related to tumour differentiation; the greater the degree of malignancy, the lower the hPL value in relation to hCG (Saxena *et al.*, 1968a; Goldstein, 1971). In some cases with active disease, hPL may disappear from the circulation while hCG remains detectable (Saxena *et al.*, 1968a).

2. Threatened Abortion

Some 15–20% of all pregnancies end in abortion and most of these patients require hospital admission. Furthermore, the outcome for the foetus is uncertain in many cases of vaginal bleeding in early gestation and such patients may require several days of hospital admission before the final

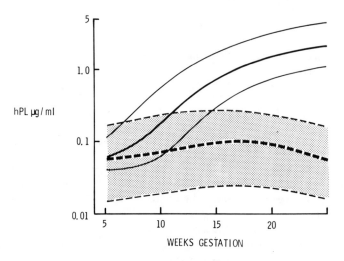

Fig. 8. Plasma hPL levels in 141 subjects who aborted on first admission (dashed lines and hatched area). The mean and range of normal subjects is also shown (solid lines) (Niven, Landon and Chard, 1972).

diagnosis is apparent. There is general agreement that low maternal hPL levels after the 8–10th week indicate that the outcome is likely to be unsatisfactory, and thus provide a valuable guide to prognosis in this condition (Genazzani, Aubert, Fioretti and Felber, 1969; Niven, Landon and Chard, 1972; Gartside and Tindall, 1975) (Fig. 8). This applies whether or not a sonogram is also abnormal (Vorster, Pannall and Slabber, 1977). Low levels, and particularly serial low levels after the 10th week, would be an indication for evacuation of the uterus without further delay unless there are contraindicating factors such as advanced maternal age or infertility.

3. Low Birth Weight Infants

Placental lactogen levels are correlated with the weight of the placenta (Sciarra, Sherwood, Varma and Lundberg, 1968; Cramer, Beck and Makowski, 1971; Lindberg and Nilsson, 1973a), and of the foetus (Letchworth *et al.*, 1971b; Lindberg and Nilsson, 1973a; Boyce, Schwartz, Hubert, Cedard and Dreyfus, 1975). The latter relationship is secondary to that between the weight of the placenta and foetus, and there is disagreement as to whether hPL levels are an efficient guide to foetal growth and the prediction of delivery weight in an individual patient. However, low levels have been described in association with severe intra-uterine growth retardation (Lindberg and Nilsson, 1973b; Hensleigh, Cheaton and Spellacy, 1977), particularly in cases of maternal hypertension (Granat, Sharf, Diengott, Spindel, Kahana and Ebrad, 1977). Increased levels occur in twin pregnancies (Garoff and Seppala, 1973) but because of the lack of a normal range for this condition clinical interpretation is difficult.

4. Pre-eclampsia and Hypertension

Spellacy and his colleagues (1971) described a "foetal danger zone" for subjects with hypertension: values of less than 4 µg/ml after the 30th week indicated a foetal mortality of 24%. The levels are generally lower in multigravidae than in primigravidae (Letchworth and Chard, 1972a; Spellacy, Buhi, Birk and McCreary, 1974), and it has been suggested that the greatest risk and lowest levels are associated with chronic vascular disease. Other workers have shown a similar clear association between low hPL levels and foetal outcome (Keller, Baertschi, Bader, Gerber, Schmid, Solterman and Kopper, 1971; Lindberg and Nilsson. 1973b; Christensen, Frayshav and Fylling, 1974). Kelly *et al.* (1975) showed a 75% foetal risk (growth retardation or perinatal asphyxia) for subjects developing hypertension after the 28th week and having hPL concentrations less than two standard deviations below the normal mean. However, Letchworth and Chard (1972a), while agreeing that hPL levels were generally reduced in pre-eclampsia, were unable to show a significant difference between cases in which foetal outcome was satisfactory and those in which it was not.

The somewhat confusing literature on hPL levels in pre-eclampsia can be attributed to two factors. First, that the condition itself is very heterogeneous and is often not clearly defined. Second, that it is all too common for authors not to distinguish between pre-eclampsia *per se*, and the foetal risk arising from the pre-eclampsia.

5. Diabetes Mellitus

Since diabetes mellitus is associated with a large placenta it would be expected that hPL would be generally elevated in this condition. This has been confirmed by numerous workers (Selenkow, Varma, Younger, White and

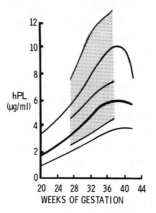

Fig. 9a. hPL levels in pregnancies complicated by diabetes mellitus in which there was no evidence of placental dysfunction.

Emerson, 1969; Cohen, Haour, Dumont and Bertrand, 1973; Ursell, Brudenell and Chard, 1973; Soler, Nicholson and Malins, 1975; Hertogh, Thomas, Hoet and Vanderkeyden, 1976) (Fig, 9a). The levels are reduced in cases in which foetal outcome is unsatisfactory (Fig. 9b). Thus hPL

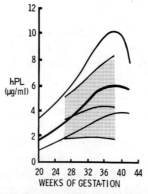

Fig. 9b. hPL levels in pregnancies complicated by diabetes mellitus in which there was evidence of placental dysfunction. The normal range is shown by solid lines (Ursell, Brudenell and Chard, 1973).

levels in diabetic pregnancies must be interpreted in relation to the elevated
range for "normal diabetics". While, under most circumstances, a level of
4 μg/ml is a useful dividing line for the diagnosis of abnormality, in patients
with diabetes the critical level becomes 5 μg/ml.

Some conflicting results on the clinical value of hPL levels can be attributed
to a number of factors, including the definition of the severity of the condition,
the failure to appreciate that abnormality should be judged in relation to
the general elevation of levels in this condition, and the fact that perinatal
death may occur due to metabolic dysfunction in the absence of notable
placental deficiency.

6. Rhesus Iso-immunisation

Most workers have agreed that hPL levels are generally elevated in this
condition, but few have found this to be of significant clinical value. However,
two groups have shown that the levels are most elevated in cases in which

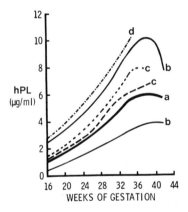

Fig. 10. Mean hPL levels in pregnancies complicated by rhesus isoimmunisation
(a = normal range; b = mildly affected cases; c = moderately affected cases;
d = severely affected cases) (Ward, Letchworth, Niven and Chard, 1974).

the child is severely affected (Lindberg and Nilsson, 1973b; Ward, Letchworth,
Niven and Chard, 1974) (Fig. 10). Before the 26th week, a value which is
greater than two standard deviations above the normal mean indicates a
90% likelihood that the case will be severe. Similar elevations are seen in
amniotic fluid hPL (Niven, Ward and Chard, 1974). Thus, the test may
provide an additional diagnostic aid at a stage when other parameters, such
as liquor bilirubin, may be equivocal.

7. Foetal Death

In many case hPL levels fall before foetal death occurs (Ward, Rochman, Varnavides and Whyley, 1973). This is in agreement with the fact that in many stillbirths the primary cause is placental insufficiency; only rarely does the primary cause lie within the foetus itself.

8. Foetal Distress and Neonatal Asphyxia

In about 12% of pregnancies with no clinical abnormalities in the antenatal period, foetal complications occur either during labour or at the time of delivery. A proportion of these cases can be diagnosed in advance by means of serial estimations of hPL (Letchworth and Chard, 1972b; England, Lorrimer, Ferguson, Moffatt and Kelly, 1974); a patient who is otherwise normal and who has three or more levels below 4 μg/ml in the last 6 weeks of pregnancy has a 71% risk of foetal complications. Similar observations have been made in a mixed group of "at risk" pregnancies, including patients with a clinical suspicion of foetal growth retardation, hypertension, pre-eclampsia, *ante partum* haemorrhage, and chronic renal disease (Edwards, Diver, Davis and Hipkin, 1976). The latter study emphasised the value of combined estimation of plasma hPL and oestriol. These findings indicate that serial estimation of hPL and/or oestriol might become a routine screening test in all pregnancies.

9. Prolonged Pregnancy

Maternal blood and amniotic fluid levels of hPL decrease in prolonged pregnancy (43 weeks and more) (Lolis, Konstandimidis, Paparangelou and Kaskarelis, 1977). Whether they serve to define a special "at risk" group is uncertain.

10. Miscellaneous Conditions

Maternal blood hPL levels are generally lower in smokers than in non-smokers, though the heaviest smokers may have slightly elevated levels (Moser, Hollingsworth, Carlson and Lamotte, 1974; Boyce *et al.*, 1975; Spellacy, Buhi and Birk, 1977). hPL levels are lower in mothers exposed to continuous aircraft noise (Ando and Hattori, 1977).

CONCLUSIONS

hPL is only one of an extensive range of specific biochemical products of the foeto-placental unit any of which might, in principle, serve as a diagnostic marker of foetal well-being. Two factors explain its present acceptance and use. First, the method of measurement is simple and widely available. Second, and following from this, there is an extensive literature on its clinical applications so that interpretation is also relatively simple. In routine obstetric practice the use of hPL or oestriol (blood or urine) determinations should provide as much information as is likely to be achieved from this field of biochemical diagnosis, and the combination of the two may be superior to either alone. Furthermore, it should be appreciated that negative information can in many cases be as valuable as positive information: a value in the upper part of the normal range indicates, almost regardless of the clinical situation, that the foetus carries a relatively low risk.

Finally, the question may be asked "is placental function testing worthwhile?" What is the value of an hPL result in relation to other parameters recorded as part of antenatal care, and can the information lead to a significant reduction in morbidity and mortality? The first question has been answered in a recent study from Gordon, Lewis, Pendlebury, Leighton and Gold (1978). Using a "relative risk factor" we demonstrated that low hPL levels, observed as part of a routine screening programme on an entire obstetric population, were as effective a predictor of poor foetal outcome as the occurrence of severe pre-eclampsia, low maternal weight at 32 weeks, and heavy smoking by the mother. All were superior to many other factors which are widely considered to be of great value in antenatal diagnosis. The second question has been answered by a pioneering study from Spellacy, Buhi and Birk (1975). Placental lactogen estimations were carried out on a large number of "at-risk" subjects; the patients were divided into two randomised groups, one in which the results were reported to the clinician and the other in which they were not. In the first group the perinatal death rate was 3·4%, in the second 15%, a clear indication of the real practical value of these determinations. Given the fact that a substantial proportion of perinatal mortality and morbidity cannot be identified by existing clinical procedures, there must be a good argument for the routine application of hPL measurement or a comparable determination in all pregnancies.

REFERENCES

Ando, Y. and Hattori, H. (1977). *Br. J. Obst. Gynaec.* **84**,115.

Beck, P., Parker, M. L. and Daughaday, W. H. (1965). *J. clin. Endocr. Metab.* **25**, 1457.

Beck, P. and Daughaday, W. H. (1967). *J. clin. Invest.* **46**, 103.

Bewley, T. A. and Li, C. H. (1974). *In* "Lactogenic Hormones, Fetal Nutrition, and Lactation" (J. B. Josimovich, ed.), p. 19. Wiley, New York.

Boyce, A., Schwartz, D., Hubert, C., Cedard, L. and Dreyfus, J. (1975). *Br. J. Obst. Gynaec.* **82**, 964.

Burgos, M. H. and Rodriguez, E. M. (1966). *Am. J. Obstet. Gynec.* **96**, 342.

Burt, R. L., Leake, N. H. and Pruitt, A. B. (1966). *Am. J. Obstet. Gynec.* **95**, 579.

Burt, R. L., Leake, N. H. and Rhyne, A. L. (1970). *Obstet. Gynec.* **36**, 233.

Buttle, H. L., Forsyth, I. A. and Knaggs, G. S. (1972). *J. Endocr.* **53**, 483.

Chard, T. (1972). Medical Monograph 8. The Radiochemical Centre, Amersham.

Chard, T. (1974). *In* "Fetal Medicine" (R. W. Beard, ed.). Saunders, London.

Chard, T. (1976). *In* "Plasma Hormone Assays in Evaluation of Fetal Wellbeing". (A. Klopper, ed.), pp. 1–19. Churchill Livingstone, Edinburgh.

Chard, T. (1978). "An Introduction to Radioimmunoassay and Related Techniques". North Holland, Amsterdam.

Christensen, A., Frayshov, D. and Fylling, P. (1974). *Acta endocr., Copenh.* **77**, 344.

Cohen, H., Grumbach, M. M. and Kaplan, S. L. (1974). *Proc. Soc. exp. Biol. Med.* **117**, 438.

Cohen, M., Haour, F., Dumont, M. and Bertrand, J. (1973). *Am. J. Obstet. Gynec.* **115**, 202.

Contractor, S. F. and Davies, H. (1973). *Nature, Lond.* **243**, 284.

Cotes, P. M. and Das, R. E. G. (1978) *Br. J. Obstet. Gynaec.* **85**, 451.

Cramer, D. W., Beck, P. and Makowski, E. L. (1971). *Am. J. Obstet. Gynec.* **109**, 649.

Crosignani, P. G., Nencioni, T. and Brambati, B. (1972). *J. Obstet. Gynaec. Br. Comm.* **79**, 122.

Currie, A. R., Beck, J. S., Ellis, S. and Reed, C. H. (1966). *J. path. Bact.* **92**, 395.

Edwards, R. P., Diver, M. J., Davis, J. C. and Hipkin, L. J. (1976). *Br. J. Obstet. Gynaec.* **83**, 229.

El-Tomi, A. E. F., Crystle, C. D. and Stevens, V. C. (1970). *Am. J. Obstet. Gynec.* **108**, 345.

England, P., Lorrimer, D., Fergusson, J. C., Moffatt, A. and Kelly, A. (1974). *Lancet*, **i**, 5.

Florini, J. R., Tonelli, G., Breuer, C. B., Coppola, J., Ringler, I. and Bell, P. H. (1966). *Endocrinology*, **79**, 692.

Frantz, A. G., Rabkin, M. T. and Friesen, H. (1965). *J. clin. Endocr. Metab.* **25**, 1136.

Friesen, H. (1965). *Endocrinology*, **76**, 369.

Gardner, J., Bailey, G. and Chard, T. (1974). *Biochem. J.* **137**, 469.

Garoff, L. and Seppala, M. (1973). *J. Obstet. Gynaec. Br. Comm.* **80**, 695.

Gartside, M. W. and Tindall, V. R. (1975). *Br. J. Obstet. Gynaec.* **82**, 303.

Gaspard, U., Goulart, M. and Franchimont, P. (1971). *C. r. Séanc. Soc.* **164** 2381.

Genazzani, A. R., Aubert, M. L., Casoli, M., Fioretti, P. and Felber, J-P. (1969). *Lancet*, **ii**, 1385.

Gillard, M., Letchworth, A. T. and Chard, T. (1973). *Obstet. Gynec.* **41**, 774.

Goldstein, D. P. (1971). *Am. J. Obstet. Gynec.* **110**, 583.

Gordon, Y. B. and Chard, T. (1979). *In* "Human Placental Proteins" (A. Klopper and T. Chard, eds). Springer-Verlag, Amsterdam.

Gordon, Y. B., Lewis, J. D., Pendlebury, D. J., Leighton, M. and Gold, J. (1978). *Lancet*, i, 1001.

Granat, M., Sharf, M., Diengott, D., Spindel, A., Kahana, L. and Elrad, H. (1977). *Am. J. Obstet. Gynec.* **129**, 647.

Grumbach, M. M. and Kaplan, S. L. (1964). *Trans. N. Y. Acad. Sci.* **27**, 167.

Gusdon, J. P. (1969). *Obstet. Gynec.* **33**, 397.

Handwerger, S., Crenshaw, C., Maurer, W. F., Barrett, J. M., Hurley, T. W., Golander, A. and Fellows, R. E. (1977). *J. Endocr.* **72**, 27.

Handwerger, S., Fellows, R. E., Crenshaw, M. C., Hurley, T., Barrett, J. and Maurer, W. F. (1976). *J. Endocr.* **69**, 133.

Handwerger, S. and Sherwood, L. M. (1974). *In* "Lactogenic Hormones, Fetal Nutrition, and Lactation (J. B. Josimovich, ed.), pp. 33–47. Wiley, New York.

Haour, R. (1971). *Horm. Met. Res.* **3**, 131.

Haour, F., Cohen, M. and Bertrand, J. (1970). *C. r. Soc. Biol. Lyon.* **66**, 821.

Hartog, M. (1972). *Clin. Endocr.* **1**, 209.

Hensleigh, P. A., Cheaton, S. G. and Spellacy, W. N. (1977). *Am. J. Obstet. Gynec.* **129**, 675.

Hertogh, R. de, Thomas, K., Hoet, J. J. and Vanderheyden, I. (1976). *Diabetologia*, **12**, 455.

Ikonicoff, L. K. de, and Cedard, L. (1973). *Am. J. Obstet. Gynec.* **116**, 1124.

Ito, Y. and Higashi, K. (1961). *Endocr. Jap.* **8**, 279.

Jepson, J. H. & Friesen, H. G. (1968). *Br. J. Haematol.* **15**, 465.

Josimovich, J. B. (1966). *Endocrinology*, **78**, 707.

Josimovich, J. B. and Archer, D. F. (1977). *Am. J. Obstet. Gynec.* **129**, 777.

Josimovich, J. B. and Brande, B. L. (1964). *Trans. N.Y. Acad. Sci.* **27**, 161.

Josimovich, J. B., Kosor, B., Boccella, L., Mintz, D. H. and Hutchinson, D. (1970). *Obstet. Gynec.* **36**, 244.

Josimovich, J. B. and MacLaren, J. A. (1962). *Endocrinology*, **71**, 209.

Josimovich, J. B., Stock, R. J. and Tobon, H. (1974) *In* "Fetal Nutrition and Lactation" (J. B. Josimovich, ed.), pp. 335–350. Wiley, New York.

Kalkhoff, R. K., Richardson, B. L. and Beck, P. (1969). *Diabetes*, **18**, 153.

Kaplan, S. L. and Grumbach, M. M. (1965). *J. clin. Endocr. Metab.* **25**, 1370.

Kaplan, S. L., Gurpide, E., Sciarra, J. J. and Grumbach, M. M. (1968). *J. clin. Endocr. Metab.* **28**, 1450.

Keller, P. J., Baertschi, U., Bader, P., Gerber, C., Schmid, J., Solterman, R. and Kopper, E. (1971). *Lancet*, ii, 729.

Keller, P. J., Gerber, C., Greub, H. and Schreiner, W. E. (1970). *Horm. Metab. Res.* **2**, 265.

Kelly, A. M., England, P., Lorrimer, J. D., Fergusson, J. C. and Govan, A. D. T. (1975). *Br. J. Obstet. Gynaec.* **82**, 272.

Kim, Y. J. and Felig, P. (1971). *J. clin. Endocr. Metab.* **32**, 864.

Klopper, A., Masson, G. and Wilson, G. (1977). *Br. J. Obstet. Gynaec.* **84**, 648–655.

Leake, N. H. and Burt, R. L. (1964). *Obstet. Gynec.* **34**, 471.

Letchworth, A. T. (1976). *In* "Plasma Hormone Assays in Evaluation of Fetal Well-being (A. Klopper, ed.), pp. 147–173. Churchill Livingstone, Edinburgh.

Letchworth, A. T. and Chard, T. (1972a). *J. Obstet. Gynaec. Br. Comm.* **79**, 680.

Letchworth, A. T. and Chard, T. (1972b). *Lancet*, i, 704.

Letchworth, A. T., Boardman, R. J., Bristow, C., Landon, J. and Chard, T. (1971a). *J. Obstet. Gynaec. Br. Comm.* **78**, 535.

Letchworth, A. T., Boardman, R. J. Bristow, C., Landon, J. and Chard, T. (1971b). *J. Obstet. Gynaec. Br. Comm.* **78**, 542.

Li, C. H., Grumbach, M. M., Kaplan, S. L., Josimovich, J. B., Friesen, H. and Catt, K. J. (1968). *Experientia*, **24**, 1288.

Lindberg, B. S. and Nilsson, B. A. (1973a). *J. Obstet. Gynaec. Br. Comm.* **80**, 619.

Lindberg, B. S. and Nilsson, B. A. (1973b). *J. Obstet. Gynaec. Br. Comm.* **80**, 1046.

Lolis, D., Konstantinidis, K., Paparangelou, G. and Kaskarelis, D. (1977). *Am. J. Obstet. Gynec.* **128**, 724.

Martin, J. M. and Friesen, H. (1969). *Endocrinology*, **84**, 619.

Moser, R. J., Holingsworth, D. R., Carlson, J. W. and Lamotte, L. (1974). *Am. J. Obstet. Gynec.* **120**, 1080.

Niall, H. D., Hogan, M. L., Tregear, G. W., Segre, G. V., Hwang, P., and Friesen, H. G. (1973). *Rec. Prog. Horm. Res.* **29**, 387.

Niven, P. A. R., Landon. J. and Chard, T. (1972). *Br. med. J.* **iii**, 799.

Niven, P. A. R., Ward, R. H. T. and Chard, T. (1974). *J. Obstet. Gynaec. Br. Comm.* **81**, 988.

Pavlou, C., Chard, T. and Letchworth, A. T. (1972). *J. Obstet. Gynaec. Br. Comm.* **79**, 629.

Pavlou, C., Chard, T., Landon, J. and Letchworth, A. T. (1973). *Eur. J. obstet. Gynec. reprod. Biol.* **3**, 45.

Riggi, S. J., Boshart, C. R., Bell, P. H. and Ringler, I. (1966). *Endocrinology.* **79**, 709.

Samaan, N. A., Yen, S. C. C., Friesen, H. and Pearson, O. H. (1966). *J. clin. Endocr. Metab.* **26**, 1303.

Saxena, B. N., Emerson, K. and Selenkow, H. A. (1969). *New Engl. J. Med.* **281**, 225.

Saxena, B. N., Goldstein, D. P., Emerson, K. and Selenkow, H. A. (1968a). *Am. J. Obstet. Gynec.* **103**, 115.

Saxena, B. N., Refetoff, S., Emerson, K. and Selenkow, H. A. (1968b). *Am. J. Obstet. Gynecol.* **101**, 874.

Sciarra, J. J., Sherwood, L. M., Varma, A. A. and Lundberg, W. B. (1968). *Am. J. Obstet. Gynec.* **101**, 413.

Selenkow, H. A., Varma, K., Younger, D., White, P. and Emerson, K. (1969). *Diabetes*, **20**, 696.

Seppala, M. and Ruoslahti, E. (1970). *Acta obstet. gynec. scand.* **49**, 143.

Sherwood, L. M., Handwerger, S., McLaurin, W. D. and Lanner, M. (1971). *Nature New Biol.* **233**, 59.

Shiu, R. P. C. and Friesen, H. G. (1973). *Science*, **180**, 968.

Shome, B. and Parlow, A. F. (1977). *J. clin. Endocr. Metab.* **45**, 1112.

Soler, N. G., Nicholson, H. O. and Malins, J. M. (1975). *Lancet*, **ii**, 54.

Spellacy, W. N. (1972). *In* "Lactogenic Hormones" (G. E. W. Wolstenholme and J. Knight, eds), p. 223. Churchill Livingstone, London.

Spellacy, W. N., Buhi, W. C. and Birk, S. A. (1975). *Am. J. Obstet. Gynec.* **121**, 835.

Spellacy, W. N., Buhi, W. C. and Birk, S. A. (1977). *Am. J. Obstet. Gynec.* **127**, 232.

Spellacy, W. N., Buhi, W. C., Birk, S. A. and McCreary, S. A. (1974). *Am. J. Obstet. Gynec.* **120**, 214.

Spellacy, W. N., Buhi, W. C., Schram, J. D., Birk, S. A. and McCreary, S. A. (1971). *Obstet. Gynec.* **96**, 1164.

Spellacy, W. N., Carlson, K. L. and Birk, S. A. (1966). *Obstet. Gynec.* **96**, 1164.

Spencer, T. S. (1971). *J. Obstet. Gynaec. Br. Comm.* **78**, 232.

Spona, J. and Janisch, H. (1971). *Acta endocr., Copenh.* **68**, 401.

Teoh, E. S., Spellacy, W. N. and Buhi, W. C. (1971). *J. Obstet. Gynaec. Br. Comm.* **78**, 673.

Turtle, J. R., Beck. B. and Daughaday, W. H. (1966). *Endocrinology*, **79**, 197.

Tyson, J. E., Austin, K. L. and Farinholt, J. W. (1971). *Am. J. Obstet. Gynec.* **109**, 1080.

Ursell, W., Brudenell, J. and Chard, T. (1973). *Br. med. J.* **ii**, 80.

Varma, S. K., Varma, K., Selenkow, H. A. and Emerson, K. (1970). *Am. J. Obstet. Gynec.* **107**, 472.

Vorster, C. S., Pannall, P. R. and Slabber, C. F. (1977). *Am. J. Obstet. Gynec.* **128**, 879.

Walsh, S. W., Wolf, R. C., Meyer, R. K., Aubert, M. L. and Friesen, H. (1977). *Endocrinology*, **100**, 851.

Ward, H., Rochman, H., Varnavides, L. A. and Whyley, G. A. (1973). *Am. J. Obstet. Gynec.* **116**, 1105.

Ward, R. H. T., Letchworth, A. T., Niven, P. A. R. and Chard, T. (1974). *Br. med. J.* **i**, 347.

Ylikorkala, O., Haapalahti, J. and Jarvinen, P. A. (1973). *J. Obstet. Gynaec. Br. Comm.* **80**, 546.

Zuckerman, J. E., Fallon, V., Tashjian, A. H., Levine, L. and Friesen, H. G. (1970). *J. clin. Endocr. Metab.* **30**, 769.

VIII. Human Chorionic Gonadotrophin

K. D. BAGSHAWE, F. SEARLE and M. WASS

INTRODUCTION

The presence of large amounts of a hormone with luteinising gonadotrophic activity in human pregnancy urine was first discovered in 1927 by Aschheim and Zondek. Although it was initially considered that this hormone was produced by the pituitary, Philipp (1930) suggested that it was not of pituitary but of placental origin. This was confirmed by Kido (1937) and Gey, Seegar-Jones and Hellman (1938). Stewart, Sano and Montgomery (1948) demonstrated experimentally with placental tissue cultures that the hormone was produced by the placenta. The hormone was named human chorionic gonadotrophin (hCG). The evidence for the placental origin of hCG was reviewed by Loraine (1956) and Diczfalusy and Troen (1961).

After implantation of the blastocyst about seven days after fertilisation the concentration of hCG in plasma and urine rises continuously during the first 10–12 weeks of pregnancy after which it declines to a lower level which is maintained during the latter half of pregnancy (Loraine, 1967). It is considered that its primary function in pregnancy is the maintenance of the production of oestrogen and progesterone by the corpus luteum, and the prevention of the decline in luteal function which normally occurs in an infertile menstrual cycle (Ross, Cargille, Lipsett, Rayford, Marshall, Strott and Rodbard, 1970; Van de Wiele, Bogumil, Dyrenfurth, Ferin, Jewelewicz, Warren, Rizkallah and Mikhail, 1970). The large amounts of hCG secreted in pregnancy, in excess of the amount apparently required to sustain luteal function, has prompted inquiries into its possible additional functions in pregnancy. hCG is found not only in the urine, blood and the trophoblast tissue of pregnant women, but also patients with trophoblastic tumours.

hCG is a glycopeptide composed of two non-identical subunits designated α and β. hCG shares this structure with pituitary glycoprotein hormones LH, FSH and TSH. Moreover, the α-subunit of all glycoprotein hormones is interchangeably identical. The β-subunit differs between the hormones and confers on the hormone its unique biological activity. Since the crude material for the isolation and purification is available in large amounts, this hormone has been the subject of numerous studies which have resulted in the elucidation of its molecular structure. The significant structural similarity of hCG with other glycoprotein trophic hormones has made it a suitable model for the study of structure-function relationships in this group of hormones.

A. CHEMISTRY OF hCG

1. Preparation

The most commonly used source of hCG for purification has been the urine of women between the 9th and 12th weeks of pregnancy. In this period 2–3 mg hCG are excreted daily. Urine specimens from patients with trophoblastic disease occasionally contain considerably larger amounts than the pregnancy urine, and they have also served as sources.

The first purification steps generally utilise adsorption techniques, and benzoic acid (Gurin, Bachman and Wilson, 1939), kaolin (Albert, 1956), tannic acid (Johnsen, 1958), or attapulgite (Salhanick, 1961) have been used. A review of the early methods of extraction, with special reference to yields, has been presented by Loraine and Mackay (1961).

Crude hCG was first prepared commercially by the method of Katzman, Godfrid, Cain and Doisy (1943), by using adsorption on permutit, elution with an alcoholic solution of ammonium acetate and subsequent precipitation by an increased concentration of alcohol. The resulting preparation had a biological potency of 2000–3000 u/mg., and has served to establish the Second International Standard for hCG (Bangham and Grab, 1964).

Methods yielding hCG preparations of high purity have been reported by several laboratories (Van Hell, Matthijsen and Homan, 1968; Goverde, Veenkamp and Homan, 1968; Bahl, 1969a; Bell, Canfield and Sciarra, 1969; Mori, 1970; Brossmer, Dörner, Hilgenfeldt, Leidenberger and Trude, 1971; Ashitaka, Tokura, Tane, Mochizuki and Tojo, 1970; Grässlin, Czygan and Weise, 1972; Qazi, Mukherjee, Javidi, Pala and Diczfalusy, 1974). The majority used the commercial crude hCG from pregnancy urine as starting material. The purification methods used were generally based on gel filtration, ion-exchange chromatography and isoelectric focusing yielding hCG preparations with activity in the range of 13,000–20,000 u/mg.

Urine of patients with trophoblastic tumours has also been used as a source of highly purified hCG and preparations, with activities up to 19,000 u/mg have been reported (Morris, 1955; Reisfeld and Hertz, 1960; Wilde and Bagshawe, 1965). Ashitaka, Mochizuki and Tojo (1972) reported the preparation of hCG of high purity from the trophoblastic tissue of hydatidiform mole. Purification of hCG from human term placenta has been reported by Lee, Wong, Lee and Ma (1977). By using affinity chromatography they achieved a 57 fold purification in a single step, and presented evidence that the purified product contained intact hormone as well as its free α-subunit.

The highly purified preparations of hCG showed considerable heterogeneity of charge, while being homogeneous in molecular size. It has now

N

been established that the charge heterogeneity is largely based on variations in the sialic acid content. Merz, Hilgenfeldt, Dörner and Brossmer (1974) demonstrated that the highly purified hCG can be separated by isoelectric focusing into fractions which lie in the isoelectric point range 4·0–5·2, and the fraction with the highest sialic acid content exhibited the highest biological activity. Goverde *et al.* (1968) found earlier that increasing sialic acid content of purified hCG correlated with increased biological activity. The complete desialylation of hCG by the action of neuraminidase gave a homogeneous hormone product with isoelectric point 10·0 (Gershey and Kaplan, 1974). On the other hand, the protein moiety of the hCG molecule was found to be fairly constant, and good agreement existed between the amino acid composition of hCG prepared by different laboratories.

2. Chemical Composition

Early work on the chemical composition of hCG established that it was a glycoprotein. Preparations of high purity by biochemical and immunological criteria have enabled investigations to derive analytical data of the amino acid and carbohydrate composition of the hormone. The amino acid composition of hCG derived from sequence studies of its subunits is shown in Table 1. Quantitative estimations of carbohydrate, from four laboratories,

Table 1

Amino acid residues per molecule of hCG subunits (Morgan *et al.*, 1975).

	hCG-α	hCG-β
Alanine	5	8
Arginine	3	12
Aspartic acid/asparagine	6	11
Cystine (half)	10	12
Glutamic acid/glutamine	9	9
Glycine	4	8
Histidine	3	1
Isoleucine	1	5
Leucine	4	12
Lysine	6	4
Methionine	3	1
Phenylalanine	4	2
Proline	7	22
Serine	8	13
Threonine	8	10
Tyrosine	4	3
Valine	7	12

Table 2

Carbohydrate composition of hCG and its subunits (g/100 g).

	Native hCG[a,b,c,d,e]					hCG-α[e,f]		hCG-β[e,f]	
Galactose	4·9	3·9	5·3	5·0	5·7	3·2	3·2	6·3	6·3
Mannose	4·9	2·9	5·3	4·8	5·3	6·6	6·6	3·0	3·0
Fucose	1·2	0·6	0·6	0·6	trace	ND	ND	trace	trace
N-acetylglucosamine	7·0	7·3	8·9	8·8	7·9	9·0	8·5	7·0	7·0
N-acetylgalactosamine	1·7	1·8	2·1	1·8	2·6	ND	ND	3·4	2·5
Sialic acid	8·5	8·2	9·0	8·4	9·1	7·3	3·5	8·3	7·3

[a] Got, R., Bourrillon, R. and Michon, J. (1960) (recalculated)
[b] Goverde, B. C., Veen Kamp, F. J. N. and Homan, J. D. H. (1968)
[c] Bahl, O. (1969a)
[d] Mori, K. F. (1970)
[e] Canfield, R. E., Birken, S., Morse, J. H. and Morgan, F. J. (1976)
[f] Morgan, F. J., Birken, S. and Canfield, R. E. (1974)
[g] ND = Not detected

are presented in Table 2. The most salient feature of the amino acid composition of hCG is a very high proline content. Proline is known to prohibit the formation of α-helix, and indeed the optical rotatory dispersion studies of hCG revealed little evidence of α-helix (Canfield, Morgan, Kammerman, Bell and Agosto, 1971).

hCG purified from the urine of patients with choriocarcinoma or hydatidiform mole has similar immunological properties to pregnancy hCG (Lewis, Dray, Genuth and Schwartz, 1964). Although electrophoretic differences were demonstrable in hCG preparation from two different sources, (Reisfeld Bergenstal and Hertz, 1959; Reisfeld and Hertz, 1960) the presence of similar electrophoretic heterogeneity in preparations of pregnancy hCG (Van Hell et al., 1968) argued against electrophoretic mobility as a criterion of difference. In their study of hCG from choriocarcinoma, Canfield, Bell and Agosto (1970) established that these preparations of hCG had high biological potency and that the amino acid analysis of the protein moiety was essentially the same as in pregnancy hCG. However, the carbohydrate composition of some choriocarcinoma hCG preparations was reported to be different (Ashitaka et al., 1972).

The absolute specificity of hCG as a marker of pregnancy and of trophoblastic tumours has been questioned as a result of recent findings. Braunstein, Rasor and Wade (1975) reported that extracts of human testis contain a substance with physical and immunological properties of hCG. Evidence for a gonadotrophin in the urine from postmenopausal women and in pituitary extracts which has physical, immunological and biological similarities to hCG has been obtained by Chen, Hodgen, Matsuura, Lin, Gross, Reichert, Birken, Canfield and Ross (1976).

3. Subunit Structure

The non-identity of the subunits of hCG was first established by two groups of investigators, Canfield *et al.* (1970) and Swaminathan and Bahl (1970). The published procedures for the preparation of subunits are generally based on two methods:

(i) dissociation in urea followed by ion-exchange chromatography (Swaminathan and Bahl, 1970; Morgan and Canfield, 1971);

(ii) dissociation in propionic acid followed by gel filtration (Morgan, Canfield, Vaitukaitis and Ross, 1973).

The characterisation of subunits has culminated in the elucidation of the primary structure of their protein moiety. Two proposals have been published (Bellisario, Carlsen and Bahl, 1973; Carlsen, Bahl and Swaminathan, 1973; Morgan, Birken and Canfield, 1973). They agreed in the sequence of the α-subunit, but contained significant differences in the amino acid sequence at the COOH-terminus of the β-subunit and the concomitant differences in the proposed sites for the carbohydrate attachment.

The COOH-terminus of hCG-β contains 30 amino acids which are not present in the β-subunit of hLH. This extra sequence of hCG-β is potentially of great value for providing an immunological means for distinguishing between hCG and LH. Morgan, Birken and Canfield (1975) re-examined their original proposal and confirmed it while at the same time establishing amide assignments. Birken and Canfield (1977) re-investigated only the 27-residue peptide, from position 115 through 141. Quantitative Edman sequence degradation of this peptide, of another peptide produced by thermolysin digestion which contained residues 142–145, and of two tryptic peptides (residues 123–145 and 134–145) has yielded an amino acid sequence for this region which has also confirmed the initial proposal by Morgan *et al.* (1973). At the same time they confirmed the positions of attachment of carbohydrate chains to serine residues 121, 127, 132 and 138. Keutmann and Williams (1977), in an independent study, employing a different type of enzymic cleavage and a different method of identifying carbohydrate–serine residues, obtained results which agreed completely with the findings of Birken and Canfield (1977). The synthesis of 31- and 35-amino acid fragments of the C-terminus of hCG-β has been reported by Fischer, Chang, Howard and Folkers (1977). The amino acid sequence of the α- and β-subunits of hCG, according to Morgan *et al.* (1975) is shown in Fig. 1.

Each subunit is highly cross-linked by disulphide bonds, of which there are five in the α-subunit, and the six in the β-subunit. The pairing of the half-cystine residues has not yet been established with certainty.

When their half-cystine residues are placed in juxtaposition, the linear sequence of hCG-α exhibits marked homology with the subunits of hLH

Ala-Pro-Asp-Val-Gln-Asp-Cys-Pro-Glu-Cys-Thr-Leu-Gln-Glu-Asp-Pro-Phe-
              10

Phe-Ser-Gln-Pro-Gly-Ala-Pro-Ile-Leu-Gln-Cys-Met-Gly-Cys-Cys-Phe-Ser-Arg-
      20   30

                                                          CHO
Ala-Tyr-Pro-Thr-Pro-Leu-Arg-Ser-Lys-Lys-Thr-Met-Leu-Val-Gln-Lys-Asn-
          40   50

Val-Thr-Ser-Glu-Ser-Thr-Cys-Cys-Val-Ala-Lys-Ser-Tyr-Asn-Arg-Val-Thr-Val-
                  60   70
                              CHO
Met-Gly-Gly-Phe-Lys-Val-Glu-Asn-His-Thr-Ala-Cys-His- Cys-Ser-Thr-Cys-Tyr-
                              80

Tyr-His-Lys-Ser.
    90

                                              CHO
Ser-Lys-Glu-Pro-Leu-Arg-Pro-Arg-Cys-Arg-Pro-Ile-Asn-Ala-Thr-Leu-Ala-
                              10

                                              CHO
Val-Glu-Lys-Glu-Gly-Cys-Pro-Val-Cys-Ile-Thr-Val-Asn-Thr-Thr-Ile-Cys-Ala-
      20   30

Gly-Tyr-Cys-Pro-Thr-Met–Thr-Arg-Val-Leu-Gln-Gly-Val-Leu-Pro-Ala-Leu-
          40   50

Pro-Gln-Val-Val-Cys-Asn-Tyr-Arg-Asp-Val-Arg-Phe-Glu-Ser-Ile-Arg-Leu-Pro-
                  60   70

Gly-Cys-Pro-Arg-Gly-Val-Asn-Pro-Val-Val-Ser-Tyr-Ala-Val-Ala-Leu-Ser-Cys-
                              80

Gln-Cys-Ala-Leu-Cys-Arg-Arg-Ser-Thr-Thr-Asp-Cys-Gly-Gly-Pro-Lys-Asp-
    90   100

                                                          CHO
His-Pro-Leu-Thr-Cys-Asp-Asp-Pro-Arg-Phe-Gln-Asp-Ser-Ser-Ser-Ser-Lys-
            110   120
            CHO   CHO   CHO
Ala-Pro-Pro-Pro-Ser-Leu-Pro-Ser-Pro-Ser-Arg-Leu-Pro-Gly-Pro-Ser-Asp-
                              130

Thr-Pro-Ile-Leu-Pro-Gln.
140

Fig. 1. The amino acid sequence of the α- (top) and β-(bottom) subunits of hCG, according to Morgan *et al.* (1975). The sites of attachment of oligosaccharide chains (CHO) are indicated.

(Dufau and Catt, 1973; Liu, Nahm, Sweeney, Lamkin, Baker and Ward, 1972; Maghuin-Rogister, Combarnous and Hennen, 1972; Sairam, Papkoff and Li, 1972a, b), human FSH (Rathnam and Saxena, 1975) and human TSH (Liao and Pierce, 1971). The sequence of LH-α differs from hCG-α only in a two-residue inversion and in a deletion of three amino acids at the NH_2-terminus. Considerable homology also exists between the primary sequence of the α-subunit of hCG/LH and the LH-α from different species, indicating great conservation of its structure during evolution. Approximately 70%

of the residues are identical, and an additional 21 % can be regarded as replaced by a single base change in the codon (Liu *et al.*, 1972; Maghuin-Rogister *et al.*, 1972).

Homologies exist, but to a lesser extent, between hCG-β and hLH-β (Closset, Hennen and Lequin, 1973; Shome and Parlow, 1973). As already mentioned, hCG-β has a 30-residue peptide at the COOH-terminus which is not present in the β-subunits of any other pituitary glycoprotein hormones. Much less homology exists between hCG-β and the β-subunits of human TSH and FSH (Saxena and Rathnam, 1976; Shome and Parlow, 1974).

4. Recombination of Subunits

When separated α- and β-subunits are incubated under the appropriate conditions, they reassociate to form hCG (Canfield *et al.*, 1971). Poly-acrylamide gel electrophoresis and gel filtration confirmed that the majority of the reassociated hCG behaved as native hCG. The reassociation also resulted in the significant restoration of biological activity, which is essentially absent in isolated subunits.

The rates of dissociation and reassociation of subunits of hCG have been studied by Aloj, Edelhoch, Ingham, Morgan, Canfield and Ross (1973). They used the method of analysing the hormone in the presence of its sub-units based on a large change in the quantum yield of the fluorescent probe 1·8-anilino-naphthalene sulphonate (ANS) which is produced when it combines with the native hormone, but not with its subunits. They followed the rates of reassociation by ANS fluorescence and by bioassay and found good agreement between the two methods. The rate of subunit association was significantly affected by temperature, pH and ionic strength.

It has been proposed (Ingham, Aloj and Edelhoch 1974; Reichert, Trowbridge, Bhalla and Lawson, 1974) that the mechanism of formation of the native hormone from its subunits involves at least two steps: a bi-molecular association of the subunits to form a complex αβ, followed by a first order rearrangement in which this complex assumes the conformation of the native hormone. The study of the effect of subunit concentration on subunit recombination (Ingham, Weintraub and Edelhoch, 1976a) confirmed the two-step mechanism.

The reversible folding of hCG at acid pH and upon the recombination of subunits was reported by Garnier, Salesse and Pernollet (1974). They followed the conformational changes by measuring the maximum of the difference spectra and by enhancement of ANS fluorescence and suggested a possible reaction scheme for reassociation consisting first of a fast equilib-rium, possibly diffusion controlled, which is followed by a rate-limiting first-order step yielding the native state. They concluded that this low rate of formation of native hormone might necessitate the storage of the hormone in secretory cells.

It has been reported that the dissociation of subunits results in the exposure of buried tyrosyl residues, as measured by difference absorption spectra (Ingham *et al.*, 1974) by reactivity towards iodine (Canfield, Morgan, Kammerman and Ross, 1973) and by chemical reagents specific for tyrosine (Hum, Botting and Mori, 1976). Studies of hCG and its subunits using tyrosine fluorescence (Ingham, Tylenda and Edelhoch, 1976a) suggested that isolated subunits possess little tertiary structure beyond that which is stabilised by numerous disulphide bonds. They stressed the important role of the disulphide bond in maintaining the rigidity of tyrosyl residues but added that other factors, such as hydrogen bonding or hydrophobic interactions might be contributing to this rigidity.

As with other gonadotrophins, the forces involved in subunit–subunit interaction of hCG appear to be conformational, electrostatic and hydrophobic, but the relative contributions of each to the total free energy change for the process $\alpha + \beta \rightarrow \alpha\beta$ under physiological conditions is not known at present.

5. Carbohydrate Composition and Structure

hCG contains approximately 30% carbohydrate, which is made up of six different monosaccharide units: sialic acid, L-fucose, D-galactose, D-mannose, *N*-acetylglucosamine, and *N*-acetylgalactosamine (Table 2). hCG is unique among glycoprotein hormones in its high content of sialic acid and its consequent long circulatory half life.

The first tentative proposal for the arrangement of monosaccharides in hCG has been presented by Bahl (1969b). He showed evidence for the presence in hCG of both types of carbohydrate–protein linkages commonly found in glycoproteins, namely the *N*-glycosidic linkage between *N*-acetylglucosamine and an asparagine residue, and the O-glycosidic linkage involving *N*-acetylgalactosamine and a serine residue. By stepwise cleavage of sugar residues using specific glycosidases he derived the sequence of monosaccharide units within each carbohydrate chain. He proposed two structures for large chains, (structures I and II, Fig. 2) and another structure for the short serine-linked chains (structure III, Fig. 2). In a later communication Bahl (1971) assigned structure I and structure II to the α- and β-subunits respectively. Subsequent work (Bellisariò *et al.*, 1973) showed that the α-subunit of hCG contained two large carbohydrate chains attached to asparagine residues, 52 and 78. The oligosaccharide chains in the β-subunit are of two types, two large chains attached to asparagine residues 13 and 30, and at the COOH-terminus four small carbohydrate chains linked to

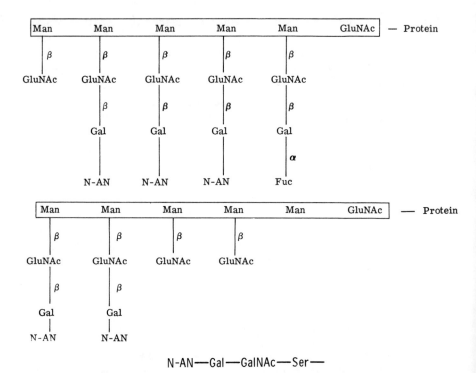

N-AN—Gal—GalNAc—Ser—

Fig. 2. Structures for the oligosaccharide chains of HCG proposed by Bahl (1969b). Top = structure I, middle = structure II, bottom = structure III. Man = mannose; Gal = galactose; Fuc = fucose; GluNAc = *N*-acetylglucosamine; GalNAc = *N*-acetylgalactosamine; N-AN = *N*-acetylneuraminic acid (sialic acid).

serine residues 121, 127, 132 and 138 (Morgan *et al.*, 1975; Birken *et al.*, 1977). As in the case of other glycoproteins (Spiro, 1970) the sites of attachment of large oligosaccharide chains to asparagine residues and in α- and β-subunits possess the invariant Asn – × – Ser/Thr sequence.

The structure of the carbohydrate chains of hCG-α has been studied more recently by Kennedy and Chaplin (1976). In contrast to studies of Bahl (1969b) which used the carboxamidomethylated derivative of hCG, Kennedy and Chaplin used as starting material the similarly modified isolated hCG-α. Proteolysis with trypsin gave rise to various peptides and glycopeptides which were identified. By subjecting the two glycopeptides to component analysis they found that these represented the two carbohydrate chains of the parent molecule. By sequential removal with specific glycosidases of monosaccharide units from these two glycopeptides they demonstrated that:

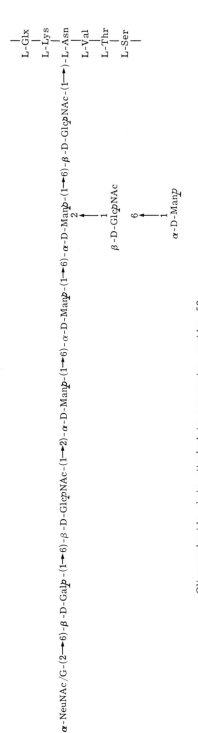

α-NeuNAc/G-(2→6)-**β**-D-Gal*p*-(1→6)-**β**-D-Glc*p*NAc-(1→2)-**α**-D-Man*p*-(1→6)-**α**-D-Man*p*-(1→6)-**α**-D-Man*p*-(1→6)-**β**-D-Glc*p*NAc-(1→)-L-Asn

|—L-Glx
|—L-Lys
|—L-Asn
|—L-Val
|—L-Thr
|—L-Ser
|—

β-D-Glc*p*NAc
2
↑
1
6
↑
1
α-D-Man*p*

Oligosaccharide chain attached to asparagine residue 52

α-NeuNAc/G-(2→6)-**β**-D-Gal*p*-(1→2)-**α**-D-Man*p*-(1→6)-**β**-D-Glc*p*NAc-(1→6)-**α**-D-Man*p*-(1→6)-**β**-D-Glc*p*NAc-(1→)-L-Asn

|—L-Val
|—L-Glx
|—L-Asn
|—L-His
|—L-Thr
|—L-Ala
|—

β-D-Glc*p*NAc
2
↑
1
6
↑
X

Oligosaccharide chain attached to asparagine residue 78

Fig. 3. Structures for oligosaccharide chains of hCG-α subunit, according to Kennedy and Chaplin (1966). NeuNAc = *N*-acetylneuraminic acid; Neu NG = *N*-glycollylneuraminic acid; Glc *p* NAc = *N*-acetylglucosamine (pyranose form); Man *p* = mannose (pyranose form); Gal *p* = galactose (pyranose form); X = unknown substituent.

(i) galactose, mannose, glucosamine, and sialic acid possess the D-con-figuration;

(ii) glucosamine units were N-acetylated;

(iii) in the oligosaccharide chain, sialic acid units were furthest from the peptide backbone, followed by D-galactose units.

They also demonstrated that the D-galactose, D-mannose, and N-acetyl-glucosamine units were present in the pyranose form; that the D-galacto-pyranose units were linked in the 1 and 6 positions; and that the D-manno-pyranose units were present in several forms, i.e. one in a terminal non-reducing position, one as a 1,2-linked residue, some as 1,6-linked residues and some as 1,2,6-linked branch points. The N-acetylglucosamine units were 1,6-linked. On the basis of the data the authors proposed structures for the two carbohydrate chains of hCG-α (Fig. 3). They also compared and contrasted the structures derived for the α-subunit of hCG with those derived for hFSH (Kennedy and Chaplin, 1972) pointing out that despite the immunological and peptide sequence similarities of the α-subunits of human gonadotrophins and of TSH, their carbohydrate structures differed not only in the monosaccharide sequences, but also in the linkage positions between units.

6. Physico-chemical Properties

Molecular weight determinations of hCG have given a wide range of values. Van Hell et al. (1968) derived a value of about 62,000 by sedimentation equilibrium. Bahl (1969a) reported a value of approximately 59,000 by gel filtration and 47,000 by sedimentation equilibrium. The higher value obtained by gel filtration is consistent with the results obtained with other glyco-proteins. (Whitaker, 1963).

The calculated molecular weight of hCG, from the composition of sub-units, is 38,000, 15,000 for the α-subunit (Bellisario et al., 1973) and 23,000 for the β-subunit (Carlsen et al., 1973).

Other physical constants of hCG are presented in Table 3.

B. BIOLOGICAL PROPERTIES

1. Biosynthesis

Chorionic gonadotrophin production by placenta has been confirmed only in humans and other primates. Tullner (1974) has reviewed data available for primates. The site of biosynthesis of hCG is now accepted to be pre-dominantly in the syncytiotrophoblast of the placenta (Midgley and Pierce, 1962; Mason, Phifer, Spicer, Swallow and Dreskin, 1969; Okudaira,

Table 3

Physicochemical properties of hCG and its subunits.

Property	hCG	hCG-α	hCG-β	References
Sedimentation coefficient, $S20$, $w(S)$	2·7			Got and Bourrillon (1965)
	2.89			Bahl (1969a)
	3·07			Mori and Hollands (1971)
Diffusion constant, $D20$ (sec^{-1})	$8·2 \times 10^{-7}$			Got and Bourrillon (1965)
Partial specific volume (ml/g)	0·727			Got and Bourrillon (1965)
Extinction coefficient $E_{1cm}^{1mg/ml}$ at 278 nm	0·425			Got and Bourrillon (1965)
	0·388			Bahl (1969a)
	0·547			Mori and Hollands (1971)
E(M^{-1} cm^{-1}) 280 nm	$1·41 \times 10^4$	$0·64 \times 10^4$	$0·56 \times 10^4$	Morgan, Canfield, Vaitukaitis and Ross (1973)
Frictional ratio $f:f_0$	1·28			Got and Bourrillon (1965)
Viscosity (η) 25	3·4			Mori and Hollands (1971)

Hashimoto, Hamanaka and Yoshinara, 1971). The mechanisms controlling biosynthesis, storage and release of hCG are not known.

2. Biological Polymorphism

Studies of the molecular forms of hCG in plasma, urine and placental extracts (Franchimont and Reuter, 1972; Vaitukaitis, 1974; Vaitukaitis, Ross, Braunstein and Rayford, 1976) indicated the presence in all three biological materials of native hCG and of the α-subunit which was immunologically similar to hCG-α. In addition to native hCG, placental extracts in the second trimester of pregnancy, contained a larger molecular form of the α-subunit. Little β-subunit was detected in the plasma and in placental extracts but a low molecular weight substance was found in urine which reacted in a radioimmunoassay for hCG-β. These findings were confirmed by Good, Ramos-Uribe, Ryan and Kempers (1977), who reported in addition, the presence in placental extracts of a large-molecular weight substance, eluted in the void volume during G-100 Sephadex gel filtration, which reacted in radioimmunoassays specific for native hCG, hCG-α and hCG-β, as well as in the radioreceptor assay. This large molecular species could not be dissociated into subunits, and the authors suggested that it may represent a single-chain prohormone for hCG.

A large immunological species of hCG was also reported by Tojo, Ashitaka, Maruo and Ohashi (1977) in extracts of chorionic tissue cultivated *in vitro* and in culture media. This large species of hCG, also eluted in the void volume during G-100 Sephadex chromatography, could not be distinguished immunologically from purified hCG, but had low biological activity in the radioreceptor assay. Since the large immunological species was the predominant form in chorionic tissue cultivated for a short period, and the authentic hCG was the predominant form in the media, the authors suggested that the large hCG, possibly a prohormone, synthesised initially in the placenta, may be converted to the active form before secretion into the media.

The question of a hCG prohormone is still unresolved, but the finding (Landefeld, McWilliam and Boime, 1976) of a mRNA in placental tissue which in an *in vitro* system gave rise to a peptide of mw 16,000 which was very similar to hCG-α, argues against the concept of a single chain prohormone for hCG.

3. Mechanism of Action

It is generally thought that the binding of hormones to membrane receptors is the initial event leading to activation of adenylate cyclase and subsequent production of a specific target tissue response. hLH and hCG appear to bind to the same receptors in a variety of species. The binding is principally localised to the plasma membranes, as evidenced by subcellular fractionation techniques (Rajaniemi, Hirshfield and Midgley, 1974; Roa, 1973) and electron microscopic radiography (Han, Rajaniemi, Cho, Hirschfield and Midgley, 1974). The binding of hCG and hLH to common receptors in rat testis and ovary has been studied extensively (Catt and Dufau, 1973b; Dufau et al., 1973; Catt, Tsuruhara, Mendelson, Ketelslegers and Dufau, 1974). Similar binding sites have been demonstrated in porcine granulosa cells in vitro and in vivo (Channing and Kammerman, 1974).

Experiments in vitro with particulate fractions from luteinised rat ovaries (Lee and Ryan, 1971, 1972) indicated that the binding of labelled hCG was specific, saturable and dependent on time, temperature, and ionic strength. Binding is of high affinity with dissociation constant of 10^{-11} M.

Whereas during in vitro studies there is a high specificity of binding of hCG to gonadal tissue, labelled hCG administered in vivo is not bound exclusively to gonads, but liver and kidney have been found to incorporate significant amounts of hCG label (Ashitaka and Koide, 1974; Kazeto and Hreshchyshyn, 1970; Rao and Saxena, 1973; Kammerman and Canfield, 1972).

A number of studies have been reported on the isolation and characterisation of hCG receptors from different target organs (Lee and Ryan, 1974; Charreau, Dufau and Catt, 1973; Haour and Saxena, 1974). Studies of gonadotrophin receptors in plasma membranes of bovine corpus luteum (Azhar·and Menon, 1976; Azhar, Hajra and Menon, 1976) indicated that changes in the phospholipid environment can alter the conformation of the gonadotrophin-receptor complex so as to decrease the binding capacity.

Bellisario and Bahl (1975) isolated and solubilised the hCG-receptor complexes from the subcellular fractions of ovarian and testicular tissues of rats that had been injected with radioactivity labelled hCG. By this method they showed that the in vivo uptake of radioactivity by gonadal tissues represents hCG rather than dissociated subunits or the degradation products of the hormone. The hCG-receptor complex was the same size as that isolated in vitro, and similar yields were obtained by both methods.

hCG appears to stimulate the synthesis of its own receptor. Pandian, Bahl and Segal (1975) showed that hCG stimulated the incorporation of [^{14}C] N-acetyl-D-glucosamine in rat ovary in vitro and that an appreciable amount of radioactivity was incorporated in the cell surface receptor for hCG.

In addition to detergent-solubilised gonadotrophin receptors, soluble gonadotrophin-binding factors have been isolated from rat testis (Bhalla, Haskell, Grier and Mahesh, 1976). The dissociation constant of ^{125}I-hCG binding to soluble factors was similar to that derived for membrane-bound or detergent-solubilised receptors. In contrast to detergent-solubilised receptors the soluble factors were thermostable and they lacked absolute tissue specificity. A possible role of soluble factors in regulation of gonadotrophic activity has been suggested by the authors.

Evidence that hCG may regulate the number of its own receptors has been presented by Sharpe (1976). His studies with immature rat testis *in vitro* and *in vivo* suggested that the binding of hCG to specific gonadotrophin receptors in the testis affected the subsequent availability of these receptors.

A close correlation was observed in luteinised rat ovaries between the number of gonadotrophin receptors and the ability of adenylate cyclase to be stimulated by the hormone (Conti, Harwood, Hsueh, Dufau and Catt, 1976). Their studies demonstrated that the exposure of ovarian cells to high concentrations of the hormone *in vivo* caused a parallel loss of binding capacity and of the hormonal stimulation of adenylate cyclase. The recovery phase following the receptor loss was relatively slow, suggesting that restoration of binding sites probably depended upon receptor synthesis. The disappearance of receptor sites after occupancy implied that any given receptor may be used only once during hormonal action.

Moyle, Bahl and März (1975) studied the effect of the carbohydrate part of hCG on its binding to rat Leydig cells *in vitro*. Whereas the sequential removal of sialic acid, galactose, *N*-acetyl-glucosamine and mannose residues led to a progressive increase in the effective dose of the hormone required to stimulate steroidogenesis, it resulted in an abrupt loss in the ability of the hormone to stimulate cAMP accumulation. The authors suggested that these differences could be explained by assuming that "steroidogenic receptor" and "cAMP receptor" are independent when assayed functionally.

C. QUANTITATION OF hCG

1. Assay Methods

Much the commonest application of knowledge of human chorionic gonadotrophin is its detection in body fluids as evidence of pregnancy. For this purpose, urinary concentrations > 500 u/l can be determined with adequate reliability by haemagglutination inhibition reactions (Wide and Gemzell, 1960), or latex particle agglutination (Henry and Little, 1962). An antibody-sensitised haemagglutination reaction for assaying urinary hCG and LH has been developed (Tanizawo, Miyake, Kinugasa, Yamagi and Kurachi, 1975) which detects as little as 5 u/l of hCG and 12·5 u/l of LH. The method, which depends on coating sheep erthrocytes with guinea-pig anti-hCG, extends to 150,000 u/l before encountering problems due to antigen excess. Such methods have clear advantages where radioisotopes are not available for radioimmunoassay. A development of latex particle agglutination using laser light scattering (von Schulthess, Cohen and Benedek, 1976) has achieved a sensitivity of about 15 u hCG/LH/l in urine.

In early or ectopic pregnancy, where determinations of serum hCG in the range of 10–100 u/l are necessary (Kosasa, Taymor, Goldstein and Levesque, 1973b) and in the management of patients with hCG-producing tumours, assays with maximum sensitivity are required. The rate of secretion by hCG by normal trophoblast has been estimated at $1·4 \times 10^{-2}$ u/cell/day. (Braunstein, Grodin, Vaitukaitis and Ross, 1973a). For choriocarcinoma cells *in vivo* the rate of secretion was estimated at 5×10^{-5} u/cell/day, but both estimates are subject to wide errors.

One method of measuring small quantities of hCG in sera (1 u of hCG is the activity contained in 0·001279 mg of the Second International Standard, see later) is by radioimmunoassay. The general principle of radioimmunoassay is competitive inhibition of the binding of isotopically-labelled purified antigen to specific antibody by unlabelled antigen. Known amounts of unlabelled antigens as reference standards are added to a series of reaction tubes to provide a calibration curve against which biological fluids such as serum, urine or spinal fluid are assayed. The reliability of the assay depends upon many factors. The precision, the difference observed in radioactive counts bound by the antibody for a small increase in the antigen to be measured, depends on the equilibrium constant of the reaction between the antigen and antibody. The sensitivity, or limit of detection, is that amount of antigen added which warrants the assertion that the counts to which it corresponds on the standard curve are significantly different from those when only labelled antigen is present. The cross-reactivity is the extent of interference in the assay of other materials present in biological fluids with which the antibody may partially react.

2. Antisera

Radioimmunoassays for the detection of hCG in the presence of LH are limited by the extent of the anti-LH cross-reaction of the antibodies directed at the hCG molecule. Since this molecule shares an immunologically identical α-subunit with LH and comprises a β-subunit which differs only in 12 of 115 of the constituent amino acids with an additional sequence of 30 amino acids at the C-terminal end of the protein chain, many of the antibodies raised to whole hCG will cross-react with LH.

In 1970 Franchimont characterised an antiserum raised to intact hCG, one of 43 screened, which discriminated between hCG and LH (Franchimont, 1970). An increasing number of radioimmunoassays specific for hCG at levels of detection of 2–10 u/l in serum are being developed. Methods have been directed at dissociating the production of antibodies to the common α-determinants of hCG and LH from those reacting specifically with intact hCG, or with the hCG-β subunit. Vaitukaitis and her colleagues (Vaitukaitis, Robbins, Nieschlag and Ross 1971) produced specific antisera to hCG subunits CR 100α and CR 100β (Morgan and Canfield, 1971). One of four rabbits immunised with 20 μg of CR 100 α bound 50% of ^{125}I-CR 100α at a final antiserum dilution of 1/500, while all five rabbits immunised with 50 μg of CR 100β produced sera which bound 50% of ^{125}I-CR 100β at a final dilution of 1/10,000.

On the homologous α-system (i.e. anti-α-antiserum, ^{125}I-α-hCG), 500 times more CR 100β was necessary for inhibition equivalent to the CR 100α, corresponding to a less than 1% cross-contamination of the β-subunit with hCG-α or intact hCG. On the homologous assay for the β-subunit, the inhibition curve of CR 100α required 500–1000 times more mass for equivalent percentage inhibition when compared to CR 100β. This could be accounted for by cross-contamination of CR 100α with either intact hCG, CR 100β or both. The inhibition curve for CR 100 hCG (intact) differed in slope from that of its β-subunit, implying masking of some antigenic sites by recombinant α. Chromatography of hCG secreted by tumours further validated the assays (Vaitukaitis, 1973). The α-subunit with an elution/void volume (Ve/Vo) ratio of 1·9 on Sephadex G-100 failed to cross-react significantly on homologous hCG-β and hCG assays. The hCG-β-subunit (Ve/Vo = 1·4) cross-reacted approximately 15% in an hCG radio-immunoassay (Vaitukaitis, 1973; Vaitukaitis, Braunstein and Ross, 1972a) in which ^{125}I-hCG was used as tracer. The elution/void volume for hCG was 1·25. Intact hCG cross-reacted approximately 15% in the homologous assay for the β-subunit (Vaitukaitis, 1974). Non-parallelism between hCG and hCG-β versus the anti-β-hCG antiserum SB 6 (Vaitukaitis et al., 1971) was encountered (Good et al., 1977) with intact ^{125}I-hCG CR 117 as tracer.

Presumably the non-parallelism between the intact hCG and β-subunit in an homologous assay for the β-subunit, coupled with the different extent to which the cold antigen displaces its labelled opponent argues that antisera raised to the β-moiety of the hCG molecule (specific for hCG vs LH) may react with several sites. If the antigenicity is mainly dependent on the sequence of components in the β-subunit, it might be possible for the antibodies to react equally well with hCG and hCG-β when corrected for relative masses. If the sites are mainly conformationally-dependent, whose reactivity may alter when the β-moiety forms part of the intact hCG molecule, it is conceivable that, if the intact hCG is more conformationally stable than the β-subunit in assay solution, binding of ^{125}I-hCG and its displacement by hCG may be more favoured than displacement by the hCG-β-subunit from antibodies originally obtained by injection of β-subunit. Where the antibodies are directed at sites which are normally unavailable in intact hCG due to the presence of the α-subunit, binding of hCG might be impaired in relation to hCG-β itself. If more than one of these factors is operating in a given antiserum raised to the β-subunit, the cross-reaction perceived will depend on the relative "diluting-out" of the titre of the less predominant antibodies under the assay conditions used.

Franchimont and co-workers (Reuter, Schoonbrood and Franchimont, 1976) have developed radioimmunoassays with antisera rendered specific for hCG, hCG-α and hCG-β by absorption. Rabbit antiserum against hCG, neutralised by incubation with 125 ng LH/ml of antiserum diluted at 1/75,000 had residual interferences of 3% for hCG-α, 2% for LH, and 15% for hCG-β (Reuter, Franchimont and Schoonbrood, 1976). Antiserum, raised against hCG-β, neutralised by incubation with LH at a concentration of 100 ng/ml of antiserum diluted at 1/50,000 had residual interferences of 5% and 0·4% for hCG and LH. When antiserum against hCG-α was neutralised with hCG at a concentration of 200 ng/ml of antiserum diluted at 1/10,000, the residual interference for hCG was 1%. The specificity of these systems was assessed by analysis of the inhibition curves and detection of immunoreactivity in the specific elution zones for intact hCG and its subunits on Sephadex G-100.

Bahl, Pandian and Ghai (1976) have suggested that hCG-specific (i.e. non-LH-reactive) determinants reside particularly in the 32-residue carboxyl-terminal peptide but are predominantly conformational rather than sequential. The problem of ensuring the production of avid and specific antisera may therefore not be necessarily resolved by the injection of suitably coupled carboxyl-terminal fragments, but, towards this end, the 31 and 35 amino acid carboxyl terminal fragments have been synthesised by the Merrifield resin technique (Fisher et al., 1977).

It should be borne in mind when comparing the binding of iodinated hCG or its subunits to a particular antiserum that when hCG is labelled by the chloramine-T method, most of the isotopic iodine is present on the α-subunit. The β-subunit possesses at least one site that is more readily iodinated in the free β-subunit than in the intact hormone (Canfield et al., 1973). If the immunological activity of a given antibody required the integrity of this site, there might be three differing equilibria involved for the iodinated hCG-β, the hCG-β and the intact hCG.

In 1974, the original double antibody method specific for hCG vs LH (Vaitukaitis et al., 1972a) was modified to form a rapid 18-hr assay based on a solid phase Sepharose-coupled anti-β-antiserum and tracer quantities of labelled β-subunit (Goldstein, Pastorfide, Osathanondh and Kosasa, 1974b). There was no cross-reaction with LH in 300 serum samples within the limit of detection of the assay, depicted as 5 u/l. An 18-hr preincubated double antibody assay for hCG in the presence of LH using labelled hCG and an antiserum raised to the β-subunit has been developed (Kardana and Bagshawe, 1976) and automated (Bagshawe, 1975). The dose-response curve was found to be linear on a log-logit transformation in the region of 0·68–87 uhCG/l.

The potential difficulty in hCG measurement relating to the choice of labelled antigen is illustrated by the following work (Tyrey and Hammond, 1976). Samples from patients with trophoblastic malignancies were assayed on double-antibody systems dependent on anti-β-hCG antisera, but with either ^{125}I-hCG or ^{125}I-hCG-β as tracer. Although most sera assayed consistently on either system, serious discrepancies in 4 of 31 patients' samples were noted in which displacement of the β-tracer resulted in a 4 fold higher results than when ^{125}I-hCG was used. When β-subunit served as the labelled antigen, the inhibition curves with purified hCG and hCG-β were distinctly different. If intact ^{125}I-hCG was used, parallelism between the preparations and the Second International Reference preparation of hCG was maintained. The authors inferred that these labelled antigens select antibody populations differing in their relative affinities for the hCG and hCG-β. They recommended that, for a given antibody, it may be necessary to use hCG-^{125}I to maintain consistent results on dilution of samples of patients' sera. However, other investigators (Jacobs, Vanthuyne and Ekins, 1974) found that when ^{125}I-hCG-β was used with their anti-hCG serum, the inhibition lines generated by hCG-β and native hCG became superimposable after weight corrections were made. Full characterisation of antisera raised to subunits is essential.

Such considerations in measurement will be particularly relevant in determining the secretion of subunits of hCG not only in trophoblastic-derived tumours but also ectopic secretion in other malignancies.

3. Assays for Subunits of hCG

Hussa (1977) has studied the production of hCG and its subunits in cultures of the human malignant trophoblast cell line BeWo, following earlier work by Vaitukaitis (1973) on the characterisation of hCG secreted by tumours. Calibrated Sephadex G-200 gel filtration of the BeWo cell homogenate and culture fluid suggested that, whereas the predominant form of hCG within the cell was hCG-β, there was approximately twice as much intact hCG in the culture fluid as of either subunit, measurements being obtained on homo-logous assays. Hussa's contention, borne out by the stimulation of secretion rates of hCG, hCG-β and a large form of hCG-α by dibutyryl cAMP, was that the bulk of hCG is present in this cell line at least, in the form of its subunits and there is little or no storage of hCG in the cell. Discordant release of the subunits is therefore a rational possibility for other neoplastic cells. Goldstein, using iodinated β-subunit (Goldstein *et al.*, 1974b) and antiserum to the β-subunit, has detected a positive response in patients with a variety of malignancies but fluctuations of serum-hCG of only about 10 u/l are depicted over seven months for a patient with metastatic bronchogenic carcinoma on treatment. Serum specimens from patients with islet-cell tumours were studied closely by Kahn, Rosen, Weintraub, Fajans and Gorden (1977) using three independent radioimmunoassays. The hCG-α assay measured also the free α-subunits of the other cross-reactive glycoprotein hormones, but was insensitive to hCG-β or intact hCG. The hCG-β assay measured free hCG-β and intact hCG equally well but was insensitive to hCG-α. The assay for intact hCG distinguished between this and the β-subunit. Of 27 patients with functioning islet-cell carcinomas, 14 displayed increased serum α-subunit, six increased serum β-subunit and three increased hCG; thus in most patients the secretion of the α- and β-subunits was discordant. The circulating levels encountered were in the range 3–25 ng/ml serum.

Clonal cell lines of a bronchogenic carcinoma (Cha Go) and a choriocarcinoma (JEG), (Lieblich, Weintraub, Krauth, Kohler, Robson and Rosen, 1976) have been studied for their production of hCG subunits measured by separate assays. In the intact hCG assay, hCG-α and hCG-β cross-reacted insignificantly. The cross-reaction of hCG in the hCG-α assay was about 5 % and that of hCG in the hCG-β assay about 70 % for which corrections were made. The lung cancer clones ChaGo-K$_1$ and Cha-GoCs secreted α-subunit but no detectable complete hCG, while the choriocarcinoma clone JEG-3 secreted intact hCG but no detectable α-subunit. While the growth curves rose steadily to a plateau, the secretory rates of both α-hCG and hCG decreased during the early part of the growth cycle and then increased again.

In vivo, the measurement of hCG in the serum may not always reflect the discordance of the subunits of hCG in the tissue of origin. Ashitaka, Nishimura, Futamara and Tojo (1977) collected the fluid from molar vesicles and determined hCG and its subunits in homologous radioimmunoassays, and found that although hCG-α was hardly measurable in serum, significant amounts (~100 ng/ml) were found in the vesicle fluids. This immunoreactive hCG-α could be combined with iodinated hCG-β to be taken up by the superovulated rat ovary, suggesting that the hCG-α was not deficient in combining power, but its accumulation depended upon some other factor.

The foregoing discussion has emphasised that the measurement of hCG by radioimmunoassay, particularly at low levels, depends not only on excluding cross-reaction by LH but also on taking account of the possible presence of free subunits whose contribution to the numerical answer will depend on the particular antiserum used.

The role of gonadotrophin inhibiting substances should perhaps be considered in comparing assays for hCG in serum and urine. A crude material isolatable from urine and human pineal extracts (Landau, Schwartz and Soffer, 1960; Banerji, Kothari and Shah, 1977) can inhibit mouse uterine response to hCG stimulation. If such a substance interfered with the immunological assessment of hCG on a given assay, its effect might vary in the serum and urine of a given patient inconsistently with the expected clearance rate of the hCG.

4. Enzyme Immunoassays

The assays discussed so far have relied upon employing isotopically-labelled antigens. Joshi, Raghavan and Sheth (1977) have conjugated hCG with alkaline phosphatase using glutaraldehyde; the conjugate was stable for six months. The method has the distinct advantage that it is cheap, and a sensitivity of 10 u hCG/l could be obtained.

5. Bioassays and Receptor Assays

An alternative method to immunoassay is the radioreceptor assay of human chorionic gonadotrophin, a technique which generally agrees well with bioassay results but is more precise and sensitive. Bioassay determinations have been reviewed recently (Mitchell and Bagshawe, 1976; Ross, 1973) and are summarised in Table 4. In 1974, Saxena, Hasan, Haour and Schmidt-Gollwitzer established a rapid, sensitive radioreceptor assay for hCG,

Table 4

Bioassays for human chorionic gonadotrophin/luteinising hormone.

Dose range (u)	Assay	References
0·4–8·0	Depletion of ascorbic acid of ovaries of pseudopregnant rats	Parlow (1961)
0·5–3·0	Uterine weight increments in mice	Diczfalusy and Loraine (1955); Umberger and Grass (1959)
18–36	Ovarian weight increase of mice and rats	Diczfalusy and Loraine (1955)
2·0–8·0	Seminal vesicle weight increase in rats	Van Hell, Matthijsen and Overbeck (1964)
0·4–12·0	Ventral prostate weight increase in hypophysectomised rats	Diczfalusy and Loraine (1955); Christiansen (1967); McArthur (1968)

using plasma membranes of bovine corpora lutea of early pregnancy to bind biologically active ^{125}I-labelled hCG. The receptor did not discriminate between LH and hCG. Plasma membranes were obtained by sucrose gradient ultracentrifugation of a tris-HCl homogenate. Lactoperoxidase iodination of hCG was employed to maintain its biological activity at 8923 u/mg. The assay was performed on plasma samples in the presence of the enzyme inhibitor Trasylol. The log-logit transformation indicated a sensitivity of 3 ng/ml hCG/LH and there was no cross-reactivity with FSH, TSH or hGH.

This radioreceptor assay has been extended to detect hCG/LH in urine. In the presence of 50 µl of dialysed urine and 30 µg of receptor protein, a sensitivity of 1·5 ng hCG/ml with an average precision of $\pm 10\%$ was achieved (Saxena, Saito, Said and Landesman, 1977). The radioreceptor assay in general gave results 2–3 times those given by the same specimen by radioimmunoassay, and required a 1 hr reaction time compared with the 72 hr needed for their radioimmunoassay.

The method of Saxena et al. (1974) has been used by other workers (Roy, Klein, Scott, Kletzky and Mishell, 1977) to compare the statistical differences between the radioreceptor assay and a radioimmunoassay. The assay employed an antiserum which was 5% cross-reactive with LH at 90% of maximum binding, i.e. would not distinguish below 3 u hCG/l. 557 women were followed with serum measurements by radioimmunoassay and radioreceptor assay to determine pregnancy. For the receptor assay, in the interval from last menstrual period to 35 days, there were 12 "false negative" results among 196 determinations; between 36–42 days there were 10 "false negative" results in 207 determinations; greater than 42 days, 2/107 of the negative results were false, while one "false positive" was encountered in a menopausal woman with an elevated LH. The limit of sensitivity of this radioreceptor assay $(95 \pm 10 \text{ u/l})$ inclines towards a higher "false negative" rate for ectopic pregnancies than those radioimmunoassays which can measure to 5 u/l.

Bahl has purified the receptor (Pandian and Bahl, 1977) from bovine corpus luteal plasma membranes by an ingenious method comprising protection of the hCG/LH receptor with hCG, enzymatic iodination of the other membrane proteins with potassium iodide, removal of the bound hCG with rabbit anti-hCG, and iodination of the now exposed receptor on the membranes with Na ^{131}I. The radio-labelled receptor itself can then be solubilised with Triton X-100 and purified by affinity-chromatography and electrophoresis. Study of the receptor complex and partially degraded hCG molecules has shown that the three monosaccharide residues from the non-reducing terminus of the carbohydrate chains are not involved in the binding of the hormone to the receptor, but removal of mannosyl residues, which may affect the conformation of hCG, or may be integral parts of the binding requirement to the receptor, does reduce binding activity. An interesting point made by Bahl is that the immunological and receptor binding sites of the hCG molecule are presumably different since the antibody can dissociate the receptor-hCG complex despite similar affinities.

Weintraub, Stannard and Rosen (1977) have investigated the immunological and receptor-binding properties of various recombinant hCG molecules derived from standard α-subunits, ectopic α-subunits derived from a gastric carcinoid tumour and a bronchogenic carcinoma cell line and standard β-subunit. The radioreceptor assay followed the method of Catt (Catt, Dufau and Tsuruhara, 1972) employing a crude rat testis homogenate. There were considerable differences in the combining activity of α-preparations with the same β-subunit but the radioimmunoassay for hCG measured a substantially higher proportion of apparent intact hCG molecules than did the radioreceptor assay for a given α–β combination. The two ectopic α-subunits had very low combining activities.

6. Standardisation of hCG

For comparison of assays it is essential to have a reliable international standard. The Second International Standard for hCG was prepared in 1961 and assayed both immunologically and biologically in a number of centres. The ampoules prepared contained hCG plus lactose, and the potency was defined as 5300 u/ampoule, one International Unit of Chorionic Gonadotrophin being the activity contained in 0·001279 mg of the Second International Standard (Bangham and Grab, 1964). Further preparations CR 119-hCG and CR 119-hCG-α and CR 119-hCG-β have been established under the auspices of the World Health Organisation (Canfield and Ross, 1976). An International Reference Preparation of hCG for Immunoassay has recently been prepared with a unitage of 650 u/ampoule by WHO and the National Institute of Biological Standards, Holly Hill, London NW3 6RB.

D. hCG IN PHYSIOLOGICAL AND PATHOLOGICAL PREGNANCY

1. Concentration of hCG and Subunits in Placental Tissue

Bioassay estimates of the concentration of hCG in first trimester placenta gave values in the range 100–650 u/g of wet tissue, and average values were lower in the last trimester (Diczfalusy, 1953). More recent studies by Vaitukaitis (1974) showed that all the placental extracts studied contained hCG and hCG-α but the concentrations of the two glycoproteins varied qualitatively and quantitatively during progression of pregnancy. The absolute amount of hCG and hCG-α decreased after the first trimester but the relative quantity of hCG-α compared with intact hCG increased by more than 10 fold in the last two trimesters. An additional species of hCG-α was identified in the second trimester.

2. Distribution of hCG in Body Fluids

Although a correlation betweeen individual maternal and foetal concentrations of hCG have been found, the concentration is much higher in maternal blood than in foetal blood. A mean ratio of maternal to foetal concentration of 344:1 was found by Geiger, Kaiser and Franchimont (1971) and the mean value for maternal antecubital vein plasma in 18 women at delivery was 22·3 ± 18·8 u/ml. with corresponding values for foetal umbilical artery and vein of 0·056 ± 0·041 and 0·065 ± 0·050 u/ml respectively. Somewhat higher values for the material/foetal ratio were found by Midgley, Fong and Jaffe (1967) and Crosignani, Nencioni and Branbati (1972), although a much lower value was reported by Faiman, Ryan, Zwirek and Rubin (1968).

Amniotic fluid concentrations also show a correlation with plasma concentrations and the evidence suggests that values are higher in early pregnancy than at term. Mishell, Wide and Gemzell (1963) found values ranging from 1·25–5·0 u/ml. between the 17th and 20th weeks of pregnancy, using a haemaglutination inhibition method. Crosignani *et al.* (1972) found a mean amniotic fluid concentration at term of 0·380 ± 0·389 u/ml and the mean serum-amniotic fluid ratio on this study was 41·6:1.

The concentration of hCG in extracellular fluid has not been reported. Concentration in cerebrospinal fluid (CSF) remains substantially lower than the plasma concentration even when plasma values have been at a high level for long periods of time. In patients with trophoblastic tumours who had no evidence of intracranial metastases the plasma/CSF ratio was between 60/1 and 600/1 for a wide range of plasma values, with a mean value in excess of 200/1 (Bagshawe, Orr and Rushworth, 1968b). There was a significan time lag between changes in the plasma concentration and changes in the CSF concentration of hCG.

3. Renal Clearance

Renal clearance rates for hCG by bioassay range from 0·18–1·19 ml/min (Gastineau, Albert and Randall, 1949; Loraine, 1950). Using radioimmunoassay Crosignani, Brambati and Nencioni (1971) obtained values of 0·94, 0·66 and 0·85 during the first, second and third trimesters of pregnancy respectively. The bioassay clearance rate of 0·36 ml/min and the corresponding value of 0·7 ml/min by immunoassay were reported by Wide, Johannison, Tillingen and Diczfalusy (1968). Radioimmunoassay estimates of clearance values on more than 100 patients with trophoblastic tumours came in the range 0·5–1·8 ml/min for a wide range of plasma concentrations. As a result of a clearance rate of approximately 1 ml/min, plasma and urine concentrations tend to be similar at normal rates of urine flow.

4. Metabolic Clearance in Man

Early studies indicated that about 20% of an i.v. administered preparation of hCG could be recovered from the urine (Friedman and Weinstein, 1937) and a similar figure was obtained when hCG was administerd i.v. or i.m. to amenorrhoeic women (Wide et al., 1968). A metabolic clearance rate of 3·38 for men and 3·86 for women was found with initial fast component half lives of 5·1 hr and 5·6 hr and slow component half lives of 23·6 hr and 23·9 hr in men and women respectively after i.v. injection (Rizkallah, Gurpide and Van de Wiele, 1969).

5. Distribution and Clearance in Experimental Animals

When hCG is administered to other species the pattern of distribution and excretion may be influenced by a variety of factors which do not operate in man. About 75% of hCG administered i.v. to rabbits was recovered from the urine between 4 and 24 days, using unspecified immunoassay methods (Hisley and Fesche, 1966).

When ^{3}H-labelled hCG, hCG-α and hCG-β-subunits were administered to immature female rats, Braunstein, Vaitukaitis and Ross (1972) found biphasic plasma disappearance curves with fast and slow components having $T_{\frac{1}{2}}$ of 141, 6·2 and 11·1 min for the fast phase, and 725, 58 and 81 min for the slow phase, respectively.

6. Receptors and Physiological Action of hCG

The distribution of ^{125}I hCG was studied by Kazeto et al. (1970) in female mice and preferential concentration occurred in ovarian tissue 2–4 hr after injection and hypophysectomised mice showed less uptake as had been suggested by the earlier experiments of Evans, Meyer and Simpson (1932) and of Figarova, Presl and Horsky (1969) with hypophysectomised rats. Tsuruhara, van Hall, Dufau and Catt (1972) observed that desialylated ^{125}I hCG had only 3% of the activity of the intact hormone when competing for uptake by rat ovarian tissue against intact hormone in vivo. However, when tested in vitro on ovarian tissue homogenate its direct uptake was slightly increased as compared with the intact hormone. It therefore appears that desialylated hCG is fully active biologically at the ovarian receptor site and its relative ineffectiveness when injected i.v. is due to rapid clearance by the liver as also shown by Morell, Gregoriadis, Scheinberg, Hickman and Ashwell (1971). Many of the discrepancies observed between earlier studies of biological and immunological activity of hCG can be accounted for by these observations. Braunstein *et al.* (1972) found that intact hCG was concentrated in the ovaries but the subunits were not. Similarly monkey granulosa cells in culture treated with asialo-hCG responded with luteinisation and progesterone synthesis but they did not respond to hCG subunits (Channing and Kammerman, 1973). Receptor sites in the ovary for hCG do not appear to be distinct from those for luteinising hormone (Han *et al.*, 1974; Mills, McPherson and Mahesh, 1974; Rao, 1974). Refractoriness of the immature rat ovary is apparently due to the lack of the specific receptor (Siebers, Schmidtke and Engel, 1977). In contrast, the rat testis does not appear to lack specific hCG receptors in the postnatal period although it is insensitive to hCG action (Engel and Frowein, 1974). Receptor sites in the testis have been localised to Leidig cells (Catt *et al.*, 1971; Ashitaka and Koide, 1974). It has also been suggested that there may be receptors for hCG in placenta and placental steroid synthesis may be under the control of hCG (Cédard, Alsat, Urtasun and Varangot, 1970).

The first step in the action of the hormone appears to involve binding to the membrane-bound receptor and it has been observed that the number of receptors in testicular tissue greatly exceeds the number which must be occupied to achieve a maximum response (Catt and Dufau, 1973a). The next step is probably mediated by cAMP (Menon, 1972; Jungman, Hiestand and Schweppe, 1974; Sulimovici and Lunenfeld, 1974) with involvement of cytochrome P_{450} in steroidogenesis (Purvis, Canick, Rosenbaum, Hologgitas and Latif, 1973). hCG subunits administered *in vivo* increased progesterone synthesis and increased concentrations of ovarian adenylate cyclase and cAMP. However, hCG-β increased the ovarian content of a second, so-called "messenger" molecule, cGMP and hCG-α also had an effect (Rao and Carmen, 1973). The incorporation of ^{14}C-cAMP into a minced preparation of placenta was stimulated by hCG, suggesting that the hormone may have a cAMP-mediated role in the placenta although adenylate cyclase was not directly stimulated *in vitro* (Mennon and Jaffe, 1973). The only major role so far defined for hCG is to sustain the corpus luteum of early pregnancy. Evidence which suggested that hCG had an effect on adrenal glands and adrenal steroidogenesis (Perloff and Jacobsohn, 1963) has not been confirmed. Winter, Tarasaka and Faiman (1972) indicated that there was no rise in plasma testosterone after hCG stimulation in four anorchic males.

Early studies suggested that the primary site of action of hCG was the ovary and evidence that the secondary effects of hCG were mediated by oestrogen and progesterone was provided by Gospadarowicz (1964) and Aakvag, Norman and Vogt (1965).

Since hCG appears to bind to the same receptors as luteinising hormone it would be expected that their endocrinological actions would be similar if not identical. Marked synergism between hCG and FSH in bioassay systems has been observed (Yamashita and Tohoku, 1965) but any intrinsic follicle-stimulating hormone-like activity of hCG may depend on the similarity of their α-subunit structures.

The hypophysectomised immature female rat responds to hCG with the repair of interstitial cells and minimal enlargement of the ovaries, uterus and adrenal zona fasciculata. The intact animal stimulated with hCG shows the formation, hypertrophy and hyperaemia of ovarian follicles and corpea lutea, uterine hypertrophy and vaginal cornification (Velardo, 1959). Ovulation occurs in the toad, rabbit, pseudo-pregnant rat and pregnant mouse. The expulsion of spermatozoa by amphibia after injection with hCG was noted by Galli-Mainini (1947) and this formed the basis of a widely used pregnancy test for several years. Various other effects attributed to hCG include growth promotion action (Schapiro, 1930; Gregorio and Buda, 1964). These actions have not been confirmed in controlled studies. Evidence that hCG was efficacious in weight reduction programmes was disproved by the early double-blind random cross-over study performed (Young, Fuchs and Voltjen, 1976). Evidence has been presented by Lemaire, Comly, Moffett, Spelasy, Cleveland and Savard (1971) that the corpus luteum is maintained and continues to function throughout pregnancy and that in the puerperium administered hCG can maintain the function of the corpus luteum.

7. Cross-reactivity of hCG in Different Species

Cross-reactivity of hCG between different species is important not only for the inherent interest in the molecular structures but also to determine suitable models for studying immunological means of fertility control by suppressing particular stages in the reproductive process.

Plasma from various species have been checked for parallelism in a radio-immunoassay for hCG/LH (Bagshawe, Orr and Godden, 1968a). Plasma from hens gave dilution curves which approached parallelism with hCG more closely than some other species examined. The curves obtained for horse, donkey, mare, pregnant donkey and pregnant mare serum gonado-trophin were parallel to each other but not to hCG: a horse pituitary gonado-trophin, probably LH, could have contributed largely to this last cross-reaction. The slight inhibition produced on the assay by plasma from mice, rats, dogs, cows and a monkey might well have been non-specific. Inhibition by chicken-LH of some other hCG assays seems to be smaller (Scanes, Follett and Goos, 1972).

While some indication for cross-reactivity between human and rat gonadotrophin was demonstrated by immunofluorescence localisation of antibodies on sections of fixed rat pituitaries (Leleux and Robyn, 1970) Zondek, Hochman and Sulmar (1939) earlier explained the lack of interruption of rat pregnancy by injection of goat anti-human gonadotrophin antiserum as owing to species specificity. In contrast, injections of rabbit antisera raised to cross-linked hCG into mice, previously rendered tolerant to rabbit γ-globulins, produced prolongation of oestrus and a prolonged phase of sterility. The dosage and catabolic rate of exogenous antibodies in the animal system under study is important for comparisons to be drawn (Schlumberger and Anderer, 1969). A high post-implantation mortality has been observed in the rat and hamster by administration of hCG on days 1–3 after conception suggesting some disturbance of the endometrium though a possible increase in oestrogen production was not ruled out as being responsible for the failure of the pregnancy (Yang and Chang, 1968). Beagles immunised with hCG, one injection, produced antibodies in their serum capable of binding about 40% of ^{125}I-hCG at 1/400 dilution between 2–24 weeks after treatment. While these antibodies were capable of abrogating the mouse uterine weight response to hCG, no impairment of reproductivity function was demonstrated in either dogs or bitches (Al-Kafawi, Hopwood, Pineda and Faulkner, 1974).

The immunological basis for within and between species cross-reactivity of hCG has been studied (Vaitukaitis, Ross, Reichert and Ward, 1972b). An antiserum reacting with the α-subunit of hLH and hCG showed no response with ovine, bovine or rat α-LH subunits, whereas an antiserum reacting to the β-subunit of hLH cross-reacted completely with ovine, bovine and rat LH-β, and cross-reacted partially with hCG-β. When interspecies combinations of subunits were investigated for biological activity the biological activity of the hybrids in the ovarian ascorbic acid depletion assay was characteristic of the β-subunit but dependent on α-β hybridisation (Vaitukaitis, Ross and Reichert, 1973). Similarities of antigenic determinants in urinary chorionic gonadotrophins from man, gorilla and chimpanzee have been demonstrated, by the behaviour of the chorionic gonadotrophins in homologous assays for the α- and β-subunits of hCG. The effect on rat uterine weight of hCG and gorilla-CG was partially neutralised by an antiserum raised to β-hCG. Rhesus monkey-CG appeared to be ineffective on radioimmunoassay for α- and β-hCG and independent of neutralisation in bioassay by anti-β-hCG antiserum (Hodgen, Nixon, Vaitukaitis, Tullner and Ross, 1973). By determining the maximal immunological cross-reactivity of a series of synthetic peptides based on the hCG-β-carboxyl terminal chain against an antiserum raised to residues 123–145 of β-hCG, it was found, for this antiserum, that the antibody site resided totally in the final 15 residues (Chen and Hodgen, 1976). The full cross-reactivity towards this antiserum observed with hCG, chimpanzee CG and gorilla CG indicate a marked molecular analogy for the terminal carboxypeptide in these species, singling out the chimpanzees as the most suitable laboratory animal in which to simulate fertility control in women.

Immunological activity is not necessarily sufficient to denote that the antiserum will be effective biologically. Four rabbit antisera raised to the carboxyl-terminal hCG-β tryptic peptide consisting of residues 123–145 (Louvet, Ross, Barker and Canfield, 1974), though capable of binding hCG, failed to neutralise its biological activity in a ventral prostate weight bioassay. In order to produce an hCG-specific, biological activity neutralising antibody, it may be necessary to select not so much for a "β-tail-specific" antibody as for one which masks the receptor-directed site of the hCG, but, in so doing, does not cross-react with allied receptor-directed sites for the other closely-related glycoprotein hormones. Such an endeavour requires a clear understanding of the exact parts of the hCG molecule which are involved in receptor binding, how far these are homologous with parts of hLH and how far the animal model receptors in use in radioreceptor assays mimic the hCG-responsive human tissue.

8. hCG Values in Normal Pregnancy

(a) Detection of pregnancy

The time at which pregnancy can be detected by standard tests depends on the sensitivity of the method used. Haemagglutination inhibition and latex agglutination methods are generally positive at about 33 days following the previous menstrual phase, that is about 19 days post-ovulation (Morris and Udry, 1967; Kosasa et al., 1973a). With urine hCG/LH radioimmuno-assay, hCG values above the normal LH range can be detected about the 9th or 10th day after ovulation and sensitive specific assays for hCG on serum detect hCG about 48 hr earlier. It is not yet clear whether hCG is in fact present in the serum before implantation occurs, but at any event it appears detectable within a few hours of implantation of the blastocyst.

(b) Doubling time

The urinary excretion rate of hCG increases at a rapid rate in early pregnancy with a doubling time of 36–48 hr and the values fall within closely defined limits. Serum values measured by hCG-β assay show a comparable rapid increase with a peak between 56 and 68 days, followed by falling values until the 18th week. Peak values are in the range 42–53 u/ml and after the 18th week values fall in the range 7–18 u/ml. A rise in serum values in the third trimester was not observed (Braunstein, Rasor, Adler, Danzer and Wade, 1976) in contrast to the rise in the third trimester observed with hCG/LH assays on urine and with serum assays using less specific antisera. These discrepancies may be attributable to heterogeneity in the sialylation of the hCG. Typical results by the rat prostate assay on urine were reported by Loraine (1957) and for radioimmunoassay by Varma, Larraga and Sclenkow (1971).

In the rhesus monkey, chorionic gonadotrophin values increased 8–12 days after the estimated day of conception and serum progesterone was significantly elevated within 24–48 hr of the appearance of CG in the serum, suggesting that the appearance of CG at the time of implantation maintains the viability of the corpus luteum and temporarily enhances progesterone secretion immediately after implantation (Hodgen, Tullner, Vaitukaitis, Ward and Ross, 1974).

(c) hCG subunits in pregnancy

During the course of normal pregnancy Reuter, Gaspard, De Ville, Gevaert-Vrindts and Franchimont (1977) found that β-subunit values followed a pattern very similar to that of intact hCG with peak values of 180–240 ng/ml, followed by a fall to about the 18th week of pregnancy, after which values remained relatively constant. The concentration of α-subunit increased progressively throughout pregnancy, reaching values between 300 and 400 ng/ml by the 37th week. α-subunit concentrations therefore appear to be higher than β-subunit and intact hCG concentrations in the placenta and in the serum in the latter half of pregnancy.

(d) Multiple pregnancy

Many anecdotal reports indicate that high values of hCG are associated with multiple pregnancy. Jovanovic, Landesman and Saxena (1977) found nine patients in a group of 590 who had high levels of hCG by radioreceptor assay and all nine cases subsequently proved to have twin pregnancies. Franchimont, using radioimmunoassay, confirmed statistically high levels of hCG in maternal serum throughout multiple pregnancies with a parallel increase in α- and β-subunits so that the ratios between the glycoproteins were unchanged from normal pregnancy (Reuter et al., 1977).

(e) Ectopic pregnancy

Ectopic pregnancy is frequently associated with negative pregnancy tests because the amount of hCG produced is below the limit of detection of these methods (Jones, 1966; Halpin, 1970). Sensitive quantitive methods reveal values above the normal luteal phase levels but below the level associated with normally progressing pregnancy (Kosasa, Levesque, Taymor and Goldstein, 1974). However, published data with reliable quantitative methods for hCG are few and one report appears to question the association of low hCG levels with ectopic pregnancy (Milwidsky, Adoni, Segal and Palti, 1977).

(f) Threatened and habitual abortion

Delfs and Jones (1948) concluded that low serum gonadotrophin values had some predictive value for impending abortion and Wide (1962) using a haemagglutination inhibition method, found that low levels of hCG in early pregnancy were generally associated with abortion later. Failure of hCG values to increase within the normal limits during the first eight weeks of pregnancy has invariably been associated with abortion or with ectopic pregnancy in patients being monitored in this laboratory by radioimmuno-assay.

(g) Genetic sex

Brody and Carlstrom (1965) suggested that in women with low hCG values there was a predominance of male foetuses, and Wide and Hobson (1974) found a decrease in the immunoreactive hCG of male placentae and an increase in the biologically active hCG in female placentae, but when the concentration and total amount of hCG was related to foetal sex, no significant difference was observed.

9. Action of Releasing Hormones

There is no evidence at present to indicate that either luteinising hormone-releasing hormone or thyrotrophin-releasing hormone have any effect on the rate of secretion of hCG by trophoblast. Thyrotrophin-releasing hormone was administered to pregnant women by Hersham and Burrow (1976). There was no significant change in the serum hCG during the ensuing 90 min.

10. hCG Values Following the End of Pregnancy

Several factors influence the length of time which elapses between the removal of all trophoblastic tissue and the disappearance of hCG from the blood and urine. The principle factors are the concentration of hCG in body fluids at the time of uterine evacuation, the clearance rate of hCG in the individual and the sensitivity of the test method. Midgley and Jaffe (1968) found an initial fast phase of $T_{\frac{1}{2}}$ of about 8 hr, and this was followed by a slower phase where $T_{\frac{1}{2}}$ increased to over 30 hr. Geiger (1973) found the mean $T_{\frac{1}{2}}$ of the first day to be 9 hr and for the second day to be 22 hr. By radio-immunoassay in this laboratory of urine for hCG/LH, hCG was detectable for 8–14 days after the end of term pregnancies and for 23 days after surgical terminations of normal first trimester pregnancies. With hCG-β assay on serum, hCG has been detectable for 3–4 days longer than by the urine assay, and Pastorfide, Goldstein, Kosasa and Levesque (1974) have also reported hCG detectable by hCG-β assay 27 days after suction curettage.

E. hCG IN NEOPLASTIC DISEASE

1. Trophoblastic and Other Tumours

In classical hydatidiform mole there is generally an excess of trophoblast in comparison with normal pregnancy. The villi are hydropic and there is little if any foetal tissue proper. Partial degrees of mole can also occur. In contrast to normal pregnancy the trophoblast of hydatidiform mole has a greater proclivity for myometrial invasion; gross degrees of myometrial invasion, sufficient to constitute a tumour mass, are described as invasive mole. The trophoblast of hydatidiform mole or that of a normal non-mole pregnancy may give rise to the malignant tumour, choriocarcinoma. Choriocarcinoma also arises in malignant teratomas, at various sites. All these lesions are regularly associated with the production of hCG. Until recently it has been thought that the detection of hCG in the body fluids of anyone who is not pregnant and who has not recently had hydatidiform mole is indicative of a malignant tumour. In the case of patients who have recently had hydatidiform mole the persistence of hCG in body fluids indicates the presence of either invasive mole or choriocarcinoma. The frequent use of radioimmunoassays for tumour markers has resulted in identifying very rare subjects in whom hCG and α-fetoprotein are raised without evidence of malignant disease.

2. Evidence for Tumour-associated Variants of hCG

Evidence that hCG produced by tumours showed different electrophoretic characteristics from that of pregnancy hCG has been previously reviewed (Bagshawe, 1969). However, hCG changes during the course of pregnancy (see above) and almost certainly some of the heterogeneity seen in tumour preparations was explicable on the basis of different degrees of sialylation.

Nevertheless, modified forms of hCG may be present in tumour tissue (Vaitukaitis, 1973).

3. Hydatidiform Mole

Zondek (1929) recognised the production of hCG by hydatidiform moles and further notable contributions were made by Hamburger (1944) and by Delfs (1959). Concentrations of hCG in molar vesicle fluid have been reported between 10,000 and 40,600 ng/ml, with corresponding values for hCG-α of 1200 to 2160 ng/ml with undetectable concentrations of hCG-β in a small group of hydatidiform moles (Ashitaka et al., 1977).

Although it is widely thought that hCG values in plasma and urine are usually above the normal pregnancy range when a mole is in situ in the uterus this appears to be true in only about half of all cases (Campbell, Brown, Fortune, Pepperell and Beischer, 1970). Values within the normal pregnancy range are found, and in some instances, may be below the normal values for that stage of pregnancy. In general the concentrations of hCG-α and hCG-β are much lower than the corresponding concentrations of intact hCG. However, the number of subjects studied has been small and exceptions may occur (Gaspard, Reuter, De Ville, Gevaert-Vrindts and Franchimont, 1977). hCG values of 53,000 $\pm$ 9000, hCG-β 1800 $\pm$ 270, and hCG-α 284 $\pm$ 45 ng/ml were reported. Values of the same order of magnitude were reported by Dawood, Saxena and Landesman (1977).

One of the main applications of hCG assays is in the follow-up of patients after evacuation of mole. The risk of choriocarcinoma after mole is about 1000 times higher than following normal term pregnancy and the risk is largely, although not completely, confined to the first two years. Even so, the risk of choriocarcinoma after mole appears to be only 2–3% in European populations studied before the introduction of chemotherapy. Although it is possible that this is a slight underestimate it is unlikely that the risk of true choriocarcinoma exceeds 5% after mole. In the majority of patients the trophoblast of hydatidiform mole dies out spontaneously but it commonly takes much longer for this to be complete than after normal pregnancy, and molar trophoblast may persist for many months as invasive mole (Bagshawe, 1969). It is common for the concentration of hCG in body fluids to fall below that detectable by pregnancy tests and to remain low for months or years before increasing again when progressive disease from a choriocarcinoma is manifested. This can also happen when follow-up by radioimmunoassay is carried out, but with the greater sensitivity of this method the risk of undetectable disease is greatly reduced. In approximately 2500 patients with hydatidiform mole followed up at this centre by hCG/LH radioimmunoassay, 0·3% had normal values for more than two months before increasing values indicated the presence of a progressive tumour. It seems likely that with hCG-β radioimmunoassay on serum the risk of undetectable disease will be further reduced but it is unlikely that it will be eliminated altogether.

Analysis of a small part of this series showed that 70% of patients were still excreting hCG 1 month after evacuation of the mole and this figure had fallen to 20% by 4 months postevacuation (Bagshawe, Wilson, Dublon, Smith, Baldwin and Kardana, 1973). Spontaneously falling values of hCG have been observed to continue up to 6–7 months after evacuation of mole. However, when hCG production continues 5–6 months after evacuation of mole, spontaneous resolution is less likely and it has been found advisable to initiate treatment at this time in those continuing to produce detectable levels of hCG. With this criteria about 9% of all mole patients have been found to require treatment by chemotherapy. Although histological criteria are not always obtained it seems likely that about half these patients have choriocarcinoma and the others invasive mole.

In addition to continued hCG production 5–6 months after evacuation of the mole, measurements of hCG values provide other indications for initiating treatment. One of these is a persisting high serum or urinary excretion rate of hCG (greater than 40,000 u hCG per day in the urine or 20,000 u/l in the serum by hCG-β assay) more than 3–4 weeks post-mole, since such patients are candidates for perforation of the uterus by aggressive lesions. Similarly, patients whose values fall after evacuation of the mole and then show a progressive increase also require treatment. (These two groups of indications are also included in the 9% mentioned above.)

Because of these considerations it is necessary that patients who have hydatidiform mole should be followed up on a regular basis and this has frequently proved difficult to achieve on locally based arrangements. In the UK, a national mole registration scheme has been introduced by the Department of Health and Social Security and the Royal College of Obstetricians and Gynaecologists so that patients with hydatidiform mole are registered with one of three central laboratories which then send to the patient the necessary requisites and instructions for providing 5 ml aliquots from measured 12 or 24 hr urines with 100 mg of merthiolate added to the collecting bottle as a preservative. Assays for LH are carried out every 2 weeks until normal values are obtained, then monthly for one year and three monthly during the second year of follow-up. In addition serum is requested for hCG-β assay after the first normal LH value has been obtained. These are continued until hCG-β becomes undetectable. In general, however, it has proved more satisfactory and more reliable to assay urine rather than serum, owing to the usual difficulty of obtaining regular blood samples.

Patients who have had hydatidiform moles appear to have an increased risk of developing choriocarcinoma after a subsequent pregnancy, and it has

o

therefore been the standard practice in this laboratory to request a further specimen of serum for hCG-β assay 3 weeks and 3 months after the end of any subsequent pregnancy. Where radioimmunoassay is not available, haemagglutination inhibition tests such as "Luteonosticon" (Organon), which is sensitive enough to detect normal LH values, can be used in conjunction with a standard pregnancy test system as described by Persijn, Korsten, Engelsman and Cleton (1972). There is no evidence to suggest that specific assays for hCG-α or hCG-β would add materially to the information provided by assays for intact hCG in the follow-up of hydatidiform mole patients. Similar considerations apply to other placental products, including human placental lactogen, placental alkaline phosphatase and the glycoprotein $\beta_1 SP_1$.

Serial hCG assays in the follow-up of patients with hydatidiform mole have revealed that if such women take oral contraceptives before complete regression of the mole, as judged by hCG values, this significantly delays the rate of decline of hCG in body fluids and doubles the risk of requiring treatment (Stone, Dent, Kardana and Bagshawe, 1976).

4. Choriocarcinoma

Although hCG values in serum vary widely, none of the 600 cases of choriocarcinoma and invasive mole with active disease investigated at this Centre has failed to produce detectable levels. Urinary excretion rates have been in the range 10^2-10^7 u/24 hr and serum values in the range 10^1-10^7 u/ml. Although there is some individual variation between tumours, some producing relatively little, and others relatively large amounts of hCG, there is in general a close correlation between the amount of hCG produced and the total mass of tumour. Since it is important to diagnose these tumours at the earliest possible time, it is essential to recognise that a small amount of hCG may be of diagnostic importance. The notion that high values are always found in choriocarcinoma is false. High values relate to advanced disease, and it is important to recognise that the chances of therapeutic success are greatest when the tumour mass is smallest. Thus the magnitude of the hCG concentration at the time treatment is started is one of several powerful prognostic factors defined for this disease (Bagshawe, 1976). Serial measurements of hCG during treatment provide a reliable guide to the course of the disease. Sustained reductions in values have invariably been followed by other evidence of tumour regression and increasing values have been accompanied or followed by other evidence of progression of the disease. When values remain elevated but relatively constant, progression of the disease usually occurs. For a given course of treatment, the change in hCG value between the time of starting a course of chemotherapy and the time when the subsequent course of chemotherapy can be initiated is a quantitative measure of the response. Such measurements provide a relatively precise means for comparing the responses of hCG-producing tumours to a particular drug regimen and it allows comparisons to be made with comparatively small numbers of patients in contrast to the large numbers required to obtain significant values using standard clinical trial procedures.

If treatment is discontinued as soon as hCG becomes undetectable, the disease relapses within days or weeks. At the limit of detection by radioimmunoassay for hCG/LH, about 10^5-10^6 choriocarcinoma cells have been judged to be present. With the hCG-β assay detecting 1–2 u/l, the limit of detection is of the order of 10^4-10^5 tumour cells. These values may be compared with the limit of sensitivity of standard pregnancy tests which is in the range 10^7-10^9 tumour cells. It is evident that the treatment must be continued well beyond the time of first attaining undetectable hCG values and a variety of factors are involved in this (Bagshawe, 1976).

hCG measurements thus provide for patients with gestational choriocarcinoma a situation where precise measurements can be made relating to the total tumour burden of the patient and providing data comparable to those obtainable in the best experimental animal work.

After completion of treatment, choriocarcinoma patients should be followed up with regular hCG assays, preferably on serum and preferably indefinitely. If relapse occurs it is almost always detectable by increasing hCG values before symptoms or signs occur.

The possibility of using radioimmunoassay with urine concentrates has been briefly described by Schreiber, Rebar, Chen, Hodgen and Ross (1976). Whilst 10–100 times the existing sensitivity in hCG assays would be valuable, the possible loss of specificity due to interfering factors in urine and urine concentrates, loss of precision in recovery of hCG from urine concentrates and the possibility of detecting hCG from non-tumour sources remain potential limitations to this approach.

Measurements of hCG-α in patients with choriocarcinoma do not appear to add any useful information to that provided by hCG. It has been suggested (Vaitukaitis et al., 1976) that hCG-β production is unfavourable prognostically. The numbers of patients studied, however, so far has been small and the complex factors involved in the prognosis of these patients are such that it might be premature to accept this evidence.

5. Malignant Teratoma

Malignant teratomas of the testis, ovary, mediastinum or other sites frequently show histological differentiation with trophoblastic or trophoblast-like cells either in the primary or secondary growths and these produce various amounts of hCG (Golding, Elston, Levison and Bagshawe, 1968). In contrast to gestational trophoblastic tumours hCG is often only a partial marker for these tumours, since other malignant elements may be present. When a diagnosis of malignant teratoma is suspect it is essential to assay for α-fetoprotein (AFP) as well as hCG. Again, AFP is generally only a partial marker for these tumours, and there may be non-marker-producing elements present. Some patients with extensive disease harbour tumours which produce only a few hundred units of hCG but others are predominantly or exclusively trophoblastic in nature and hCG is then comparable to hCG in gestational tumours. It is important to recognise that although trophoblast may not be seen in the primary tumour, hCG production by metastases is frequent. More than 80% of samples from teratoma patients sent to this department for analysis contain detectable levels of hCG and similar values have been observed by others (Höffken and Schmidt, 1976). It is advisable to obtain serum for hCG and AFP estimation by radioimmunoassay from any patient with a testicular swelling before, as well as after gonadectomy.

About 25% of patients with seminoma also produce hCG. In some cases this is associated with teratomatous change (Hobson, 1965; Braunstein, Vaitukaitis, Carbone and Ross, 1973b). In our own series we have seen a small number of patients where hCG and AFP values have become normal after treatment for malignant teratoma but where clinical and radiological evidence of progressive disease has occurred as a result of non-marker producing elements.

6. Ectopic Production of hCG by Non-trophoblastic Tumours

Gonadotrophin production by patients with carcinoma of the lung was described by Fusco and Rosen (1965).

Braunstein et al. (1973c) studied hCG values in 828 patients with non-testicular tumours and 60 had detectable levels of hCG. Carcinomas of the stomach, pancreas or breast, multiple myeloma and melanoma were those most likely to give positive response. Goldstein, Kosasa and Skarim (1974) found results positive for hCG in 44 out of 118 patients. In patients with islet cell tumours, hCG and its subunits were found only in those with islet cell carcinoma (Kahn et al., 1977). hCG production was also found to occur in 13·6% of 125 Ugandan patients with hepatocellular carcinoma (Braunstein, Vogel, Vaitukaitis, and Ross, 1973c).

The high incidence of hCG production and detection in the serum in patients with tumours not thought to contain trophoblastic elements is clearly of considerable interest, and has been attributed to the phenomenon of genetic derepression. It is, however, important to recognise that in the majority of patients with ectopic hCG production, the concentration of hCG in the serum is generally small and in only a few cases exceeds 100 u/l. Moreover, when assays are used close to the limits of their reliability, false positives can occur. The study of tumour markers by Williams, McIntire, Waldmann, Feinleib, Go, Kannel, Dawber, Castelli and MacNamara (1977) was therefore salutary. Although 10–26 months elapsed between detecting elevated carcinoembryonic antigen and/or hCG levels before tumours were diagnosed clinically, the 20% incidence of false positive results at the levels of sensitivity used would create grave problems were these markers to be used for a screening. Thus, in contrast to the situation where hCG is produced as a marker by gestational and non-gestational trophoblastic tumours, the clinical benefit so far attributable to measurements of hCG as an ectopic product has been small.

7. Cerebro-spinal Fluid hCG in Patients with CNS Metastases from Choriocarcinoma

Some early workers suggested that choriocarcinoma and hydatidiform mole could be distinguished from pregnancy by the ability to detect hCG in the cerebro-spinal fluid (CSF) (McCormick, 1954). Later it was observed that hCG values in CSF was high in patients with intracranial metastases from choriocarcinoma (Tashima, Timberger, Burdick, Leavy and Rawson, 1965). The relationship between the concentration of hCG in CSF and serum or urine has been described above and it was only when this had been established that the value of hCG measurements in CSF could be interpreted (Rushworth, Orr and Bagshawe, 1968). In patients without CNS metastases the concentration of hCG in CSF is proportional to the plasma concentration and results from diffusion of hCG across the blood/brain barrier. In patients with hCG-producing metastases in the CNS, the CSF value is determined partly by diffusion of the hormone from the systemic body fluids and also from the contribution produced within the CNS.

In general, patients with intracranial metastases producing hCG have serum:CSF values less than 60:1. Where most of the active tumour is confined to the CNS, the CSF concentration may then exceed the serum concentration. Changes in serum concentration of hCG are only slowly reflected in changes in the CSF concentration but repeated estimations may be used to monitor the course of the CNS metastases. It is advisable to take into account both the serum:spinal fluid ratio and the absolute concentration of hCG in the CSF (Bagshawe and Harland, 1976). Although the same principles apply to hCG production by malignant teratomas which have metastasised to the CNS, it is important to recognise that metastases from non-trophoblastic elements may occur in this tumour.

REFERENCES

Aakvaag, A., Norman, N. and Vogt, J. H. (1965). *Acta endocr., Copenh.* (Suppl.) **100**, 111.

Albert, A. (1956). *Rec. Prog. Horm. Res.* **12**, 227.

Al-Kafawi, A. A., Hopwood, M. L., Pineda, M. M. and Faulkner, L. C. (1974). *Am. J. vet. Res.* **35**, 261.

Aloj, S. M., Edelhoch, H., Ingham, K. C., Morgan, F. J., Canfield, R. E. and Ross, G. T. (1973). *Arch. biochem. Biophys.* **159**, 497.

Aschheim, S. and Zondek, B. (1927). *Klin. Wchnschr.* **6**, 1322.

Ashitaka, Y. and Koide, S. S. (1974). *Fert. Steril.* **25**, 177.

Ashitaka, Y., Mochizuki, M. and Tojo, S., (1972). *Endocrinology*, **90**, 609.

Ashitaka, Y., Nishimura, Y., Futamara, K. and Tojo, S. (1977). *Endocrinology*, (*Jap.*), **24**, 115.

Ashitaka, Y., Tokura, Y., Tane, M., Mochizuki, M. and Tojo, S. (1970). *Endocrinology*, **87**, 233.

Azhar, S., Hajra, A. K. and Menon, K. M. J. (1976). *J. biol. Chem.* **251**, 7405.

Azhar, S. and Menon, K. M. J. (1976). *J. biol. Chem.* **251**, 7398.

Bagshawe, K. D. (1969. "Choriocarcinoma: the Clinical Biology of the Trophoblast and its Tumours." Edward Arnold, London.

Bagshawe, K. D. (1975). *Lab Prac.* 573.

Bagshawe, K. D. (1976). *Cancer*, **38**, 1373.

Bagshawe, K. D. and Harland, S. (1976). *Cancer*, **38**, 112.

Bagshawe, K. D., Orr, A. H. and Godden, J. (1968a). *J. Endocr.* **42**, 513.

Bagshawe, K. D., Orr, A. H. and Rushworth, A. G. J. (1968b). *Nature, Lond.* **217**, 950.

Bagshawe, K. D., Wilson, H., Dublon, P., Smith, A., Baldwin, M. and Kardana, A. (1973). *J. Obstet. Gynec. Cwlth*, **80**, 461.

Bahl, O. P. (1969a). *J. biol. Chem.* **244**, 567.

Bahl, O. P. (1969b). *J. biol. Chem.* **244**, 575.

Bahl, O. P. (1971). *In* "Structure–Activity Relationships of Protein and Polypeptide Hormones" (M. Margoulies and F. C. Greenwood, eds), Part 1, p. 99. Excerpta Medica, Amsterdam.

Bahl, O. P. (1977). *Fed. Proc.* **36**, 2119.

Bahl, O. P., Pandian, M. R. and Ghai, R. D. (1976). *Biochem. biophys. Res. Commun.* **70**, 525.

Bangham, D. R. and Grab, B. (1964). *Bull. World Health Org.* **31**, 111.

Banerji, A. P., Kothari, L. S. and Shah, P. N. (1977). *Endokrinologie*, **69**, 274.

Bell, J. J., Canfield, R. E. and Sciarra, J. J. (1969). *Endocrinology*, **84**, 298.

Bellisario, R. and Bahl, O. P. (1975). *J. biol. Chem.* **250**, 3837.

Bellisario, R., Carlsen, R. B. and Bahl, O. P. (1973). *J. biol. Chem.* **248**, 6796.

Bhalla, V. K., Haskell, J., Grier, H. and Mahesh, V. B. (1976). *J. biol. Chem.* **251**, 4947.

Birken, S. and Canfield, R. E. (1977). *J. biol. Chem.* **252**, 5386.

Braunstein, G. D., Grodin, J. M., Vaitukaitis, J. L. and Ross, G. T. (1973a). *Am. J. Obstet. Gynec.* **115**, 447.

Braunstein, G. D., Rasor, J., Adler, D., Danzer, H. and Wade, M. E. (1976). *Am. J. Obstet. Gynec.* **126**, 678.

Braunstein, G. D., Rasor, J. and Wade, M. E. (1975). *New Engl. J. Med.* **293**, 1339.

Braunstein, G. D., Vaitukaitis, J. L. and Ross, G. T. (1972). *Endocrinology*, **91**, 1030.

Braunstein, G. D., Vaitukaitis, J. L., Carbone, P. P. and Ross, G. T. (1973b). *Ann. int. Med.* **78**, 39.
Braunstein, G. D., Vogel, C. L., Vaitukaitis, J. L. and Ross, G. T. (1973c). *Cancer*, **32**, 223.
Brody, S. and Carlstrom, G. (1965). *J. clin. Endocr. Metab.* **25**, 792.
Brossmer, R., Dörner, M., Hilgenfeldt, V., Leidenberger, F. and Trude, E. (1971). *FEBS Lett.* **15**, 33.
Campbell, D. G., Brown, J. B., Fortune, D. W., Pepperell, R. and Beischer, N. A. (1970). *J. Obstet. Gynec. Br. Cwlth*, **77**, 410.
Canfield, R. E., Bell, J. J. and Agosto, G. M. (1970). In "Gonadotropins and Ovarian Development" (W. R. Butt, A. C. Crooke and M. Ryle, eds), pp. 161–170. Livingstone, Edinburgh.
Canfield, R. E., Birken, S., Morse, J. H. and Morgan, F. J. (1976). In "Peptide Hormones" (J. A. Parsons, ed.), pp. 299–315. Macmillan, London.
Canfield, R. E., Morgan, F. J., Kammerman, S., Bell, J. J. and Agosto, G. M. (1971). *Rec. Prog. Horm. Res.* **27**, 121.
Canfield, R. E., Morgan, F. J., Kammerman, S. and Ross, G. T. (1973). In "Structure-Activity Relationships of Protein and Polypeptide Hormones" (M. Margoulies and F. C. Greenwood, eds), pp. 337–339. Excerpta Medica, Amsterdam.
Canfield, R. E. and Ross, G. T. (1976). *Bull. WHO*, **54**, 463.
Carlsen, R. B., Bahl, O. P. and Swaminathan, N. (1973). *J. biol. Chem.* **248**, 6810.
Catt, K. J. and Dufau, M. L. (1973a). *Nature New Biol.* **244**, 219.
Catt, K. J. and Dufau, M. L. (1973b). In "Receptors for Reproductive Hormones" (B. W. O'Malley and A. R. Means, eds), pp. 379–418. Plenum Press, New York.
Catt, K. J., Dufau, M. L. and Tsuruhara, T. (1971). *J. clin. Endocr. Metab.* **32**, 860.
Catt, K. J., Dufau, M. L. and Tsuruhara, T. (1972). *J. clin. Endocr. Metab.* **34**, 123.
Catt, K. J., Tsuruhara, T., Mendelson, C., Ketelslegers, J. M. and Dufau, M. L. (1974). "Hormone Binding and Target Cell Activation in the Testis" (M. L. Dufau and A. R. Means. eds), pp. 1–30. Plenum Press, New York.
Cédard, L., Alsat, E., Urtasun, M. J. and Varangot, J. (1970). *Steroids*, **16**, 361.
Channing, C. P. and Kammerman, S. (1973). *Endocrinology*, **93**, 1035.
Channing, C. P. and Kammerman, S. (1974). *Biol. Reprod.* **10**, 179.
Charreau, E. H., Dufau, M. L. and Catt, K. J. (1973). *J. biol. chem.* **249**, 4189.
Chen, H-C. and Hodgen, G. D. (1976). *J. clin. Endocr. Metab.* **43**, 1414.
Chen, H-C., Hodgen, G. D., Matsuura, S., Lin, L. J., Gross, E., Reichert, L. E. Jr., Birken, S., Canfield, R. E. and Ross, G. T. (1976). *Proc. natn. Acad. Sci. USA*, **73**, 2885.
Christiansen, P. (1967). *Acta endocr. Copenh.* **56**, 608.
Closset, J., Hennen, G. and Lequin, R. M. (1973). *FEBS Lett.* **29**, 97.
Conti, M. Harwood, J. P., Hsueh, A. J. W., Dufau, M. L. and Catt, K. J. (1976). *J. biol. Chem.* **251**, 7729.
Crosignani, P. G., Brambati, B. and Nencioni, T. (1971). *Am. J. Obstet. Gynec.* **109**, 985.
Crosignani, P. G., Nencioni, T. and Branbati, B. (1972). *J. Obstet. Gynec. Br. Cwlth*, **79**, 122.
Dawood, M. Y., Saxena, B. B. and Landesman, R. (1977). *Obstet. Gynec.* **50**, 172.
Delfs, E., (1959). *Ann. N.Y. Acad. Sci.* **80**, 125.
Delfs, E. and Jones, G. E. S. (1948). *Obstet. Gynaec. Surv.* **3**, 680.
Diczfalusy, E. (1953). *Acta endocr., Copenh.* **12**, 7.
Diczfalusy, E. and Loraine, J. A. (1955). *J. clin. Endocr.* **15**, 424.

Diczfalusy, E. and Troen, P. (1961). *Vitam. Horm.* **19**, 229.

Dufau, M. L. and Catt, K. J. (1973). *Nature New Biol.* **242**, 246.

Engel, W. and Frowein, J. (1974). *Cell*, **2**, 75.

Evans, H. M., Meyer, K. and Simpson, M. E. (1932). *Am. J. Physiol.* **100**, 141.

Faiman, C., Ryan, R. J., Zwirek, S. J. and Rubin, M. E. (1968). *J. clin. Endocr. Metab.* **28**, 1323.

Figarova, V., Presl, J. and Horsky, J. (1969). *Physiol. Bohemoslov.* **18**, 477.

Fisher, G. H., Chang, D., Howard, G. and Folkers, K. (1977). *J. org. Chem.* **42**, 3341.

Franchimont, P. (1970). *Eur. J. clin. Invest.* **1**, 65.

Franchimont, P. and Reuter, A. (1972). *In* "Structure Activity Relationships of Protein and Polypeptide Hormones", Part II, pp. 381–387. Excerpta Medica Int. Cong. Ser. 241, Amsterdam.

Friedman, M. H. and Weinstein, G. L. (1937). *Endocrinology*, **21**, 489.

Fusco, F. D. and Rosen, S. W. (1965). *New Engl. J. Med.* **275**, 507.

Galli-Mainini, C. (1947). *J. clin Endocr.* **7**, 653.

Garnier, J., Salesse, R. and Pernollet, J. C. (1974). *FEBS Lett.* **45**, 166.

Gaspard, U., Reuter, A. M., De Ville, J. C., Gevaert-Vrindts, Y. and Franchimont, P. (1977). *Acta endocr., Copenh.* (Suppl.) **212**, 33.

Gastineau, C. F., Albert, A. and Randall, L. M. (1949). *J. clin. Endocr. Metab.* **9**, 615.

Geiger, W. (1973). *Horm. Metab. Res.* **5**, 342.

Geiger, W., Kaiser, R. and Franchimont, P. (1971). *Acta endocr., Copenh.* **68**, 169.

Gershey, E. L. and Kaplan, I. (1974). *Biochem. biophys. Acta.*, **342**, 322.

Gey, G. O., Seegar-Jones, G. E. and Hellman, L. M. (1938). *Science*, **88**, 306.

Golding, P. R., Elston, C. W., Levison, V. B. and Bagshawe, K. D. (1968). *Br. J. Surg.* **55**, 508.

Goldstein, D. P., Kosasa, T. S. and Skarim, A. T. (1974a). *Surg. Gynec. Obstet.* **138**, 747.

Goldstein, D. P., Partorfide, G. B., Osathanondh, R. and Kosasa, T. S. (1974b). *Obstet. Gynec.* **45**, 527.

Gospodarowicz, D. (1964). *Acta endocr., Copenh.* **47**, 293.

Got, R. and Bourrillon, R. (1965). *Biochim. biophys. Acta*, **39**, 241.

Got, R. Bourrillon, R. and Michon, J. (1960). *Bull Soc. chim. biol.* **42**, 41.

Goverde, B. C., Veenkamp, F. J. N. and Homan, J. D. H. (1968). *Acta endocr., Copenh.* **59**, 105.

Grässlin, D. Czygan, P-J and Weise, H. C. (1973). *In* "Structure-Activity Relationships of Protein and Polypeptide Hormones" (M. Margoulies and F. C. Greenwood, eds), pp. 366–368. Excerpta Medica, Amsterdam.

Gregorio, de G. and Buda, A. (1964). *Boll. Soc. ital. Biol. sper.* **40**, 1718.

Gurin, S., Bachman, C. and Wilson, D. W. (1939). *J. biol. Chem.* **128**, 525.

Halpin, T. F. (1970). *Am. J. Obstet. Gynec.* **106**, 227.

Hamburger, C. (1944). *Acta obstet. gynec. scand.* **24**, 45.

Han, S. S., Rajaniemi, H. J., Cho, M. I., Hirshfield, A. M. and Midgley, A. R., Jr. (1974). *Endocrinology*, **95**, 589.

Haour, F. and Saxena, B. B. (1974). *J. biol. Chem.* **249**, 2195.

Henry, J. B. and Little, W. A. (1962). *J. Am. med. Assoc.* **182**, 230.

Hershman, J. M. and Burrow, G. N. (1976). *J. clin. endocr. Metab.* **44**, 970.

Hisley, J. C. and Fesche, H. (1966). *Proc. Soc. exp. Biol. Med.* **121**, 235.

Hobson, B. M. (1965). *Acta endocr., Copenh.* **49**, 337.

Hodgen, G. D., Nixon, W. E., Vaitukaitis, J. L., Tullner, W. W. and Ross, G. T. (1973). *Endocrinology*, **92**, 705.

Hodgen, G. D., Tullner, W. W., Vaitukaitis, J. L., Ward, D. N. and Ross, G. J. (1974). *J. clin. Endocr. Metab.* **39**, 457.

Höffken, K. and Schmidt, C. G. (1976). *Z. Krebsforsch.* **87**, 37.

Hum, V. G., Botting, H. and Mori, K. F. (1976). *Endocr. Res. Commun.* **3**, 145.

Hussa, R. O. (1977). *J. clin. Endocr. Metab.* **44**, 1154.

Ingham, K. C., Aloj, S. M. and Edelhoch, H. (1974). *Arch. biochem. Biophys.* **163**, 589.

Ingham, K. C., Tylenda, C. and Edelhoch, H. (1976a). *Arch. biochem. Biophys.* **173**, 680.

Ingham, K. C., Weintraub, B. D. and Edelhoch, H. (1976b). *Biochemistry*, **15**, 1720.

Jacobs, H. S., Vanthuyne, C. and Ekins, R. P. (1974). *In* "Radioimmunoassay and related procedures in medicine" Vol. 1, pp. 237–243. International Atomic Energy Agency, Vienna.

Johnsen, S. G. (1968). *Acta endocr., Copenh.* **28**, 69.

Jones, D. H. (1966). *Br. J. clin. Prac.* **20**, 377.

Joshi, U. M., Raghavan, V. and Sheth, A. R. (1977). *Indian J. med. Res.* **65**, 807.

Jovanovic, L., Landesman, R. and Saxena, B. B. (1977). *Science*, **198**, 738.

Jungmann, R. A., Hiestand, P. C. and Schweppe, J. S. (1974). *Endocrinology*, **94**, 168.

Kahn, C. R., Rosen, S. W., Weintraub, B. D., Fajans, S. A. and Gorden, P. (1977). *New Engl. J. Med.* **297**, 565.

Kammerman, S. and Canfield, R. E. (1972). *Endocrinology*, **90**, 384.

Kardana, A. and Bagshawe, K. D. (1976). *J. immunol. Meth.* **9**, 297.

Katzman, P. A., Godfrid, M., Cain, C. K. and Doisy, E. A. (1943). *J. biol. Chem.* **148**, 501.

Kazeto, S. and Hreshchyshyn, M. M. (1970). *Am. J. Obstet. Gynec.* **106**, 1229.

Kennedy, J. F. and Chaplin, M. F. (1972). *Biochem. J.* **115**, 225.

Kennedy, J. F. and Chaplin, M. F. (1976). *Biochem. J.* **155**, 303.

Keutman, H. T. and Williams, R. M. (1977). *J. biol. Chem.* **252**, 5393.

Kido, I. (1937). *Zentralbl. Gynäk.* **61**, 1551.

Kosasa, T. S., Levesque, L. A., Goldstein, D. P. *et al.* (1973a). *J. clin. Endocr. Metab.* **36**, 622.

Kosasa, T. S., Levesque, L. A., Taymor, M. L. and Goldstein, D. P. (1974). *Fert. Steril.* **25**, 211.

Kosasa, T. S., Taymor, M. L., Goldstein, D. P. and Levesque, L. A. (1973b). *Obstet. Gynaec.* **42**, 868.

Landau, B., Schwartz, H. S. and Soffer, L. J. (1960). *Metabolism*, **9**, 85.

Landefeld, T. D., McWilliam, D. R. and Boime, I. (1976). *Biochem. biophys. Res. Commun.* **72**, 381.

Lee, C. Y. and Ryan, R. J. (1971). *Endocrinology*, **89**, 1515.

Lee, C. Y. and Ryan, R. J. (1972). *Proc. natn. Acad. Sci. USA*, **69**, 3520.

Lee, C. Y. and Ryan, R. J. (1974). *In* "Gonadotropins and Gonadal Function" (N. R.

Lee, C. Y., Wong, S., Lee, A. S. K. and Ma, L. (1977). *Hoppe-Seyler's Z. Physiol. Chem.* **358**, 909.

Mougdal, ed.), pp. 444–459. Academic Press, New York and London.

Leleux, P. and Robyn, C. (1970). *Ann. endocr.* **31**, 181.

Lemaire, W. J., Comly, P. W., Moffett, A., Spelasy, W. N., Cleveland, W. W. and Savard, K. (1971). *Am. J. Obstet. Gynec.* **110**, 612.

Lewis, J. Jr., Dray, S., Genuth, S. and Schwartz, H. S. (1964). *J. clin Endocr. Metab.* **24**, 197.

Liao, T. H. and Pierce, J. G. (1971). *J. biol. Chem.* **246**, 850.

Lieblich, J. M., Weintraub, B. D., Krauth, G. H., Kohler, P. O., Rabson, A. S. and Rosen, S. W. (1976). *J. Natn. Cancer Inst.* **56**, 911.

Liu, W. K., Nahm, H. S., Sweeney, C. M., Lamkin, W. M., Baker, H. N. and Ward, D. N. (1972). *J. biol. Chem.* **247**, 4351.

Loraine, J. A. (1950). *Q. J. exp. Physiol.* **36**, 11.

Loraine, J. A. (1956). *Vit. Horm.* **14**, 307.

Loraine, J. A. (1957). *In* "Ciba Foundation Colloquia on Endocrinology", pp. 19–37. Churchill, London.

Loraine, J. A. (1967). *In* "Hormones in Blood" (C. H. Gray and A. L. Bacharach, eds), pp. 313–332. Academic Press, London and New York.

Loraine, J. A. and Mackay, M. A. (1961). *J. Endocr.* **22**, 277.

Louvet, J. P., Ross, G. T., Barker, S. and Canfield, R. E. (1974). *J. clin. Endocr. Metab.* **39**, 1155.

Maghuin-Rogister, G., Combarnous, Y. and Hennen, G. (1972). *FEBS Lett.* **25**, 57.

Mason, T. E., Phifer, R. F., Spicer, S. S., Swallow, R. A. and Dreskin, R. B. (1969). *J. Histochem. Cytochem.* **17**, 563.

Menon, K. M. (1972). *J. biol. Chem.* **248**, 494.

Menon, K. M. and Jaffe, R. B. (1973). *J. clin. Endocr. Metab.* **36**, 1104.

Merz, W. E., Hilgenfeldt, V., Dörner, M. and Brossmer, R. (1974). *Hoppe-Seyler's Z. Physiol. Chem.* **355**, 1035.

Midgley, A. R., Fong, I. F. and Jaffe, R. B. (1967). *Nature, Lond.* **213**, 733.

Midgley, A. R. and Jaffe, R. B. (1968). *J. clin. Endocr. Metab.* **28**, 1712.

Midgley, A. R. and Pierce Jr., G. B. (1962). *J. exp. Med.* **115**, 289.

Mills, T. M. and McPherson, J. C. and Mahesh, V. B. (1974). *Proc. Soc. exp. Biol. Med.* **145**, 446.

Milwidsky, A., Adoni, A., Segal, S. and Palti, Z. (1977). *Obstet. Gynec.* **50**, 145.

Mishell, D. R., Wide, L. and Gemzell, C. A. (1963). *J. clin Endocr.* **23**, 125.

Mitchell, H. D. C. and Bagshawe, K. D. (1976). *In* "Hormone Assays and their Clinical Application" (J. A. Loraine and E. T. Bell. eds), pp. 142–170, 4th edition. Churchill, Livingstone, Edinburgh, London and New York.

Morell, A. G., Gregoriadis, G. P. H., Scheinberg, I. H., Hickman, J. and Ashwell, G. (1971). *J. biol. Chem.* **246**, 1461.

Morgan, F. J., Birken, S. and Canfield, R. E. (1973). *Mol. Cell. Biochem.* **2**, 97.

Morgan, F. J., Birken, S. and Canfield, R. E. (1974). *In* "Gonadotropins and Gonadal Function" (N. R. Mougdal, ed.), pp. 79–92. Academic Press, London and New York.

Morgan, F. J., Birken, S. and Canfield, R. E. (1975). *J. biol. Chem.* **250**, 5247.

Morgan, F. J. and Canfield, R. E. (1971). *Endocrinology*, **88**, 1045.

Morgan, F. J., Canfield, R. E., Vaitukaitis, J. L. and Ross, G. T. (1973). *In* "Methods in Investigative and Diagnostic Endocrinology" (S. A. Berson and R. S. Yalow, eds), p. 736, Part III. North Holland Publishing Co., Amsterdam.

Mori, K. F. (1970). *Endocrinology*, **86**, 97.

Mori, K. F. and Hollands, T. R. (1971). *J. biol. Chem.* **246**, 7223.

Morris, C. J. O. R. (1955). *Br. med. Bull.* **11**, 101.

Morris, N. M. and Udry, J. R. (1967). *Am. J. Obstet. Gynec.* **98**, 1148.

Moyle, W. R., Bahl, O. P. and März, L. (1975). *J. biol. Chem.* **250**, 9163.

McArthur, J. W. (1968). *In* "Gonadotrophins" (E. Rosemberg, ed.), p. 71. Geron-X, Los Altos, California.

McCormick, J. B. (1954). *Obstet. Gynaec.* **3**, 58.

Okudaira, Y., Hashimoto, T., Hamanaka, N. and Yoshinara, S. (1971). *J. Electron Microsc.* **20**, 93.

Orr, A. H., Rushworth, A. G. J. and Bagshawe, K. D. (1968). *Nature, Lond.* 217, 950.
Pandian, M. R. and Bahl, O. P. (1977). *Arch biochem. Biophys.* 182, 420.
Pandian, M. R., Bahl, O. P. and Segal, S. J. (1975). *Biochem. biophys. Res. Commun.* 64, 1199.
Parlow, A. F. (1961). *In* "Human Pituitary Gonadotrophin" (A. Albert, ed.), pp. 300–310. C. C. Thomas, Springfield.
Pastorfide, G. B., Goldstein, D. P., Kosasa, T. S. and Levesque, L. (1974). *Am. J. Obstet. Gynec.* 118, 293.
Perloff, W. H. and Jacobsohn, G. (1963). *J. clin. Endocr. Metab.* 23, 1177.
Persijn, J. P., Korsten, C. B., Engelsman, E. and Cleton, F. J. (1972). *Z. Klin. Chem. Klin. Biochem.* 10, 403.
Philipp, E. (1930). *Zentralbl. Gynäk.* 54, 1858.
Purvis, J. L., Canick, J. A., Rosenbaum, J. H., Hologgitas, J. and Latif, S. A. (1973). *Arch. biochem. Biophys.* 159, 31.
Qazi, M. H., Mukherjee, G., Javidi, K., Pala, A. and Diczfalusy, E. (1974). *Eur. J. Biochem.* 47, 219.
Rajaniemi, H. J., Hirshfield, A. N. and Midgley, A. R., Jr. (1974). *Endocrinology*, 95, 557.
Rao, C. V. (1973). *In* "Symposium on Advances in Chemistry, Biology and Immunology of Gonadotropins" (Bangalore).
Rao, C. V. (1974). *J. biol. Chem.* 249, 2864.
Rao, C. V. and Carmen, F. (1973). *Biochem. biophys. Res. Commun.* 54, 744.
Rao, C. V. and Saxena, B. B. (1973). *Biochim. biophys. Acta.* 313, 372.
Rathnam, P. and Saxena, B. B. (1975). *J. biol. Chem.* 250, 6735.
Reichert, L. E. Jr., Trowbridge, C. G., Bhalla, V. K. and Lawson, G. M., Jr. (1974). *J. biol. Chem.* 249, 6472.
Reisfeld, R. A., Bergenstal, D. M. and Hertz, R. (1959). *Arch. biochem. Biophys.* 81, 456.
Reisfeld, R. A. and Hertz, R. (1960). *Biochem. biophys. Acta*, 43, 540.
Reiss, M., Hillman, J., Pearse, J. J., Reiss, J. M., Daley, N. and Suwalski, R. (1965). *Acta endocr., Copenh.* 49, 349.
Reuter, A. M., Franchimont, P. and Schoonbrood, J. (1976). *In* "Protides of Biological Fluids" (H. Peeters, ed.), pp. 583–589, 24th Colloquium. Pergamon Press, London.
Reuter, A. M., Gaspard, U., De Ville, J. C., Gevaert-Vrindts, Y. and Franchimont, P. (1977). *Acta endocr., Copenh.* (Suppl.) 212, 32.
Reuter, A. M., Schoonbroodt, J. and Franchimont, P. (1976). *In* "Cancer Related Antigens" (P. Franchimont, ed.), pp. 237–249. North Holland Publishing Co., Amsterdam.
Rizkallah, T., Gurpide, E. and Van de Wiele, R. L. (1969). *J. clin Endocr. Metab.* 29, 92.
Ross, G. T. (1973). *In* "Methods in Investigative and Diagnostic Endocrinology" (S. A. Berson and R. S. Yalow, eds), pp. 749–756. North Holland Publishing Co., Amsterdam.
Ross, G. T., Cargille, C. M., Lipsett, M. B., Rayford, P. L., Marshall, J. R., Strott, C. A. and Rodbard, D. (1970). *Rec. Prog. Horm. Res.* 26, 1.
Roy, S., Klein, T. A., Scott, J. Z., Kletzky, O. A. and Mishell, D. R. (1977). *Obstet. Gynec.* 50, 401.
Rushworth, A. G. J., Orr, A. H. and Bagshawe, K. D. (1968). *Br. J. Cancer*, 22, 253.
Sairam, M. R., Papkoff, H. and Li, C. H. (1972a). *Arch. biochem. Biophys.* 153, 554.
Sairam, M. R., Papkoff, H. and Li, C. H. (1972b). *Biochem. biophys. Res. Commun.* 48, 530.

Salhanick, H. A. (1961). *In* "Human Pituitary Gonadotropins" (A. Albert, ed.), pp. 37–42. C. C. Thomas, Springfield.

Saxena, B. B., Hasan, S. H., Haour, F. and Schmidt-Gollwitzer, M. (1974). *Science*, **184**, 793.

Saxena, B. B and Rathnam, P. (1976). *J. biol. Chem.* **251**, 993.

Saxena, B. B., Saito, T., Said, N. and Landesman, R. (1977). *Fert. Steril.* **28**, 163.

Scanes, C. G., Follett, B. K. and Goos, H. J. T. (1972). *Gen. comp. Endocr.* **19**, 596.

Schapiro, B. (1930). *Dtsch. Med. Wschr.* **56**, 1605.

Schlumberger, H. D. and Anderer, F. A. (1969). *Acta endocr, Copenh.* **60**, 681.

Schreiber, J. R., Rebar, R. W., Chen. H. C., Hodgen, G. D. and Ross, G. T. (1976). *Am. J. Obstet. Gynec.* **125**, 705.

Sharpe, R. M. (1976). *Nature, Lond.* **264**, 644.

Shome, B. and Parlow, A. F. (1973). *J. clin. Endocr. Metab.* **36**, 618.

Shome, B. and Parlow, A. F. (1974). *J. clin. Endocr. Metab.* **39**, 203.

Siebers, J. W., Schmidtke, J. and Engel, W. (1977). *Experientia*, **33**, 689.

Spiro, R. G. (1970). *Ann. Rev. Biochem.* **39**, 599.

Stewart, H. L. Jr., Sano, M. E. and Montgomery, T. L. (1948). *J. clin. Endocr.* **8**, 175.

Stone, M., Dent, J., Kardana, A. and Bagshawe, K. D. (1976). *Br. J. Obstet. Gynec.* **83**, 913.

Sulimovici, S. and Lunenfeld, B. (1974). *FEBS Lett.* **41**, 345.

Swaminathan, N. and Bahl, O. P. (1970). *Biochem. biophys. Res. Commun.* **40**, 422.

Tanizawo, O., Miyake, A., Kinugasa, T., Yamagi, K. and Kurachi, K. (1975). *Acta obstet. Gynec. Jap.* **22**, 150.

Tashima, C. K., Timberger, R., Burdick, R., Leavy, M. and Rawson. R. W. (1965). *J. clin. Endocr. Metab.* **25**, 1493.

Tojo, S., Ashitaka, Y., Maruo, T. and Ohashi, M. (1977). *Endocr. jap.* **24**, 351.

Tsuruhara, T., van Hall, E. V., Dufau, M. L. and Catt, K. J. (1972). *Endocrinology*, **91**, 463.

Tullner, W. W. (1974). *Contrib. Primatol.* **3**, 235.

Tyrey, L. and Hammond, C. B. (1976). *Am. J. Obstet. Gynec.* **2**, 160.

Umberger, E. J. and Grass, G. H. (1959). *Science*, **129**, 1738.

Vaitukaitis, J. L. (1973). *J. clin. Endocr. Metab.* **37**, 505.

Vaitukaitis, J. L. (1974). *J. clin. Endocr. Metab.* **38**, 755.

Vaitukaitis, J. L., Braunstein, G. D. and Ross, G. T. (1972a). *Am. J. Obstet. Gynec.* **113**, 751.

Vaitukaitis, J. L., Robbins, J. B., Nieschlag, E. and Ross, G. T. (1971). *J. clin. Endocr.* **33**, 988.

Vaitukatis, J. L., Ross, G. T., Braunstein, G. D. and Rayford, P. L. (1976). *Rec Prog. Horm. Res.* **32**, 289.

Vaitukaitis, J. L., Ross, G. T and Reichert, L. E. (1973). *Endocrinology*, **92**, 411.

Vaitukaitis, J. L., Ross, G. T., Reichert, L. E. and Ward, D. N., (1972b). *Endocrinology*, **91**, 1337.

Van de Wiele, R. L., Bogumil, J., Dyrenfurth, I., Ferin, M., Jewelewicz, R., Warren, M., Rizkallah, T. and Mikhail, G. (1970). *Rec. Prog. Horm. Res.* **26**, 63.

Van Hell, H. R., Matthijsen, R. and Homan, J. D. H. (1968). *Acta endocr., Copenh.* **59**, 89.

Van Hell, H. R., Matthijsen, R. and Overbeck, G. A. (1964). *Acta endocr., Copenh.* **47**, 409.

Varma, K., Larraga, L. and Sclenkow, H. A. (1971). *Obstet. Gynec.* **37**, 10.

Velardo, J. T. (1959). *Ann N.Y. Acad. Sci.* **80**, 65.

von Schulthess, G. K., Cohen, R. J. and Benedek, G. B. (1976). *Immunochemistry*, **13**, 963.

Weintraub, B. D., Stannard, B. S. and Rosen, S. W. (1977). *Endocrinology*, **101**, 225.

Whitaker, J. R. (1963). *Anal. chem.* **35**, 1950.

Wide, L. (1962). *Acta endocr., Copenh.* (Suppl.) **70**, 11.

Wide, L. and Gemzell, C. A. (1960). *Acta endocr, Copenh.* **35**, 261.

Wide, L. and Hobson, B. (1974). *J. Endocr.* **61**, 75.

Wide, L., Johannison, E., Tillingen, K. G. and Diczfalusy, E. (1968). *Acta endocr., Copenh.* **59**, 579.

Wilde, C. E. and Bagshawe, K. D. (1965). *In* "Ciba Foundation Study Group No. 22. Gonadotropins: Physio-chemical and Immunological Properties" (G. E. W. Wolsenholme and J. Knight, eds), pp. 46–55. Little, Brown, Boston.

Williams, R. R., McIntire, K. R., Waldmann, T. A., Feinleib, M., Go, V. L. W., Kannel, W. B., Dawber, T. R., Castelli, W. R. and McNamara, P. M. (1977). *J. natn. Cancer Inst.* **58**, 1547.

Winter, J. S., Tarasaka, S. and Faiman, C. (1972). *J. clin. Endocr.* **34**, 348.

Yamashita, K. (1965). *Tohoku J. exp. Med.* **87**, 105.

Yang, W. H. and Chang, M. C. (1968). *Endocrinology*, **83**, 217.

Young, R. L., Fuchs, R. J. and Voltjen, M. J. (1976). *J. Am. Med. Assoc.* **236**, 2495.

Zondek, B. (1929). *Endocrinologie*, **5**, 425.

Zondek, B., Hochman, A. and Sulmar, F. (1939). *Proc. Soc. exp. Biol.* **42**, 338.

IX. Gonadotrophins

W. R. BUTT

INTRODUCTION

In recent years specific methods of assay for the pituitary gonadotrophins in blood have become available, and they have been applied extensively to a large number of clinical problems. In addition, human pituitary prolactin has been isolated and assay systems developed and there have also been notable advances in research into hypothalamic regulating hormones. As a result our knowledge of the relationships between the hypothalamus, pituitary and the gonads has increased considerably. Notable advances have been made in methods for the diagnosis of disorders of the reproductive system, particularly for anovulatory conditions and this had led to improved methods for the treatment of infertility in the female.

The two pituitary gonadotrophins, follicle stimulating hormone ("follitropin"; FSH) and luteinizing hormone ("lutropin"; LH) circulate in blood and are excreted in urine. The term interstitial cell stimulating hormone (ICSH) for LH is still used in some centres and is retained in the titles of international reference preparations and standards.

The best known urinary gonadotrophin is prepared from the urine of postmenopausal women (human menopausal gonadotrophin, hMG). In early pregnancy the trophoblast produces another gonadotrophin, human chorionic gonadotrophin (hCG) which is described in another chapter. It resembles LH in biological properties and in some structural details.

A. CHEMISTRY

1. Sources

The best starting material for the extraction and purification of FSH and LH is the pituitary. Preparations from animal sources have been available for many years, but there has been a steady increase in demand for human gonadotrophins for clinical use and for radioimmunoassays. Successful methods have been described using fresh frozen glands or glands which have been preserved in acetone. A secondary source has been large volumes of urine from postmenopausal women for which preparations of FSH mixed with LH have proved useful for clinical use and to act as standards.

(a) Pituitary FSH

Several satisfactory methods have been described for the initial extraction and purification of human pituitary FSH. Fresh frozen glands may be extracted in solutions of phosphate buffer (Roos, 1968) and acetone-dried glands by mixtures of ammonium acetate and ethanol (Butt, Crooke and Cunningham, 1961; Hartree, 1966; Saxena and Rathnam, 1971).

The separation of FSH from LH and other contaminants is then possible by fractional precipitation from ammonium sulphate (Roos, 1968) or by chromatography on CM- and DEAE-celluloses. A good primary separation of FSH from LH (and from thyroid stimulating hormone, TSH) is achieved on CM-cellulose, FSH being eluted at low salt concentration, while LH is retained (Hartree, 1966).

Preparations of very high potency have been obtained by Roos (1968) starting with fresh frozen pituitaries. After chromatography on DEAE-cellulose, Sephadex G-100 and hydroxylapatite, the products were subjected to electrophoresis on a vertical column of polyacrylamide gel. The LH contamination by bioassay or radioimmunoassay appeared to be very low.

Table 1

Outline of method for the preparation of FSH suitable for use in radioimmunoassay (Bluck, Reay, Lynch and Butt, in preparation).

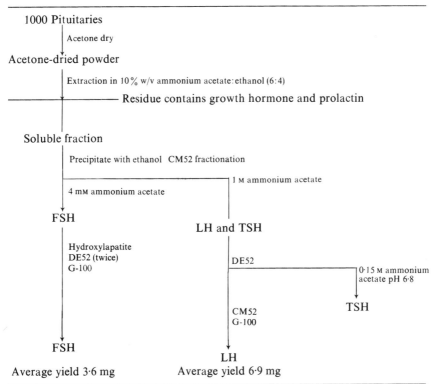

Other preparations of high potency have been described by Reichert, Kathan and Ryan (1968), Peckham and Parlow (1969), Saxena and Rathnam (1971) and Butt and Lynch (1972) all making use of the same general methods. The biological activity of the product has been reported to be as high as 14,400 u (2nd IRP-HMG)/mg when freshly prepared, but the best stable preparations contain between 7000 and 8000 u/mg. A method which has been found to give good yields of FSH of high potency and biological purity and which is suitable for labelling in radioimmunoassay is shown in Table 1.

Reichert and Ramsey (1977) have isolated a large molecular weight fraction, not retarded by Sephadex G-100, during the preparation of FSH from acetone-dried pituitaries. This fraction showed no evidence of dissociation on refiltration or electrophoresis. It was biologically active and cross-reacted immunologically with FSH. It resembles therefore a prohormone but as yet there is no evidence of its conversion to native FSH.

(b) Pituitary LH

The methods described for the purification of human pituitary LH include chromatography on the ion-exchange celluloses, electrofocusing and gel filtration. Hartree (1966; 1975) extracted acetone dried pituitaries in a mixture of ammonium acetate and ethanol and used fractionation on CM-cellulose, DEAE-cellulose and Amberlite IRC-50. Rathnam and Saxena (1970) used the same initial extraction and purification followed by iso-electric focusing and gel filtration on Sephadex G-75: they obtained three species of LH with different isoelectric points. The potencies of the products obtained by these methods were given in terms of an ovine standard: by conversion they range from about 3000–6000 u (2nd IRP-HMG)/mg.

Roos (1968) obtained an LH preparation of very high potency starting with fresh frozen glands. The procedure employed ammonium sulphate fractionation, DEAE-cellulose, Sephadex G-100 and SE-Sephadex C-50 chromatography and finally preparative polyacrylamide electrophoresis at pH 8·8. The yield of LH before electrophoresis was about 1·3 mg/100 g fresh pituitary tissue. Roos et al. (1975) later isolated four components by poly-acrylamide gel electrophoresis each with biological activity. Potencies ranged from 1700–8100 u (2nd IRP-HMG)/mg.

Several other methods employing similar principles have been described recently (Torjesen et al., 1974; Loeber, 1977). A method which has proved suitable for the preparation of LH for use in radioimmunoassays is outlined in Table 1.

(c) Urinary gonadotrophins

Many methods have been proposed for the extraction of gonadotrophins from urine, chiefly for subsequent use in clinical studies. Precipitation from alcohol or acetone was used in the earlier methods, but clearly these methods are impractical for dealing with large volumes of urine, since up to five volumes of solvent are required to one of urine for efficient precipitation. The most popular methods have been those depending on adsorption, usually on to kaolin (Scott, 1941). The adsorption is most efficiently carried out at pH 4·0 and the gonadotrophins eluted at about pH 11·0. They may then be precipitated by ethanol or acetone at pH 5·5. Acidification is usually carried out with acetic acid and elution with ammonium hydroxide (Albert et al., 1958). The highest yields of gonadotrophin are obtained from the urine of post-menopausal women (human menopausal gonadotrophin, hMG) or from castrates.

Early attempts to purify hMG were designed to separate the FSH and LH components and to remove toxic impurities from the crude extracts. Methods which showed promise were fractional precipitation from ammonium sulphate (Johnsen, 1955) and chromatography on calcium phosphate (Butt and Crooke, 1953). Some separation of FSH and LH was claimed for the latter method but it eventually proved of use chiefly for the removal of toxic material and was subsequently adopted for the preparation of the first reference preparation, hMG 24.

An increase in the specific activity was achieved by use of fractionation by ethanol and ion-exchange materials (Johnsen, 1955; Bourrillon, Got and Marcy, 1960; Donini, Montezemolo and Puzzuoli, 1964). The second international standard for hMG was prepared in this way and Roos (1968), Donini et al. (1970), and Van Hell, Schuurs and Hollander (1972) purified such material by similar methods to those used for the pituitary gonadotrophins. In this way both FSH (about 5000 u/mg) and LH (1000 u/mg and above) have been prepared from hMG. The two hormones proved rather more difficult to separate on CM-cellulose than did the corresponding pituitary materials, and Van Hell et al. (1972) employed affinity chromatography to remove the LH from the major FSH fraction using an antiserum to HCG coupled to Sepharose 4B. The LH was subsequently recovered by a buffer at low pH or by 4M-MgCl$_2$.

(d) Gonadotrophins in blood

Although many studies have been made on the circulating levels of gonadotrophin, relatively little information is available about its nature, mainly because of the technical difficulties of investigating the small amounts present. Antoniades et al. (1957) concentrated the plasma of post-menopausal women by means of cold ethanol fractionation procedures and precipitation with zinc salts. Simpler methods have been devised for clinical use, using ethanol or acetone precipitation (Apostolakis, 1960; Keller and Rosemberg, 1965).

The nature of circulating LH was investigated by Graesslin et al. (1976). Samples of sera were submitted to gel filtration on Sephadex G-200 and two main components were observed by radioimmunoassay and in vitro bioassays. One was of mw 30,000 and the other between 140,000 and 180,000. These components showed no change on treatment with 6 M urea, 0·1% mercaptoethanol, exposure to different pH values, changes of salt concentration or on rechromatography. The amount of the low molecular weight species increased after administration of LH-RH. The two components did not separate on ion-exchange chromatography or isoelectric focusing and appeared to have the same charge. An additional small molecular weight species (about 1000) recognised by all assay systems, appeared in dialysates of the serum samples: the nature of this component is at present unclear.

Similar studies on post-menopausal sera by Prentice and Ryan (1975) revealed a species of LH eluted from Sephadex G-100 in the position of native pituitary LH, a variable amount of a larger species which cross-reacted in radioimmunoassays for LH and its subunits and material which eluted in the position of subunits and gave reactions mainly for the α-subunits.

2. Standard Preparations

The first standards for human gonadotrophins were prepared from the urine of post-menopausal women and were designed for use in biological assays. Later, pituitary preparations became available and these have been widely used as standards both in biological assays and in radioimmunoassays.

The international standard for human urinary FSH and LH (ICSH) for bioassay was prepared from post-menopausal urine and is coded 70/45. It has replaced the earlier standard known as the Second International Reference Preparation (2nd IRP-hMG) for bioassay. The potency has been defined as 54 u FSH/ampoule and 46 u LH/ampoule (Storring, Dixon and Bangham, 1976). Like the earlier reference preparation this standard is stable but not highly purified and contains less than 5% FSH and LH.

Pituitary standards are available for both bioassay and radioimmunoassay. The First International Reference Preparation (1st IRP) for FSH and LH, coded 69/104, for bioassay, contains 10 u FSH and 25 u LH ampoule (Bangham et al., 1973). Again the purity is not high (FSH 0·25%, LH 0·33%, with 60 mu TSH/ampoule by bioassay), but, using specific reagents it is a widely used and satisfactory standard for radioimmunoassays in serum.

A purified preparation of human pituitary LH (ICSH), 68/40 has been established as the International Reference Preparation for Immunoassay.

The agreed potency is 77 u/ampoule. The preparation is 95 % pure containing < 0·9 u FSH/ampoule and 0·1 min TSH/ampoule by an *in vitro* assay.

The 2nd IRP-hMG was widely used as a standard for radioimmunoassays of urinary gonadotrophins in clinical trials. In the absence of an international standard preparation of serum gonadotrophins, the pituitary standards are used for most studies on serum and where possible results given in this chapter will be in these terms.

B. PROPERTIES OF THE GONADOTROPHINS

Many purified preparations of pituitary gonadotrophins show some degree of microheterogeneity of the terminal amino acids and of the attached carbohydrates. Their mw have generally been estimated to be between 28,000 and 32,000 although Roos (1968) reported his preparation of FSH from frozen pituitary glands to have a mw nearer 40,000, based on ultra-centrifugal data. The carbohydrate content is about 15 % in LH and nearer 30 % in FSH. These carbohydrates are covalently bonded to the protein chain and consist of sialic acid (*N*-acetylneuraminic acid), L-fucose, D-galac-tose, D-mannose, 2-acetamido-2-deoxy-D-glucose (glucosamine) and 2-aceta-mido-2-deoxy-D-galactose (galactosamine). Qualitative and quantitative differences in the carbohydrates in the two hormones reported in early studies are not apparent in later publications (Table 2).

Table 2

Carbohydrates in FSH and LH. Results expressed as percentage of the total molecules and as residues/molecule. Results collected from Barker *et al.* (1969) and (a) from the range of results in four electrophoretic fractions prepared by Roos *et al.* (1975).

	FSH		LH		
	% by weight:	No. of residues (mw 30,000)	% by weight (a)		No. of residues (mw 30,000) (a)
Fucose	1·0	2	1·0	0·5–1·5	1– 3
Galactose	4·5	7	⎫ 5·6	3·4– 3·8	6–7
Mannose	9·6	16	⎭	7·5– 9·0	13–16
N-acetylglucosamine	11·5	15	⎫ 6·5	9·6–10·6	14–15
N-acetylgalactosamine	0·6	1	⎭	1·3– 2·5	3– 3
N-acetylneuraminic acid	5·0	5	2·1	4·8– 6·9	5– 7

Each hormone, in common with the other glycoprotein hormone of the pituitary, TSH, and the placental gonadotrophin HCG, can be reversibly dissociated into two dissimilar subunits by treatment with reagents which do not rupture covalent bonds. Early evidence for dissociation was afforded from work on ovine LH, a hormone which readily dissociates in acid pH. The method more commonly used to prepare subunits is by incubation of the native hormone in the presence of 8–10 M urea at 40° for 1 hr. The dissociated material is separated by gel filtration or by ion-exchange chromatography (Swaminathan and Bahl, 1970; Parlow and Shome, 1974; Hartree, 1975; Wallis, 1975; Bishop, Nureddin and Ryan, 1976; Saxena and Rathnam, 1976) in the presence of a dissociating agent or by means of affinity chromatography using specific antisera to the subunits (Vaitukaitis et al., 1973). The separated subunits designed α and β, reassociate if concentrated mixtures are incubated together in buffer of neutral pH at 37°.

The separate subunits possess negligible biological activity, but when they are reassociated the activity is restored, the type of activity being dependent on the β-subunit. The α-subunits in all the glycoprotein hormones including TSH, are similar and possess identical amino acid sequences (Fig. 1). They contain up to 92 residues, there being some heterogeneity at the N-terminus:

```
         1                                  10
H–Ala–Pro–Asp–Val –Glu–Asp–Cys–Pro–Glu–Cys–
                                           20
    Thr–Leu–Gln–Glu–Asn–Pro–Phe–Phe–Ser–Gln–
                                           30
    Pro –Gly–Ala–Pro– Ile –Leu–Gln–Cys–Met–Gly–
                                           40
    Cys–Cys–Phe–Ser–Arg–Ala–Tyr–Pro–Thr–Pro–
                                           50
    Leu–Arg–Ser–Lys–Lys–Thr–Met–Leu–Val –Gln–
                                           60
    Lys–Asn–Val –Thr–Ser–Glu–Ser–Thr–Cys–Cys–
                         I
                      (CHO)
                                           70
    Val –Ala–Lys–Ser–Tyr–Asn–Arg–Val –Thr–Val –
                                           80
    Met–Gly–Gly–Phe–Lys–Val –Glu–Asn–His–Thr–
                                   I
                                (CHO)
                                           90
    Ala– Cys–His–Cys–Ser–Thr–Cys–Tyr–Tyr–His–
         92
    Lys –Ser– OH
```

Fig. 1. Amino acid sequence in the α-subunits of the human gonadotrophins (Rathnam and Saxena, 1975).

carbohydrate residues are linked through the asparagine residues at positions 52 and 78 (Shome and Parlow, 1974a; Rathnam and Saxena, 1975). The β-subunits of FSH and LH show considerable differences (Fig. 2) but if the structures are adjusted so that the first residue of FSH (Asn) is aligned against the seventh (Pro) in LH there is some homology in the first 32 residues (Saxena and Rathnam, 1976). Carbohydrates are attached at residues 7 and

```
                                      (CHO)
                                        |              10
FSH     H–Asn–Ser–Cys–Glu–Leu–Thr–Asn– Ile –Thr– Ile –
LH      H– Ser–Arg–Glu–Pro–Leu–Arg–Pro– Trp–Cys–His–
                                                       20
FSH     Ala– Ile –Glu–Lys–Glu–Glu–Cys–Arg–Phe–Cys–
LH      Pro– Ile –Asn–Ala– Ile –Leu–Ala–Val –Gln–Lys–
                                      (CHO)
                                        |              30
FSH     Leu–Thr– Ile –Asn–Thr–Thr–Trp–Cys–Ala–Gly–
LH      Glu–Gly–Cys–Pro–Val–Cys– Ile –Thr–Val –Asn–
                                                        |
                                                      (CHO)
                                                       40
FSH     Tyr–Cys–Tyr–Thr–Arg–Asp–Leu–Val –Tyr–Lys–
LH      Thr–Thr– Ile –Cys–Ala–Gly–Tyr–Cys–Pro–Thr–
                                                       50
FSH     Asn–Pro–Ala–Arg–Pro–Lys– Ile –Glu–Lys–Thr–
LH      Met–Arg–Val –Leu–Glu–Ala–Val –Leu–Pro–Pro–
                                                       60
FSH     Cys–Thr–Phe–Lys–Glu–Leu–Val –Tyr–Glu–Thr–
LH      Leu–Pro–Gln–Val –Cys–Thr–Tyr –Arg–Asp–Val –
                                                       70
FSH     Val –Arg–Val –Pro–Gly–Cys–Ala–His–His–Ala–
LH      Arg–Phe–Glu–Ser– Ile –Arg–Leu–Pro–Gly–Cys–
                                                       80
FSH     Asp–Ser–Leu–Tyr–Thr–Tyr–Pro–Val –Ala–Thr–
LH      Pro–Arg–Gly–Val –Asp–Pro–Val –Val –Ser–Phe–
                                                       90
FSH     Gln–Cys–His–Cys–Gly–Lys–Cys–Asp–Ser–Asp–
LH      Pro–Val –Ala–Leu–Ser–Cys–Arg–Cys–Gly–Pro–
                                                      100
FSH     Ser–Thr–Asp–Cys–Thr–Val –Arg–Gly–Leu–Gly–
LH      Cys–Arg–Arg–Ser–Tyr–Ser–Asp–Cys–Gly–Gly–
                                                      110
FSH     Pro–Ser–Tyr–Cys–Ser–Phe–Gly–Glu–Met–Lys–
LH      Pro–Lys–Asn–His–Pro–Leu–Thr–Cys–Asn–Gln–
                                                118
FSH     Gln–Tyr–Pro–Thr–Ala–Leu–Ser–Tyr–OH
LH      Pro–His–Ser–Lys–Gly–OH
```

Fig. 2. Amino acid sequences in the β-subunits of human gonadotrophins.

24 in the β-subunit of FSH, while in LH there is only one at position 30 (Shome and Parlow, 1974b; Saxena and Rathnam, 1976). The disulphide bonds and the type of folding within the LH molecule have been investigated in the ovine hormone (Ward *et al.*, 1973; Holladay and Puett, 1975; Garnier *et al.*, 1975). There is considerably more β-pleated sheet structure than α-helix in the intact hormone and the rigidity of the structure is lower in the subunits. Reassociation of the subunits appears to take place in two stages, the initial combination being followed by a slow rearrangement of molecular conformation (Bewley, Sairam and Li, 1974; Salesse *et al.*, 1975).

1. Structure/Activity Relationships

Even slight chemical modifications to structure may lead to loss of *in vivo* biological activity (Butt, 1969, 1975; Rathnam and Saxena, 1972). There are many examples however, where *in vitro* receptor activity or immunological activity is retained. The FSH molecule is easily oxidised: photo-oxidation which affects histidine and tyrosine residues or reaction with chloramine-T which oxidises cysteine and methionine, both destroy *in vivo* activity, but radioimmunological activity is preserved. Not all the disulphide groups seem to be essential however, since activity is retained after reduction with mercaptoethanol followed by alkylation with iodoacetamide (Rathnam and Saxena, 1972).

The reagent, chloramine-T, which is widely employed for protein iodinations must therefore, be used with caution when the iodinated product is to be applied to biological studies, e.g. radioreceptor assays. The usual reaction has been modified to avoid extensive damage by decreasing the concentration of reagents and the time of reaction (Reichert, Leidenberger and Trowbridge, 1973). Contact between chloramine-T and the hormone may be avoided by using the reagent to generate chlorine gas from sodium chloride which then releases iodine from sodium iodide (Butt, 1972). The products are biologically active and suitable for radioimmunoassays. Marchalonis (1969) used lactoperoxidase to catalyse the oxidation of iodide in the presence of very small amounts of hydrogen peroxide. The method is suitable for gonadotrophins (Miyachi *et al.*, 1972) and immunological and biological activities are retained (Miyachi and Chrambach, 1972). It is likely that in future Iodo-Gen (Pierce and Warriner Ltd.) will be the reagent of choice. It gives excellent incorporation of iodine with minimal damage and the products are stable (Butt, Lynch, Robinson and Williams, in preparation).

Modifications to the sugar residues of FSH and to those of the placental gonadotrophin HCG have been studied extensively. Removal of terminal sialic acid residues results in loss of *in vivo* biological activity, while immunological activity remains (Ryle *et al.*, 1970; Vaitukaitis and Ross, 1971). The loss of biological activity appears to be related to the decreased time the molecule remains in the circulation. The half life of intact FSH is reported to be about 90 min, but when sialic acid is removed it is reduced to a few minutes (Vaitukaitis and Ross, 1971). The liver contains receptors for glycoproteins with exposed terminal non-reducing galactosyl residues. When these are blocked by sialic acid, binding and subsequent clearing from the circulation does not occur and the plasma half life is prolonged (Morell et al., 1971).

The biological activity of LH is retained after methylation of up to 70% of the lysine residues (Ascoli and Puett, 1974; de la Llosa, 1974): acylation of α- and ε-amino groups with maleic anhydride or with cyanate results in loss of activity however (Liu et al., 1974). The methionine residues in bovine LH at positions 8 and 33 in the α-subunit and at 52 in the β-subunit are preferentially carboxymethylated (Cheng 1976a, b). Since the modified subunits reassociate these residues do not appear to be essential for interaction between the subunits. Immunological activity is retained but when a total of three residues is alkylated, biological activity in a radioreceptor assay is reduced to less than 5% of the original. As a result of these experiments Cheng (1976b) concluded that while methionine at position 8 is not essential for biological activity, the residues at α-33 and β-52 are important for optimal binding by the LH to receptors. When the β-subunit of LH is acylated to modify amino groups (Liu and Ward, 1975; Sairam and Li, 1975) or coupled with glycine methyl ester to modify carboxyl groups (Faith and Pierce, 1975), substantial activity can be regenerated on recombination with the α-subunit. In general it appears that modifications to the α-subunit more seriously affect recombination than do similar modifications to the β-subunit.

In contrast to the loss of biological activity on removal of sialic acid in the FSH molecule, little or no inactivation of LH was reported to occur after treatment with neuraminidase (Papkoff, 1973). This is probably because of the lower sialic acid content of this hormone and the nature of its action which does not depend on having a long biological half life.

The purified subunits are biologically inert and early reports that they were active probably arose because of inefficient separation of the two subunits. When pure α-subunits are incubated under conditions in which reassociation of α- and β-subunits occur, no biological activity is recovered (Reichert et al., 1973). Likewise β-subunits do not generate any biological activity on incubation, but when α is mixed with β, biologically active molecules are produced, the type of activity being that of the β-subunits.

The separate α- and β-subunits bind only weakly to target sites in vitro (Canfield et al., 1971; Catt, Dufau and Tsuruhara, 1973) and do not stimulate steroid synthesis (Braunstein, Vaitukaitis and Ross, 1972; Channing and Kammerman, 1973; Morgan et al., 1974). This suggests that the binding sites of the intact molecules include part of both subunits or that they depend on the tertiary conformation. Combarnous and Hennen (1974) treated LH with carbodiimide to link the subunits covalently, and when 0·01 M reagent was used there was no loss of activity. This suggests that after binding to the receptor no dissociation of the subunits is required to elicit biological activity.

2. Biological Properties

The sequence of ovarian changes occurring during the normal menstrual cycle is governed by the release of gonadotrophins from the pituitary, which is dependent on hypothalamic control and modulation by gonadal steroids. FSH stimulates the growth of the primordial follicle which in turn produces oestrogen and stimulates endometrial growth in the uterus. Then LH, possibly in combination with FSH, induces the final stages of follicular ripening, release of the ovum and transformation of the follicular remnant to a functional corpus luteum.

In the male it has usually been considered that FSH stimulates growth of the seminiferous tubules and maintains spermatogenesis, while LH promotes the secretion of androgen by the interstitial (Leydig) cells (hence the alternative terminology ICSH). A major difficulty in defining the exact physiological roles of these hormones has been the lack of purity of the preparations available.

Although in the adult, LH is the predominant factor stimulating the secretion of androgens by the Leydig cells, a synergism between FSH and LH probably exists in the immature male. In the sexually immature hypophysectomised rat, LH alone, even in large doses, has little or no effect on Leydig cells (Odell et al., 1974; Davies and Lawrence, 1978; Odell and Swerdloff, 1978). If FSH is given for several days before LH however, there is a marked rise in testosterone secretion: FSH given alone produces no change in serum testosterone levels. Odell and Swerdloff (1976) consider that FSH stimulates the production of LH receptors in the experimental animals and that it may also be an important factor in the process of sexual maturation in boys.

It is probable that the transformation of spermatogonia to mature spermatozoa is also under the synergistic control of LH and FSH. FSH stimulates a testicular androgen-binding protein and possibly increases tubular permeability to the binding protein and testosterone (Hansson et al., 1975). Thus there is increased local concentration of testosterone and this induces spermatogenesis.

C. BIOLOGICAL ASSAYS

1. *In vivo* Assays

(a) *LH*

The assay of Greep, van Dyke and Chow (1941) depends on the increase in the weight of the ventral prostate of hypophysectomised immature male rats which had been given an LH preparation over several days. The assay depending on the increase in the weight of the seminal vesicles in hypophysectomised immature rats (Watts and Adair, 1943) can be carried out in intact animals but is less sensitive (Diczfalusy and Loraine, 1955; Van Hell, Matthijsen and Overbeek, 1964).

The ovarian ascorbic acid depletion assay (OAAD) is carried out in immature rats pretreated with pregnant mares' serum gonadotrophin PMSG and hCG (Parlow, 1961). In contrast to the other assays in which the test material is administered over several days, this is an acute assay in which the ovaries are dissected for ascorbic acid determinations 4 hr after the injection of LH. Some interference has been reported in the assay from vasopressin (McCann and Teleisnik, 1960) and from the serum of hypophysectomised rats (De Groot, 1967).

(b) *FSH*

Steelman and Pohley (1953) described an ovarian augmentation assay in immature rats and this was modified for use in mice by Brown (1955). The animals are given an excess of LH (in the form of hCG) simultaneously with the test material, and the end-point is the ovarian weight. The assay is specific, being unaffected by LH in the test material, and is reasonably precise.

The OAAD and ovarian augmentation assays have been widely applied to the biological assay of standard materials and of urinary extracts in clinical studies. They are not sufficiently sensitive to apply to small volumes of serum. They measure the complete hormonal activity of the gonadotrophins, however, and should be used when the preparations are designed for therapeutic applications.

2. *In vitro* Assays

The high affinity of gonadal target sites for gonadotrophins offers the possibility of sensitive *in vitro* bioassays. Radioreceptor assays depend on the competition for binding sites on ovarian or testicular preparations between the test material and a tracer amount of the labelled (usually iodinated) hormone. As in radioimmunoassay, the high purity of the gonadotrophin used for labelling is important for high specificity. A metabolic end-point may be used instead: the tissue and the hormone are incubated in a suitable medium and the steroid or other product produced is measured, usually by radioimmunoassay. A third type of assay depends on a cytochemical reaction and this again measures a biological function of the hormone, e.g. the depletion of ascorbic acid in the ovary.

(a) Radioreceptor assays (radioligand)

Homogenates of rat testes contain binding sites suitable for the assay of both LH (Catt, Dufau and Tsuruhara, 1972; Leidenberger and Reichert, 1972) and FSH (Reichert and Bhalla, 1974). In the assay for LH (Leidenberger et al., 1976; Schlamowitz et al., 1976) the homogenate is incubated with ^{125}I-labelled LH for 2 hr at 37° and then centrifuged. The radioactivity of the pellet isolated gives a measure of the bound fraction. The homogenate is prepared from rats weighing between 250–300 g: first the tunica albuginea is removed and after homogenising in buffer at pH 7·5 the mixture is filtered through glass wool. One rat provides sufficient for 120–150 tubes and the homogenate can be kept on ice for 12–16 hr without loss of binding capacity. The labelling of LH has to be carried out under mild conditions to avoid damage to the hormone, and so preserve binding activity (Reichert et al., 1973).

When applied to serum, non-specific components tend to interfere in this assay and it is necessary to include a preliminary extraction. The method preferred by Leidenberger et al. (1976) was an ethanol extraction: the serum was mixed with ethanol to about 8 % v/v and the precipitate forming after 1 hr at 0° was removed by centrifuging. The supernatant was redissolved in buffer at pH 7·4 after freeze drying. The sensitivity of these assays is comparable with radioimmunoassay, the detection limit reported being of the order of 15 mu LH in terms of 2nd IRP-hMG.

In a similar way the specific uptake of labelled FSH by testicular tubules (Means and Vaitukaitis, 1972) has been adopted for an in vitro assay method (Reichert and Bhalla, 1974). Adult rat testes are homogenised gently and filtered through gauze (Brown et al., 1976). The tubular material is trapped by the gauze and is then rehomogenized to give a satisfactory preparation for the assay.

Solubilised receptors for LH from rat testes have been prepared (Charreau, Dafau and Catt, 1974) by the use of detergents and affinity chromatography and have been partially characterised (Dufau et al., 1975). Solubilised receptors for FSH have been prepared from calf (Abou-Issa and Reichert, 1977) or porcine testes (Closset et al., 1977). Testes were treated with non-ionic detergents and iodine-labelled FSH was used as a marker. The solubilised receptor retained its high affinity and specificity for FSH. The association constant (K_a) was 4.7×10^{10} M and the mw was about 244,000.

(b) In vitro assays depending on steroidogenesis

The steroidogenic response of gonadal tissue stimulated by gonadotrophin has been utilised for the in vitro bioassay of LH. Progesterone production from ovarian tissue (Watson, 1971; Shirley and Stephenson, 1973) or more commonly testosterone production from interstitial cells of the testis (Moyle and Ramachandran, 1973; Van Damme, Robertson and Diczfalusy, 1974; Qazi, Romani and Diczfalusy, 1974; Dufau et al., 1976; Dufau et al., 1977) are suitable end-points. Dispersed interstitial cells are prepared by incubating decapsulated rat testes with collagenase at 37° for 15–20 min. After centrifuging, the cells are dispersed in a suitable medium containing 1 mg/ml bovine serum albumin. Incubations with the test material proceed for 3 hr at 37° after which the testosterone produced is measured by radioimmunoassay. The dose response range in serum in terms of the 2nd IRP-hMG has been reported to be between 0.1 and 5.0 mu. Parallel standard curves are given with LH from many different species.

Van Damme et al. (1974) used isolated mouse Leydig cells. The incubation period of 3 hr was carried out at 34°. The assay was very sensitive and measured as little as 50 µu LH in 0.1 ml samples and was suitable for application to serum.

(c) Cytochemical methods

A method for LH has been described based on a combination of the OAAD technique and a histochemical method. The reducing activity of ovarian slices treated with LH was estimated by microdensitometry after staining with Prussian blue (Rees et al., 1973). The method is extremely sensitive, capable of detecting between 5 µu of LH/ml in terms of the standard 68/40 but the standard curve was biphasic in some of the assays (Holdaway et al., 1974). When applied to serum the dose–response curves were usually parallel to that of the standard hormone but the levels estimated in samples taken from normal menstrual cycles in three subjects did not correspond to the usual pattern obtained by radioimmunoassay.

The α- and β-subunits of LH had only low activity in this assay as in in vivo bioassays.

3. Radioimmunoassays of FSH and LH

The specificity of antisera to FSH and LH depends greatly on the purity of the immunogen used, and when highly purified preparations are employed they give excellent results (Lynch and Shirley, 1975; Wide *et al.*, 1973; Torjesen *et al.*, 1974). Cross-reactions between FSH and LH or with the other glycoprotein, TSH, are negligible in the best systems, but cross-reactivity between LH and hCG is common. Urinary FSH and LH may be assayed using antisera raised to the pituitary hormones as well as by using antisera raised to FSH and LH prepared from hMG.

The antisera to the native gonadotrophins cross-react to various degrees with the α- and β-subunits (Parlow and Shome, 1974). The subunits themselves may also be used as immunogens. The α-subunits from any of the glyco-protein hormones are immunologically similar, but the β-subunits differ as would be expected from their structures (Prentice and Ryan, 1975).

Iodinated tracers for use in radioimmunoassays are usually prepared by the chloramine-T method. Alternative methods are the lactoperoxidase and chlorine gas techniques referred to on p. 420.

Solid phase systems using antibody coupled to Sepharose particles (Wide, 1969), polypropylene tubes (Catt and Tregear, 1967) or second antibody coupled to Sepharose (den Hollander and Schuurs, 1971), have been described for the separation of free and bound fractions, but by far the most common method is by the double antibody technique. A system which has been used for several years for clinical applications is outlined in Table 3.

4. Applications of Assay Systems to Serum Samples: Comparative Results

The *in vivo* biological assay methods for gonadotrophins are not sufficiently sensitive to apply to small samples of blood and a direct comparison with other methods is therefore difficult. Monroe *et al.* (1968) used the OAAD assay and a radioimmunoassay to determine LH in a small number of samples of serum from rats. The bioassay invariably gave higher results than radio-immunoassay, but the relative differences between samples were similar. The same pattern has emerged from several other studies in which *in vitro* bioassays have been compared with radioimmunoassays. Qazi *et al.* (1974) determined LH in samples of blood taken from normal women at each stage of the menstrual cycle and from post-menopausal women. The method was the *in vitro* technique of Van Damme *et al.* (1974) based on testosterone production. The *in vitro* technique was applied directly to the samples of serum without any chemical manipulations and the ratio of biological to immunological activity ranged from 2·1–14·0. When the samples were passed through a column of Sephadex G-100 the biological activity was eluted essentially as a single peak, whereas the immunological activity was spread over many fractions. Romani, Robertson and Diczfalusy (1977) extended these observations to samples obtained throughout the cycle from 12

Table 3
Procedures for the radioimmunoassay of FSH and LH.

Diluent for all reagents:
 10 mM phosphate (pH 7·5) containing NaCl (9 g/l), bovine serum albumin (5 g/l) and thiomersal (0·1 g/l).
 The buffer may also contain EDTA (1 mM) with a final concentration of 10 mM–NaOH to maintain the pH.

Standards:
 FSH (69/104: 10 u/ampoule): 50 mu/ml and seven doubling dilutions.
 LH (68/40: 77 u/ampoule): 240 mu/ml and seven doubling dilutions.

Antisera:
 FSH (rabbit antiserum M93–2; Lynch and Shirley, 1975). Dilution for assay 1:3 million.
 LH (rabbit antiserum F87–2; Lynch and Shirley, 1975). Dilution for assay 1:4 million.

Antigens for iodination:
 FSH (CPDS batches of Bluck et al., in preparation).
 LH (2/3: Bluck et al., in preparation).

Ioination by standard methods or by:
 (a) Gonadotrophins (1 μg in 5 μl) mixed with 200 μCi Na^{125}-I (5 μl) in pointed polypropylene tube with lid (Sarstedt Ltd: 0·7 ml size: 30/8). 50 μg NaCl (5 μl) and 50 μg chloramine-T (5 μl) are placed on 1 cm square filter paper (Green's 401) and clamped by lid in top of vial. Chlorine generated diffuses into mixture which is vibrated gently at intervals for 5 min. Filter paper is discarded and reaction stopped by metabisulphite (Butt. 1972).
 (b) Gonadotrophin (1 μg in 5 μl) mixed with 100 μ Ci Na^{125}-I (5 μl) and phosphate buffer to 20 μl, in glass tube containing 0·2 μg Iodo-Gen (see page 420). After 5 min separate labelled protein from free iodine on Sephadex G-25″.

Assay procedure:
 Add 100 μl sample or standard to 0·7 ml of diluted antiserum.
 Incubate 6 hr (FSH; room temp) or 24 hr (LH; 0°).
 Add 100 μl ^{125}I-FSH or ^{125}I-LH (10,000 cpm).
 Incubate 18 hr (FSH; 4°) or 24 hr (LH; 4°).
 Add second antibody (donkey anti-rabbit γ-globulin) at dilution determined by titration containing normal rabbit serum (1:100) in total volume of 100 μl.
 Incubate 18 hr at 4° in both systems.
 Centrifuge at 4000 rpm for 30 min.
 Decant supernatant and count precipitate.

menstruating women. Again the patterns by *in vitro* bioassay and radio-immunoassay were similar, but the bioassay results were 5–6 times higher throughout. Leidenberger et al. (1976) using testicular receptors and Saito and Saxena (1976) using receptors from bovine corpora lutea, compared results with radioimmunoassays on samples taken throughout menstrual cycles. The levels in the follicular phase were low by both methods, but the mid-cycle surge was clearly indicated by both, although there were differences in some cycles for the days on which the peak values were observed by the two methods. The decline in concentration following the peak was rapid by radioimmunoassay, but extended over 4–5 days by the *in vitro* methods in most cycles. Throughout, the radioreceptor estimates were higher than the radioimmunoassay results.

A similar study for FSH determined by testicular receptor assay and by radioimmunoassay was reported by Reichert, Ramsey and Carter (1975). Samples of sera from post-menopausal women were extracted before assay by the *in vitro* technique to remove inhibiting substances. Again the results were invariably higher than radioimmunoassay, the average ratio being 5·4. Both methods indicated the reduction in levels following the administration of oestrogen and there were undetectable levels in samples from a hypophysectomised patient.

D. CONTROL OF GONADOTROPHIN SECRETION

1. Hypothalamus–Pituitary

The evidence from many observations on animals suggested that the release of gonadotrophins is influenced by the central nervous system and the hypothalamus, and this research culminated in the isolation of the hypothalamic gonadotrophin-releasing hormone in 1971 (Schally *et al.*, 1971). This releasing hormone, generally known as luteinising hormone releasing hormone (LH-RH, gonadorelin, gonadoliberin) was originally isolated from porcine hypothalamic tissue and later from ovine (Amoss *et al.*, 1971) and bovine tissue (Currie *et al.*, 1971). This hormone is a decapeptide and the natural and synthetic compounds appear to release both LH and FSH and to play a part in the synthesis of the gonadotrophins. The main sources of LH-RH in the hypothalamus are the arcuate nucleus and the ventromedial nucleus (Wheaton, Krulich and McCann, 1975). It is also produced outside the hypothalamus in the pineal, mid-brain, cerebral and cerebellar cortices and brain stem (White *et al.*, 1974; Wilber *et al.*, 1976). There is as yet no firm evidence for the existence of a separate FSH-RH but the action of LH-RH is modulated by a number of factors including the gonadal steroids.

The hypothalamic–pituitary portal system was described by Popa and Fielding (1933) and the work which followed clearly demonstrated that the hypothalamus was involved in the control of anterior pituitary function (Green and Harris, 1947). Many observations have been made on the effects of electrical stimulation of various areas of the hypothalamus and brain on the surge of LH at oestrus in experimental animals. The recent study of Cáceres and Taleisnik (1976) showed that the LH surge is blocked by electrical stimulation of the anterior, mediodorsal and posterior median nuclei but not by stimulation of the lateral, central or other nuclei in the thalamus. Carillo *et al.* (1977) demonstrated that the amygdala is involved both in release and inhibition. Stimulation of the corticomedial amygdala just before the critical period led to synchronisation in the time of the LH surge: the surge was delayed and reduced by stimulation of the basolateral amygdala and blocked by stimulation of the dorsal hippocampus.

Studies on drugs date back to the observation that barbiturates completely inhibit the neurogenic stimulus for LH release (Everett, 1948). Among recent experiments Pang *et al.* (1977) have shown that animals treated with morphine (which blocks ovulation in rats if given before the critical period on the afternoon of pro-oestrus, Barraclough and Sawyer, 1955) still respond normally to LH-RH. The drug evidently interrupts the neurogenic stimulus of the hypothalamus which triggers the ovulatory discharge of gonadotrophin. Clinical studies showing that narcotics affect menstrual function have been described by Santen *et al.* (1975).

Gonadotrophins are released in pulses and the control mechanisms are not well understood. Catecholamines are present in high amounts in the hypothalamus and they serve as neurotransmitters for critical steps in the regulation of LH-RH (Fuxe and Hökfelt, 1969; Kamberi, Mical and Porter, 1971). The mechanisms involved have been investigated by the use of adrenergic blocking agents. Pulsatile LH release is abolished by α, but not by β blocking agents in animals (Knobil, 1974) and not by the doses that have been used in humans. The many neural inputs from the CNS are thought to operate through transmitters which converge upon the medial basal hypothalamus leading to the release of LH-RH by the neurosecretory neurones (Wurtman, 1971; Halasy, 1972; Yen *et al.*, 1972). Modifications in the pulsatile release of LH are noted in patients with hypothalamic dys-function (see p. 457).

Depletion of brain catecholamines and of serotonin by reserpine blocks ovulation (Barraclough and Sawyer, 1959) and many later studies have further indicated that the hypothalamic monoamines play an important role in cyclical changes of the gonadotrophins. The rate of synthesis of these amines increases during pro-oestrus possibly by a direct action of steroids on the hypothalamic neurones (Zschaeck and Wurtman, 1973). Although intraventricular administration of serotonin blocks gonadotrophin release, there is evidence for a stimulating effect on the cyclical release of LH (Héry *et al.*, 1976). Furthermore, serotonin antagonists such as LSD and methysergide inhibit PMS-induced ovulation in mice (Brown, 1967).

Prostaglandins are involved in the process of gonadotrophin release at the pituitary and/or the hypothalamic level (Patrono *et al.*, 1976). Prosta-glandins of the E series particularly can act centrally to stimulate LH release (Harms *et al.*, 1973, 1974) while inhibitors of prostaglandin synthesis can block

P

LH release (Carlsen *et al.*, 1974; Ojeda *et al.*, 1975). Ojeda, Jameson and McCann (1977a) showed that PGE_2 implanted in the preoptic area or in the anterior ventral portion of the anterior hypothalamus was an effective stimulant. Since these areas contain LH-RH the results suggest that prostaglandins activate LH-RH-secreting neurones. In a further study PGE_2 injected into the postchiasmic region and other sites clearly elevated FSH levels (Ojeda, Jameson and McCann, 1977b). Most sites affecting the release of FSH were similar to the LH areas but enhanced release of FSH was noted from the dorsal area.

There is experimental evidence that acetylcholine is involved in the mechanism triggering LH-RH release (Libertun and McCann, 1973; Dickey and Marks, 1974; Martini, 1977). When anterior pituitary tissue and hypothalamic tissue were incubated together a small amount of LH was released: there was a significant increase when acetylcholine was added (Martini, 1977). The anticholinergic drug atropine inhibited this release and anti-acetylcholinesterase antibody produced a 3-fold increase in LH output. Similar experimental evidence for the release of FSH influenced by acetylcholine was afforded by Simonovic, Motta and Martini (1974).

The pineal factors melatonin (Axelrod, 1975) and the nonapeptide, 8-arginine vasotocin (Cheesman, Osland and Forsham, 1977; Osland, Cheesman and Forsham, 1977; Reiter and Vaughan, 1977) have been shown to inhibit LH release, thereby preventing ovulation in some animals. Serum levels of melatonin fluctuate during the menstrual cycle with lowest levels at the time of the LH surge (Wetterberg *et al.*, 1976). Melatonin itself has not been shown to affect LH levels and it seems more likely that it antagonises the action of serotonin and inhibits LH release which has been triggered or facilitated by serotonin pathways (Smythe, 1977). Arginine vasotocin, in pg amounts, inhibits the pro-oestrus surge of LH, but does not affect the tonic secretion of LH during the period of dioestrus. The LH release by LH-RH, prostaglandin or electrical stimulation is not affected however, and it seems likely that the nonapeptide acts via the CNS to suppress selectively the cyclical release of LH.

Interest in the role of prolactin in anovulation has prompted recent work on the effect of dopamine and dopaminergic agonists on gonadotrophin release. Administration of prolactin itself partially blocks the postcastration rise in serum LH and FSH (Gudelsky *et al.*, 1976) suggesting that prolactin can inhibit the release of gonadotrophin. In these experiments prolactin also selectively enhanced dopamine turnover in the median eminence and anterior hypothalamus, which suggests that hypothalamic dopaminergic neurones may mediate the effect on LH and FSH release (Fuxe *et al.*, 1976). Experiments with dopamine have sometimes given contradictory results, possibly because of different conditions used: there is pharmacological evidence that dopamine can trigger the release of LH-RH but other evidence that dopamine inhibits LH release. Rotsztejn *et al.* (1977) have produced evidence that the effects of dopamine may depend on the steroid environment. Beck and Wuttle (1977) administered apomorphine, a dopamine agonist to ovariectomised rats and this reduced LH in a dose-dependent way and it was concluded from this evidence that dopamine inhibited LH release, probably by reducing hypothalamic LH-RH. Leblanc *et al.* (1976) observed a significant fall in serum LH levels during infusions of dopamine with a marked rebound at the end of the infusions. Lachelin, Leblanc and Yen (1977) extended this study to the dopamine agonist L-dopa and bromocriptine. Again LH was suppressed: L-dopa taken orally produced the greatest suppression within between 1 and 4 hr, and there was a rebound between 7 and 10 hr, but there was no change in FSH. The bromocriptine experiments were carried out in hyperprolactinaemic women and again both LH and FSH were suppressed during the 10 hr of the experiment. The suppression of L-dopa may be due to the rapid conversion of this compound to dopamine within the hypothalamic-pituitary system. The longer action of bromocriptine and apparent difference from L-dopa in the suppression of FSH is interesting, but the observations were not obtained in normal women. The experiments suggest however, that dopaminergic activity may play a role in the regulation of LH secretion in humans, although the mechanism of action remains uncertain.

Evidence that a short feedback mechanism exists whereby gonadotrophins control the further release of gonadotrophins has come from experiments in animals receiving gonadotrophin or being given implants of gonadotrophin in the median eminence area. In a recent study Molitch *et al.* (1976) administered hCG to castrated rabbits and showed that there was a reduction in serum LH levels. This experiment was possible because rabbit LH does not cross-react with hCG. A similar observation has been made in human subjects by Miyake *et al.* (1976). They administered 10,000 u hCG to eight castrated women and observed a suppression of endogenous LH levels by using a specific β-LH subunit assay. The effect was extended over 24 hr and there was no corresponding suppression of FSH.

2. Gonadal Factors

(a) Androgens

The control of gonadotrophin secretion exerted by the gonadal steroids is complex. In the human male there is good evidence for negative feedback control of testosterone on LH (Lee *et al.*, 1972; Capell *et al.*, 1973; Sherins and Loriaiux, 1973; Stewart-Bentley, Odell and Horton, 1974; Mauss *et al.*, 1975; Santen, 1975) but the effect on FSH secretion is more contradictory.

Most studies have indicated that FSH is less easily suppressed by androgen than is LH.

The LH and FSH responses to LH-RH are reduced following the administration of testerone, but the effect is delayed. Caminos-Torres, Ma and Snyder (1977) showed that in normal males an increase to 150% above the mean normal level of circulating testosterone was required for 28 days for the effect to be observed, and considerably longer was required in patients with primary hypogonadism.

Changes in the binding of testosterone to sex hormone binding globulin (SHBG) are important since it is only the 1% unbound testosterone circulating which exerts the control on gonadotrophin release (Anderson, 1974). It is likely that testosterone is converted to another steroid, possibly a 5α reduced metabolite such as 5α-dihydrotestosterone which exerts its effect at the hypothalamus or the pituitary. Conversion to oestradiol is also possible, although Davis, Lipsett and Korenman (1965) showed that non-aromatizable synthetic androgens can suppress FSH.

(b) Inhibin

An alternative mechanism for the control of FSH has been suggested by postulating the existence of a substance known as inhibin. This substance is thought to be secreted by the tubules, probably the Sertoli cells, and is non-steroidal in nature. Evidence for the existence of such a controlling substance is afforded by the observation that there is a selective increase in FSH levels where there is extensive tubular damage (Rosen and Weintraub, 1971; Franchimont et al., 1972; De Kretser et al., 1972; Leonard et al., 1972; Bramble et al., 1974; Hunter et al., 1974).

Inhibin has been extracted from ram and boar rete-testis fluid (Setchell and Sirinathsinghji, 1972) and from human (Franchimont et al., 1974b) and bull (Chari, Duraiswami and Franchiment, 1978) seminal plasma. It appears to be a peptide and from gel filtration data appears in two mw species of about 20,000 and 5000. Chari et al. (1978) isolated a single component of 19,000.

Inhibin probably exerts its control at the pituitary level. The high basal levels of FSH found in cases of germinal cell aplasia (Zarate et al., 1974) and cryptorchidism (Bramble et al., 1974, 1975) are associated with augmented FSH response to LH-RH with a normal LH response. The possibility that inhibin also acts at the hypothalamus by, for instance, inhibiting the release or action of LH-RH has not been excluded.

Inhibin activity may be measured by in vivo bioassay depending on the reduction of the postcastration rise in serum FSH in rats (Franchimont et al., 1975) or by the reduction of HCG-stimulation of ovarian weight in rats (Setchell and Sirinathsinghji, 1972; Setchell and Wallace, 1972; Chari *et al.*, 1976). In the latter assay the injected hCG is believed to act in synergism with endogenous FSH, the release of which is inhibited by inhibin. *In vitro* systems using pituitary cell cultures (Baker *et al.*, 1975) or half pituitaries (Setchell and Sirinathsinghji, 1972) have also been described. Pituitary cells are incubated with LH-RH and LH and FSH released into the medium are measured after 6 hr. With some preparations LH release is suppressed but only at higher doses than are required to suppress FSH.

Arguments for the presence of an inhibin-like substance in ovarian follicular fluid have been put forward by Sherman and Korenman (1975). This would help to explain the relatively greater increase in serum FSH compared with LH in post-menopausal women. Oestrogens appear to affect both hormones equally. Furthermore, the presence or absence of follicles in women with amenorrhoea was shown to be related to the FSH levels in the studies of Goldenberg *et al.* (1973). Experimental evidence for follicular inhibin has been afforded by studies in animals: porcine follicular fluid contains a substance which inhibits the spontaneous maturation of isolated rabbit oocytes (Tsafiri, Pomerantz and Channing, 1976). It appears to be a peptide with a mw of about 2000. Marder, Channing and Schwartz (1977) found that after removal of steroids, follicular fluid from porcine ovaries reduced FSH levels in ovariectomised rats and De Jong and Sharpe (1976) obtained similar evidence from bovine follicular fluid.

(c) Ovarian steroids

The negative feedback exerted by oestrogens on gonadotrophin secretion is illustrated by the decreasing concentrations of FSH in the follicular phase of the normal menstrual cycle at a time when oestrogen levels are rising. In the luteal phase when both oestrogens and progesterone are secreted from the corpus luteum FSH and LH are suppressed to their lowest levels in the cycle. In post-menopausal women and young women with premature ovarian failure, oestrogen production falls and gonadotrophins increase. Treatment of post-menopausal women with oestrogens decreases the serum gonadotrophin concentration (Odell and Swerdloff, 1968; Nillius and Wide, 1971a; Moore, 1976; Studd, Chakravarti and Oram, 1977: Fig. 3). Nillius and Wide (1971a) showed that 100 µg ethinyloestradiol daily for four weeks brought the levels within the normal range for fertile women. Progesterone (10 mg or 100 mg) however, did not cause any major change in either FSH or LH.

Experimental demonstration of the negative feedback of ovarian steroids in normal young women is more difficult as the basal concentrations of gonadotrophin are already low. However, the effect of oestrogen, particularly on FSH, can be demonstrated after the administration of natural or synthetic oestrogens. Shaw *et al.* (1975d) administered 1 mg oestradiol benzoate to normal women in the follicular phase of the cycle and showed that levels of both gonadotrophins were suppressed by 8 hr and remained low until 24 hr later (Fig. 4). Similar results were obtained by using ethinyloestradiol (Tsai and Yen, 1971b; Van Look *et al.*, 1977).

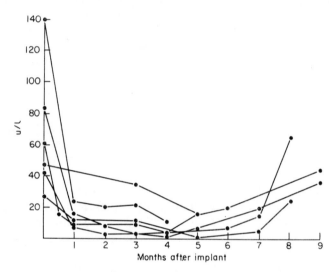

Fig. 3. Plasma FSH levels in six oophorectomised women following an implant of 100 mg oestradiol (Studd *et al.*, 1977. Reproduced by permission of the authors and editors of *Clin. Obstet. Gynaecol.*).

The negative feedback of oestrogen may be demonstrated in another way by determining the gonadotrophin response to a standard 100 µg dose of LH-RH before and after the administration of oestrogen. Shaw, Butt and London (1975b) showed that by 4 hr after giving 2·5 mg oestradiol benzoate the LH response was suppressed, returning to normal by about 24 hr. This suggests that oestrogens exert a direct effect on pituitary sensitivity to LH-RH but endogenous LH-RH cannot be measured and therefore an action at this level cannot be excluded.

The so-called "positive" feedback of gonadal steroids on gonadotrophin secretion is demonstrated by the release of both LH and FSH at mid-cycle following the preovulatory rise of oestrogens from the maturing follicle. This can be demonstrated experimentally by administering oestrogen to normal subjects in the follicular phase of the cycle (Nillius and Wide, 1971b; Tsai and Yen, 1971a, b; Monroe *et al.*, 1972; Cargille *et al.*, 1973; Shaw *et al.*, 1975d; Baird *et al.*, 1977). There is a surge of LH and FSH similar to that seen at mid-cycle usually within 72 hr after the administration of oestradiol benzoate (Fig. 4).

The positive effect may also be demonstrated by determining gonado-trophin responses to a standard dose of LH–RH at intervals after the administration of oestrogen (Shaw *et al.*, 1975b;Yen *et al.*, 1975; Butt *et al.*, 1978; Kandeel *et al.*, 1978). Yen *et al.* (1975) observed a transitory increased release of FSH and LH to LH–RH after chronic administration of ethinyl

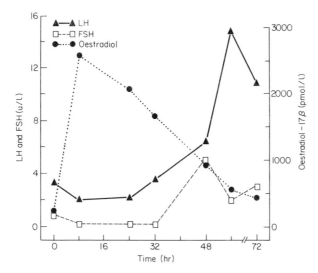

Fig. 4. Demonstration of negative and positive influences of oestrogen (oestradiol benzoate, 1 mg at time 0 hr) on serum concentrations of LH and FSH (Shaw, 1976. Reproduced by permission of the author and editors of *Clin. Obstet. Gynaecol.*).

oesradiol. Shaw *et al.* (1975b) reported that many normal subjects in the early follicular phase show a biphasic effect: up to 20 hr after receiving 0·5 mg oestradiol benzoate the response to LH–RH tended to be suppressed, but by 44 hr after the administration of 2·5 mg oestradiol benzoate the response was amplified. Butt *et al.* (1978) and Kandeel *et al.* (1978) demon-strated that the effect was even greater at 92 hr and all normal subjects investigated showed an amplified response at this time (Fig. 5).

The effect of progesterone on positive feedback appears to depend on the level of circulating oestrogen. Leyendecker, Wardlaw and Nocke (1972) showed that progesterone induced a discharge of LH in women receiving oral oestrogen each day. The discharge occurred immediately and terminated

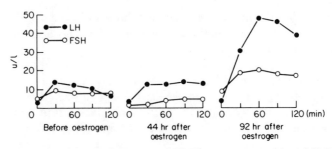

Fig. 5. Oestrogen amplification of LH and FSH responses to 100 μg LH-RH at 44 and 92 hr (Kandeel *et al.*, 1978). The first LH-RH test was performed on a normal subject on the 4th day of the menstrual cycle. Oestradiol benzoate (2·5 mg) was administered 4 hr later and further LH-RH tests were performed after 44 and 92 hr.

abruptly: the duration of the surge decreased with increase in dose of the steroid. It was suggested that oestrogen is responsible for the initial stimulus leading to an LH surge at mid-cycle: preovulatory luteinisation of the theca interna results in an increase in progesterone which regulates the final

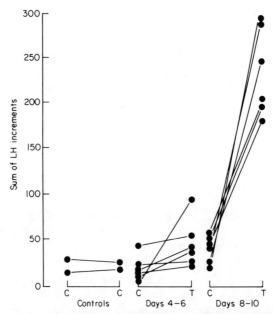

Fig. 6. Changes in LH release after 100 μg LH-RH (expressed as sum of LH increments) induced by progesterone (12·5 mg) given 20 hr previously at two stages of the menstrual cycle (days 4–6 and days 8–10). C = control response; T = after progesterone (Shaw *et al.*, 1975c. Reproduced by permission of the authors and editors of *Clin. Endocr.*).

discharge of LH to complete ovulation. The balance of oestrogen and progesterone may therefore be one of the factors preventing multiple ovulation. Progesterone also blocks the cyclic centre and therefore prevents further stimulation in the luteal phase. Further information on the joint action of progesterone and oestrogen was obtained by Shaw *et al.* (1975c) who administered 12·5 or 25 mg progesterone to normal women in the follicular phase of the cycle. They noted that the LH response to LH-RH was amplified 20 hr afterwards and amplification became more marked in the late follicular phase of the cycle when the basal oestrogen level was greater (Fig. 6). Lasley *et al.* (1975) further showed that progesterone given after oestradiol had a quicker and more marked effect on the amplitude of gonadotrophin release to LH-RH than oestradiol alone.

Some of these control mechanisms for the release of gonadotrophins are illustrated diagrammatically in Fig. 7.

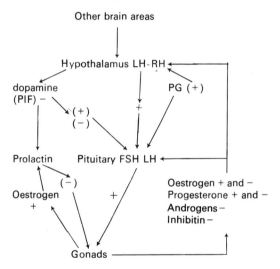

Fig. 7. Diagram illustrating some of the factors controlling release of gonadotrophins. Negative and positive influences indicated by − and + respectively or (−) and (+) where mechanism is not firmly established. PIF = prolactin inhibiting factor, PG = prostaglandins.

E. GONADOTROPHINS IN SERUM: NORMAL SUBJECTS

1. In Foetal Life

In early pregnancy there are high concentrations of hCG in foetal serum until about 12 weeks of gestation when the levels start to decline. In order to measure LH it is necessary to use radioimmunoassays for the specific β-subunit to avoid interference from the hCG. It has been established that the foetal pituitary is capable of synthesising and secreting gonadotrophins by about the 70th day of gestation and the content then rises rapidly. Clements *et al.* (1976) were unable to detect FSH and LH in foetal serum before about 70 days, but afterwards concentrations rose rapidly. In accordance with these observations Kaplan and Grumbach (1976) and Kaplan, Grumbach and Aubert (1976a, b) reported high concentrations of gonadotrophins in foetal serum from 80–150 days gestation similar to the concentrations found in postmenopausal women. Significantly higher values were found for FSH (but not for LH) in the female than in the male foetus. In the last trimester the concentrations decreased and by term became undetectable.

Assays for α- and β-subunits in foetal serum indicated that the α form predominated (Kaplan *et al.*, 1976a). The β-subunit of LH was also detected in low concentration at mid-gestation. The presence of α-subunit is in accordance with the observations of Franchimont and Pasteels (1972) who demonstrated a preponderance of α-subunits secreted *in vitro* from foetal pituitaries. Hagen and McNeilly (1975) also observed that the α-subunit was the principal glycoprotein in umbilical cord serum. Kaplan *et al.* (1976a, b) fractionated sera on Sephadex in order to separate the intact gonadotrophins from the subunits and found that the intact gonadotrophin components for both FSH and LH were present in higher concentrations in the female foetus.

2. Normal Children

(a) Infancy

Winter *et al.* (1975) were unable to detect FSH in cord blood, but observed a rapid rise in serum concentration postnatally in boys within a week, which persisted for three months. Serum concentrations then declined to the low values found in older children. In girls the postnatal rise was even more marked and by 2–3 months reached about three times the concentration found in boys. The concentrations remained somewhat elevated until about the age of four years. Serum LH in boys reached the adolescent range by one week with maximum values by about one month and the concentration then declined at four months. The pattern for girls was similar but the levels attained were somewhat lower.

The elevated concentrations of serum gonadotrophins in early life have also been recognised by Forest *et al.* (1974) and Penny *et al.* (1974) in normal subjects, and by Ryle *et al.* (1975) who determined gonadotrophin levels in a large series of children admitted to hospital for various non-endocrine diseases.

(b) Prepubertal and puberty

There have been many studies on gonadotrophin levels in older children and there is general agreement that concentrations of both FSH and LH remain low and fairly constant until puberty (Johanson et al., 1969; Yen, Vivic and Kearchner, 1969; Burr et al., 1970; Lee, Midgley and Jaffe, 1970; Roth et al., 1970; Sizonenko et al., 1970; Yen and Vivic, 1970; Blizzard et al., 1972; Winter and Faiman, 1972; 1973; Widholm et al., 1974; Kantero, Wide and Widholm, 1975; Sizonenko, 1975; Sizonenko and Paunier, 1975). The serum concentrations in boys for both LH and FSH are about 40% of the adult levels, while in girls FSH concentrations are only about 25% of the adult levels.

The concentrations of both hormones rise at the beginning of puberty. In a series of over 100 boys Sizonenko and Paunier (1975) related the values to bone age and androgen production. The major increase in testosterone was preceded by the rise in LH and FSH. At a bone age of five years, the concentration of FSH averaged 1·8 u/l with a range of 1–3·4 u/l, and this remained steady until eight years, when it rose to 2·4 u/l and continued to rise to an average of 4·2 (1·0–6·4) u/l at 14–15 years. The level of LH averaged 3·2 u/l at five years and remained constant until about 11 years, when it began increasing, reaching a plateau at 13 years at 9·1 (6·1–13·7) u/l.

When the results were arranged according to the stages of puberty (Tanner, 1962) of the boys, the average concentration of FSH increased from 2·4 u/l at Stage I to 3·2 u/l for Stage III, while LH increased from 3·5 u/l in Stage I to 6·6 u/l in Stage IV.

In a group of 123 girls testosterone levels rose concurrently with LH and FSH after 10 years of age, but dehydroepiandrosterone levels rose before those of the gonadotrophins. The average concentration of FSH for a bone age of five years was 2·4 u/l and this remained fairly constant until 10 years, after which the level rose steadily to 4·3 (1·9–9·7) u/l at 13 years. The concentration of LH at five years was 3·7 u/l and this also began to rise after 10 years, reaching 9·8 (5·9–16·1) u/l by 13 years. When related to the stages of puberty, FSH averaged 2·2 u/l for Stage I and 4·3 u/l for Stage III and then remained constant to Stage V. LH averaged 4·1 u/l for Stage I and rose to levels of between 8·7 and 10·0 u/l at Stages III–V.

Penny et al. (1977b) studied the patterns of gonadotrophins and steroids in girls through Stages I to IV of puberty relating them to the menstrual history. They observed that the initial menses probably resulted from oestrogen withdrawal, but cycles with ovulatory peaks of gonadotrophin were established within a few months of the menarché.

The detection of small changes in gonadotrophin secretion when serum concentrations are low is difficult because of the inherent errors in assays.

Penny *et al.* (1977a) however, were able to show an episodic pattern of LH secretion in samples taken at 15 min intervals over a 4 hr period in pre- and post-pubertal girls and boys aged 9–17 years. There were about three episodes in the 4 hr period in both the girls and boys, the increase at each pulse being about 2·5 u (2nd IRP-hMG)/l. The increments increased with advancing age but the frequency of episodes remained constant. Minor fluctuations in FSH were also observed, but were probably more difficult to detect because of the longer half life. Significant differences in LH concentrations have been shown in early puberty associated with sleep (Boyar *et al.*, 1972a; 1974; Judd *et al.*, 1974). No such changes were noted in pre-pubertal children or in adults. Gonadotrophins and testosterone were measured at 20 min intervals throughout 24 hr in six pubertal boys by Boyar *et al.* (1974). In each an increase in LH occurred with the onset of Stage IV sleep and the secretion was episodic. The changes in testosterone were not so marked but every major secretory episode of LH was followed about 20 min later by an increase in testosterone. Although testosterone concentrations decreased during the day, no major increase of LH was observed. In mid-puberty similar but smaller changes occurred and in sexually mature young men no increases in LH were associated with sleep and testosterone concentrations remained relatively constant throughout the 24 hr. LH is usually considered to be controlled by a negative feedback exerted by the gonadal steroids, but these observations suggest that the central nervous system may exert a more important regulatory influence in puberty.

3. Normal Adults

(a) Males

The secretion of gonadotrophins in adult men is by an episodic process which has been demonstrated by measuring serum levels every 15–20 min over 24 hr (Nankin and Troen, 1971; Boyar *et al.*, 1972b; Naftolin, Yen and Tsai, 1972; Alford *et al.*, 1973; Naftolin, Judd and Yen, 1973a; Santen and Bardin, 1973; Mortimer *et al.*, 1974a; Baker *et al.*, 1975). Pulses of LH occur every 2–4 hr (Nankin and Troen, 1971; Boyar *et al.*, 1972b) with peak concentrations between two and three times the mean value. Fluctuations in FSH also occur but they are less pronounced (Alford *et al.*, 1973). In spite of some early reports of a possible diurnal rhythm in FSH most authors have reported fairly constant mean levels of this gonadotrophin throughout the 24 hr (Krieger *et al.*, 1972; Odell, Ross and Rayford, 1967).

The circulating gonadotrophin levels in serum rise progressively after the age of 40–50 years corresponding to a fall in testosterone and 5α-dihydrotestosterone levels (Baier, Biro and Weinges, 1974; Hammond *et al.*, 1977). Wide *et al.* (1973) found that the FSH concentration in normal men aged 57–76 years was significantly higher than in younger subjects aged 17–36 years, but the change in LH was not significant.

(b) Females

The mid-cycle surge of LH and FSH was first recognised by bioassays performed on extracts of urine. The techniques were not sufficiently sensitive to apply to small volumes of serum and the fluctuations in serum therefore, were not described until radioimmunoassays became available. These assays have now been very widely applied and the patterns for FSH and LH are well documented (see Sherman and Korenman, 1974 for further references). When specific systems have been used the mid-cycle peak of LH is easy to recognise, accompanied by a smaller peak in FSH, and at the beginning of the cycle FSH is usually elevated and shows a decrease subsequently during the days preceding ovulation. Quantitatively however, results vary between laboratories (Taymor and Miyata, 1969) and the range in LH values at mid-cycle is considerable. These discrepancies are probably explained by differences in reagents used, the conditions for carrying out the assay and the standards. In the absence of standards prepared from serum itself, urinary or pituitary preparations are substituted.

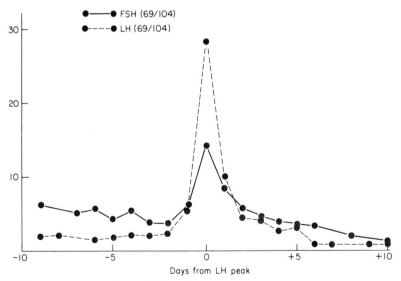

Fig. 8. Serum concentrations of LH and FSH (u 69/104/l) throughout the menstrual cycle. The mean values from 23 ovulatory cycles have been adjusted so that the LH peak in each coincides and is indicated as day 0.

Recently *in vitro* bioassay techniques have been developed for LH sufficiently sensitive to apply to small samples of sera so that an independent check has become possible (p. 424). Romani *et al.* (1977) studied 12 subjects aged from 23–29 years and the pattern for the average results adjusted to the LH peak as day 0 was similar to the pattern obtained by radioimmunoassay. The lowest values were on days 3–5 preceding menstruation, after which there was a gradual rise to a plateau level 8–3 days before the mid-cycle peak. There was a very steep rise on the day before the peak and a similar decrease on the day after. The ratio of the highest to the lowest values ranged from 22–38. As with radioimmunoassays, in most cycles there were secondary LH peaks ranging from 10–60 % of the height of the mid-cycle peak, and these occurred most frequently 6 days before or 5 days after the mean peak.

The typical pattern for FSH and LH throughout the cycle is shown in Fig. 8 and the inter-relationships with fluctuations in steroid hormones in Fig. 9. A mathematical model of the hormonal changes taking account of the pulsatile secretion of LH, the mid-cycle surges of LH and FSH triggered by a significant fall of oestrogen after secretion has been maintained for a critical

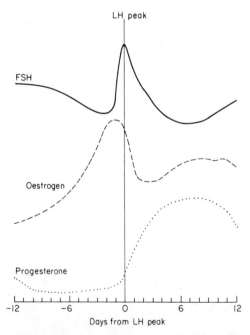

Fig. 9. Schematic representation of the changes in the serum concentrations of FSH, oestrogen and progesterone during the normal menstrual cycle, related to the day of the LH peak. Reproduced by permission of the editors, from Butt (1978).

period of time and the sensitivity of the pituitary to oestrogen, etc., has been described (Feng *et al.*, 1977).

As in males, the secretion of LH and probably of FSH occurs in pulses (Midgley and Jaffe, 1971; Yen *et al.*, 1972; Kapen *et al.*, 1973; Wide *et al.*, 1973). There are 10–15 secretory episodes in LH during 24 hr in the early follicular phase: at the time of the LH peak the pulses are superimposed on an increasing baseline (Weitzman *et al.*, 1975). Pulses of LH are rapid in onset followed by a slower decline with a halflife of 30–90 min. The pulses vary in frequency and magnitude according to the phase of the cycle. Yen *et al.* (1972) observed a periodicity of 1–2 hr during the early follicular phase, early luteal phase and the mid-cycle surge, but a periodicity of 4 hr in the mid and late luteal phase. The pulsatile release continues during sleep (Kapen *et al.*, 1973; Naftolin *et al.*, 1973b) and is not abolished by anaesthesia (Yen *et al.*, 1974).

Treloar *et al.* (1967) showed that there was a wide variability in cycle length for 5–7 years after the menarché and for 6–8 years before the menopause. Sherman and Korenman (1975) found that there were long follicular phases with delayed follicle maturation in young women of 18–21 years with gonadotrophin levels within the expected normal range for women with normal cycles. Changes in gonadotrophin secretion, particularly in FSH have been recognised in the years just before the menopause (Sherman, West and Korenman, 1976; Reyes, Winter and Faiman, 1977). Reyes *et al.* (1977) demonstrated that there is a steady rise in FSH with increasing age in pre-menopausal women in the early follicular phase of the cycle. Occasionally high concentrations were found in women between 34 and 39 years and by 40–44 years the increase became significant. Older premenopausal women (45–50 years) showed high FSH throughout the cycle. The changes in LH were not so marked and a slight but significant increase occurred in the follicular phase only in the 45–50 year olds. A corresponding decrease in oestrogen levels was not recognised, so that the differential changes in the two gonadotrophins are interesting. There may be a different sensitivity in negative feedback for FSH and LH or a decline in production of follicular inhibin (Franchimont, 1977).

There is a marked increase in serum concentrations of FSH and to a lesser degree in LH at the menopause (Wide *et al.*, 1973). Again pulsatile secretion occurs (Yen *et al.*, 1972) with a frequency of 1–2 hr, and the FSH and LH pulses are usually coincident. In a study where samples were taken at 1 min intervals in three post-menopausal women (Medina *et al.*, 1976) rapid oscillations in serum levels of both FSH and LH were shown to occur. The changes in FSH and LH were not coincident. Analysis of the results showed that in addition to these fluctuations there were periodic changes with a frequency of about 2 hr. The concentration of FSH rises more than

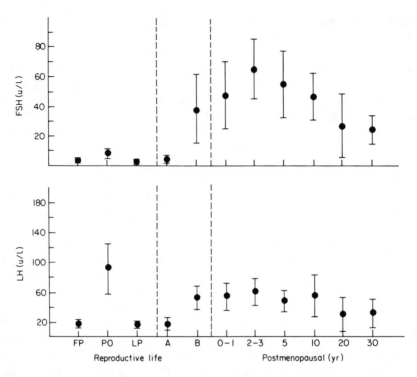

Fig. 10. Plasma concentrations of FSH and LH (M. ± s.d.) at different ages. FP = follicular phase; PO = peak ovulatory phase; LP = luteal phase; A = perimenopausal women; B = perimenopausal women complaining of vascomotor symptoms (Studd *et al.*, 1977. Reproduced by permission of the authors and editors of *Clin. Obstet. Gynaecol.*).

that of LH (Fig. 10): Wide *et al.* (1973) found an average increase in FSH of 8 fold while LH increased on average no more than at the time of ovulation in the normal menstual cycle. The loss of negative feedback exerted by ovarian steroids helps to explain the rise in gonadotrophins, but the excessive increase in FSH may again be due to the lack of inhibin. The increased secretion of gonadotrophins persists for 25 years or more after the menopause, but there is a slight decline in average levels of both hormones after the age of 65.

(c) Pregnancy

The basal serum concentrations of FSH fall progressively during the first weeks of pregnancy (Jaffe, Lee and Midgley, 1969; Parlow, Daane and Dignam, 1970; Jeppson *et al.*, 1977a; Jeppson, Rannivek and Thorell, 1977b) and from the third week onwards remain low until the later stages of pregnancy (Jeppson and Rannevic, 1976). The concentrations found are at or below the lower limit of normal for the follicular phase of the cycle (Jeppson *et al.*, 1977b).

The determination of LH in pregnancy is complicated by the presence of HCG and few radioimmunoassay systems are capable of differentiating the two hormones. Using a specific system Jeppson *et al.* (1977b) observed a decrease during the first two weeks of gestation and the levels remained within the luteal phase range thereafter.

F. DRUGS AFFECTING GONADOTROPHIN SECRETION

1. LH-RH

(a) Responses in children

Both FSH and LH are released in response to LH-RH throughout childhood (Job *et al.*, 1972; Kastin *et al.*, 1972; Roth *et al.*, 1972; Thomas, Malvaux and Ferin, 1972; Franchimont *et al.*, 1974a; Sizonenko, 1975). 25 µg (Franchimont *et al.*, 1974a) or 100 µg (Job *et al.*, 1972) given intravenously produced a significant increase in LH in both sexes before and during puberty. The responses, particularly the FSH responses, are greater in girls than in boys before puberty, although the levels of the sex steroids are comparable. There is a striking increase in LH responsiveness with the onset of puberty, but the FSH responsiveness is not significantly altered (Fig. 11, Sizonenko, 1975).

(b) Adult males

The LH responsiveness to LH-RH is greater than the FSH responsiveness in normal males (Besser *et al.*, 1972; Rebar *et al.*, 1973; Mortimer *et al.*, 1974b). The LH levels begin to rise within 2–3 min of an i.v. injection, and maximum concentrations up to 5 or 6 fold above the basal levels are attained by 20–30 min in response to 100 µg. The elevated levels persist for 5–7 hr (Mortimer *et al.*, 1974b). The FSH response is slower and the increase is about 2 fold (Franchimont *et al.*, 1974a) and the levels remain elevated for between 3–5 hr. There is a relationship between the doses of LH-RH and the responses. Haug and Torjesen (1973) investigated doses of 12·5–400 µg and in spite of much variation in response there was a linear relationship between the FSH responses and the log dose of LH-RH and an approximately linear relationship for LH. The LH responses also tended to correlate with

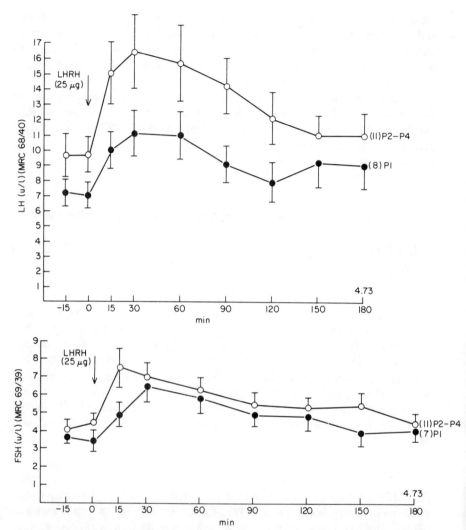

Fig. 11. Responses of plasma LH and FSH (M. ± s.e.) to LH-RH in normal boys. The stages of puberty = P1 and P2–P4: number of subjects in brackets. (Sizonenko, 1977. Reproduced by permission of the author and editors of *Clin. Endocr. Metab.*)

the basal values (Isurugi *et al.*, 1973). Haug *et al.* (1974) demonstrated a reduction in mean response after the age of 70 and particularly in the 80–89 year age group at a time when serum testosterone concentrations also fall.

A daily variation in gonadotrophin responsiveness to a standard (50 µg) dose of LH-RH has been reported (Schwarzstein *et al.*, 1975). Normal male subjects showed maximum responses at 06.00 and 18.00 hours and minimum responses at 12.00 at which time the FSH response was insignificant.

Various routes of administration have been investigated: 100 µg LH-RH is equally effective given intravenously, intramuscularly or subcutaneously (Arimura *et al.*, 1973; Mortimer *et al.*, 1974a). It is also effective when given intranasally, but 2·5 mg is required to produce the same responses as 100 µg intravenously (London *et al.*, 1973a). This route is however, useful for self administration and when taken every 2 hr elevated levels of LH and FSH are maintained (London *et al.*, 1973b; Butt *et al.*, 1974).

Mortimer *et al.* (1974a) observed that exaggerated, pulsatile, asynchronous release of LH and FSH persisted during a continuous infusion of LH-RH. Whether this is because there are short periods of time when the pituitary cells are refractory to the action of LH-RH, or that the action of the deca-peptide is augmented by endogenous hypothalamic hormone secreted inter-mittently, cannot be answered from these experiments. It is unlikely that the episodes are related to the periods required for resynthesis since large amounts of gonadotrophin appear to be available in the pituitary cells ready for release according to the immunohistological experiments of Phifer *et al.* (1973).

(c) Adult females

The gonadotrophin responses to a standard dose of LH-RH vary according to the stage of the menstrual cycle (Nillius and Wide, 1972; Yen and Tsai, 1972; Shaw *et al.*, 1974; Wang *et al.*, 1976). The release of LH, and to a lesser extent of FSH, is greatest at mid-cycle when oestrogen levels reach their preovulatory peak, and is lowest in the early follicular phase, when serum oestrogen concentrations are low. The response is also increased during the luteal phase when both oestrogens and progesterone are increased (Fig. 12).

Jewelewicz *et al.* (1977) gave a constant infusion of 12·5–25 µg per hour of LH-RH over 24 hr to normal subjects in the early follicular, late follicular and luteal phases. The same quantitative pattern was demonstrated but relatively more FSH was released in the early follicular phase and more LH at mid-cycle.

Faure and Olivier (1978) compared the effects of repeated administration of small (5 µg) doses of LH-RH with a single infusion of 100 µg. In the early follicular phase the release of LH was about equal for the two regimes, but the FSH response was more prominent and sustained. In the late follicular phase the release of LH increased progressively after repeated administration of 5 µg, while the larger dose induced a more pronounced and sustained response.

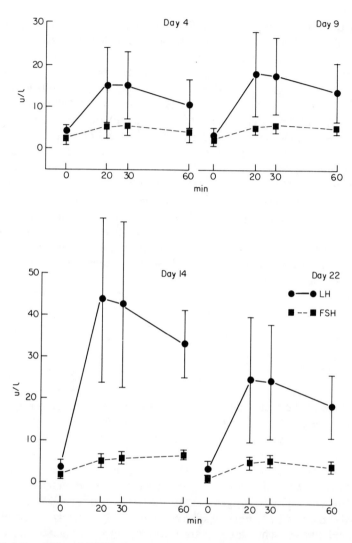

Fig. 12. Mean LH and FSH responses ($\pm$ s.D.) to 100 µg LH-RH given at time 0 min at different stages of the menstrual cycle in four normal subjects. (Reproduced by permission of Shaw, R. W.)

The magnitude of the response therefore appears to be related to the changes in endogenous oestrogen and progesterone levels. In many experiments the effects of the steroids on LH-RH response have been investigated (Jaffe and Keye, 1974; Shaw *et al.*, 1975b; Kandeel *et al.*, 1978). When oestrogens are administered in the follicular phase of the cycle, the immediate effect is to reduce the response to LH-RH. Shaw *et al.* (1975b) administered 2·5 mg oestradiol benzoate intramuscularly to normal women on days 4–6 of the cycle. LH-RH (100 μg) tests were performed 4 hr before and at intervals after giving the oestrogen. The release of both LH and FSH in tests carried out 4 and 24 hr afterwards was reduced. At 44 hr however, the responses were amplified and increased still more by 92 hr (Kandeel *et al.*, 1978; Fig. 5).

There are many animal experiments which show similar effects of oestrogen. Before and during the preovulatory surge of LH in the rat there is increased responsiveness to LH-RH (Aiyer, Fink and Grieg, 1974; Cooper, Fawcett and McCann, 1974; Gordon and Reichlin, 1974; Martin *et al.*, 1974). Henderson, Baker and Fink (1977) produced "rectangular pulses" of oestradiol in rats by the use of silastic capsules containing crystalline oestradiol. When these experiments were performed in animals ovariectomised at dioestrus, the capsules produced serum levels of oestradiol similar to those reached during the preovulatory surge of oestrogen. The LH response to LH-RH was first reduced, but after 7 hr the response increased significantly to reach a peak by 12 hr. The FSH response was also greatest at 12 hr.

Shaw *et al.* (1975c) demonstrated that exogenous progesterone also amplified the response to LH-RH. They administered 25 mg in oil and after 24 hr the release of both LH and FSH was amplified. The magnitude of the effect appeared to be related to the level of endogenous oestrogen, and therefore was greatest at the time of the preovulatory surge of oestrogen.

The experiments of Wang *et al.* (1976), Hoff *et al.* (1977) and Jewelewicz *et al.* (1977) suggest that there are two pools of gonadotrophin available for release during the menstrual cycle termed the "acutely releasable" and the "reserve" pools. The first is released within the first hour of starting a continuous infusion of LH-RH and the second is released when supplemented by additional separate injections of small amounts (10 μg) of LH-RH given at two hourly intervals. The initial release probably represents stored gonadotrophin while the later one reflects newly synthesised gonadotrophin. The two pools are present at all stages of the cycle, but the comparative pool sizes are influenced by the ovarian steroids. In the follicular phase the size of the second pool is preferentially augmented. There is a small increase in the first pool in the late follicular phase accompanied by a 5 fold increase in the second. At the mid-cycle surge however, there is a marked increase in the first pool relative to the second. During the luteal phase the first pool is small and the second pool remains larger.

Römmler (1978) studied the effects of repeated injections of 25 μg LH-RH at intervals ranging from 30 min–24 hr. At 30 min and 6 hr the effect of a second injection was significantly less than the response following the first injection, but it was significantly greater at 1–3 hr with a maximum increment at 2 hr. It may be that this represents increased synthesis at this time. The effect was noted only in women during the menstrual cycle and not in post-menopausal women or men.

Regular menstrual cycles and ovulation do not resume immediately after parturition and several studies indicate that hypothalamic–pituitary function is implicated. The response to LH-RH is unusual up to about 30 days after parturition there being little or no release of LH but a significant release of FSH (Canales *et al.*, 1974; Friedman *et al.*, 1976; Jeppson *et al.*, 1977c). Later in the puerperium a normal response pattern is re-established.

The failure to release LH early after parturition has also been demonstrated in sheep (Chamley *et al.*, 1974) and may be related to the progressive decrease in pituitary LH content throughout pregnancy (Chamley *et al.*, 1976). In the human also there is evidence that the LH content of the pituitary decreases during pregnancy (de la Lastra and Llados, 1977) and failure to respond to LH–RH in the puerperium may be related to this deficiency.

2. Anti-oestrogens

Anti-oestrogens related to the non-steroidal oestrogen trianisylchloro-ethylene are widely used in the treatment of infertility and are useful for the investigation of hypothalamic and pituitary function. They include clomiphene, tamoxifen and cyclofenil. The exact mechanisms of action are unknown, but these drugs are generally considered to bind to steroid receptors in the hypothalamus and so block the negative feedback control on the release of gonadotrophins exerted by androgens in the male and by oestrogens in the female. The anti-oestrogens themselves do not block the release of LH and FSH and hence the circulating levels of these hormones rise. The effect is prolonged and gonadotrophins may remain elevated for some days after treatment is stopped.

(a) *Effects in males*

Several diagnostic test procedures have been described. Marshall (1975) recommended 200 mg/day clomiphene citrate for 10 days for adults and 3 mg/kg body weight for adolescents. Within 9 or 10 days in normal males there is an increase in LH of between 70 % and 250 % and in FSH of between 40 % and 130 %. Although these increases are small they are similar to those occurring in a similar period of time after castration (Walsh, Swerdloff and Odell, 1973).

In children a response is seen only after Stage III of puberty. Anti-oestrogens may therefore be useful in the assessment of patients with partial or delayed pubertal development as a positive response indicates that normal puberty will ensue.

(b) Effects in females

Anti-oestrogens are frequently used in the treatment of infertility. They are usually administered for five days starting near the beginning of a menstrual period if the patient has anovular cycles. Changes in gonadotrophin secretion during treatment are small but often effective in stimulating follicular development. Ravid et al. (1977) administered 150 mg clomiphene daily to normal ovulating women and noted a 78% increase in LH and 82% increase in FSH levels by the fourth day.

Clomiphene or tamoxifen administered to menopausal or oophorectomized women reduces rather than increases serum concentrations of gonadotrophin. Ravid et al. (1977) treated oophorectomized patients with 150 mg clomiphene for four days and found a 22% suppression of LH and an 11% suppression of FSH within four days. Similar findings were reported by Ishizuka (1973). Willis et al. (1977b) measured LH and FSH at intervals during the treatment of post-menopausal women with recurrent breast cancer with 20 mg tamoxifen daily. Basal LH levels were reduced from 20–13 u/l within two weeks and the level then remained constant throughout 12 weeks treatment. FSH levels fell from 59–40 u/l within two weeks and remained at this level for 12 weeks. In these studies therefore, clomiphene and tamoxifen appear to act as oestrogens rather than anti-oestrogens, although there may be other explanations. In the study of Willis et al. (1977b) the responsiveness to LH-RH was not changed during treatment so the explanation does not appear to be a decreased sensitivity at the pituitary level.

3. Anti-androgens

The anti-androgen cyproterone and its acetate have been used experimentally but their mode of action is imperfectly understood. Angeli et al. (1976) treated girls with idiopathic precocious puberty with the acetate and noted that there was a significant reduction in the LH response but not in the FSH response to LH-RH. This action was not considered to be solely anti-gonadotrophic and the possibility remains of an effect on steroid biosynthesis. Donald et al. (1976) used doses of 100–150 mg daily in the treatment of eight boys with excessive libido. Again in three months LH and this time also FSH responses to LH-RH were reduced. The reductions correlated with a fall in serum testosterone levels and this fall was attributed to the suppression of LH release rather than to an anti-androgen effect on the testes.

G. CONDITIONS IN WHICH SERUM GONADOTROPHINS ARE RAISED

Some of these conditions are listed below:
    Males: Primary testicular failure
        Anorchia
        Klinefelter's syndrome
        Complete testicular feminisation, FSH sometimes normal
        Incomplete male pseudohermaphroditism, FSH often normal LH usually
            elevated
        Tumours secreting gonadotrophin (lung, liver, etc.)
        Bonnevie-Ullrich syndrome
        Noonan's syndrome
        Precocious puberty not caused by adrenal or gonadal abnormality
        Severe impairment of spermatogenesis, gonadotrophins sometimes
            normal
    Females
        Primary ovarian failure (premature menopause, resistant ovary syn-
            drome, Turner's syndrome)
        Pituitary adenomas secreting gonadotrophin

1. Gonadal Failure

In both sexes primary gonadal failure is associated with high circulating levels of FSH and LH and the determination of these hormones offers a useful diagnostic procedure to differentiate this condition from hypo-thalamic–pituitary defects.

High concentrations of FSH and LH circulate long before puberty in individuals lacking functional ovaries as in Turner's syndrome (Suwa, Maesaka and Matsui, 1974; Illig et al., 1975). The concentrations increase still further at a time when puberty would have been expected (Grumbach et al., 1974). Gonadotrophins are also usually elevated in Turner's syndrome in the male (Bonnevie-Ullrich syndrome; London, 1975) and in a variant of this condition referred to as Noonan's syndrome (Bolton et al., 1974; Noonan and Ehrake, 1963; Char et al., 1972). The patient described by Bolton et al. (1974) was fertile, although serum FSH, LH and androgens were high which raises the possibility of an end organ resistance.

In the male, lesions of the testis may result from X-irradiation, orchitis, or Klinefelter's syndrome (Paulsen, 1974), a condition where there is hyalin-isation of the seminiferous tubules, small testes and azospermia. Damage to the germinal epithelium, for example by irradiation, may be associated with normal Leydig cell function, in which case FSH may rise independently of LH. The level of LH depends on the production of androgens and a correlation between the stage of maturation of the germinal epithelium and the serum levels of FSH has been reported (Franchimont et al., 1972), but the exact relationship is doubtful and the interpretation of elevated levels of FSH in sub-fertile males remains uncertain (De Kretser, Burger and Hudson, 1974; Marshall, 1975). In Klinefelter's syndrome FSH is elevated, while the level of LH depends on the concentration of androgens.

In these conditions with elevated basal gonadotrophins there is also an excessive response to LH-RH. In Klinefelter's syndrome when the abnormality is mainly of the tubules and in other conditions where only basal FSH is elevated, the LH response may be normal but the FSH response increased (Lipshultz et al., 1977). The elevated basal gonadotrophins do not increase further however, after the administration of clomiphene. This is probably because the secretion is already maximal in the absence of any androgen feedback (Anderson et al., 1972; Marshall, 1975).

Elevated basal serum levels of LH in the presence of normal or elevated testosterone are associated with the condition of complete male pseudohermaphroditism (complete testicular feminisation) (Faiman and Winter, 1974; Nusynowitz and Strader, 1975; Aono et al., 1978). This condition may present as a problem of indeterminate sex at birth, as apparent inguinal hernia found to contain testes, or as a problem of primary amenorrhoea in a superficially normal female (London, 1975). The underlying cause may be an abnormality of a cytosol androgen-binding protein which is necessary for testosterone to exert its cellular effects. An absence of positive feedback by oestrogen on LH release as in normal males and in contrast to normal females has been reported (Aono et al., 1978). FSH concentrations are usually normal (Judd et al., 1972) but are sometimes elevated (Aono, et al., 1978). There are various forms of incomplete male pseudohermaphroditism and these may be associated with abnormalities of androgen receptors, and lack of 5α-reductase necessary for the conversion of testosterone to dihydrotestosterone, the biosynthesis of testosterone or the lack of the hypothetical Müllerian inhibitor which is said to be responsible for preventing the development of the female internal genitalia (Brook et al., 1973). Hormone levels may be variable (Wilson et al., 1974): LH concentrations are usually elevated with testosterone in the upper normal range and FSH is often normal.

In association with deficient secondary sexual development high levels of gonadotrophin may indicate the absence of testes (anorchia). Maldescent of the testes may be associated with deficiency of gonadotrophin and more rarely with a primary testicular abnormality. Swerdloff et al. (1971) showed that rats with cryptorchidism developed Leydig cell damage leading to elevated LH as well as FSH concentrations. In some patients high FSH levels alone are found, a consequence of a defect in spermatogenesis (Bramble *et al.*, 1974).

In primary ovarian failure in young women, the increase in FSH is considerably greater than that of LH as it is in the normal menopause. The condition is sometimes associated with other deficiencies, e.g. with Addison's disease (Irving *et al.*, 1968). Elevated levels of gonadotrophin usually persist but sometimes they revert to normal at a later date and treatment for infertility with gonadotrophins may then be successful.

In the "Resistant Ovary syndrome" high levels of gonadotrophin are associated with the presence of ovaries with apparently normal primordial follicles (Starup, Sele and Henriksen, 1971; Van Campenhout, Vauclair and Maraghi, 1972; Kim, 1974; Koninckx and Brosens, 1977). The aetiology is unknown. Gonadotrophins are usually measured by radioimmunoassay, but the possibility that these methods are detecting biologically inactive hormone is unlikely as the condition was reported when bioassays were commonly used, and recently Lucky *et al.* (1977) checked this possibility by an *in vitro* testosterone production assay as well as by radioimmunoassay. If anti-gonadotrophins are circulating and explain the condition, they have not yet been detected (Koninckx and Brosens, 1977). Again, lack of feedback control by oestrogen seems unlikely as a normal suppression of FSH by ethinyloestradiol and norethisterone and by other steroid preparations has been reported (Koninckx and Brosens, 1977; Lucky *et al.*, 1977). In view of some recent evidence for the possible existence of ovarian inhibin (p. 433) a lack of this substance could explain the elevated levels. It seems more probable however, that there is increased ovarian resistance to gonadotrophins, possibly because of antibodies to gonadotrophin receptors, as has been shown for other hormone receptors.

Abnormalities of ovarian function become increasingly common in women approaching the menopause (Treloar *et al.*, 1976). Van Look *et al.* (1977) determined gonadotrophin levels in women in this age group with dysfunctional uterine bleeding under basal conditions and during dynamic diagnostic procedures, and recognised several different patterns. Usually gonadotrophins were in the normal range, but there were defects in oestrogen feedback mechanisms. In some patients with regular or irregular cycles, circulating FSH was raised but not LH, as in the studies on normal women of this age group (Sherman *et al.*, 1976; Reyes *et al.*, 1977). This was in spite of the fact that oestrogen was present in concentrations associated with the levels at mid-cycle. Again the possibility is raised of a decrease in the hypothetical "inhibin-like" substance produced in the follicular fluid.

2. Gonadotrophin-secreting Tumours

Pituitary adenomas secreting FSH and LH are rare. Gordon and Moses (1965), Bower (1968) and Woolf and Schenk (1974) reported FSH-secreting pituitary tumours in male subjects with hypogonadism and Demura *et al.* (1977) noted grossly elevated FSH but only slightly elevated LH levels in a 50-year-old man with a pituitary adenoma and no evidence of hypogonadism. There was no response to LH-RH and the levels were not suppressed by steroids but were reduced after hypophysectomy. A tumour secreting both FSH and LH was reported by Snyder and Sterling (1976) while a chromophobe adenoma secreted FSH and prolactin but not LH (Cunningham and Huckins, 1977). Ectopic production of FSH and LH from non-endocrine tumours has been reported and the subject reviewed by Rees (1978).

H. CONDITIONS IN WHICH GONADOTROPHIN LEVELS ARE NORMAL OR LOW

1. Disorders of the Hypothalamus and Pituitary

In the absence of a direct measure of circulating levels of LH-RH it is difficult to distinguish between disorders of the hypothalamus and of the pituitary. Dynamic diagnostic procedures, making use of LH-RH, oestrogen, progesterone and anti-oestrogens, help to clarify the situation.

In children constitutional sexual precocity may be associated with adult levels of FSH and LH. Idiopathic precocious puberty is generally not accompanied by any observable lesion of the central nervous system, pituitary or gonads, and changes in the sensitivity of the gonadal-hypothalamic feedback mechanism has usually been considered to be responsible. Angeli *et al.* (1976) found an augmented LH response to LH-RH compared with controls of the same chronological age which suggests premature activation of the neuro-endocrine mechanism responsible for sexual development. Possibly there may be some defect in the hypothalamic control of gonadotrophin release, but the precise mechanism underlying the condition is not clear.

A response to anti-oestrogens is seen in children only after stage 3 of puberty. Tests using anti-oestrogens may therefore be useful in the assessment of children with partial or delayed pubertal development as a positive response indicates that normal puberty will ensue. Snoep *et al.* (1977) described a test to distinguish delayed puberty from hypogonadotrophic hypogonadism by measuring the response to LH-RH before and after the administration of clomiphene. Basal determinations of LH, FSH or androgens and the response to LH-RH or to hCG failed to distinguish these conditions. After receiving 200 mg of clomiphene/day for seven days, patients with delayed puberty showed a diminished response to LH-RH, while those with hypogonadotrophic hypogonadism showed a greater response. In the former condition there is a block in LH secretion and diminished reserve in the pituitary, while in the latter condition clomiphene induces an increase in pituitary LH reserve, and therefore an increased response.

In males, changes in testicular size are largely controlled by FSH, while penile and scrotal development depend on androgens stimulated by LH. Dissociation of FSH and LH release during puberty may lead to irregular development of genitalia. Dickerman *et al.* (1977) studied 19 boys with discrepancies between the development of genitalia and pubic hair and found abnormalities of LH and FSH secretion. The LH response to LH-RH was lower than normal when results were plotted against the pubertal stage for genitalia, but both LH and FSH responses were higher than normal when plotted against pubertal stage for pubic hair.

There are a number of conditions in which defective hypothalamic or pituitary function is associated with hypogonadism. In Kallman's syndrome (Kallman, Schonfald and Barrera, 1944) there is diminished secretion of FSH and LH, but not necessarily of other pituitary hormones. The primary cause lies in the hypothalamus and successful treatment may be achieved by the prolonged administration of LH-RH (Mortimer *et al.*, 1974b). There is gonadotrophin deficiency also in the Prader-Willi syndrome but patients respond to treatment with anti-oestrogens (Hamilton, Scully and Kliman, 1974) or with LH-RH (Morgner *et al.*, 1974).

Isolated FSH deficiency in the male has not been convincingly demonstrated, but isolated LH deficiency is well recognised ("Fertile-Eunuch syndrome"). Santen and Paulsen (1973) reported normal FSH levels, but low concentrations of LH and androgens in this syndrome. Bell *et al.* (1975) described an isolated deficiency of FSH in a young woman. There was no release of FSH in response to LH-RH but there was a rapid release of LH suggesting that the defect is probably at the pituitary level. The α-subunit was detected and the level increased after LH-RH. It appears therefore, that the deficiency is in the synthesis of the β-subunit of FSH. Another interesting finding was the presence of antibody to FSH in the serum of this woman after treatment with hMG.

Idiopathic oligospermia is a common cause of infertility. Gonadotrophin levels are usually within the normal range. Attempts have been made to treat the condition with hMG (Lytton and Mroueh, 1966; Lunenfeld, Mor and Mani, 1967), anti-oestrogens (Foss, Tindall and Birkett, 1973; Paulsen *et al.*, 1975; Comhaire, 1976; Willis *et al.*, 1977a) and LH-RH (Zarate *et al.*, 1973; Mortimer *et al.*, 1974b). Although serum levels of gonadotrophin are increased the effects on spermatogenesis have not been remarkably successful.

Hypogonadism is common in the condition of haemochromatosis in which iron is deposited in various tissues of the body. There is some doubt as to the cause of the hypogonadism. Tourniaire *et al.* (1974) and Bezwoda *et al.* (1977) reported that gonadotrophin concentrations tended to be low and there was a subnormal response to anti-oestrogens or to LH-RH. Simon *et al.* (1972), on the other hand, found elevated FSH levels.

The condition of anorexia nervosa in the male is rare but in the female is more common. Patients usually have low serum concentrations of oestradiol and show a poor gonadotrophin response to LH-RH (Palmer *et al.*, 1975). There is a virtual absence of pulsatile release of gonadotrophins (Yen *et al.*, 1973). Patients are unresponsive to anti-oestrogens during the acute stage of the disease, but a response is shown after regain of body weight (Marshall and Fraser, 1971). The response to LH-RH correlates directly with the severity of the condition, those who are worst affected having the poorest response.

The abnormality may be related to a lack of LH-RH production. Shaw, Butt and London (1975a) showed that there was a failure to release gonadotrophins in response to oestrogen (positive feedback effect), a response which probably depends on the release of endogenous LH-RH. Nillius *et al.* (1975) demonstrated that administration of LH-RH over a period of time resulted in the re-establishment of menstrual function.

An association of amenorrhoea and lactation is well recognised: serum prolactin concentrations are usually elevated and the hormone has been implicated as a possible cause for the absence of cyclical release of gonadotrophins. Basal gonadotrophins tend to be lower than normal in women with hyperprolactinaemia and the absence of the typical episodic LH fluctuations has been noted (Bohnet *et al.*, 1975). The response to LH-RH is variable: it may be blunted (Asfour *et al.*, 1977), normal (Jacobs *et al.*, 1976) or even exaggerated (Glass *et al.*, 1976). Suppression of the elevated concentrations of prolactin with bromocriptine restores an abnormal gonadotrophin response to a normal response (Asfour *et al.*, 1977). The response to oestrogen is abnormal and patients usually fail to respond to anti-oestrogens (Bohnet *et al.*, 1975). Glass *et al.* (1975) demonstrated a failure to release LH in response to oestrogen although the negative feedback effect was normal. There was also a failure to show the normal amplifying effect of oestradiol on LH response to LH-RH 44 hr after administration of oestrogen (Glass *et al.*, 1976) and the FSH response was inhibited at this time. Butt *et al.* (1978) however, showed that at 92 hr after the administration of oestrogen, most of the patients showed some amplification of LH response, so it appears that the response to oestrogen is not absent but delayed. From such evidence it may be concluded that the positive feedback of oestrogen on gonadotrophin release is abnormal and this may help to explain the anovulation frequently observed in this condition.

Elevated but variable levels of serum LH with normal or low serum FSH concentrations have usually been reported in women with polycystic ovary (PCO) disease (Yen, Vela and Rankin, 1970; Gordon et al., 1972; Daane et al., 1973; Friedman, 1973; Baird et al., 1977). Pulsatile release of LH in these patients occurs every 4 hr as in normal control subjects, and the frequency of pulses is reduced by oestrogen (Baird et al., 1977). The mean pulse height however, is greater in anovulatory PCO patients than in normal controls (4·94 u 68/40/l compared to 2·16 u/l). Pulses of FSH occur less frequently (every 12 hr) than in controls (every 4 hr) but the amplitude is not significantly different.

Several attempts have been made to classify these patients. It seems likely that there are certain abnormalities of hypothalamic pituitary function in this condition which may be related to the frequently observed elevated levels of androgen. Shaw et al. (1975e) and Baird et al. (1977) used oestrogen provocation tests to show that most patients had a normal release of LH, although this release occurred earlier than in most normal controls. The amplification of LH response to LH-RH 44 hr after the administration of oestrogen tended to be lower than in normal women in the early follicular phase of the cycle (Shaw et al., 1976). Kandeel et al. (1978) extended this study and were able to classify patients into two categories based on the LH responses to LH-RH 44 and 92 hr after the administration of oestradiol benzoate. Normal controls and one group of patients showed a greater amplification at 92 hr than at 44 hr, but the other group of patients showed a greater amplification at 44 hr (Fig. 13). Serum concentrations of androgen and of oestrone were greatest in the second group of patients. This classification was useful as it served as a guide to subsequent therapy. Only the first group of patients with the lower androgen levels responded satisfactorily to clomiphene. Raj et al. (1977) reported similar findings using the classification of Patton et al. (1975) which depended on ovarian morphology. They found that corticosteroids were more successful in the treatment of those patients with elevated androgens which were considered to be of adrenal origin. Katz and Carr (1976) used a classification depending on the basal LH levels and the response to LH-RH: Type 1 had elevated LH and an excessively prolonged response to LH-RH.

Aono et al. (1977) and Kandeel et al. (1978) showed that the LH/FSH ratio was significantly higher in PCO patients than in normal women in the follicular phase of the cycle. An appropriate ratio of LH to FSH is necessary to initiate the menstrual cycle since a relative deficiency of FSH during the follicular phase is associated with poor follicular development and subsequent inadequate luteinisation (Strott *et al.*, 1970). The high ratio of LH to FSH in these patients may therefore contribute to the anovular condition frequently associated with this syndrome.

There remains a large number of infertile patients who appear to ovulate regularly and in whom the gonadotrophin patterns are usually considered

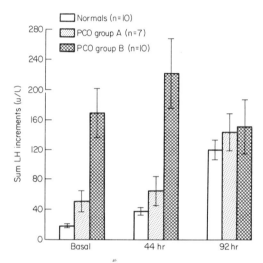

Fig. 13. Oestrogen amplification of LH responses to 100 μg LH-RH in a group of 10 normal subjects and in two groups (A and B) of women with polycystic ovary syndrome. Results are expressed as mean sum of increments with s.e. (Kandeel *et al.*, 1978).

to be normal. Defective luteal phases have been implicated but there are few detailed studies reported. The luteal phase may be short, i.e. less than 10 days (Sherman and Korenman, 1974a), "inadequate" as seen in obese oligomenorrhoeic women (Sherman and Korenman, 1974b) or "defective" but of normal length (Lenton, Adams and Cooke, 1978). In the second group FSH was found to be low at the time preceding the LH/FSH surge. In the third group the only hormonal abnormality was in the serum progesterone level during the first half of the luteal phase, but FSH and LH were normal. Stimulation with anti-oestrogens or gonadotrophin corrected the progesterone deficiency, but even so none of the patients conceived. Pepperell *et al.* (1976) used gonadotrophin measurements in the hope of predicting the response of patients to anti-oestrogens. They found that in secondary amenorrhoea treatment was unsuccessful if FSH levels were less than 1·4 mu/l and in oligomenorrhoea if LH was less than 0·8 mu/l.

REFERENCES

Abou-Issa, H. and Reichert Jr., L. E. (1977). *J. biol. Chem.* **252**, 4160.

Aiyer, M. S., Fink, G. and Grieg, F. (1974). *J. Endocr.* **60**, 47.

Albert, A., Derner, T., Stellmacher, V., Leiferman, J. and Barnum, J. (1958). *J. clin. Endocr. Metab.* **18**, 600.

Alford, F. P., Baker, H. W. G., Patel, Y. C., Rennie, G. C., Youalt, G., Burger, H. and Hudson, B. (1973). *J. clin. Endocr. Metab.* **36**, 108.

Amoss, M., Burgus, R., Blackwell, R., Vale, W., Fellows, R. and Guillemin, R. (1971). *Biochem. biophys. Res. Comm.* **44**, 205.

Anderson, D. C. (1974). *Clin. Endocr.* **3**, 69.

Anderson, D. C., Marshall, J. C., Young, J. L. and Fraser, T. R. (1972). *Clin. Endocr.* **1**, 127.

Angeli, A., Boccuzzi, G., Bisbocci, D., Fonzo, D., Frajria, R., de Sanctis, C. and Ceresa, F. (1976). *J. clin. Endocr. Metab.* **42**, 551.

Antoniades, H. N., Pennell, R. B., McArthur, J. W., Ingersoll, F. M., Ulfelder, M. and Oncley, J. L. (1957). *J. biol. Chem.* **228**, 863.

Aono, T., Miyake, A., Kinugasa, T., Kurachi, K. and Matsumoto, K. (1978). *Acta endocr., Copenh.* **87**, 259.

Aono, T., Miyazaki, M., Miyake, A., Kinugasa, T., Kurachi, K. and Matsumoto, K. (1977). *Acta endocr., Copenh.* **85**, 840.

Apostolakis, M. (1960). *J. Endocr.* **19**, 377.

Arimura, A., Saito, M., Yaoi, Y., Kumasaka, T., Sato, N., Koyama, T., Nishi, N., Kastin, A. J. and Schally, A. V. (1973). *J. clin. Endocr. Metab.* **36**, 385.

Ascoli, M. and Puett, D. (1974). *Biochim. biophys. Acta*, **371**, 203.

Asfour, M., L'Hermite, M., Hedouin-Quincampoix, M. and Fossati, P. (1977). *Acta endocr., Copenh.* **84**, 738.

Axelrod, J. (1975). *Rec. Prog. Horm. Res.* **31**, 1.

Baier, H., Biro, G. and Weinges, K. F. (1974). *Horm. Metab. Res.* **6**, 514.

Baird, D. T., Corker, C. S., Davidson, D. W., Hunter, W. M., Michie, E. A. and van Look, P. F. A. (1977). *J. clin. Endocr. Metab.* **45**, 798.

Baker, H. W. G., Bremner, W. J., Burger, H. G., de Kretser, D. M., Dulmanis, A., Eddie, L. W., Hudson, B., Keogh, E. J., Lee, V. W. K. and Rennie, G. C. (1975). *Rec. Prog. Horm. Res.* **32**, 429.

Bangham, D. R., Berryman, I., Burger, H., Cotes, P. M., Furnival, B. E., Hunter, W. M., Midgley, A. R., Mussett, W. V., Reichert, L. E., Rosemberg, E., Ryan, R. J. and Wide, L. (1973). *J. clin. Endocr. Metab.* **36**, 647.

Barker, S. A., Gray, C. J., Kennedy, J. F. and Butt, W. R. (1969). *J. Endocr.* **45**, 285.

Barraclough, C. A. and Sawyer, C. H. (1955). *Endocrinology*, **57**, 329.

Barraclough, C. A. and Sawyer, C. H. (1959). *Endocrinology*, **65**, 563.

Beck, W. and Wuttle, W. (1977). *J. Endocr.* **74**, 67.

Bell, J., Beneviste, R., Spitz, T. and Rabinowitz, D. (1975). *J. clin. Endocr. Metab.* **40**, 790.

Besser, G. M., McNeilly, A. S., Anderson, D. C., Marshall, J. C., Harsoulis, P., Hall, R., Ormston, B. J., Alexander, L. and Collins, W. P. (1972). *Br. med. J.* **3**, 267.

Bewley, T. A., Sairam, M. R. and Li, C. H. (1974). *Arch. biochem. Biophys.* **163**, 625.

Bezwoda, W. R., Bothwell, T. H., Van der Walt, L. A., Kronheim, S. and Pimstone, B. C. (1977). *Clin. Endocr.* **6**, 377.

Bishop, W. H., Nureddin, A. and Ryan, R. J. (1976). "Peptide Hormones", p. 273, Macmillan, London.

Blizzard, R. M., Penny, R., Foley Jr., T. P., Baghdassarian, A., Johanson, A. and Yen, S. S. C. (1972). "Gonadotropins", p. 502. Wiley–Interscience, New York.

Bohnet, H. G., Dahlén, H. G., Wuttke, W. and Schneider, H. P. G. (1975). *J. clin. Endocr. Metab.* **42**, 132.

Bolton, M. R., Pugh, D. M., Mattioli, L. F., Dunn, M. I. and Schimke, R. N. (1974). *Ann. int. Med.* **80**, 626.

Bourrillon, R., Got, R. and Marcy, R. (1960). *Acta endocr., Copenh.* **35**, 225.

Bower, B. F. (1968). *Ann. int. Med.* **69**, 107.

Boyar, R. M., Finkelstein, J. W., Roffwarg, H., Weitzman, E. and Hellman, L. (1972a). *New Engl. J. Med.* **287**, 582.

Boyar, R. M., Parlow, A. F., Hellman, L., Kapen, S. and Weitzman, E. (1972b). *J. clin. Endocr. Metab.* **35**, 73.

Boyar, R. M., Rosenfield, R. S., Kapen, S., Finkelstein, J. W., Roffwarg, H. P., Weitzman, E. D. and Hellman, L. (1974). *J. clin. Invest.* **54**, 609.

Bramble, F. J., Houghton, A. L., Eccles, S., Murray, M. A. F. and Jacobs, H. S. (1975). *Clin. Endocr.* **4**, 443.

Bramble, F. J., Houghton, A. L., Eccles, S., O'Shea, A. and Jacobs, H. S. (1974). *Lancet*, **ii**, 311.

Braunstein, G. D., Vaitukaitis, J. L. and Ross, G. T. (1972). *Endocrinology*, **91**, 1030.

Brook, C. G. D., Wagner, H., Zachmann, M., Prader, A., Armendares, S., Frenk, S., Aleman, P., Najjar, S. S., Slim, M. S., Genton, N. and Bozic, C. (1973). *Br. med. J.* **1**, 771.

Brown, P. S. (1955). *J. Endocr.* **13**, 59.

Brown, P. S. (1967). *J. Endocr.* **37**, 327.

Brown, P. S., Sharpe, R. M., Hartog, M. and Shahmanesh, M. (1976). *Acta endocr., Copenh.* **82**, 673.

Burr, I. M., Sizonenko, P. C., Kaplan, S. L. and Grumbach, M. M. (1970). *Pediat. Res.* **4**, 25.

Butt, W. R. (1969). *Acta endocr., Copenh.* (Suppl. 142), 13.

Butt, W. R. (1972). *J. Endocr.* **55**, 453.

Butt, W. R. (1975). "Hormone Chemistry", 2nd edition, Vol. 1, p. 140. Ellis Horwood, Chichester.

Butt, W. R. (1978). "Control of Ovulation", p. 357. Butterworths, London.

Butt, W. R. and Crooke, A. C. (1953). *Ciba Found. Coll. Endocr.* **5**, 44.

Butt, W. R., Crooke, A. C. and Cunningham, F. J. (1961). *Biochem. J.* **81**, 596.

Butt, W. R., Kandeel, F., Lane, J. and London, D. R. (1978). "Clinical Psycho-neuro-endocrinology in Reproduction" p. 153. Academic Press, London and New York.

Butt, W. R., London, D. R., Lynch, S. S., Marshall, J. C. and Shaw, R. W. (1974). "Recent Progress in Reproductive Endocrinology", p. 389. Academic Press, London and New York.

Butt, W. R. and Lynch, S. S. (1972). "Hormones Glycoprotéiques Hypophysaire", p. 82. Inserm, Paris.

Cáceres, A. and Taleisnik, S. (1976). *Neuroendocrinology*, **22**, 30.

Caminos-Torres, R., Ma, L. and Snyder, P. J. (1977). *J. clin. Endocr. Metab.* **44**, 1142.

Canales, E. S., Zárate, A., Garrido, J., Léon, C., Soria, J. and Schally, A. V. (1974). *J. clin. Endocr. Metab.* **38**, 1140.

Canfield, R. E., Morgan, F. J., Kammerman, S., Bell, J. S. and Agosto, G. M. (1971). *Rec. Prog. Horm. Res.* **27**, 121.

Capell, P. T., Paulsen, C. A., Derleth, D., Skoglund, R. and Plymate, S. (1973). *J. clin. Endocr. Metab.* **37**, 752.

Cargille, C. M., Vaitukaitis, J. L., Bermudez, J. A. and Ross, G. T. (1973). *J. clin. Endocr. Metab.* **36**, 87.

Carillo, A. J., Rabii, J., Carrer, M. F. and Sawyer, C. M. (1977). *Brain. Res.* **128**, 81.

Carlson, J. L., Barcikowski, B., Cargill, V. and McCracken, J. A. (1974). *J. clin. Endocr. Metab.* **39**, 399.

Catt, K. J., Dufau, M. L. and Tsuruhara, T. (1972). *J. clin. Endocr. Metab.* **34**, 123.

Catt, K. J., Dufau, M. L. and Tsuruhara, T. (1973). *J. clin. Endocr. Metab.* **36**, 73.

Catt, K. J. and Tregear, G. W. (1967). *Science*, **158**, 1570.

Chamley, W. A., Findlay, J. K., Cumming, I. A., Buckmaster, J. M. and Goding, J. R. (1974). *Endocrinology*, **94**, 291.

Chamley, W. A., Jones, H. A. and Parr, R. A. (1976). *Endocrinology*, **98**, 1535.

Channing, C. P. and Kammerman, S. (1973). *Endocrinology*, **93**, 1035.

Char, F., Rodriguez-Fernandez, H. L., Scott, C. I., Borgaenhar, D. S., Bell, B. B. and Rowe, R. D. (1972). *Birth. Def.* **8**, 110.

Chari, S., Duraiswami, S. and Franchimont, P. (1976). *Horm. Res.* **7**, 129.

Chari, S., Duraiswami, S. and Franchimont, P. (1978). *Acta endocr., Copenh.* **87**, 434.

Charreau, E. M., Dufau, M. L. and Catt, K. J. (1974). *J. biol. Chem.* **249**, 4189.

Cheesman, D. W., Osland, R. B. and Forsham, P. H. (1977). *Endocrinology*, **101**, 1194.

Cheng, K. W. (1976a). *Biochem. J.* **159**, 71.

Cheng, K. W. (1976b). *Biochem. J.* **159**, 79.

Clements, J. A., Reyes, F. I., Winter, J. S. D. and Faiman, C. (1976). *J. clin. Endocr. Metab.* **42**, 9.

Closset, J., Maghuin-Rogister, G., Ketelslegers, J. M. and Hennen, G. (1977). *Biochem. biophys. Res. Comm.* **79**, 372.

Combarnous, Y. and Hennen, G. (1974). *FEBS Lett.* **44**, 224.

Comhaire, F. (1976). *Int. J. Fertil.* **21**, 232.

Cooper, K. J., Fawcett, C. P. and McCann, S. M. (1974). *Endocrinology*, **95**, 1293.

Cunningham, G. R. and Huckins, C. (1977). *J. clin. Endocr. Metab.* **44**, 248.

Currie, B. L., Sievertsson, H., Bogentoft, C., Chang, J. K., Folkers, K., Bowers, C. Y. and Doolittle, R. F. (1971). *Biochem. biophys. Res. Comm.* **42**, 1180.

Daane, T. A., Dignam, W. J., Frankland, M. V., Simmer, H. M. and Parlow, A. F. (1972). *Am. J. Obstet. Gynec.* **117**, 392.

Davies, A. G. and Lawrence, N. R. (1978). "The Gonadotropins: Structure and Function." Plenum Press, New York.

Davis, T. E., Lipsett, M. B. and Korenman, S. G. (1965). *J. clin. Endocr. Metab.* **25**, 456.

de Jong, F. F. and Sharpe, R. M. (1976). *Nature, Lond.*, **263**, 71.

de Kretser, D. M., Burger, H. G., Fortune, D., Hudson, B., Long, A. R., Paulsen, C. A. and Taft, H. P. (1972). *J. clin. Endocr. Metab.* **35**, 392.

de Kretser, D. M., Burger, H. G. and Hudson, B. (1974). *J. clin. Endocr. Metab.* **38**, 787.

de la Lastra, M. and Llados, C. (1977). *J. clin. Endocr. Metab.* **44**, 921.

de la Llosa, Durosay, M., Tertrin-Clary, C. and Jutisz, M. (1974). *Biochim. biophys. Acta*, **342**, 97.

Demura, R., Kubo, O., Demura, H. and Shizume, K. (1977). *J. clin. Endocr. Metab.* **45**, 653.

den Hollander, F. C. and Schuurs, A. H. W. M. (1971). "Radioimmunoassay Methods", p. 419. Churchill-Livingstone, Edinburgh and London.

Dickerman, Z., Bar-Haim, Y., Prager-Lewin, R., Kaufman, H. and Laron, Z. (1977). *Acta endocr., Copenh.* **85**, 454.

Dickey, R. P. and Marks, B. H. (1974). *Fed. Proc.* **33**, 253.

Diczfalusy, E. and Loraine, J. (1955). *J. clin. Endocr. Metab.* **15**, 424.

Donald, R. A., Espiner, E. A., Cowles, R. J. and Fazacherley, J. E. (1976). *Acta endocr., Copenh.* **81**, 680.

Donini, P., Montezemolo, R. and Puzzuoli, D. (1964). *Acta endocr., Copenh.* **45**, 321.

Donini, P., Puzzuoli, D., d'Alessio, I., Bergazi, G. and Donini, S. (1970). "Gonadotrophins and Ovarian Development", p. 39. Livingstone, Edinburgh.

Dufau, M. L., Hodgen, G. D., Goodman, A. L. and Catt, K. J. (1977). *Endocrinology*, **100**, 1557.

Dufau, M. L., Pock, R., Neubauer, A. and Catt, K. J. (1976). *J. clin. Endocr. Metab.* **42**, 958.

Dufau, M. L., Ryan, D. W., Baukal, A. J. and Catt, K. J. (1975). *J. biol. Chem.* **250**, 4822.

Everett, J. W. (1948). *Endocrinology*, **43**, 389.

Faiman, C. and Winter, J. D. (1974). *J. clin. Endocr. Metab.* **39**, 631.

Faith, M. R. and Pierce, J. G. (1975). *J. biol. Chem.* **17**, 6923.

Faure, N. and Olivier, G. C. (1978). *Horm. Res.* **9**, 12.

Feng, L.-J., Rodbard, D., Rebar, R. and Ross, G. T. (1977). *J. clin. Endocr. Metab.* **45**, 775.

Forest, M. G., Sizonenko, P. C., Cathiard, A. M. and Bertrand, J. (1974). *J. clin. Invest.* **53**, 819.

Foss, G. I., Tindall, V. R. and Birkett, J. P. (1973). *J. Rep. Fertil.* **32**, 167.

Franchimont, P. (1977). "Clinics in Endocrinology and Metabolism", Vol. 6, p. 101. Saunders, London, Philadelphia and Toronto.

Franchimont, P., Becker, H., Ernould, Ch., Thys, Ch., Demoulin, A., Bourguignon. J. P., Legros, J. J. and Valcke, J. C. (1974a). *Clin. Endocr.* **3**, 27.

Franchimont, P., Chari, S., Hagelstein, M. T. and Duraiswami, S. (1975). *Nature, Lond.* **257**, 402.

Franchimont, P., Legros, J. J., Demoulin, A. and Burger, H. (1974b). "The Endocrine Function of the Human Testis", p. 221. Academic Press, New York and London.

Franchimont, P., Millet, D., Vendrely, E., Letawe, J., Legros, J. J. and Netter, A. (1972). *J. clin. Endocr. Metab.* **34**, 1003.

Franchimont, P. and Pasteels, J.-L. (1972). *C.r. Hebd. Séance Acad. Sci.* **257**, 1799.

Friedman, C., Galki, M. E., Fang, V. and Kim, M. H. (1976) *Am. J. Obstet. Gynec.* **124**, 75.

Friedman, S. (1973). *Obstet. Gynec.* **41**, 809.

Fuxe, K. and Hökfelt, T. (1969). "Frontiers of Neuroendocrinology", p. 47. Oxford University Press, London and New York.

Fuxe, K., Hökfelt, T., Agonosti, C., Lofström, A., Everitt, B. J., Johansson, O., Jonsson, G., Wuttke, W. and Goldstein, M. (1976). "Neuroendocrine Regulation of Fertility", p. 124. Karger, Basel.

Garnier, J., Pernollet, J. C., Tetrin-Clay, C., Salesse, R., Custaing, M., Barnavon, M., de la Llosa, P. and Jutisz, M. (1975). *Eur. J. Biochem.* **53**, 243.

Glass, M. R., Shaw, R. W., Butt, W. R., Logan Edwards, R. and London, D. R. (1975). *Br. med. J.* **iii**, 274.

Glass, M. R., Shaw, R. W., Williams, J. W., Butt, W. R., Logan Edwards, R. and London, D. R. (1976). *Clin. Endocr.* **5**, 521.

Goldenberg, R. L., Grodin, J. M., Rodbard, D. and Ross, G. T. (1973). *Am. J. Obstet. Gynec.* **116**, 1003.

Gordon, G. G., Southren, A. L., Calang, A., Olivo, J. and Rafii, F. (1972). *J. clin. Endocr. Metab.* **35**, 444.

Gordon, J. H. and Reichlin, S. (1974). *Endocrinology*, **94**, 974.

Gordon, S. J. and Moses, A. M. (1965). *Ann. Int. Med.* **63**, 313.

Graesslin, D., Leidenberger, F. A., Lichtenberg, V., Glismann, D., Hess, N., Czygan, P. J. and Bettendorf, G. (1976). *Acta endocr., Copenh.* **83**, 466.

Green, J. D. and Harris, G. W. (1947). *J. Endocr.* **5**, 136.

Greep, R. O., van Dyke, H. B. and Chow, B. F. (1941). *Proc. Soc. exp. Biol. Med.* **46**, 644.

Groot, C. A. de (1967). *Acta endocr., Copenh.* **55**, 611.

Grumbach, M. M., Roth, J. E., Kaplan, S. L. and Kelch, R. P. (1974). "Control of the Onset of Puberty", p. 115. Wiley, New York.

Gudelsky, G. A., Simpkins, J., Mueiler, G. P., Meites, J. and Moore, K. E. (1976). *Neuroendocrinology*, **22**, 206.

Hagen, C. and McNeilly, A. S. (1975). *Am. J. Obstet. Gynec.* **121**, 926.

Halasy, B. (1972). *Prog. Brain Res.* **38**, 97.

Hamilton Jr., C. R., Scully, R. E. and Kliman, B. (1972). *Am. J. Med.* **52**, 322.

Hammond, G. L., Kontturi, M., Maattala, P., Puukka, M. and Vihko, R. (1977). *Clin. Endocr.* **7**, 129.

Hansson, V., Weddington, S., Petrusz, P., Martin-Ritzen, E., Nayfeh, S. N. and French, F. S. (1975). *Endocrinology*, **97**, 469.

Harms, P. G., Ojeda, S. R. and McCann, S. M. (1973). *Science*, **181**, 760.

Harms, P. G., Ojeda, S. R. and McCann, S. M. (1974). *Endocrinology*, **94**, 1459.

Hartree, A. Stockell (1966). *Biochem. J.* **100**, 754.

Hartree, A. Stockell (1975). *Meth. Enzymol.* **37**, 380.

Haug, E., Aakvaag, A., Sand, T. and Torjesen, P. A. (1974). *Acta endocr., Copenh.* **77**, 625.

Haug, E. and Torjesen, P. A. (1973). *Acta endocr., Copenh.* **73**, 465.

Henderson, S. R., Baker, C. and Fink, G. (1977). *J. Endocr.* **73**, 441.

Héry, M., Laplante, E. and Kordon, C. (1976). *Endocrinology*, **99**, 496.

Hoff, J. D., Lasley, B. L., Wang, C. F. and Yen, S. S. C. (1977). *J. clin. Endocr. Metab.* **44**, 302.

Holdaway, I. M., Kramer, R. M., McNeilly, A. S., Rees, L. T. and Chard, T. (1974). *Clin. Endocr.* **3**, 383.

Holladay, L. and Puett, D. (1975). *Arch. biochem. Biophys.* **171**, 708.

Hunter, W. M., Edmond, P., Watson, G. S. and McLean, N. (1974). *J. clin. Endocr. Metab.* **39**, 740.

Illig, R., Tolksdorf, M., Mürset, G. and Prader, A. (1975). *Helv. paed. Acta*, **30**, 221.

Irving, W. J., Chan, M. M. W., Scarth, L., Kolb, F. O., Hartog, M., Bayliss, R. I. S. and Drury, M. I. (1968). *Lancet*, **ii**, 883.

Ishizuka, N., Mizutani, S., Narita, O. and Tomoda, Y. (1973). *Endocr. Jap.* **20**, 51.

Isurugi, K., Wakabayashi, K., Fukutani, K., Takayasu, H., Tamaoki, B. I. and Okada, M. (1973). *J. clin. Endocr. Metab.* **37**, 533.

Jacobs, H. S., Franks, S., Murray, M. A. F., Hull, M. G. R., Steele, S. J. and Nabarro, J. D. N. (1976). *Clin. Endocr.* **5**, 439.

Jaffe, R. B. and Keye, W. R. (1974). *J. clin. Endocr. Metab.* **39**, 850.

Jaffe, R. B., Lee, P. A. and Midgley, A. R. Jr. (1969) *J. clin. Endocr. Metab.* **29**, 1281.

Jeppson, S. and Rannevik, G. (1976). *Am. J. Obstet. Gynec.* **125**, 480.

Jeppson, S., Rannevik, G., Liedholm, P. and Thorell, J. I. (1977a). *Am. J. Obstet. Gynec.* **127**, 32.

Jeppson, S., Rannevik, G. and Thorell, J. I. (1977b). *Acta endocr., Copenh.* **85**, 177.

Jeppson, S., Rannevik, G., Thorell, J. I. and Wide, L. (1977c). *Acta endocr., Copenh.* **84**, 713.

Jewelewicz, R., Dyrenfurth, I., Ferin, M., Bogumil. J. and Van de Wiele, R. L. (1977). *J. clin. Endocr. Metab.* **45**, 662.

Job, J. C., Garnier, P. E., Chaussain, J. L. and Milhaud, G. (1972). *J. clin. Endocr. Metab.* **35**, 473.

Johanson, A. J., Guyda, H., Light, C., Migeon, C. J. and Blizzard, R. M. (1969). *J. Pediat.* **74**, 416.

Johnsen, S. G. (1955). *Acta endocr., Copenh.* **20**, 101.

Judd, H. L., Hamilton, C. R., Barlow, J. J., Yen., S. S. C. and Kliman, B. (1972). *J. clin. Endocr. Metab.* **34**, 229.

Judd, H. L., Parker, D. C., Siler, Th. M. and Yen, S. S. C. (1974). *J. clin. Endocr. Metab.* **38**, 710.

Kallman, F., Schonfeld, W. A. and Barrera, S. E. (1944). *Am. J. Ment. Def.* **48**, 203.

Kamberi, I. A., Mical, R. S. and Porter, J. C. (1971). *Endocrinology*, **89**, 1042.

Kandeel, F. R., Butt, W. R., London, D. R., Lynch, S. S., Logan Edwards, R. and Rudd, B. T. (1978). *Clin. Endocr.* **9**, 429.

Kantero, R.-L., Wide, L. and Widholm, O. (1975). *Acta endocr., Copenh.* **78**, 11.

Kapen, S., Boyar, R., Hellman, L. and Weitzman, E. C. (1973). *J. clin. Endocr. Metab.* **36**, 724.

Kaplan, S. L. and Grumbach, M. M. (1976) *Acta endocr., Copenh.* **81**, 808.

Kaplan, S. L., Grumbach, M. M. and Aubert, M. L. (1976a). *J. clin. Endocr. Metab.* **42**, 995.

Kaplan, S. L., Grumbach, M. M. and Aubert, M. L. (1976b). *Rec. Prog. Horm. Res.* **32**, 161.

Kastin, A. J., Schally, A. W., Schalch, D. S., Korenman, S. G., Miller, M. C., Gual, C. and Perez-Pasten, E. (1972). *Pediat. Res.* **6**, 481.

Katz, M. and Carr, P. J. (1976). *J. Endocr.* **70**, 163.

Keller, P. J. and Rosemberg, E. (1965). *J. clin. Endocr. Metab.* **25**, 1050.

Keye, W. R. and Jaffe, R. B. (1974). *J. clin. Endocr. Metab.* **38**, 805.

Kim, M. H. (1974). *Am. J. Obstet. Gyec.* **120**, 257.

Knobil, E. (1974). *Rec. Prog. Horm. Res.* **30**, 1.

Koninckx, Ph. R. and Brosens, I. A. (1977). *Fertil. Steril.* **28**, 926.

Krieger, D. T., Ossowski, R., Fogel, M. and Allen, W. (1972). *J. clin. Endocr. Metab.* **35**, 619.

Lachelin, G. C. L., Leblanc, H. and Yen, S. S. C. (1977). *J. clin. Endocr. Metab.* **44**, 728.

Leblanc, H., Lachelin, G. C. L., Abu-Fadil, S. and Yen, S. S. C. (1976). *J. clin. Endocr. Metab.* **43**, 668.

Lee, P. A., Jaffe, R. B., Midgley, A. R., Kohen, F. and Niswender, G. D. (1972). *J. clin. Endocr. Metab.* **35**, 633.

Lee, P. A., Midgley, Jr., A. R. and Jaffe, R. B. (1970). *J. clin. Endocr. Metab.* **31**, 248.

Leidenberger, F. L. and Reichert, Jr., L. E. (1972). *Endocrinology*, **91**, 901.

Leidenberger, F. L., Willaschek, R., Pahnke, V. G. and Reichert, Jr., L. E. (1976). *Acta endocr., Copenh.* **81**, 54.

Lenton, E. A., Adams, M. and Cooke, I. D. (1978). *Clin. Endocr.* **8**, 241.

Leonard, J. M., Leach, R. B., Couture, M. and Paulsen, C. A. (1972). *J. clin. Endocr. Metab.* **34**, 209.

Leyendecker, G., Wardlow, S. and Nocke, W. (1972). *Acta endocr., Copenh.* **71**, 160.

Libertun, C. and McCann, S. M. (1973). *Endocrinology*, **92**, 1714.

Lipshultz, L. I., Greenberg, S. H., Caminos-Torres, R. and Snyder, P. J. (1977). *Clin. Endocr.* **7**, 103.

Liu, W. K. and Ward, D. N. (1975). *Biochim. biophys. Acta*, **405**, 522.

Liu, W. K., Yang, K. P., Nakagawa, Y. and Ward, D. N. (1974). *J. biol. Chem.* **249**, 5544.

Loeber, J. G. (1977). *Acta endocr., Copenh.* (Suppl.) **210**, 85.

London, D. R. (1975). "Clinics in Endocrinology and Metabolism", Vol. 4, p. 597. Saunders, London, Philadelphia and Toronto.

London, D. R., Butt, W. R., Lynch, S. S., Marshall, J. C., Owusu, S., Robinson, W. and Stephenson, J. M. (1973a). *J. clin. Endocr. Metab.* **37**, 829.

London, D. R., Butt, W. R., Lynch, S. S., Marshall, J. C., Owusu, S., Robinson, W. and Stephenson, J. M. (1973b). *J. Endocr.* **59**, xiii.

Lucky, A. W., Rebar, R. W., Blizzard, R. M. and Goren, E. M. (1977). *J. clin. Endocr. Metab.* **45**, 673.

Lunenfeld, B., Mor, A. and Mani, M. (1967). *Fertil. Steril.* **18**, 581.

Lynch, S. S. and Shirley, A. (1975). *J. Endocr.* **65**, 127.

Lytton, B. and Mroueh, A. (1966). *Fertil. Steril.* **17**, 696.

Marchalonis, J. J. (1969). *Biochem. J.* **113**, 299.

Marder, M. L., Channing, C. P. and Schwartz, N. B. (1977). *Endocrinology*, **101**, 1639.

Marshall, J. C. (1975). "Clinics in Endocrinology and Metabolism", Vol. 4, p. 545. Saunders, London, Philadelphia and Toronto.

Marshall, J. C. and Fraser, T. R. (1971). *Br. med. J. iv*, 590.

Martin, J. E., Tyrey, L., Everett, J. W. and Fellows, R. E. (1974). *Endocrinology*, **94**, 556.

Martini, L. (1977). *Acta endocr., Copenh.* (Suppl.) **214**, 85, 19.

Mauss, J., Börsch, G., Bormacher, K., Richter, E., Leyendecker, G. and Nocke, W. (1975). *Acta endocr., Copenh.* **78**, 373.

McCann, S. M. and Teleisnik, S. (1960). *Am. J. Physiol.* **199**, 847.

Means, A. and Vaitukaitis, J. (1972). *Endocrinology*, **90**, 39.

Medina, M., Scaglia, H. E., Vázquez, G., Alatorre, S. and Pérez-Palacios, G. (1976). *J. clin. Endocr. Metab.* **43**, 1015.

Midgley, Jr., A. R. and Jaffe, R. B. (1971). *J. clin. Endocr. Metab.* **33**, 962.

Miyachi, Y. and Chrambach, A. (1972). *Biochem. biophys. Res. Comm.* **46**, 1213.

Miyachi, Y., Vaitukaitis, J. L., Nieschlag, E. and Lipsett, M. B. (1972). *J. clin. Endocr. Metab.* **34**, 23.

Miyake, A., Tanizawa, O., Aono, T., Yasuda, M. and Kurachi, K. (1976). *J. clin. Endocr. Metab.* **43**, 928.

Molitch, M., Edmonds, M., Jones, E. E. and Odell, W. D. (1976). *Am. J. Physiol.* **230**, 907.

Monroe, S. E., Jaffe, R. B. and Midgley, Jr., A. R. (1972). *J. clin. Endocr. Metab.* **34**, 342.

Monroe, S. E., Parlow, A. F. and Midgley, Jr., A. R. (1968). *Endocrinology*, **83**, 1004.

Moore, B. (1976). *Post. Med. J.* (Suppl. 6), **52**, 39.

Morell, A. G., Gregoriadis, G., Scheinberg, I. H., Hickman, J. and Ashwell, G. (1971). *J. biol. Chem.* **246**, 1461.

Morgan, F. J., Canfield, R. E., Vaitukaitis, J. L. and Ross, G. T. (1974). *Endocrinology*, **94**, 1601.

Morgner, K. D., Geisthovel, W., Niedergerke, V. and Mühlen, A. (1974). *Dt. med. Wschr.* **99**, 1196.

Mortimer, C. H., Besser, G. M., Hook, J. and McNeilly, A. S. (1974a). *Clin. Endocr.* **3**, 19.

Mortimer, C. H., McNeilly, A. S., Fisher, R. A., Murray, M. A. F. and Besser, G. M. (1974b). *Br. med. J.* **iv**, 617.

Moyle, W. R. and Ramachandran, J. (1973). *Endocrinology*, **93**, 127.

Naftolin, F., Judd, H. L. and Yen, S. S. C. (1973a). *J. clin. Endocr. Metab.* **36**, 285.

Naftolin, F., Yen, S. S. C., Perlman, O., Tsai, C. C., Parker, D. C. and Vargo, T. (1973b). *J. clin. Endocr. Metab.* **37**, 6.

Naftolin, F., Yen., S. S. C. and Tsai, C. C. (1972). *Nature, Lond.* **236**, 82.

Nankin, H. R. and Troen, P. (1971) *J. clin. Endocr. Metab.* **33**, 558.

Nillius, S. J. and Wide, L. (1971a). *Acta endocr., Copenh.* **67**, 362.

Nillius, S. J. and Wide, L. (1971b). *J. Obstet. Gynaec. Br. Comm.* **78**, 822.

Nillius, S. J. and Wide, L. (1972). *J. Obstet. Gynaec. Br. Comm.* **79**, 865.

Nillius, S. J. and Wide, L. (1975). *Br. med. J.* **iii**, 405.

Noonan, J. A. and Emhke, D. A. (1963). *J. Pediat.* **63**, 468.

Nusynowitz, M. L. and Strader, W. J. (1975). *Am. J. Med. Sci.* **270**, 491.

Odell,W. D., Ross, G. T. and Rayford, P. L. (1967). *J. clin. Invest.* **46**, 248.

Odell, W. D. and Swerdloff, R. S. (1968). *Proc. natn. Acad. Sci. USA*, **61**, 529.

Odell, W. D. and Swerdloff, R. S. (1976). *Rec. Prog. Horm. Res.* **32**, 245.

Odell, W. D. and Swerdloff, R. S. (1978). *Clin. Endocr.* **8**, 149.

Odell, W. D., Swerdloff, R. S., Bain, J., Wollesen, F. and Grover, P. (1974). *Endocrinology*, **95**, 1380.

Ojeda, S. R., Harms, P. G. and McCann, S. M. (1975). *Endocrinology*, **97**, 843.

Ojeda, S. R., Jameson, H. E. and McCann, S. M. (1977a). *Endocrinology*, **100**, 1585.

Ojeda, S. R., Jameson, H. E. and McCann, S. M. (1977b). *Endocrinology*, **100**, 1595.

Osland, R. B., Cheesman, D. W. and Forsham, P. H. (1977). *Endocrinology*, **101**, 1203.

Palmer, R. L., Crisp, A. H., McKinnon, P. C. B., Franklin, M., Bonnar, J. and Wheeler. M. (1975). *Br. med. J.* **i**, 179.

Pang, C. M., Zimmermann, E. and Sawyer, C. H. (1977). *Endocrinology*, **101**, 1726.

Papkoff, H. (1973). "Hormonal Proteins and Peptides", Vol. 1, p. 59. Academic Press, New York and London.

Parlow, A. F. (1961). "Human Pituitary Gonadotropins", p. 300. C. C. Thomas, Illinois.

Parlow, A. F., Daane, T. A. and Dignam, W. J. (1970). *J. clin. Endocr. Metab.* **31**, 213.

Parlow, A. F. and Shome, B. (1974). *J. clin. Endocr. Metab.* **39**, 195.

Patrono, C., Serra, G. B., Ciabattori, G., Grossi-Belloni, D. and Soler, R. C. (1976). "The Endocrine Function of the Human Ovary", p. 47. Academic Press, London and New York.

Patton, W. C., Berger, M. J., Thompson, I. E., Chong, A. P., Grimes, E. M. and Taymor, M. L. (1975). *Am. J. Obstet. Gynec.* **121**, 382.

Paulsen, C. A. (1974). "The Testes: Textbook of Endocrinology", p. 323. Saunders, Philadelphia.

Paulsen, C. A., Wackman, J., Hammond, C. B. and Wiese, H. R. (1975). *Fertil. Steril.* **26**, 982.

Peckham, W. D. and Parlow, A. F. (1969). *Endocrinology*, **84**, 953.

Penny, R., Olatunji-Olambiwonnu, N. and Frasier, D. (1974) *J. clin. Endocr. Metab.* **38**, 320.

Penny, R., Olatunji-Olambiwonnu, N. and Frasier, D. (1977a), *J. clin. Endocr. Metab.* **45**, 307.

Penny, R., Parlow, A. F., Olatunji-Olambiwonnu, N. and Frasier, D. (1977b). *New Engl. J. Med.* **287**, 582.
Pepperell, B. J., Burger, H. C., de Kretser, D. M. and Rennie, G. C.(1976). *Br. J. Obstet. Gynaec.* **83**, 68.
Phifer, R. F., Midgley, A. R. and Spicer, S. S. (1973). *J. clin. Endocr. Metab.* **36**, 125.
Popa, G. T. and Fielding, V. (1933). *J. Anat.* **67**, 227.
Prentice, L. G. and Ryan, R. J. (1975). *J. clin. Endocr. Metab.* **40**, 303.
Qazi, M. H., Romani, P. and Diczfalusy, E. (1974). *Acta endocr., Copenh.* **77**, 672.
Raj, S. G., Thompson, I. E., Berger, H. J. and Taymor, M. L. (1977). *Obstet. Gynec.* **49**, 552.
Rathnam, P. and Saxena, B. B. (1970). *J. biol. Chem.* **245**, 3725.
Rathnam, P. and Saxena, B. B. (1972). "Gonadotropins", p. 120. Wiley-Interscience, New York.
Rathnam, P. and Saxena, B. B. (1975). *J. biol. Chem.* **250**, 6735.
Ravid, R., Jedwab, G., Persitz, E., David, M. P., Karni, N., Gil, S., Cordova, T., Harell, A. and Ayalon, D. (1977). *Clin. Endocr.* **6**, 333.
Rebar, R., Yen, S. S. C., Vandenburg, G., Naftolin, F., Ehara, Y., Engblom, S., Ryan, K. J., Rivier, J., Amoss, M. and Guillemin, R. (1973). *J. clin. Endocr. Metab.* **36**, 10.
Rees, L. H. (1978). "Topics in Hormone Chemistry", Vol. 1, p. 109. Ellis Horwood, Chichester.
Rees, L. H., Holdaway, I. M., Kramer, R., McNeilly, A. S. and Chard, T. (1973). *Nature, Lond.* **244**, 232.
Reichert, Jr., L. E. and Bhalla, V. K. (1974). *Endocrinology*, **94**, 483.
Reichert, Jr., L. E., Kathan, R. and Ryan, R. J. (1968). *Endocrinology*, **82**, 109.
Reichert, Jr., L. E., Leidenberger, F. and Trowbridge, C. G. (1973). *Rec. Prog. Horm. Res.* **29**, 487.
Reichert, Jr., L. E. and Ramsey, R. B. (1977). *J. clin. Endocr. Metab.* **44**, 545.
Reichert, Jr., L. E., Ramsey, R. B. and Carter, E. B. (1975). *J. clin. Endocr. Metab.* **41**, 634.
Reiter, P. J. and Vaughan, M. K. (1977). *Life Sci.* **21**, 159.
Reyes, F. I., Winter, J. S. D. and Faiman, C. (1977). *Am. J. Obstet. Gynec.* **129**, 557.
Romani, P., Robertson, D. M. and Diczfalusy, E.(1977). *Acta endocr., Copenh.* **84**, 697.
Römmler, A. (1978). *Acta endocr., Copenh.* **87**, 248.
Roos, P. (1968). *Acta endocr., Copenh.* (Suppl. 131), 32.
Roos, P., Nyberg, L., Wide, L. and Gemzell, C. (1975). *Biochim. biophys. Acta*, **405**, 363.
Rosen, S. W. and Weintraub, B. D. (1971). *J. clin. Endocr. Metab.* **32**, 410.
Roth, A. W., Moshang, T., Bongiovanni, A. M. and Eberlein, W. R. (1970). *Pediat. Res.* **4**, 175.
Roth, J. C., Kelch, R. P., Kaplan, S. L. and Grumbach, M. M. (1972). *J. clin. Endocr. Metab.* **35**, 926.
Rotsztejn, W. H., Charli, J. L., Patton, E. and Kordon, C. (1977). *Endocrinology*, **101**, 1475.
Ryle, M., Chaplin, S. M. F., Gray, C. J. and Kennedy, J. (1970). "Gonadotrophins and Ovarian Development", p. 98. Livingstone, Edinburgh.
Ryle, M., Stephenson, J., Williams, J. and Stuart, J. (1975). *Clin. Endocr.* **4**, 413.
Sairam, M. R. and Li, C. H. (1975). *Arch. Biochem. Biophys.* **167**, 534.
Saito, T. and Saxena, B. B. (1976). *J. clin. Endocr. Metab.* **43**, 1186.
Salesse, R., Castaing, M., Pernollet, J. C. and Garnier, J. (1975). *J. mol. Biol.* **95**, 483.
Santen, R. J. and Paulsen, C. A. (1973). *J. clin. Endocr. Metab.* **36**, 55.

Santen, R. J. and Bardin, C. W. (1973). *J. clin. Invest.* **52**, 2617.

Santen, R. J. and Paulsen, C. A. (1973). *J. clin. Endocr. Metab.* **36**, 55.

Santen, R. J., Sofsky, J., Bilic, N. and Lipsett, B. (1975). *Fertil. Steril.* **26**, 538.

Saxena, B. B. and Rathnam, P. (1971). *J. biol. Chem.* **246**, 3549.

Saxena, B. B. and Rathnam, P. (1976). *J. biol. Chem.* **251**, 993.

Schally, A. V., Arimura, A., Baba, Y., Nair, R. M. G., Matsuo, H., Redding, T. W., Debeljuk, L. and White, W. F. (1971). *Biochem. biophys. Res. Comm.* **43**, 393.

Schlamowitz, M., Cronquist, J., Esfahani, M. and Ward, D. N. (1976). *Acta endocr., Copenh.* **81**, 270.

Schwarzstein, L. de Laborde, N. P., Aparicio, N. J., Turner, D., Mirkin, A., Rodriguez, A., Llullier, F. R. and Rosner, J. M. (1975). *J. clin. Endocr. Metab.* **40**, 313.

Scott, L. D. (1941). *Br. J. exp. Path.* **21**, 320.

Setchell, B. P. and Sirinathsinghji, D. J. (1972). *J. Endocr.* **52**, ix.

Setchell, B. P. and Wallace, A. L. (1972). *J. Endocr.* **54**, 67.

Shaw, R. W., Butt, W. R. and London, D. R. (1975a). *Br. J. Obstet. Gynaec.* **82**, 337.

Shaw, R. W., Butt, W. R. and London, D. R. (1975b). *Clin. Endocr.* **4**, 297.

Shaw, R. W., Butt, W. R. and London, D. R. (1975c). *Clin. Endocr.* **4**, 543.

Shaw, R. W., Butt, W. R., London, D. R. and Marshall, J. C. (1974). *J. Obstet. Gynaec. Brit. Comm.* **81**, 632.

Shaw, R. W., Butt, W. R., London, D. R. and Marshall, J. C. (1957d). *Clin. Endocr.* **4**, 267.

Shaw, R. W., Duignan, N. M., Butt, W. R., Logan Edwards, R. and London, D. R. (1975e). *Br. J. Obstet. Gynaec.* **82**, 952.

Shaw, R. W., Duignan, N. M., Butt, W. R., Logan Edwards, R. and London, D. R. (1976). *Clin. Endocr.* **5**, 495.

Sherins, R. J. and Loriaux, D. L. (1973). *J. clin. Endocr. Metab.* **36**, 886.

Sherman, B. M. and Korenman, S. G. (1947a). *J. clin. Endocr. Metab.* **38**, 89.

Sherman, B. M. and Korenman, S. G. (1974b). *J. clin. Endocr. Metab.* **39**, 145.

Sherman, B. M. and Korenman, S. G. (1975). *J. clin. Invest.* **55**, 699.

Sherman, B. M., West, J. H. and Korenman, S. G. (1976). *J. clin. Endocr. Metab.* **42**, 629.

Shirley, A. and Stephenson, J. (1973). *J. Endocr.* **58**, 345.

Shome, B. and Parlow, A. F. (1974a). *J. clin. Endocr. Metab.* **39**, 199.

Shome, B. and Parlow, A. F. (1974b). *J. clin. Endocr. Metab.* **39**, 203.

Simon, M., Franchimont, P., Marie, N., Ferrand, B., van Cauwenberge, H. and Bowel, M. (1972). *Eur. J. clin. Invest.* **36**, 811.

Simonovic, T., Motta, M. and Martini, L. (1974). *Endocrinology,* **95**, 1373.

Sizonenko, P. C. (1975). "Clinics in Endocrinology and Metabolism", Vol. 4, p. 173. Saunders, London, Philadelphia and Toronto.

Sizonenko, P. C., Burr, I. M., Kaplan, S. L. and Grumbach, M. M. (1970) *Pediat. Res.* **4**, 36.

Sizonenko, P. C. and Paunier, L. (1975) *J. clin. Endocr. Metab.* **41**, 894.

Smythe, G. A. (1977). *Clin. Endocr.* **7**, 325.

Snoep, M. C., de Lange, W. E., Sluiter, W. J. and Doorenbos, H. (1977). *J. clin. Endocr. Metab.* **44**, 603.

Snyder, P. J. and Sterling, F. H. (1976). *J. clin. Endocr. Metab.* **42**, 544.

Starup, J., Sele, V. and Henriksen, B. (1971). *Acta endocr., Copenh.* **66**, 248.

Steelman, S. L. and Pohley, F. M. (1953). *Endocrinology,* **53**, 604.

Stewart-Bentley, M., Odell, W. D. and Horton, R. (1974). *J. clin. Endocr. Metab.* **38**, 545.

Storring, P. L., Dixon, H. and Bangham, D. R. (1976). *Acta endocr., Copenh.* **83**, 700.

Strott, C. A., Cargille, C. M., Ross, G. T. and Lipsett, M. B. (1970). *J. clin. Endocr. Metab.* **30**, 246.

Studd, J., Chakravarti, S. and Oram, D. (1977). "Clinics in Obstetrics and Gynaecology" Vol. 4, p. 3. Saunders, London, Philadelphia and Toronto.

Suwa, S., Maesaka, H. and Matsui, I. (1974). *Pediatrics*, **54**, 470.

Swaminathan, N. and Bahl, O. P. (1970). *Biochem. biophys. Res. Comm.* **40**, 422.

Swerdloff, R. S., Walsh, P. C., Jacobs, H. S. and Odell, W. D. (1971). *Endocrinology*, **88**, 120.

Tanner, J. M. (1962). "Growth and Adolescence", 2nd edition, p. 28. Blackwell Scientific Publications, Oxford.

Taymor, M. L. and Miyata, J. (1969). *Acta endocr., Copenh.* (Suppl. 142), 324.

Thomas, K., Malvaux, P. and Ferin, J. (1972). *J. clin. Endocr. Metab.* **35**, 938.

Torjesen, P. A., Sand, T., Norman, N., Trygstad, O. and Foss, I. (1974). *Acta endocr., Copenh.* **77**, 485.

Tourniaire, J., Fevre, M., Mazenod, B. and Pousin, G. (1974). *J. clin. Endocr. Metab.* **38**, 1122.

Treloar, A. E., Boynton, R. E., Benn, B. G. and Brown, B. W. (1967). *Int. J. Fertil.* **12**, 77.

Tsai, C. C. and Yen, S. S. C. (1971a). *J. clin. Endocr. Metab.* **32**, 766.

Tsai, C. C. and Yen, S. S. C. (1971b). *J. clin. Endocr. Metab.* **32**, 917.

Tsafiri, A., Pomerantz, S. H. and Channing, C. P. (1976). *Biol. Rep.* **14**, 511.

Vaitukaitis, J. L. and Ross, G. T. (1971). *J. clin. Endocr. Metab.* **33**, 308.

Vaitukaitis, J. L., Ross, G. T., Pierce, J. G., Cornell, J. S. and Reichert, Jr., L. E. (1973). *J. clin. Endocr. Metab.* **37**, 653.

Van, Campanhout, J. V., Vauclair, R. and Marghi, K. (1972). *Obstet. Gynaec.* **40**, 6.

Van Damme, M. P., Robertson, D. M. and Diczfalusy, E. (1974). *Acta endocr., Copenh.* **77**, 655.

Van Hell, H., Matthijsen, R. and Overbeek, G. A. (1964). *Acta endocr., Copenh.* **47**, 409.

Van Hell, H., Schuurs, A. H. W. M. and Hollander, F. C. den (1972), "Gonadotropins", p. 185. Wiley-Interscience, New York.

Van Look, P. F. A., Lothian, H., Hunter, W. M., Michie, E. A. and Baird, D. T. (1977). *Clin. Endocr.* **7**, 13.

Wallis, M. (1975). *Biol. Rev. Camb. Phil. Soc.* **50**, 35.

Walsh, P., Swerdloff, R. S. and Odell, W. D. (1973). *J. Urol.* **110**, 84.

Wang, C. F., Lasley, B. L., Lein, A. and Yen, S. S. C. (1976). *J. clin. Endocr. Metab.* **42**, 718.

Ward, D. N., Reichert, Jr., L. E., Wan-Kyng Liu, Nahm, H. S., Hsia, J. Lamkin, W. M. and Jones, N. S. (1973). *Rec. Prog. Horm. Res.* **29**, 533.

Watson, J. (1971). *J. Endocr.* **50**, 71.

Watts, R. M. and Adair, F. L. (1943). *Am. J. Obstet. Gynec.* **46**, 183.

Weitzman, E. D., Boyar, R. M., Kapen, S. and Hellman, L. (1975). *Rec. Prog. Horm. Res.* **31**, 399.

Wetterberg, L., Arendt, J., Paunier, L., Sizonenko, P. C., van Donselaar, W. and Heyden, T. (1976). *J. clin. Endocr. Metab.* **42**, 185.

Wheaton, J. E., Krulich, L. and McCann, S. M. (1975). *Endocrinology*, **97**, 30.

White, N. F., Hedlund, M. T., Weber, G. F., Reppel, R. W., Johnson, E. S. and Wilber, S. F. (1974). *Endocrinology*, **94**, 1422.

Wide, L. (1969). *Acta endocr., Copenh.* (Suppl. 142), 207.

Wide, L., Nillius, S. J., Gemzell, C. and Roos, P. (1973). *Acta endocr., Copenh.* **73** (Suppl. 174), 1.

Widholm, O., Kantero, F.-L., Axelson, E., Johansson, E. D. B. and Wide, L. (1974). *Acta obstet. gynec. scand.* **53**, 197.

Wilber, J. F., Montoya, E., Plotnikoff, N. P., White, N. R., Gendrich, R., Renaud, L. and Martin, J. B. (1976). *Rec. Prog. Horm. Res.* **32**, 117.

Willis, K. J., London, D. R., Bevis, M. A., Butt, W. R., Lynch, S. S. and Holder, G. (1977a). *J. Endocr.* **73**, 171.

Willis, K. J., London, D. R., Ward, H. W. C., Butt, W. R., Lynch, S. S. and Rudd, B. T. (1977b). *Br. med. J.* **1**, 425.

Wilson, J. D., Harrod, M. J., Goldstein, J. L., Hemsell, D. J. and MacDonald, P. C. (1974). *New Engl. J. Med.* **290**, 1097.

Winter, J. S. D. and Faiman, C. (1972). *Pediat. Res.* **6**, 126.

Winter, J. S. D. and Faiman, C. (1973). *Pediat. Res.* **7**, 948.

Winter, J. S. D., Faiman, C., Hobson, W. C., Prasad, A. V. and Reyes, F. I. (1975). *J. clin. Endocr. Metab.* **40**, 545.

Woolf, P. D. and Schenk, E. A. (1974). *J. clin. Endocr. Metab.* **38**, 561.

Wurtman, R. J. (1971). *Neurosci. Res. Prog. Bull.* **9**, 172.

Yen, S. S. C., Lasley, B. L., Wang, C. F., Leblanc, H. and Siler, T. M. (1975). *Rec. Prog. Horm. Res.* **31**, 321.

Yen, S. S. C., Rebar, R., VandenBerg, G. and Judd, H. (1973). *J. clin. Endocr. Metab.* **36**, 811.

Yen, S. S. C. and Tsai, C. C. (1972). *J. clin. Endocr. Metab.* **34**, 298.

Yen, S. S. C., Tsai, C. C., Naftolin, F., VandenBerg, G. and Ajabor, L. (1972). *J. clin. Endocr. Metab.* **34**, 671.

Yen, S. S. C., VandenBerg, G., Tsai, C. C. and Parker, D. C. (1974). "Biorhythms and Human Reproduction", p. 203. Wiley, New York.

Yen, S. S. C., Vela, P. and Rankin, J. (1970). *J. clin. Endocr. Metab.* **30**, 435.

Yen, S. S. C. and Vivic, W. J. (1970). *Am. J. Obstet. Gynec.* **106**, 134.

Yen, S. S. C., Vivic, W. J. and Kearchner, D. V. (1969). *J. clin. Endocr. Metab.* **29**, 382.

Zárate, A., Garrido, J., Canales, E. S., Soria, J. and Schally, A. V. (1974). *J. clin. Endocr. Metab.* **38**, 1125.

Zárate, A., Valdes-Vallina, F., Gonzales, A., Perez-Ubierna, C., Canales, E. S. and Schally, A. V. (1973). *Fertil. Steril.* **24**, 485.

Zschaeck, L. L. and Wurtman, R. J. (1973). *Neuroendocrinology*, **11**, 144.

X. Erythropoietin

P. MARY COTES and D. E. GUÈRET WARDLE

INTRODUCTION

In the intact animal, administration of erythropoietin (Van Dyke, 1960; Gordon, 1959) or increased secretion of endogenous erythropoietin normally induces polycythaemia. This effect of erythropoietin is mediated by stimulation of the formation of a new generation of pronormoblasts and of proliferation of less mature erythropoietin responsive cells (Lajtha, 1975).

Thus the erythropoietin responsive cell is not confined to one morphological type, and it is not clear whether erythropoietin affects only cells already committed to development in the red cell series or whether it has some direct effect on the pluripotential stem cell (Van Zant and Goldwasser, 1977). Intracellular effects of erythropoietin include the development of systems for synthesis of haemoglobin, not present in early red cell precursors. These include RNA synthesis (Gross and Goldwasser, 1969; Gross and Goldwasser, 1971; Terada, Cantor, Metafora, Rifkin, Banks and Marks, 1972) and stimulation of incorporation of iron, initially into the cell and then into haemoglobin (Gross and Goldwasser, 1970; Storring and Fatah, 1975) (reviewed by Nienhuis, Barker and Anderson, 1977; Goldwasser, 1975a).

A. CHEMISTRY OF ERYTHROPOIETIN

1. Extraction

Purified preparations of erythropoietin have been obtained in limited amounts by extraction of plasma of anaemic sheep (Goldwasser and Kung, 1968; Kawakita, Miyake and Kishimoto, 1975; Goldwasser and Kung, 1971a) and urine of anaemic humans (Espada and Gutnisky, 1970; Miyake, Kung and Goldwasser, 1977). The preparation obtained by Miyake et al. (1977) had higher biological activity than earlier preparations but is still not fully characterised. The hormone is a glycoprotein and recent work has demonstrated that affinity chromatography on immobilised lectins can be used to concentrate it and to diminish the toxicity of extracts of human urinary erythropoietin in tissue culture systems (Sieber, 1977). Wheat germ agglutinin and phytohaemagglutin have been used for direct purification of erythropoietin from urine (Spivak, Small and Hollenberg, 1977). Whereas yields of erythropoietin have usually been poor, Miyake et al. (1977) fractionated 2550 l of urine from patients with aplastic anaemia and recovered 21 % of the biological activity of an initial urine concentrate, an average yield of about 480 u biological activity per litre of urine. This and other recent methods show considerable improvements in yield and purification.

2. Chemical Characteristics

Sheep plasma and human urinary erythropoietins are acidic glycoproteins which are heterogeneous on isoelectric focusing. Lukowsky and Painter (1972) found that the isoelectric point of fractions which had biological activity in vivo was between pH 3·5 and 4·0. Completely asialo erythropoietin has an isoelectric point between 5·0 and 6·5. Espada, Langton and Dorado (1972) report that their most highly purified preparation of human erythropoietin contains about 29% carbohydrate which may be compared with 26% carbohydrate in sheep plasma erythropoietin (Goldwasser and Kung, 1971a). However, detailed chemical studies have not yet been made using the most highly purified human erythropoietin now available.

3. Physical Properties

Physical properties of erythropoietin from human urine are listed in Table 1. Problems in the satisfactory determination of molecular weight which is estimated to be between 27,000 and 60,000 are discussed by Goldwasser and Kung (1971b).

4. Biological Activity and Structure

Estimates of the *in vivo* biological activity of highly purified preparations of sheep erythropoietin indicate a potency of about 8000–9000 u/mg (Goldwasser and Kung, 1971a). Human urinary erythropoietin extracted by Espada and Gutnisky (1970) showed the same order of potency. Neither of these preparations was available in sufficient amounts for complete characterisation and each seemed to represent nearly homogeneous material, but, more recently Miyake *et al.* (1977) isolated a fraction from human urine with some 70,000 u/mg by bioassay *in vivo*. Although confidence limits are not given for the potency estimates, Miyake *et al.* (1977) present good evidence that this preparation of human erythropoietin has considerably higher potency than has been obtained hitherto. However, much of our information about erythropoietin is based on studies using less highly purified preparations or crude extracts of urine or plasma. The intact molecule is necessary for *in vivo* biological activity and complete or partial desialation results in loss of *in vivo* biological activity (Lowy, Keighley and Borsook, 1960) but retention of *in vitro* biological activity (Goldwasser and Kung, 1968). Oxidation of asialo-erythropoietin with galactose oxidase restores biological activity *in vivo* (Lukowsky and Painter, 1972). Thus, in common with other glycoproteins (Morrell, Gregoriadas, Scheinberg, Hickman and Ashwell, 1971), exposure of the penultimate galactose residue seems to result in rapid removal of the hormone from the circulation. Survival of erythropoietin during transport in plasma is increased by oxidation or removal of the exposed galactose residue (Lukowsky and Painter, 1972).

In vivo biological activity of erythropoietin is destroyed by a wide range of proteolytic enzymes including trypsin, pepsin, papain, chymotrypsin A, elastase, ficin, bromelin and a protease from Streptomyces griseum (see review by Espada, 1977). Other effects of structure modification on biological activity are reviewed by Goldwasser (1975b) and Espada (1977).

Table 1

Physical properties of erythropoietin from human urine.

Molecular radius Å	Molecular weight (daltons)	Sedimentation coefficient	Frictional ratio	Axial ratio	λ_{max} (nm)	Absorbance ($A_{1\,cm}^{1\%}$)	References
	24,000–30,000[a]			10			Rosse, Berry and Waldmann (1963)
	52,000–77,000[b]						Olesen and Fogh (1968)
	57,000–64,000[c]						Lukowsky and Painter (1968)
32.6[d]	60,000[c]						O'Sullivan, Chiba, Gleich and Linman (1970)
33	27,600–35,600[e]	2·63S	1·58	10–11[f]	279	9·26[g]	Espada, Langton and Dorado (1972)
	23,000[h]						Dorado, Espada, Langton and Brandon (1974)
	30,000–36,000[i] 45,000–57,000[h]						Shelton, Ichiki and Lange (1975)
	39,000[i]					8·1[j]	Miyake, Kung and Goldwasser (1977)

[a] Radiation inactivation by high energy electrons.
[b] Radiation inactivation by X-rays.
[c] Gel filtration.
[d] Calculated by O'Sullivan et al. (1970).
[e] Gel filtration and sucrose density gradient.
[f] Calculated by Goldwasser (1975).
[g] At 279 nm.
[h] SDS-polyacrylamide gel electrophoresis.
[i] Gel filtration in 6 M GuHCl.
[j] At 278 nm.

It requires emphasis that to test whether a specific structural change is accompanied by any change in biological activity, it must be shown that a sufficient proportion of the hormone (which may be associated with many impurities) has itself undergone the intended reaction and comparisons of estimates of initial and remaining biological activity must take into account fiducial or confidence limits of the potency estimates.

5. Species and Source

Erythropoietins from man, sheep and rabbit all show biological activity in rats and mice (Gordon, 1959). In man, it is not known whether heterologous erythropoietins have any biological activity if administered *in vivo* although, in *in vitro* cultures of human bone marrow, sheep erythropoietin increases haem synthesis (Krantz, 1965). There is evidence for differences between erythropoietins from different species and sources. Antisera to erythropoietin from human urine and sheep plasma may each neutralise erythropoietins from urine and plasma of man, rabbit, and sheep but Garcia (1972) prepared an antiserum which neutralised the biological activity of human but not of rabbit erythropoietin. In addition Peschle and Condorelli (1975) found an antiserum with a different capacity for neutralising the biological activity of erythropoietins from man, rat and rabbit. One ml of antiserum neutralised 125, 12 and 1·2 u of the respective erythropoietins.

Comparisons of the relative biological activity of erythropoietins are usually made in mice or rats. Tested in these species, highly purified erythropoietin from human urine shows higher potency than erythropoietin from sheep plasma (Miyake *et al.*, 1977). However, this difference would not necessarily be the same if the comparison was made in another species of test animal.

B. TISSUE OF ORIGIN AND BIOSYNTHESIS

1. Summary

The classical endocrine techniques of observation of the effects of organ excision and replacement have been used to investigate the origin of erythropoietin. Results obtained indicate that, in adult man, functioning renal tissue is essential for the normal formation of erythropoietin whereas, in the foetus, liver is the main tissue associated with erythropoietin formation (Zanjani, Poster, Mann and Wasserman, 1977). In anephric man, erythropoietin secretion is impaired but can still take place. Additionally, tumours and cysts arising in several tissues may be associated with abnormally high production of erythropoietin. Normal biosynthesis requires a renal precursor and a plasma factor, but the nature of these and of their interaction has not been elucidated.

2. The Role of the Kidney

(a) The need for functioning renal tissue

In man, the normal erythropoietic response to an hypoxic stimulus is dependent upon a normally functioning kidney. In patients with renal disease and an associated anaemia, estimates of erythropoietin in plasma by bioassay *in vivo* show undetectable or lower levels than are found in patients with anaemia of comparable severity of other aetiology (Gallagher, McCarthy and Lange, 1960; Naets and Heuse, 1962; Raich and Korst, 1978). Using *in vivo* bioassays these findings are widely confirmed. After nephrectomy, erythropoietin secretion can still occur, but is considerably diminished (see review by Krantz and Jacobson, 1970). In bilaterally nephrectomised man, haemoglobin levels are usually maintained at 7–9 g/100 ml instead of at normal levels (Nathan, Schupak and Stohlman, 1964). Such subjects respond to a further hypoxic stimulus, such as haemorrhage or a haemolytic episode, with an increase in serum erythropoietin to levels which then become detectable by *in vivo* bioassay (Naets and Witteck, 1968; Mirand, Murphy, Steeves, Weber and Retief, 1968; Mirand and Murphy, 1969; Mirand, Fisher, Stuckey, Lindhold and Abshire, 1971).

Estimates of erythropoietin by radioimmunoassay conflict with the findings from bioassay estimates *in vivo*. Thus, using a radioimmunoassay, Garcia (1974) found a mean serum level of 261 (S.E. 41) mu/ml in 10 anephric patients (mean haemoglobin 5·8 g/100 ml) and 211 (S.E. 21) mu/ml in 19 patients with renal disease maintained on dialysis and with mean haemoglobin 6·4 g/100 ml. These erythropoietin levels are respectively 56 and 46 times the levels which he found in normal subjects. Also using a radioimmunoassay, Lertora, Dargon, Rege and Fisher (1975) found 3 fold higher levels of erythropoietin in four patients with uraemia and anaemia than in five normal subjects. Although a level of 200 mu/ml should be easily detectable by bioassay, Garcia found no erythropoietin by bioassay of sera from anaemic anephric patients and this must be attributable to differences between the specificities of the bioassay and radioimmunoassay systems used.

In other species, studied during uraemia induced by nephrectomy or by ureter ligation, the effects of renal deprivation on erythropoiesis and erythropoietin secretion do not result directly from uraemia and accumulation of metabolites (Jacobson, Goldwasser, Fried and Plzak, 1957a; Naets, 1958; Reissmann, Nomura, Gunn and Brosius, 1960; Naets and Heuse, 1964) although patients maintained by repeated dialysis do show some improvement in erythroid marrow function (Esbach, Funk, Adamson, Kuhn, Scribner and Finch, 1967).

(b) Effects of renal replacement

Successful renal transplantation restores the previously depressed erythropoiesis in 80% of renoprival patients maintained by dialysis (without kidneys or with severely diseased kidneys and no significant excretory function) (Hoffman, 1968). Whereas before transplantation, plasma levels of erythropoietin were undetectable by bioassay in vivo, Abbrecht and Greene (1966) found that, after transplantation, plasma erythropoietin increased to a level which was detectable by in vivo bioassay even when at the same low haemoglobin level before transplantation, plasma erythropoietin was not detectable. Denny, Flanigan and Zukoski (1966) also found intermittently detectable (raised) levels after kidney transplantation. The mechanism of induction of the increased level is not understood. It is postulated that incipient graft rejection may be associated with renal hypoxia but this does not seem to account for all instances of raised plasma erythropoietin (and sometimes polycythaemia) occurring after renal transplantation.

(c) Kidney perfusates and renal extracts as sources of erythropoietin

Storage of erythropoietin does not seem to occur in the kidney and there has been little success in extracting erythropoietin from normal or anaemic kidney tissue from several species (Gordon, Piliero, Medici, Siegal and Tannenbaum, 1956; Rambach, Alt and Cooper, 1961; Naets, 1960 and Penington, 1963). Isolated perfused rabbit or dog kidneys seem to generate erythropoietin in response to a hypoxic stimulus (Kuratowska, Lewartowski and Michalak, 1961; Fisher and Langston, 1967) but subsequent evidence indicates that the kidney produces not erythropoietin but a precursor from which erythropoietin is generated by reaction with a plasma factor (Kuratowski, Lewartowski and Lipski, 1964). Contrera, Gordon and Weintraub (1966) found that a renal factor could be extracted in the light mitochondrial fraction of rat kidneys. This factor generates erythropoietin after incubation with serum, and has been called the renal erythropoietic factor (REF) or erythrogenin (Gordon 1971). Sherwood and Goldwasser (1978) found that extracts of normal kidneys from rat, ox, dog and rabbit contain erythropoietin and not a precursor of the hormone.

(d) The renal eruthropoietic factor (REF)

REF has been obtained from light mitochondrial fractions of kidney of rabbit, dog, sheep, pig and man (Zanjani, Cooper, Gordon, Wong and Scribner, 1967) and these findings are confirmed with kidneys from dog (Malgor and Fisher, 1970) and rat (Rodgers, Geroge and Fisher, 1972; Martelo, Toro and Hirsch, 1976). However the amounts of erythropoietin generated are small. Neither REF nor the plasma factor have yet been fully characterised. They are not species specific and REF from one species can react with plasma factor from another. In some systems the plasma factor may serve only as a non-specific carrier protein.

(e) *Immunochemical relationships between erythropoietin, REF and plasma factor*

Erythropoietin is immunochemically distinct from both REF and plasma factor. Thus, neither REF nor plasma factor react with antisera raised against erythropoietin although the biological activity of erythropoietin generated during incubation of REF and plasma factor can be neutralised by antiserum to erythropoietin (Schooley, Zanjani and Gordon, 1970). Antisera to REF do not neutralise the biological activity of erythropoietin (McDonald, Zanjani, Lange and Gordon, 1971). Erythropoietin generated in the reaction between rat REF and rabbit plasma factor was examined with an antiserum with different capacities for neutralising the biological activities of rat and rabbit erythropoietins. Generated erythropoietin was found to react as rat erythropoietin, which was the species of the REF and not that of the plasma factor (Peschle and Condorelli, 1975). Some evidence suggests that availability of the plasma factor may control generation of erythro- poietin (Zanjani, McLaurin, Gordon, Rappaport, Gibbs and Gidari, 1971) but the nature of the reaction which leads to the unmasking or production of immunologically and biologically recognisable erythropoietin is not known.

C. CONTROL OF SECRETION

1. Effects of Hypoxia and of Hyperoxia

Hypoxia of any aetiology is usually associated with increased production of erythropoietin. This effect depends not on blood oxygen tension or content nor on haemoglobin saturation but on tissue hypoxia at the site of production of erythropoietin (or its precursors) and believed normally to be the kidneys (reviewed by Krantz and Jacobson, 1970). Conversely, hyperoxia appears to be associated with cessation or a decrease in erythropoietin production. Thus Necas and Neuwirt (1969) found that erythropoietin levels in anaemic rats were decreased to undetectable levels after exposure to hyperbaric oxygen and Cotes and Lowe (1963) showed a fall in plasma erythropoietin (estimated *in vivo*) when an anaemic patient breathed 75% oxygen. Within wide limits, the degree of anaemia and the level of plasma erythropoietin are directly correlated (Fig. 1).

Enhanced affinity of haemoglobin for oxygen can result in tissue hypoxia and erythropoietin release. Conversely, diminished affinity of haemoglobin for oxygen can result in increased tissue oxygen tension and decreased erythropoietin release. The first of these mechanisms operates in patients who have an abnormal haemoglobin with high oxygen affinity (Adamson, Parer and Stamotoyannopoulos and Burger, 1972). Ascent to a high altitude

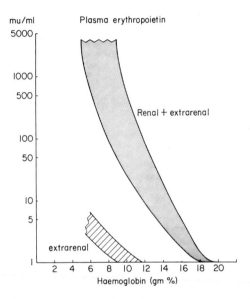

Fig. 1. The relation between haemoglobin and plasma erythropoietin estimated by bioassay in transfusion induced polycythaemic mice. The curves are based on estimates of about 50 unconcentrated plasma samples (levels > 50 mu/ml) and about 50 concentrated plasma extracts of samples from normal and anephric subjects (levels < 50 mu/ml). We are indebted to Dr A. J. Erslev who kindly provided and allows us to reproduce this figure.

from sea level can result in acute hypoxia and in man this induces an increase in levels of erythropoietin in plasma (Abbrecht and Littell, 1972 and in urine (Siri, Van Dyke, Winchell, Pollycove, Parker and Cleveland, 1966; Caremena, Garcia, de Testa and Frias, 1967) demonstrable by bioassay *in vivo*. Abbrecht and Littell (1972) found that plasma erythropoietin concentrations reached their highest values after about 18 hr at 4360 m then, during about four days, decreased towards basal levels despite continuous exposure to the same altitude. Miller, Rorth, Parving, Howard, Reddington, Valeri and Stohlman (1973) suggest that the rapid increase in plasma erythropoietin which follows hypoxia from exposure to air at a reduced pressure is triggered both by a fall in arterialised capillary oxygen saturation and by an increase in haemo-globin affinity for oxygen which results from the respiratory alkalosis induced by hyperventilation. These authors showed that, if acetazolamide is adminis-tered during exposure to a simulated altitude of 4500 m, alkalosis is prevented, the associated increase in oxygen affinity of haemoglobin does not occur and the increase in the plasma erythropoietin from simulated high altitude exposure is greatly decreased. The eventual decrease in erythropoietin level which normally follows continuous exposure to hypoxia from high altitude exposure may result from accumulation of red cell 2,3-diphosphoglycerate (2,3-DPG) which binds to deoxyhaemoglobin, decreases oxygen affinity for haemoglobin and decreases the relative hypoxia which was the initial stimulus to erythropoietin secretion (Miller *et al.*, 1973; Rorth, 1974).

The effect of an increase in erythropoietin secretion is both to increase the erythropoietin responsive cell pool and, in the long term, to increase the red cell mass and the oxygen carrying capacity of the blood. This tends to correct tissue hypoxia and a negative feedback mechanism dependent on an oxygen sensing mechanism, postulated to exist in the kidney, then operates to decrease the production of erythropoietin.

2. Cellular Regulation

At a cellular level it is suggested that stimuli such as hypoxia (Rodgers, Fisher and George, 1974a), cobalt which induces local hypoxia (Rodgers,

Table 2

Substances which have been found both to induce increases in renal adenyl cyclase or renal cAMP when added to renal tissue *in vitro* and to induce an increase in plasma erythropoietin when administered *in vivo*.

Substance	Reference to effect on renal adenylate cyclase or on renal AMP *in vitro*	Reference to effect on plasma erythropoietin *in vivo*
Parathyroid hormone	Kurokawa and Massry (1973)	Rodgers, Fisher and George (1975)
Lactate	Rodgers, Fisher and George (1974a)	Rodgers *et al.* (1974a)
β adrenergic stimuli (Salbutamol and isoprenaline)	Kurokawa and Massry (1973); Bell (1974)	Fink and Fisher (1975)
Prostaglandin E1[a]	Paulo, Wilkerson, Roh, George and Fisher (1973)	Paulo *et al.* (1973); Schooley and Mahlmann (1971)

[a] Prostaglandin PGE_1 does not occur in man. A naturally occurring prostaglandin, PGE_2, has been found by Schooley and Mahlmann (1971) to induce an increase in plasma erythropoietin *in vivo*.

George and Fisher, 1972), and the synthetic prostaglandin PGE$_1$ (Paulo, Wilkerson, Roh, George and Fisher, 1973), initiate a cascade whereby a renal protein kinase activates the renal erythropoietic factor by phosphorylation in the presence of cAMP (Rodgers, Fisher and George, 1974b; Martelo, Toro and Hirsch, 1976). This then interacts with a plasma factor to generate erythropoietin which may be detected *in vivo*. Other substances listed in Table 2 have been found *in vivo* to stimulate erythropoietin production and *in vitro* to induce an increase in renal adenylate cyclase, the enzyme mediating conversion of ATP to cAMP, or a direct increase in renal cAMP. These observations have been made in animals other than man, and stimulating agents are sometimes administered at pharmacological rather than physiological doses. It is not clear how far the suggested pathways represent normal regulatory mechanisms.

D. ESTIMATION OF ERYTHROPOIETIN IN PLASMA AND OTHER BODY FLUIDS

1. General Considerations and the International Unit

Chemical methods are not yet applicable to the estimation of erythropoietin. Estimates are made either by bioassay *in vivo* or *in vitro*, or by immunoassay (Table 3). No system is entirely specific for erythropoietin and estimates made in different systems are commonly heterogeneous. Assays are comparative and estimates are expressed in International Units (u), using as standard the second International Reference Preparation (IRP) for erythropoietin which was prepared from an extract of human urine (less than 0·01 % erythropoietin) and intended for use in bioassays (Annable, Cotes and Mussett, 1972). The IRP and the 1st IRP which preceded it (Cotes and Bangham, 1966) give *in vivo* assay dose response curves parallel to those given by erythropoietins from several species and sources (Cotes and Bangham, 1961; Camiscoli, Weintraub and Gordon, 1968) although, in some *in vivo* systems plasma and urinary forms of erythropoietin give non-parallel response curves (Dukes, Hammond and Shore, 1969; Dukes, Hammond, Shore and Ortega, 1971) and may require separate standards. In immunoassays it is not expected that plasma and urinary forms of the hormone will react identically and as in the case of the gonadotrophic hormones (Albert, 1968) each form may require a separate standard. Thus slopes of assay dose response curves for human sera and the 1st IRP (from human urine) were parallel in one radioimmunoassay system (Garcia, 1974) and non-parallel in another (Lertora, Dargon, Rege and Fisher, 1975).

Iscove, Sieber and Winterhalter (1974) have found that the IRP and other preparations of urinary erythropoietin contain granulocyte colony stimulating activity (CSA or CSF) which has been found by Van Zant and Goldwasser (1977) to suppress stimulation of haem synthesis by erythropoietin in mouse bone marrow *in vitro*. Therefore in *in vitro* bioassays it may be necessary to use a purified preparation of erythropoietin as standard and to test only preparations from which CSF has been extracted.

Table 3

Approximate amounts of erythropoietin required for assay in different test systems and lowest amounts which may be estimated.

Assay	Smallest amount of erythropoietin detectable (mu)	Lowest concentration estimatable (mu/ml)	Minimal amount of test preparation needed for an assay (approx)
In vivo bioassay			
Rat (starved) appearance of ^{59}Fe in red cells	500–1000 (per rat)	80	16 u
Mouse (polycythaemic) appearance of ^{59}Fe in red cells	20–50 (per mouse)	25	2 u
In vitro bioassay			
Foetal liver (mouse) incorporation of ^{59}Fe into haem	1–2 (per culture)	10–12	0·1 u
Bone marrow (rat or human) incorporation of ^{59}Fe into haem	75 (per culture)	50	not applicable to plasma assays
In vitro immunological assay			
Haemagglutination inhibition	2	10	0·0005 u
Radioimmunoassay	3	3	0·01 u

Assay results are sometimes expressed as the magnitude of a biological or biochemical response and not as potency relative to a standard. The latter form of expression permits comparison of estimates made in different assay systems, whereas the former varies with the strain of test animal or cell source (as well as on each occasion that the test is carried out) and the response is seldom directly related to the dose of the substance inducing it.

For activity *in vivo*, intact but not desialated forms of the hormone are needed whereas, in *in vitro* bioassays and in one radioimmunoassay both forms are active (Lukowsky and Painter, 1972; Garcia, 1977). Thus *in vivo* assays provide different information from that provided by *in vitro* systems. Both types of assay are beset by problems arising from insensitivity, poor precision and non-specificity.

2. *In vivo* Bioassays

The *in vivo* bioassays for erythropoietin are usually too insensitive to permit estimation of normal levels in plasma. However, information from them has provided a framework on which concepts of the role of erythropoietin in the physiological regulation of erythropoiesis are based, even though these assays are not specific for erythropoietin.

Assays are carried out in animals in which red cell formation and endogeneous secretion of erythropoietin are suppressed by starvation or polycythaemia to provide a low base line from which to detect stimulation of new red cell formation. Assays depend upon measurement of incorporation of ^{59}Fe into red cells as metameter of erythropoietin effect. The starved rat (Fried, Plzak and Jacobson, 1957; Hodgson, Perreta, Yudilevich and Eskuche, 1958) has the advantage of low cost and a short time for animal preparation but because it is less sensitive than the polycythaemic mouse the latter has replaced it for tests on plasma (Table 3).

Mice were initially made polycythaemic by transfusion (Jacobson, Goldwasser, Plzak and Fried, 1957b) but Cotes and Bangham (1961) found that the labour and cost of transfusion could be avoided by using a polycythaemia of each animals own red cells formed during exposure to air at a reduced pressure (Wright, 1964). Other methods for preparing polycythaemic mice include maintenance in a silicone rubber membrane enclosure with a difference in permeability for oxygen and carbon dioxide (Lange, Simmons and Dibelius, 1966; Ichiki and Lange, 1974), intermittent treatment with carbon monoxide (Fogh, 1966) and maintenance in air/nitrogen mixtures (Wagemaker, van Eijk and Leijnse, 1972). Practical detail and variants of these assays are described by Cotes (1973) and by Wagemaker *et al.* (1972) who developed a particularly sensitive assay system.

Problems and non-specificity in *in vivo* assays may arise from:

(i) stimulation of endogenous erythropoietin secretion, for example by androgens, tri-iodothyronine and prostaglandins (see reviews by Fisher, 1972; Garcia, 1977) or by anaemia from haemolysis induced by toxic constituents in test samples;

(ii) factors which inhibit or decrease stimulation of new red cell formation such as toxic components or drugs in urine or serum and specific inhibitors of erythropoiesis which may occur in nature as chalones (for discussion see Bateman, 1974).

A specific factor which modifies erythroid cell proliferation has been found in saline extracts of red blood cells (Lord, Shah and Lajtha, 1977). The relationship is not known between this factor and the erythropoiesis inhibiting factors (EIF) found in plasma from polycythaemic subjects brought from high altitude to sea level (Reynafarje, 1968) and in urine (Lindemann,

1971). The red cell factor of Lord *et al.* (1977) was active at a dose of 10 μg in normal mice but, under the conditions tested, it did not reduce erythropoietin-induced stimulation of incorporation of ^{59}Fe into red cells in the polycythaemic mouse. Plasma factor present in test extracts might generate erythropoietin by reaction with endogenous kidney factor in assay animals but, although anticipated, this has not been recognised as occurring.

3. *In vitro* Bioassays

In vitro bioassays based on stimulation of haem synthesis by intact and desialated erythropoietin acting in tissue cultures of rat or human bone marrow (Krantz, Gallien-Lartigue and Goldwasser, 1963; Gallien-Lartigue and Goldwasser, 1964; Krantz, 1968) have been used to monitor extracted erythropoietin but not for estimation of erythropoietin in plasma because the systems are sensitive to inhibitors or toxic constituents in plasma. Liver cells from 13 day mouse foetuses provide an alternative assay system in which ^{59}Fe incorporation into haem is increased by erythropoietin (Cole and Paul, 1966; Stephenson and Axelrad, 1971) and this was used by Wardle, Baker, Malpas and Wrigley (1973) to estimate erythropoietin in serum and plasma. Dunn, Jarvis and Greenman (1975) and Dunn and Napier (1975) modified this system but Napier, Dunn, Ford and Price (1977) emphasise that it does not respond to the same erythropoietic factors as are detected in *in vivo* assays.

Rudzki and Kimber (1978) showed that differences in iron levels between test sera invalidated estimates of serum erythropoietin in the foetal mouse liver system and May and Napier (1978) showed that it is also necessary to take account of different levels of human transferrin in sera. De Klerk, Kruiswijk, Hart and Goudsmit (1978b) and de Klerk, Hart, Kruiswijk and Goudsmit (1978a) estimate and correct for the effects of different levels of iron and transferrin in each serum and for interfering factors in each serum by use of an internal standard of erythropoietin added to each test serum. The method elegantly meets the criticisms of earlier applications of the foetal mouse liver system but is too complex for widespread use.

The development of erythroid colonies from human or mouse bone marrow *in vitro* is dependent upon, and increased by, erythroid colony stimulating activity (E-CSA) which during fractionation procedures remains associated with erythropoietin estimated *in vivo* in the polycythaemic mouse assay. Erythroid colony formation can be used as the basis of an assay for extracted erythropoietin (Iscove *et al.*, 1974). The method is no more sensitive than the polycythaemic mouse assay but may represent an advance in specificity. It might prove of value in assay of erythropoietin in plasma and urine after an initial extraction step (Sieber, 1977).

4. Immunochemical Assay

(a) Haemagglutination inhibition assay

Lange and co-workers (Lange, McDonald, Jordan, Trobaugh, Kretchmar and Chernoff, 1970; Lange, McDonald, Jordan, Mitchell and Kretchmar, 1971b) have developed a haemagglutination inhibition assay (HIA) using partially purified preparations of human urinary erythropoietin as the antigen both to coat red cells and to raise antisera. Specificity is introduced by adsorption of the antiserum with protein from urine of normal subjects (Lange, 1971) and it is difficult to assess the adequacy of this step. However, problems of non-specificity should be overcome when sufficiently highly purified antigen is used for red cell sensitisation.

There have been few direct comparisons of estimates of erythropoietin by HIA and by bioassay *in vivo* in polycythaemic mice but ranking samples in order of erythropoietin content did not give the same order for serum samples tested by each of these two methods (Lange *et al.*, 1970). The HIA has been applied to urinary erythropoietin as well as to serum erythropoietin and Ichiki and Lange (1974) used estimates by the HIA as a guide to select doses to be administered *in vivo* in a mouse assay.

(b) Radioimmunoassay

Two systems have been described for radioimmunoassay of erythropoietin in human serum and urine (Garcia, 1974; Lertora *et al.*, 1975). Assays are not widely available because of scarcity of highly purified human erythro-poietin for preparation of the homologous tracer. Although sheep plasma erythropoietin cross-reacts with antisera to human erythropoietin (Garcia and Schooley, 1963) no valid assay has yet been developed using a hetero-logous tracer. Assays have not yet been reported using the highly purified human urinary erythropoietin extracted in good yield by Miyake *et al.* (1977). So far tracer antigens have required considerable purification after radioiodination. Garcia removed components binding to antiserum to normal urine proteins and then obtained ^{125}I erythropoietin monomer by reaction with anti-erythropoietin antibody and subsequent acid dissociation of antibody bound tracer. Lertora *et al.* (1975) found immunoreactivity and biological activity associated with erythropoietin aggregates but not with monomer separated on Sephadex G-150 or G-100. As assay tracer, they used an ^{125}I erythropoietin aggregate separated on Sephadex G-150. Cotes (1974) found that heavy and lighter fractions of ^{125}I human erythropoietin separated by ultracentrifugation gave essentially similar radioimmunoassay dose displacement curves with a standard from human urine but this system did not distinguish between high and low levels of erythropoietin in pairs of plasma samples from subjects sampled respectively before and after correction of an anaemia (Cotes, unpublished). The validity of Garcia's assay is supported by the demonstration that in a normal subject erythropoietin levels estimated in plasma (by radioimmunoassay) and in urine (by bioassay *in vivo*) were increased after bleeding and decreased after transfusion.

(c) Immunoprecipitation assay

Goudsmit, Krugers, Dagneaux and Krijnen (1967) developed a radial immunoprecipitation assay system depending on the reaction of human plasma erythropoietin with an antiserum raised against rat serum erythropoietin. Estimates by it agreed well with estimates in an exhypoxic polycythaemic mouse assay and it was sufficiently sensitive to estimate erythropoietin in normal plasma. Although preliminary work with this system was encouraging it has not been confirmed.

E. LEVELS IN BODY FLUIDS

1. Normal Levels

(a) Plasma and serum

Estimates made in different assay systems are listed in Table 4. Attempts to estimate erythropoietin in plasma or serum samples from normal subjects using *in vivo* bioassay systems usually fail because of inadequate sensitivity.

Table 4

Estimates of erythropoietin in plasma or serum from normal subjects.

Method	No. of subjects	Estimate u/l	References
In vivo bioassay			
Polycythaemic mice	7	3·0–4·5	Wagemaker *et al.* (1972)
	3	< 3·0	
In vitro bioassay			
Foetal mouse liver	20 (male)	48	de Klerk *et al.* (1978a)
	18 (female)	29	
Radioimmunoassay	311 (male)	4·9 (s.e. 0·2)	Garcia (1974)
	457 (female)	4·2 (s.e. 0·2)	
	5 (female)	52–84	Lertora *et al.* (1975)
Haemagglutination inhibition	449	37 (s.e. 22)	Lange, Jordan, Ichiki and Chernoff (1971a)
Immunoprecipitation		0·5–2·0	Goudsmit *et al.* (1967)

Thus from experience in many laboratories using the polycythaemic mouse assay, it has been inferred (and estimates by Wagemaker *et al.* (1972) support this inference) that plasma levels in normal adults are usually below 25 or 50 u/l (from tests in which 2 ml plasma are administered to mice found to respond to 50 or 100 mu erythropoietin). It has been a common finding that some test plasmas from normal subjects induce stimulation of appearance of ^{59}Fe iron in red cells of test animals without inducing the increased response to be expected when a higher dose of plasma erythropoietin is administered (see for example Mirand, Weintraud, Gordon, Prentice and Grace, 1965). It must be inferred that these are non-specific responses not necessarily induced by erythropoietin. Using an unusually sensitive modification of the polycythaemic mouse assay *in vivo*, able to detect a dose 10 mu/mouse, Wagemaker *et al.* (1972), estimated serum levels in 10 normal human subjects. Doses of 3 ml serum/mouse give responses at the lowest end of the dose response curve, and although the authors' results cannot be taken to indicate unequivocal demonstration of erythropoietin, they suggest that normal serum levels are below 10 u/l.

Estimates by radioimmunoassay (Garcia, 1974) are essentially the same as those made by *in vivo* assay, whereas the haemagglutination inhibition assay gives slightly higher results (Lange, Jordon, Ichiki and Chernoff, 1971a). In 10% of normal subjects, estimates by the HIA are >60 u/l although not found by bioassay sufficiently sensitive to detect this level. Preliminary estimates by immunoprecipitation (Goudsmit *et al.*, 1967) are similar to those by bioassay *in vivo* and by radioimmunoassay.

(b) Urine

Urinary excretion of erythropoietin can be studied in concentrates of urine, and thus daily 24 hr excretion of erythropoietin by normal subjects can be estimated by bioassay *in vivo* using assays which are not sufficiently sensitive to estimate normal serum levels. Using an *in vivo* polycythaemic mouse assay, Adamson, Alexanian, Martinez and Finch (1966) found 1·2–9·5 u/24 hr urine for nine normal men and no recognisable pattern of diurnal or activity related change in excretion rate. Women and prepubertal boys seem to excrete less erythropoietin in urine than men but the differences reported are not significant (Alexanian, 1966a; Alexanian, Vaughn and Ruchelman, 1967).

2. Levels in Disease

References to estimates of erythropoietin levels in conditions associated with anaemia and with polycythaemia are listed in Tables 5 and 6. The insensitivity and poor precision of estimates preclude useful comparison

Table 5

Erythropoietin levels assessed by bioassay in vivo in clinical conditions associated with anaemia (+ = increased; ND = none detected; * = inappropriately low).

	Clinical conditions	Erythropoietin levels Serum/plasma	Urine	References
Normal erythropoietin response	Erythroid hypoplasia	+[a]	+[b]	Peschle, Marmont, Marone, Genovese, Scchetti and Condovelli (1975)[a]; Van Dyke, Layrisse, Lawrence, Garcia and Pollycove (1961)[b]
	Primary red cell aplasia	+		Marmont, Peschle, Sanguineti and Condorelli (1975)
	Bone marrow hypoplasia (aplastic anaemia)	+[c]	+[d]	Hammond, Shore and Movassaghi (1968)[c]; Van Dyke, Layrisse, Lawrence, Garcia and Polycove (1961)[d]
	Iron deficiency anaemia	+	+	Movassaghi, Shore and Hammond (1967)
	Megaloblastic anaemia	+	+	Penington (1961)
	Autoimmune haemolytic anaemia	+[e]	+[f]	Penington (1961)[e]; Van Dyke, Layrisse, Lawrence, Garcia and Pollycove (1961)[f]
	Thalassaemia major	+[g]	+[h]	Penington (1961)[g]; Winkert and Gordon (1960)[h]
	Sickle cell anaemia	+		Jones and Klingberg (1960)
	Paroxysmal nocturnal haemoglobinuria	+[i]	+[j]	Cotes and Lowe (1963)[i]; Van Dyke, Layrisse, Lawrence, Garcia and Pollycove (1961)[j]
	Malignant disease	+		Zucker, Friedman and Lysik (1974)
	Kwashiorkor	+		McKenzie, Friedman, Katz and Lanzkowsky (1967)
Abnormal erythropoietin response	Infant prematurity	+		Stockman, Garcia and Oski (1977)
	Renal disease	ND[k]	ND[l]	Naets and Heuse (1962)[k]; Penington (1961)[l]
Antibody to endogenous erythropoietin		*		Marmont, Peschle, Sanguineti and Condorelli (1975)

Table 6

Erythropoietin levels assessed by bioassay in vivo in clinical conditions associated with polycythaemia (+ = increased; ND = none detected; − = below normal).

Clinical conditions	Erythropoietin levels Serum/plasma	Urine	Tissue extract	References
Mediated by physiological erythropoietin response to tissue hypoxia				
Pulmonary disease		+		Alexanian (1978)
Abnormal haemoglobin with increased oxygen affinity		+		Adamson and Stamatoyannopoulos
Renal artery stenosis	+			Bourgoignie, Gallagher, Perry, Kurz, Warnecke and Donati (1968)
Autonomous bone marrow				
Polycythaemia rubra vera	ND[a,b]	−		DeGowin and Gurney (1964)[a]; Noyes, Domm and Willis (1962)[b]; Adamson and Finch (1968)[c]
Autonomous erythropoietin production				
Familial erythrocytosis	+[d,f]	+[d,e]		Kontras and Romshe (1967)[d]; Alperin, Levin, Alexanian and Houston (1968)[e]; Adamson, Stamatoyannopoulos, Kontras, Lascari and Detter (1973)[f]
Renal cyst	+		+	Gallagher and Donati (1968)
Hydronephrosis	+			Gallagher and Donati (1968)
Hypernephroma	+			Gallagher and Donati (1968)
Wilms tumour	+[g]		+[h]	Tharman, Grabstald and Lieberman (1966)[g]; Shalet, Holder and Walters (1967)[h]
Cerebellar haemangioma	+		+	Gallagher and Donati (1968)
Adrenal adenoma	+			Gallagher and Donati (1968)
Phaeochromocytoma			+	Waldman, Rosse and Swarm (1968)
Uterine fibromyoma	+		+	Ossias, Zanjani, Zalusky, Estren and Wasserman (1973)
Iatrogenic stimulus to erythropoietin production				
Hepatoma	+			Gordon, Zanjani and Zalusky (1970)
Androgens		+		Alexanian (1969)

of estimates made in different disease states except where the differences are considerable or where serial measurements are made in the same patient. In general, haemoglobin levels and erythropoietin levels are inversely related. Exceptions are:

(i) in the anaemia of renal disease when the erythropoietin level is lower than expected from the degree of anaemia and seldom detectable by *in vivo* bioassay;

(ii) in chronic iron deficiency anaemia when, unless the anaemia is severe, the increase in serum or plasma and urinary erythropoietin is usually lower than expected;

(iii) in occasional patients when a modest anaemia is accompanied by a very high level of erythropoietin in serum and urine. Figure 1 indicates the wide variation in estimates of serum erythropoietin which may be found at any one haemoglobin concentration (Erslev, 1977).

There are two instances in which the finding of a raised level of erythropoietin in plasma or serum may contribute to the clinical management of a patient. These are:

(i) In the differential diagnosis of polycythaemia rubra vera and a "secondary" polycythaemia. The latter is mediated by and may show an increased level of erythropoietin whereas polycythaemia rubra vera is not induced by erythropoietin over-production. Although a secondary polycythaemia follows increased availability of erythropoietin induced by tissue hypoxia, the resulting polycythaemia may have suppressed erythropoietin secretion to a level no longer detectable by assay *in vivo*. In polycythaemia rubra vera at a normal haemoglobin level, there is no hypoxia and no increase in erythropoietin secretion (Adamson and Finch, 1968).

(ii) In the investigation of an unexplained polycythaemia. If plasma or serum erythropoietin is increased, the search for an erythropoietin secreting lesion should be intensified.

Suppression tests are not used to demonstrate the autonomous nature of erythropoietin secretion by abnormal erythropoietin secreting lesions since the finding of a high level of erythropoietin with polycythaemia without an abnormal haemoglobin or evidence of generalised or regional hypoxia is diagnostic. Space occupying renal lesions may generate erythropoietin, and this is possibly a result of local hypoxia from pressure on adjacent renal tissue.

If a polycythaemia is attributed to abnormal secretion of erythropoietin it should be demonstrated that erythropoietin is present in plasma or urine in abnormally great amounts and that removal of the lesion or correction of the underlying condition is associated with a fall in plasma or urine erythropoietin as well as with correction of the polycythaemia. Tumours or lesions secreting erythropoietin autonomously may not store it, and a tumour extract will not necessarily contain erythropoietin except from the blood in it. It is not known whether all such lesions secrete intact erythropoietin or whether any produce precursor (perhaps REF) or plasma factor.

3. Conclusion

Estimates of erythropoietin in body fluids can provide information about the mechanism of control of erythropoiesis in normal and pathological conditions. However, before conclusions are drawn from estimates it is essential to appreciate their variable and often poor precision, and to question the specificity of the assay system.

REFERENCES

Abbrecht, P. H. and Greene, J. A. (1966). *Ann. int. Med.* **65**, 908.
Abbrecht, P. H. and Littell, J. K. (1972). *J. appl. Physiol.* **32**, 54.
Adamson, J. W., Alexanian, R., Martinez, C. and Finch, C. A. (1966). *Blood*, **28**, 354.
Adamson, J. W. and Finch, C. A. (1968). *Ann. N.Y. Acad. Sci.* **149**, 560.
Adamson, J. W., Hayashi, A., Stamatoyannopoulos, G. and Burger, W. F. (1972). *J. clin. Invest.* **51**, 2883.
Adamson, J. W., Parer, J. T. and Stamatoyannopoulos, G. (1969). *J. clin. Invest.* **48**, 1376.
Adamson, J. W. and Stamatoyannopoulos, G. (1967). *Blood*, **30**, 848.
Adamson, J. W., Stamatoyannopoulos, G., Kontras, K., Lascari, A. and Detter, J. (1973). *Blood*, **41**, 641.
Albert, A. (1968). *J. clin. Endocr*, **28**, 1683.
Alexanian, R. (1966a). *Blood*, **28**, 344.
Alexanian, R. (1966b). *Blood*, **28**, 1007.
Alexanian, R. (1978). *In* "Kidney Hormones. 2. Erythropoetin" (J. W. Fisher, ed.), p. 533. Academic Press, London and New York.
Alexanian, R., Vaughn, W. K. and Ruchelman, M. W. (1967). *J. Lab. clin. Med.* **70**, 777.
Alperin, J. B., Levin, W. C., Alexanian, R. and Houston, E. W. (1968). *Clin. Res.* **16**, 40.
Annable, L., Cotes, P. M. and Mussett, M. V. (1972). *Bull. Wld. Hlth Org.* **47**, 99.
Bateman, A. E. (1974). *Cell Tissue Kinet.* **7**, 451.
Bell, N. H. (1974). *Acta endrocr., Copenh.* **77**, 604.
Bourgoignie, J. J., Gallagher, N. I. Perry, Jr., H. M., Kurz, L., Warnecke, M. A. and Donati, R. M. (1968). *J. Lab. clin. Med.* **71**, 523.
Camiscoli, J. F., Weintraub, A. H. and Gordon, A. S. (1968). *Ann. N.Y. Acad. Sci.* **149**, 40.
Carmena, A., Garcia de Testa, N. and Frias, F. L. (1967). *Proc. Soc. exp. Biol.* **125**, 441.
Cole, R. J. and Paul, J. (1966). *J. Embryol. exp. Morph.* **15**, 245.
Contrera, J. F., Gordon, A. S. and Weintraub, A. H. (1966). *Science*, **152**, 653.
Cotes, P. M. (1973). *In* "Methods in Investigative and Diagnostic Endocrinology. 2. Peptide Hormones" (S. A. Berson and F. S. Yalow, eds), p. 1110. North Holland Publishing Co., Amsterdam.

R

Cotes, P. M. (1974). *Horm. metab. Res.* (Suppl. Ser. 5), 35.

Cotes, P. M. and Bangham, D. R. (1961). *Nature, Lond.* **191**, 1065.

Cotes, P. M. and Bangham, D. R. (1966). *Bull. Wld. Hlth Org.* **35**, 751.

Cotes. P. M. and Lowe, R. D. (1963). *In* "Hormones and the Kidney" (P. C. Williams, ed.), p. 187. Adacemic Press, London and New York.

De Gowin, R. L. and Gurney, C. W. (1964). *Arch. int. Med.* **114**, 424.

De Klerk, G., Hart, A. A. M., Kruiswijk, C. and Goudsmit, R. (1978a). *Blood*, **52**, 569.

De Klerk, G., Kruiswijk, C., Hart, A. A. M. and Goudsmit, R. (1978b). *Blood*, **52**, 560.

De Klerk, G., Otten-Kruiswijk, C. and Goudsmit, R. (1977). *Br. J. Haemat.* **35**, 672.

Denny, W. F., Flanigan, W. J. and Zukoski, C. F. (1966). *J. Lab. clin. Med.* **67**, 386.

Dorado, M., Espada, J., Langton, A. A. and Brandan, N. C. (1974). *Biochem. Med.* **10**, 1.

Dukes, P. P., Hammond, D. and Shore, N. A. (1969). *J. Lab. clin. Med.* **74**, 250.

Dukes, P. P., Hammond, D., Shore, N. A. and Ortega, J. A. (1971). *Israel J. med. Sci.* **7**, 919.

Dunn, C. D. R., Jarvis, J. H. and Greenman, J. M. (1975). *Exp. Hemat.* **3**, 65.

Dunn, C. D. R. and Napier, J. A. F. (1975). *Exp. Hemat.* **3**, 362.

Erslev, A. J. (1977). *In* "Kidney Hormones. 2. Erythropoietin" (J. W. Fisher, ed.), p.571. Academic Press, London and New York.

Esbach, J. W., Funk, D., Adamson, J., Kuhn, I., Scribner, B. H. and Finch, C. A. (1967). *New Engl. J. Med.* **276**, 653.

Espada, J. (1977). *In* "Kidney Hormones. 2. Erythropoietin" (J. W. Fisher, ed.), p. 37. Academic Press, London and New York.

Espada, J. and Gutnisky, A. (1970). *Acta physiol. Lat. Am.* **20**, 122.

Espada, J., Langton, A. A. and Dorado, M. (1972). *Biochim. biophys. Acta*, **285**, 427.

Fink, G. D. and Fisher, J. W. (1975). *Fed. Proc.* **34**, 805.

Fisher, J. W. (1972). *Pharmacol. Rev.* **24**, 459.

Fisher, J. W. and Langston, J. W. (1967). *Blood*, **29**, 114.

Fisher, J. W., Stuckey, W. J., Lindholm, D. D. and Abshire, S. (1971). *Israel J. med. Sci.* **7**, 991.

Fogh, J. (1966). *Scand. J. clin. Lab. Invest.* **18**, 33.

Fried, W., Plzak, L. F., Jacobson, L. O. and Goldwasser, E. (1957). *Proc. Soc. exp. Biol.* **94**, 237.

Gallagher, N. I. and Donati, R. M. (1968). *Ann. N. Y. Acad. Sci.* **149**, 528.

Gallagher, N. I., McCarthy, J. M. and Lange, R. D. (1960). *Ann. int. Med.* **52**, 1201.

Gallien-Lartigue, O. and Goldwasser, E. (1964). *Science*, **145**, 277.

Garcia, J. C. (1972). *In* "Regulation of Erythropoiesis" (A. S. Gordon, M. Condorelli and C. Peschle, eds), p. 132. Publishing House Ponte, Milan.

Garcia, J. F. (1974). *In* "Radioimmunoassay and Related Procedures in Medicine", Vol. I, p. 275. IAEA, Vienna.

Garcia, J. F. (1977). *In* "Kidney Hormones. 2. Erythropoietin" (J. W. Fisher, ed.), p. 7. Academic Press, London and New York.

Garcia, J. F. and Schooley, J. C. (1963). *Proc. Soc. exp. Biol.* **112**, 712.

Goldwasser, E. (1975a). *Fed. Proc.* **34**, 2285.

Goldwasser, E. (1975b). *In* "Erythropoiesis" (K. Nakao, J. W. Fisher and F. Takaku, eds), p. 75. University Park Press, Baltimore, London and Tokyo.

Goldwasser, E. and Kung, C. K. H. (1968). *Ann. N.Y. Acad. Sci.* **149**, 49.

Goldwasser, E. and Kung, C. K. H. (1971a). *Proc. natn. Acad. Sci. USA*, **68**, 697.

Goldwasser, E. and Kung, C. K. H. (1971b). *In* "Regulation of Erythropoiesis" (A. S. Gordon, M. Condorelli and C. Peschle, eds). p. 159. Il Ponte, Milan.

Gordon, A. S. (1959). *Physiol. Rev.* **39**, 1.

Gordon, A. S. and Zanjani, E. S. (1971). *Israel J. med. Sci.* **7**, 963.

Gordon, A. S., Piliero, S. J., Medici, P. T., Siegel, C. D. and Tannenbaum, M. (1956). *Proc. Soc. exp. Biol.* **92**, 598.

Gordon, A. S., Zanjani, E. D. and Zalusky, R. (1970). *Blood*, **35**, 151.

Goudsmit, R., Krugers Dagneaux, P. G. L. C. and Krijnen, H. W. (1967). *Folia. med. Neerl.* **10**, 39.

Gross, M. and Goldwasser, E. (1969). *Biochemistry*, **8**, 1795.

Gross, M. and Goldwasser, E. (1971). *J. biol. Chem.* **246**, 2480.

Hammond, D., Shore, N. and Movassaghi, N. (1968). *Ann. N.Y. Acad. Sci.* **149**, 516.

Hodgson, G., Perreta, M., Yudilevich, D. and Eskuche, I. (1968). *Proc. Soc. exp. Biol. N.Y.* **99**, 137.

Hoffman, G. C. (1968). *Ann. N.Y. Acad. Sci.* **149**, 504.

Ichiki, A. T. and Lange, R. D. (1974). *Biochem. Med.* **10**, 50.

Iscove, N. N., Sieber, F. and Winterhalter, K. H. (1974). *J. cell Physiol* **83**, 309.

Jacobson, L. O., Goldwasser, E., Fried, W. and Plzak, L. (1957a). *Nature, Lond.* **179**, 633.

Jacobson, L. O., Goldwasser, E., Plzak, L. F. and Fried, W. (1957b). *Proc. Soc. exp. Biol.* **94**, 243.

Jones, B. and Klingberg, W. G. (1960). *J. Pediatr.* **56**, 752.

Kawakita, M., Miyake, T. and Kishimoto, S. (1975). *In* "Erythropoiesis" (K. Nakao, J. W. Fisher and F. Takaku, eds), p. 55. University Park Press, Baltimore, London and Tokyo.

Kontras, S. B. and Romshe, C. (1967). *Am. J. Dis. Child.* **113**, 473.

Krantz, S. B. (1965). *Life Sci.*, **4**, 2393.

Krantz, S. B. (1968). *J. Lab. clin. Med.* **71**, 999.

Krantz, S. B., Gallien-Lartigne, O. and Goldwasser, E. (1963). *J. biol. Chem* **238**, 4085.

Krantz, S. B. and Jacobson, L. O. (1970). "Erythropoietin and the Regulation of Erythropoiesis", p. 27. University of Chicago Press, Chicago and London.

Kurokawa, K. and Massry, S. G. (1973). *Proc. Soc. exp. Biol.* **143**, 123.

Kuratowska, Z., Lewartowska, B., Lipmiski, B. (1964). *J. Lab. clin. Med.* **64**, 226.

Kuratowska, Z., Lewartowski, B. and Michalak, E. (1961). *Blood*, **18**, 527.

Lajtha, L. J. (1975). *Br. J. Haemat.* **29**, 529.

Lange, R. D. (1971). *In* "Kidney Hormones" (J. W. Fisher, ed.), p. 373. Academic Press, London and New York.

Lange, R. D., Jordon, T. A., Ichiki, A. T. and Chernoff, A. I. (1971a). *In* "Regulation of Erythropoiesis" (A. S. Gordon and M. Condorelli, eds), p. 107. Il Ponte, Milan.

Lange, R. D., McDonald, T. P., Jordan, T. A., Mitchell, T. J. and Kretchmar, A. L. (1971b). *Israel J. med. Sci.* **7**, 861.

Lange, R. D., McDonald, T. P., Jordan, T. A., Trobaugh, Jr., F. E., Kretchmar, A. L. and Chernoff, A. I. (1970). *In* "Hemopoetic Cellular Proliferation" (F. Stohlman Jr., ed.), p. 122. Grune and Stratton, New York and London.

Lange, R. D., Simmons, M. L. and Dibelius, N. R. (1966). *Proc. Soc. exp. Biol.* **122**, 761.

Lertora, J. J. L., Dargon. P. A.. Rege, A. B. and Fisher. J. W. (1975). *J. Lab. clin. Med.* **86**, 140.

Lindemann, R. (1971). *Br. J. Haemat*, **21**, 623.

Lord, B. I., Shah, G. P. and Lajtha, L. G. (1977). *Cell Tissue Kinet.* **10**, 215.

Lowy, P. H., Keighley, G. and Borsook, H. (1960). *Nature, Lond.* **185**, 102.

Lukowsky, W. and Painter, R. H. (1968). *Can. J. Biochem.* **46**, 731.

Lukowsky, W. A. and Painter, R. H. (1972). *Can. J. Biochem.* **50**, 909.

496   P. M. COTES AND D. F. GUÈRET WARDLE

Malgor, L. A. and Fisher, J. W. (1970). *Am. J. Physiol.* **218**, 1732.
Marmont, A., Peschle, C., Sanguineti, M. and Condorelli, M. (1975). *Blood*, **45**, 247.
Martelo, O. J., Toro, E. F. and Hirsch, J. (1976). *J. Lab. clin. Med.* **87**, 83.
Marver, D. and Gurney, C. W. (1968). *Ann. N.Y. Acad. Sci.* **149**, 570.
May, A. and Napier, J. A. F. (1978). *Br. J. Haemat.* **40**, 162.
McDonald, T. P., Zanjani, E. D., Lange, R. D. and Gordon, A. S. (1971). *Br. J. Haemat.* **20**, 113.
McKenzie, D., Friedman, R., Katz, S. and Lanzkowsky, P. (1967). *S. Af. med. J.* **41**, 1094.
Miller, M. E., Rorth, M., Parving, H. H., Howard, D., Reddington, I., Valeri, C. R. and Stohlman Jr., F. (1973). *New Engl. J. Med.* **288**, 706.
Mirand, E. A., Murphy, G. P., Steeves, R. A., Weber, H. W. and Retief, F. P. (1968). *Acta haemat.* **39**, 359.
Mirand, E. A. and Murphy, G. P. (1969). *J. Am. med. Assoc.* **209**, 392
Mirand, E. A., Weintraub, A. H., Gordon, A. S., Prentice, T. C. and Grace, J. T. (1965). *Proc. Soc. exp. Biol.* **118**, 823.
Miyake, T., Kung, C. K.-H. and Goldwasser, E. (1977). *J. biol. Chem.* **252**, 5558.
Morell, A. G., Gregoriadis, G., Scheinberg, I. H., Hickman, J. and Ashwell, G. (1971). *J. biol. Chem.* **246**, 1461.
Movassaghi, N., Shore, N. A. and Hammond, D. (1967). *Proc. Soc. Exp. Biol.* **126**, 615.
Naets, J.-P. (1958). *Nature, Lond.* **182**, 1516.
Naets, J.-P. (1960). *Proc. Soc. exp. Biol.* **103**, 129.
Naets, J.-P. and Heuse, A.-F. (1962). *J. Lab. clin. Med.* **60**, 365.
Naets, J.-P. and Wittek, M. (1968). *Blood*, **31**, 249.
Napier, J. A. F., Dunn, C. D. R., Ford, T. W. and Price, V. (1977). *Br. J. Haemat.* **35**, 403.
Nečas, E. and Neuwirt, J. (1969). *Life Sci.* **8**, 1221.
Nienhuis, A. W., Barker, J. E. and Anderson, W. F. (1977). *In* "Kidney Hormones. 2. Erythropoietin" (J. W. Fisher, ed.), p. 245. Academic Press, London and New York.
Noyes, W. D., Domm, B. M. and Willis, L. C. (1962). *Blood*, **20**, 9.
Olesen, H. and Fogh, J. (1968). *Scand. J. Haemat.* **5**, 211.
Ossias, A. L., Zanjani, E. D., Zalusky, R., Estren, S. and Wasserman, L. R. (1973). *Br. J. Haemat.* **25**, 179.
O'Sullivan, M. B., Chiba, Y., Gleich, G. J. and Linman, J. W. (1970). *J. Lab. clin. Med.* **75**, 771.
Paulo, L. G., Wilkerson, R. D., Roh, B. L., George, W. J. and Fisher, J. W. (1973). *Proc. Soc. exp. Biol.* **142**, 771.
Penington, D. G. (1861). *Lancet*, **i**, 301.
Penington, D. G. (1963). *In* "Hormones and the Kidney" (P. C. Williams, ed.), p. 201. Academic Press, London and New York.
Peschle, C. and Condorelli, M. (1975). *Science*, **190**, 910.
Peschle, C., Marmont, A. H., Marone, G., Genovese, A., Sachetti, L. and Condorelli, M. (1975). *In* "Erythropoisis" (K. Nakao, J. W. Fisher and F. Takaku, eds), p. 489. University Park Press, Baltimore, London and Tokyo.
Raich, P. C. and Korst, D. R. (1978). *Arch. Path. lab. Med.* **102**, 73.
Rambach, W. A., Alt, H. L. and Cooper, J. A. D. (1961). *Proc. Soc. exp. Biol.* **108**, 793.
Reissman, K. R., Nomura, T., Gunn, R. W. and Brosius, F. (1960). *Blood*, **16**, 1411.
Reynafarje, C. (1968). *Ann. N. Y. Acad. Sci.* **149**, 472.

Rodgers, G. M., Fisher, J. W. and George, W. J. (1974a). *J. Pharmacol. exp. Ther.* **190**, 542.

Rodgers, G. M., Fisher, J. W. and George, W. J. (1974b). *Proc. Soc. Exp. Biol.* **145**, ⁓ 1207.

Rodgers, G. M., Fisher, J. W. and George, W. J. (1975). *Am. J. Physiol.* **229**, 1387.

Rodgers, G. M., George, W. J. and Fisher, J. W. (1972). *Proc. Soc. exp. Biol.* **140**, 977.

Rokicinski, M., Rudzki, Z. and Kimber, R. J. (1978). *Br. J. Haemat.* **38**, 425.

Rosse, W. F., Berry, R. J. and Waldmann, T. A. (1963). *J. clin. Invest.* **42**, 124.

Schooley, J. C. and Mahlmann, L. J. (1971). *Proc. Soc. exp. Biol.* **138**, 523.

Schooley, J. C., Zanjani, E. D. and Gordon, A. S. (1970). *Blood,* **40**, 662.

Shalet, M. F., Holder, T. M. and Walters, T. R. (1967). *J. Pediatr.* **70**, 615.

Shelton, R. N., Ichiki, A. T. and Lange, R. D. (1975). *Biochem. Med.* **12**, 45.

Sherwood, J. B. and Goldwasser, E. (1978). *Endocrinology,* **103**, 866.

Sieber, F. (1977). *Biochim. biophys. Acta,* **496**, 146.

Siri, W. E., Van Dyke, D. C., Winchell, H. S., Pollycove, M., Parker, H. G. and Cleveland, A. S. (1966). *J. appl. Physiol.* **21**, 73.

Spivak, J. L., Small, D. and Hollenberg, M. D. (1977). *Proc. natn Acad. Sci. USA,* **74**, 4633.

Stephenson, J. R. and Axelrod, A. A. (1971). *Endocrinology,* **88**, 1519.

Stockman III, J. A., Garcia, J. F. and Oski, F. A. (1977). *New Engl. J. Med.* **296**, 647.

Storring, P. L. and Fatah, S. (1975). *Biochim. biophys. Acta,* **392**, 26.

Terada, M. Cantor, L., Metafora, S., Rifkind, R., Banks, A. and Marks, P. A. (1972). *Proc. natn. Acad. Sci. USA,* **69**, 3575.

Thurman, W. G., Grabstald, H. and Leberman, P. H. (1966). *Arch. int. Med.* **117**, 280.

Van Dyke, D. C. (1960). *In* "Haemopoiesis, Cell Production and its Regulation" (G. E. W. Wolstenholme and M. O'Connor, eds), p. 397. Churchill, London.

Van Dyke, D. C., Layrisse, M., Lawrence, J. H., Garcia, J. F. and Pollycove, M. (1961). *Blood,* **18**, 187.

Van Zant, G. and Goldwasser, ⌐. (1977). *Science,* **198**, 733.

Wagemaker, G., Van Eijk, H. G. and Leijnse, B. (1972). *Clin. chim. Acta,* **36**, 357.

Waldmann, T. A., Rosse, W. F. and Swarm, R. L. (1968). *Ann. N.Y. Acad. Sci.* **149**, 509.

Wardle, D. F. H., Baker, I., Malpas, J. S. and Wrigley, P. F. M. (1973). *Br. J. Haemat.* **24**, 49.

Winkert, J. W. and Gordon, A. S. (1960). *Proc. Soc. Exp. Biol.* **104**, 713.

Wright, B. M. (1964) *Br. J. Haemat.* **10**, 75.

Zanjani, E. D., Cooper, G. W., Gordon, A. S., Wong, K. K. and Scribner, V. A. (1967). *Proc. Soc. exp. Biol.* **126**, 540.

Zanjani, E. D., McLaurin, W. D., Gordon, A. S., Rappaport, I. A., Gibbs, J. M. and Gidari, A. S. (1971). *J. Lab. clin. Med.* **77**, 751.

Zanjani, E. D. Poster, J., Mann, L. I. and Wasserman, L. R. (1977). *In* "Kidney Hormones. 2. Erythropoietin" (J. W. Fisher, ed.), p. 463. Academic Press, London and New York.

Zucker, S., Friedman, S. and Lysik, R. M. (1974). *J. clin. Invest.* **53**, 1132.

XI. Pituitary Thyroid-stimulating Hormone and Other Thyroid-stimulating Substances

P. G. CONDLIFFE and B. D. WEINTRAUB

INTRODUCTION

Thyroid-stimulating hormone, thyrotrophin (TSH), is a glycoprotein found in the pituitary gland of all vertebrates which activates the thyroid in every species of vertebrate so far tested. It was discovered by Smith and Smith (1922) who found that extracts of fresh bovine pituitary glands would reactivate the atrophied thyroids of hypophysectomised tadpoles. Other thyroid-stimulating substances of non-pituitary origin have been described. Some of these, such as the thyroid stimulator found in metastasising choriocarcinomas (Odell, Bates, Rivlin, Lipsett and Hertz, 1963) are related chemically to TSH isolated from the pituitary. Others such as the long acting thyroid-stimulator (Adams and Purves, 1956) are unrelated chemically and can be sharply differentiated from the glycoprotein hormones, including TSH, by immuno-chemical techniques and other chemical and biological criteria.

Since the second edition of this book, published in 1967, our knowledge of glycoprotein hormones has been completely revolutionised. Today we know that thyroid-stimulating hormones are part of a group of hetero-polymeric glycoproteins which have two different subunits of approximately the same size. These subunits have been isolated, their amino acid sequences determined, their chemical and many of their biological properties well characterised for several vertebrate species, including man. Hybrid molecules comprised of subunits from different hormones, such as TSH or follicle-stimulating hormone (FSH) have been prepared. Interspecies hybrids have been prepared and their biological properties tested. As a result we can say that there are two distinct types of subunit now designated α and β; that the α type is shared in common by all the glycoprotein hormones; that the hormonal differences, observed as differing biological activities, depend on the β type which confers biological specificity or hormonal specificity on the molecule.

In this article the convention suggested by Fontaine (1967) and used widely by others, has been adopted in which the species of origin is designated by a lower case prefix, using the systematic Latin name of the species. Thus, human (homo) TSH is abbreviated hTSH, cattle (bos) as bTSH, sheep (oves) as oTSH, pig (sus) as sTSH, mouse (mus) as mTSH, etc.

The principal physiological effect of TSH is to stimulate the rate at which the thyroid produces its hormones. The mechanism by which this effect is accomplished involves a series of physico-chemical reactions beginning, as originally demonstrated by Pastan, Roth and Macchia (1966), with the binding of the hormone to a specific site on the surface of the thyroid cell. After the reaction of TSH with its binding site, various biochemical and morpho-logical effects quickly manifest themselves. Interference with the binding by alteration or destruction of the site, by reagents such as antibodies to

TSH or analogues of TSH without biological activity, will prevent the initiation of the biochemical events leading to increased production of thyroid hormone. For a detailed discussion of thyroid biochemistry and the internal mechanisms of thyroid cells, the reader is referred to Field (1975).

Much of the material that will be discussed in this chapter has been extensively reviewed elsewhere. Reviews by Kirkham (1966), Pierce, Carsten and Wynston (1960) and Bates and Condliffe (1960, 1966) should be mentioned. Informed reviews of the state of knowledge of LATS have appeared by Dorrington and Munro (1966) and McKenzie (1967, 1968). Pierce (1974) has reviewed the chemistry of TSH. A later paper by Pierce *et al.* (1976b) on the structure and function of the glycoprotein hormones presents a particularly valuable discussion of chemical relationships between the compounds of this class.

Several problems present themselves in any consideration of a hormone in blood. First, is the circulating form of the hormone the same as that which is found in the gland where it is synthesised and stored? Second, what is its concentration under normal circumstances and under what circumstances will this concentration vary and in what direction? Third, does the circulating form interact directly with its receptor site or is some conversion step required?

It is necessary, therefore, to consider the properties of pituitary TSH in order to discuss the available information about blood TSH in a rational manner. The importance of knowing in what chemical form the hormone may exist has been shown by the work on the long acting thyroid-stimulator (LATS) which is now known to be a 7S globulin similar to the IgG class of γ-globulins.

In evaluating data on the concentration of TSH in blood, one must examine critically the assay methods used to obtain them. The introduction of the U.S.P. reference standard of bovine origin in 1952, and the redefinition and equating of the U.S.P. and international units of thyroid-stimulating activity (Mussett and Perry, 1955) made it possible to compare results published by different investigators.

As a result of comparisons using this international reference standard of bovine origin, the marked species specificity of TSH became obvious (Bakke, 1965a, b). In order to overcome problems related to immunoassays arising from this species specificity, TSH standards of human origin are now available from the Division of Biological Standards, National Institute for Medical Research, MRC, Mill Hill, London, acting on behalf of the International Standards Committee of the World Health Organization (WHO). These various standards are described in the section below. The importance of stating results in terms of standardised units of TSH activity and of avoiding the introduction of biological units should be emphasised.

A. CHEMICAL CONSTITUTION AND PHYSICAL PROPERTIES OF TSH

The first attempts to isolate TSH came in 1931 when Janssen and Loeser (1931) used trichloroacetic acid to separate TSH from insoluble impurities. Following their work other investigators applied salt fractionation techniques to the problem as well as fractionation with organic solvents such as acetone. Albert (1949) concluded that the most active preparations of TSH made during this period, from 1931–1945, were probably about 100–300 times as potent as the starting material. Much of this early work has been reviewed by White (1944), Albert (1949), and Bates and Condliffe (1960). Developments to about 1957 have been discussed by Sonenberg (1958). Over the past 20 years the application of chromatography, gel filtration and other modern techniques has led to further purification of the hormone. The most active preparations that have been obtained in various laboratories appear to be at least 2000 times as potent as the starting material.

1. Standard Preparations and Units of Thyroid-stimulating Activity

(a) The Junkman–Schoeller unit

Before the adoption of an international reference standard preparation, thyroid-stimulating activity was expressed in terms of biological responses. Various biological units were employed. Of these the most useful and the most widely used was the Junkmann–Schoeller unit (JSU) (Junkmann and Schoeller, 1932). This was defined as the smallest daily dose of TSH required to produce a histologically detectable response in the guinea-pig thyroid. The histological response was graded as 0–3 plus after the animals had been injected with TSH for three days. A JSU produces a 2-plus response in half of the animals injected.

(b) The bovine standards

To facilitate comparison of results from different laboratories, an international unit was adopted in 1955 (Mussett and Perry, 1955). This unit was defined as the activity present in 13·5 mg of the international standard. The international unit is equipotent with the U.S.P. unit adopted in 1952 which had been defined as the activity present in 20 mg of the U.S.P. reference substance.

In terms of the international unit defined as above, the JSU appears to be approximately 0·1 international unit. Where results cited in this review were originally given in JSU they have been converted to international units on the basis of 10 JSU = 1 international bovine unit (bu) (Hays and Steelman, 1955; Bakke and Lawrence, 1956; Querido and Lameyer, 1956).

(c) *Human pituitary standards and reagents*

Because of the species specificity, human thyrotrophin standards have been adopted by the Biological Standards Expert Committee of the World Health Organization. Standardised reference preparations A and B are available from the National Institute of Biological Standard, MRC, Mill Hill, London.

The WHO standards A and B are intended as primary reference materials. For working purposes hTSH standards, calibrated in terms of the human reference standards, together with immunoassay agents are available from the Hormone Distribution Program of the National Institute of Arthritis, Metabolism, and Digestive Diseases, Bethesda, Maryland, USA. Similar working standards and kits of immunoassay materials for hTSH are available from commercial sources.

2. Chemical Constitution of TSH and its Subunits

After the discovery by Li and Starman (1964) that the sedimentation rate of oLH decreased from 3·0–2·0 when the hormone was examined in the ultra-centrifuge at pH 1·8, several groups of scientists demonstrated that under acid conditions, or in the presence of concentrated urea, luteinising hormone (LH) dissociates to yield two subunits of approximately the same mass but with different amino acid and carbohydrate compositions (Papkoff and Samy, 1967; Lamkin, Fujino, Mayfield, Holcomb and Ward, 1970). Hormonal activity disappears when the molecule is disaggregated. The hormonal activity can be regenerated from the disaggregated subunits in solution by adjusting the pH to neutrality and by removal of the urea or other disaggregating agent (de Llosa, Courte and Jutisz, 1967).

After the demonstration that LH could be dissociated, many attempts were made to demonstrate the existence of similar subunits in other glyco-proteins including TSH. In 1969 Condliffe reported that when bTSH was treated with acid the sedimentation rate decreased from 2·85–2·0. The mw of the acid-treated bTSH was estimated to be about 15,000 by density gradient centrifugation and gel filtration, or half the value found at neutral pH (Condliffe, 1969). These and other results led to the speculation that like LH, TSH was comprised of two subunits. However, this speculation could not be confirmed until Pierce and his collaborators showed that not only is TSH composed of two non-identical subunits but that one of them is either the same as or similar to, the CI subunit previously found in LH. In a brilliant series of papers Pierce and his collaborators revolutionised our ideas about the pituitary glycoprotein hormones by showing that bTSH dissociates at acid pH to yield two non-identical subunits of approximately equal mass; that one of these subunits, now termed TSH_α is either the same as or similar to the α-subunits of bLH; that the other, designated TSH_β, confers hormonal specificity on the whole TSH molecule; that under the right conditions the separated, inactive subunits will reassociate to form hormonally active TSH; that hybrid molecules can be formed between the α-subunit of one hormone and the β-subunit of another, the resulting hybrid having hormonal activity determined by the β-subunit; that the subunits are combined in the active hormone by non-covalent interactions and that the disulphide bonds are intrachain rather than interchain. A complete review of these relationships has appeared by Pierce et al. (1976b).

3. Human TSH (hTSH)

Human TSH was first isolated in purified form in 1963 (Condliffe, 1963); in terms of the bovine standard the potency of this highly purified hTSH was 20 bovine units (bu)/mg when first isolated, but the preparation was unstable (see below). This preparation was used for immunochemical studies by Utiger et al (1963) which led ultimately to development of a radioimmunoassay for hTSH. Despite the fall in biological activity the immunochemical properties of the preparation did not appear to change during the immunochemical studies. Later studies by Giudice and Pierce (1977) have shown that there are non-functional β-subunits of hTSH and bTSH which will react with antisera to TSH and to antisera against the β-subunits yet will not recombine with TSH_α subunits to yield the active hormone.

The concentration of hTSH has been reported to be ca 2×10^{-2} bu/mg dry weight in a lyophilised pool of several hundred pituitaries. These estimates were obtained by the chick assay (Bates and Condliffe, 1960). Other reports have indicated that the TSH content of human pituitaries is considerably lower. Thus Bakke and Lawrence (1959) and Bakke, Kammer and Lawrence (1964) found ca 2×10^{-3} bu/mg using the bovine slice weight technique. This kind of discrepancy is probably due to the species specificity of TSH or to differences in the handling of the glands. As pointed out by Fontaine and Fontaine (1962) and Bates and Condliffe (1966), assay of this hormone from one species can give a different result depending upon the species in which it is assayed when the unknown and the standard are prepared from different species.

(a) Isolation

Heidemann, Bakke and Lawrence (1959) were able to show with limited starting material that hTSH like bTSH could be absorbed to the synthetic cation exchange resin IRC-50. Studies by Limanova (1962a, b) also showed that hTSH could be adsorbed to carboxymethyl cellulose (CMC) and diethyl-aminoethyl cellulose (DEAEC) and then eluted in a purified state.

After these early studies, Condliffe (1963) prepared hTSH with a potency of 20 u/mg, using as starting material Reisfeld's fraction E (Reisfeld, Lewis, Brink and Steelman, 1962) obtained during the purification of human growth hormone. The method used was first equilibration on Sephadex G-50 at pH 6 in 0·01 M sodium phosphate buffer followed by adsorption to CMC. The unabsorbed fraction contained the bulk of the FSH (Parlow, Condliffe, Reichert and Wilhelmi, 1965), whereas TSH was retained on the column. The TSH was readily eluted from CMC by a linear gradient to 1 M NaCl. It emerged from the column when the conductivity reached a value of 4 ohms^{-3} in contrast to bTSH which is not displaced from CMC until the conductivity of the gradient reaches 8–10 ohms^{-3}. The bovine hormone thus appeared to be more basic than the hTSH. Later studies on the amino acid composition and primary structure of hTSH have confirmed this difference (Pierce, 1974).

This difference in behaviour during ion exchange chromatography was confirmed by experiments on DEAEC where hTSH was more tightly bound than bTSH (Condliffe, 1963; Stockell-Hartree, Butt and Kirkham, 1964). The highest potency reported for hTSH is 20 bovine u/mg (Condliffe, 1963); however the preparation lost 50% of its activity in the three months after its isolation. This loss occurred during storage as a dry powder at 2°.

After these early studies Bates et al. (1968) prepared hTSH, hLH, hFSH and human growth hormone (hGH) from acetone-dried human pituitaries by the following steps: the finely milled glands were extracted by percolation (Bates, Garrison and Howard, 1959 (50% ethanol–5% NaCl) followed by water. The 50% ethanol–5% NaCl solvent front contained most of the hTSH hLH and hFSH. hTSH and hLH were separated from hFSH and most of the contaminating hGH by adsorption of the hTSH and hLH at pH 6 on carboxymethyl-cellulose. The hTSH was then separated from hLH by adsorbing the hTSH on diethylaminoethyl cellulose at pH 9·5 at low ionic strength. A hLH fraction with a potency of 5·5 mg equivalents of NIH-LH-S-1/mg was obtained that had a hTSH activity of only 0·01 human u/mg. The hTSH preparation recovered by gradient elution, had a potency of 17 bovine u/mg and contained less than 0·165 sheep units/mg LH. About 170 mg of hTSH was recovered from 10,000 pituitaries. Using the chick assay of Bates and Cornfield (1957) and the hTSH international reference standard A the preparation had a potency of 10·4 human u/mg.

Purified hTSH has been prepared by several groups using somewhat different methods of extraction but relying on sequential chromatographic steps on cellulosic ion exchangers combined with gel filtration for final separation of hTSH from the other hormones yielding essentially similar results (Stockell-Hartree *et al.*, 1964; Cornell and Pierce, 1973; Sairam and Li, 1977a). In all these procedures the hTSH obtained is contaminated with small amounts of hLH which, while not significant from a chemical point of view, being less than 1% by weight, are troublesome in radioimmunoassay procedures. As will be described in a later section on radioimmunoassay of hTSH this difficulty can be solved in part by adsorption of the anti-hTSH antisera with hCG (Odell *et al.*, 1965a). The cross-reactivity between hTSH and other glycoproteins which share the α-subunit can also be reduced by developing antisera to the β-subunit separated and purified from disaggregated hTSH (Vaitukatis, Ross, Pierce, Cornell and Reichert, 1973).

(b) Homogeneity

Human, like bovine TSH exhibits microheterogeneity when examined by gel electrophoresis (Shome, Parlow, Ramirez, Elrick and Pierce, 1968a). The causes of this microheterogeneity is most probably variation in the amino terminal sequence of the β-subunit, differences in conformation which do not interfere with the biological activity could be variations in the subunits of a minor nature. From recent work of Giudice and Pierce (1977) it is known that there are non-functional subunits which arise during extraction and purification. An additional source of this type of heterogeneity is variation in the carbohydrate composition of the hormone e.g. between bTSH and hTSH (see below); for example there is a difference in that sialic acid is missing in bTSH, whereas hTSH has one residue. Furthermore, if this single sialic acid residue is removed there is no change in the biological activity of hTSH (Shome *et al.*, 1968b).

(c) Subunit structure of hTSH

After the demonstration of bTSH subunits by Pierce and Liao (1970), Cornell and Pierce (1973) applied the same techniques to hTSH prepared by a modification of the procedure of Stockell-Hartree (1966). After dissociation in 1 M propionic acid the subunits were separated by gel filtration on 300 × 2·5 cm columns of Sephadex G-100 in 0·126 M ammonium bicarbonate. The α- and β-subunits were isolated in the same relative positions on the column as were those from the bovine hormone.

Recombination experiments showed that TSH activity could be regenerated and that hybrids could be formed between human and bovine subunits with the regenerated activity being dependent upon the β-subunit.

Another method for separating the subunits of hTSH is that of Sairam and Li (1973) who used counter-current distribution after dissociating the hormone in 0·05 M HCl and 8 M urea (pH 2·8). The dissociated hTSH was then distributed in a two-phase system consisting of 40% $(NH_4)SO_4$ (w/v): 0·2% dichloroacetic acid: n-propanol: ethanol (60:60:27:33 by vol.). After nine transfers the β-subunit which moved with the upper mainly organic phase almost completely separated from the α-subunit which remained in the stationary or aqueous phase.

(d) Molecular weight and other properties

When examined by density gradient ultracentrifugation, hTSH had a sedimentation coefficient of 2·9 S (Condliffe, unpublished). This figure is close to that reported by Fontaine and Condliffe (1963a) for bTSH. From this single experiment a mw of 28,000 was calculated for hTSH relative to pepsinogen, the molecular weight of which is known. This result is consistent with the fact that during the purification hTSH and bTSH were indistinguishable in gel filtration on Sephadex G-100 (Condliffe, 1963).

Shome, Brown, Howard and Pierce (1968a) determined the mw of human, bovine and porcine TSH to be 28,000 by sedimentation velocity and diffusion. Some evidence of aggregation was found. Sedimentation equilibrium studies of the bovine hormone gave an extrapolated mw of 25,000 and there was evidence that bTSH behaved like a reversible aggregating system. This agreed with the experiments of Condliffe (1969) who showed that when bTSH was treated with 0·1 M HCl and then centrifuged in a sucrose density gradient the sedimentation coefficient decreased from 2·8–2·05. Sairam and Li (1977a) have redetermined the sedimentation coefficient of human TSH and report a value of 2·84 at pH 8·2. At pH 1·5 a value of 2·01S was found. The mw of hTSH was computed to be 28,900 from structural date (Sairam and Li, 1977). The computed mw of $hTSH_\alpha$ and $hTSH_\beta$ were 14,400 and 14,500 (Sairam and Li, 1977b).

The amino acid composition and primary structure of hTSH has been completely determined by Sairam and Li (1977a). Table 1 shows the amino acid composition of purified human and bovine TSH. hTSH differs from bovine and several other species in having a lower lysine content. It contains only 13 lysine residues per 28,000 mw as opposed to 19 for cattle. This together with the finding of Cornell and Pierce (1973) that hTSH, unlike bTSH, contains at least one residue of sialic acid/molecule explains the difference in isoelectric point between bovine and human thyrotrophin.

The hTSH-β-subunit has the same sequence as does bTSH-β except for differences at positions 43, 65, 67, 77, 79 and 109 as shown in Fig. 2 (taken from Pierce *et al.*, 1976a). With one or two exceptions in the amino acid sequence, the α chains from both species are identical.

Table 1

Amino acid composition of hTSH and bTSH in residues per molecule from sequence data.

Amino acid	Human (Sairam and Lee, 1977a)			Bovine (from Pierce, 1974)		
	α	β	TOTAL	α	β	TOTAL
Lysine	6	7	13	10	9	19
Histidine	3	3	6	3	3	6
Arginine	3	5	8	3	4	7
Aspartic acid	1	6	7	1	7	3
Asparagine	4	3	7	5	2	12
Threonine	8	11	19	9	11	20
Serine	8	5	13	6	5	11
Glutamic acid	3	5	8	3	5	8
Glutamine	6	2	8	5	2	7
Proline	6	7	13	7	7	14
Glycine	4	4	8	4	4	8
Alanine	4	6	10	7	6	13
Half cystine	10	12	22	10	12	22
Valine	7	4	11	5	6	11
Methionine	3	2	5	4	5	9
Isoleucine	1	9	10	2	6	8
Leucine	4	6	10	2	4	6
Tyrosine	4	11	15	5	11	16
Phenylalanine	4	4	8	5	4	9
TOTAL	89	112	201	96	113	209

(e) Carbohydrate composition

hTSH contains approximately 21·1 % carbohydrate by weight compared with 14% for bTSH (Hara, Rathnam and Saxena, 1978). Like bTSH there are three carbohydrate moieties, two attached to the α-subunit through asparagine at positions 49 and 75 and one attached to the β-subunit through the asparagine residue at position 23. hTSH contains two sialic acid residues in contrast to bTSH which has less than 0·1 residue/mole. Sairam and Li (1977a) have shown that both sialic acid residues are located in the carbohydrate attached to the α-subunit. Hara *et al.* (1978) have proposed a common structure for the glycopeptides from the α-subunits of LH, TSH and FSH in which branching occurs through a mannose residue. Removal of sialic acid from hTSH does not affect its biological or immunological activity (Shome *et al.*, 1968b).

(*f*) *Activity in human subjects*

Bovine TSH has long been known to stimulate the human thyroid (Hays, Solomon, Pierce and Carsten, 1961). hTSH has been tested in patients by the same ^{131}I uptake technique and was found to be active (Schneider, Robbins and Condliffe, 1965). In terms of the bovine reference preparation by assay in chicks (Bates and Cornfield, 1957) a unit of hTSH had the same effect in man as did a unit of bTSH.

4. Bovine TSH (bTSH)

While there is today much more known about hTSH than was the case a decade ago, most of our knowledge of the chemistry of TSH is based upon studies with the bovine hormone.

(*a*) *Extraction*

The method of Cieresko (1945) based upon extraction of pituitary glands with 2% NaCl at 2° and pH 7 has been widely used. After the initial extraction half of the TSH activity can be recovered by acetone fractionation between 50% (v/v) and 75% (v/v). Material with a potency of 1 bovine unit/mg is obtained.

Bates, Garrison and Howard (1959) devised a technique in which a filter-bed of anterior pituitary powder mixed with a filter aid is percolated with a succession of solvents starting with 95% ethanol and proceeding stepwise with solutions of increasingly aqueous character and salt concentration. TSH is extracted by the step to 57% ethanol, 5% NaCl. The procedure can be carried out at 25° and with minimal volumes of solvent. The yield is higher than in the method of Cieresko and takes less time. The potency of the bTSH prepared by percolation is between 1 and 2 bu/mg.

(*b*) *Counter-current distribution*

Counter-current distribution has been used by Pierce and his collaborators (Pierce, 1974) to remove impurities from crude fractions of TSH before purification by chromatography and gel filtration. The TSH is precipitated at the interface of the system *n*-butanol-*p*-toluene sulfonic acid (Pierce and Carsten 1957).

(*c*) *Chromatographic studies*

Early studies showed that bTSH could be adsorbed to synthetic cation exchangers at pH 6–7 from solutions of low ionic strength (Heidemann 1953; Crigler and Waugh, 1955; Condliffe and Bates 1956; Pierce and Nye, 1956).

Condliffe and Bates (1956) introduced the use of carboxymethyl cellulose (CMC) which has a greater capacity to bind TSH than does the synthetic ion exchanger IRC-50. Similar chromatographic patterns are obtained with either exchanger. bTSH is adsorbed at pH 6 on columns equilibrated with 0·01 sodium phosphate buffers. FSH activity is not adsorbed under these conditions, a finding made use of in later studies on the purification of hTSH and hFSH (Condliffe, 1963; Parlow et al., 1965). bTSH was eluted from the column together with bLH by raising the ionic strength with a gradient to 1 M NaCl or by simple stepwise elution. Preparations of 5 bu/mg were recovered. Further purification was obtained with the anion exchanger diethylaminoethyl cellulose (Condliffe and Bates, 1957). Fractions with a potency of 5 bu/mg prepared by chromatography on CMC were placed on DEAEC columns at pH 9·5 in 0·01 M glycine buffer. Most of the bLH was unadsorbed under these conditions (Condliffe, Bates and Fraps, 1959) and could be recovered in purified form by rechromatography on CMC. These procedures were subsequently exploited for the purification of hLH/hFSH and hTSH (Condliffe, 1963; Bates, Garrison, Cooper and Condliffe, 1968; Parlow, Condliffe, Reichert and Wilhelmi, 1965). This use of DEAEC for the separation of TSH and LH for several species is still the method of choice when combined with chromatography on CMC and gel filtration (Sairam and Li, 1977a).

(d) Gel filtration

The use of gel filtration for the purification of TSH was introduced by Condliffe and Porath (1962). They showed that bTSH prepared by sequential chromatography on CMC and DEAEC could be further purified by gel filtration on Sephadex G-100. Incorporation of gel filtration into purification procedures for TSH accomplishes several purposes in addition to purification of the hormone on the basis of molecular size. Solutions of the hormone can be desalted before lyophilisation and the hormone can be equilibrated with appropriate buffers in preparation for ion-exchange chromatography as described by Porath and Flodin (1959). For desalting it is necessary to use a volatile buffer such as ammonium bicarbonate since TSH is adsorbed to the Sephadex in distilled water. The volatile buffer can be subsequently removed by lyophilisation.

Pierce et al. (1971) have used gel filtration in combination with counter-current distribution to prepare bTSH which is virtually completely free of traces of active bLH. Using a solvent system which dissociates bLH the bTSH is recovered with the α-chain of bLH. The β-chain of bLH and the remaining bFSH was separated during the counter-current distribution procedure. Since the bLH_{α} is half the size of the undissociated bTSH it was separated from the bTSH by gel filtration. The disadvantage of this procedure is that it does not yield active bLH but in order to obtain bTSH free of bLH for immunochemical study the procedure has considerable utility.

(e) Electrophoresis

No systematic studies of highly purified bTSH by free electrophoresis have been reported. Many studies using gel electrophoresis have shown that highly purified bTSH preparations contain several biologically active components which can be isolated by careful rechromatography on DEAEC (Carsten and Pierce, 1960) or by recovering the separated bTSH components from polyacrylamide gels after electrophoresis at pH 8·5 (Condliffe and Mochizuki, 1965). Within the experimental error the amino acid composition of these various active components is the same (Pierce, Carsten and Wynston, 1960). Fawcett, Dedman and Morris (1969) separated the components of bTSH by electrofocusing. Preliminary analysis indicated differences in the carbohydrate composition of the different components. They also found several active components in extracts of single bovine pituitary glands so that the polymorphism is not an artefact of isolation. Immunoelectrophoresis of extracts of single glands likewise showed polymorphism (Goetinck and Pierce, 1966). Similar findings have been reported for a single whale gland by Ui and Tamura (1966). Ui has recently published a series of studies on bovine LH and thyrotrophin using electrofocusing to separate the biologically active components of bTSH that were prepared by chromatography on DEAEC. Five bTSH components were identified having isoelectric points of 7·2, 7·0, 8·32, 8·60 and 8·95. These figures differ slightly from those reported by Fawcett et al. (1969) who studied relatively crude pituitary extracts.

(f) Affinity chromatography

Several reports have appeared within the last three years using specific adsorbents for the purification of glycoprotein hormones including TSH. Ui, Yora, Takahashi and Condliffe (1977) used Concanavalin-A Sepharose to adsorb the glycoprotein hormones from crude fractions prepared by percolation. Bloomfield, Faith and Pierce (1978) have employed Concanavalin A-Sepharose in two modifications of their isolation procedures. In both, Concanavalin A-Sepharose was used to adsorb the glycoproteins from crude extracts before fractionation by ion-exchange chromatography and gel filtration. The latter authors used the method to isolate the glycoprotein hormones from a single gland. Again, as with other studies of single glands there was evidence of polymorphism in the final product although the degree was variable.

Following their earlier work on Concanavalin A, Yora and Ui (1978) used the lectin for group separation of the glycoprotein hormones obtaining fractions which yielded five fractions with immunological reactivity in a radioimmuno assay for bTSH. Final purification of the bTSH was achieved by removing immunologically reactive bLH by affinity chromatography on a Sepharose 4 B column to which had been coupled anti-LH antibodies. The separated components prepared by isoelectric focusing (see Section A.4.e) were individually chromatographed on the affinity column. 80%–95% of the TSH activity measured by immunoassay was recovered while the LH contamination was reduced by a factor of a thousand or more. Clearly the development of a similar bioaffinity procedure for TSH will be useful for the study of the individual components of active TSH in all species.

(g) Composition and structure

Ten years ago virtually nothing was known about the structure of TSH. Today (as discussed earlier) the hormone is known to be comprised of two different subunits. The primary structure of each subunit has been determined except for the location of the disulphide bonds within each chain.

(1) *Amino acid composition.* The amino acid composition of the complete hormone is given for hTSH and bTSH in Table 1. Included are the compositions of the individual subunits. The data are taken from sequence data rather than from amino acid analysis. Significant differences are apparent. The bovine hormone has five more basic residues than does the human. Overall the human hormone has seven fewer amino acid residues than the bovine and this difference is entirely due to the α-chain. Notwithstanding this difference in length of the chain, hybrids between hTSH and bTSH have been prepared as have hybrids between bTSH and hTSH.

(2) *Primary structure and amino acid sequence.* The sequences of the α-subunit from bovine and human TSH are shown in Fig. 1. The α-subunits from other glycoprotein hormones bear a close resemblance to hTSHα and bTSHα. From the fact that, so far as can be determined, any α-subunit can substitute for another in recombination and hybridisation experiments to regenerate hormonal activity, it can be presumed that all the α-subunits from various hormones have a very similar secondary and tertiary structure for recombination to take place.

In contrast to the α-subunits, the β-subunits from different hormones differ considerably as is seen in Fig. 2. In this figure taken from Pierce (1976) the ordering of the various chains is relative to bovine and ovine LHβ in order to maximise the homology. In particular the half cystine residues are aligned and blank spaces are inserted for the same reason. Parentheses indicate uncertainty or alignment based on composition only.

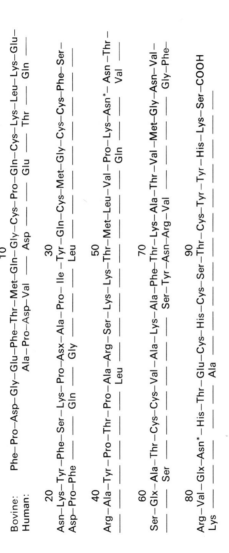

Fig. 1. Amino acid sequences of α-subunits of glycoprotein hormones. From Pierce (1976). The sequence of ovine LH-α is the same as that of bovine α; that of porcine LH-α differs in three positions from that of the bovine ovine subunit (–Leu–Glu– at 25–26 and Ala at 78); —— indicates identical residues in the human and bovine ovine sequences.

```
                        10                                              20
hTSH-β    Phe —  Ile —  Thr-Glx-Tyr-(Met, Thr, His, Val,-  )Arg-Arg-Glx —— Ala-
pTSH-β    Phe —  Ile —  Thr-Glu-Tyr-Met-Met-His-Val ——  Arg-Lys-Glu —— Ala-
bTSH-β    Phe —  Ile —  Thr-Glu-Tyr-Met-Met-His-Val ——  Arg-Lys-Glu —— Ala-
b,oLH-β   Ser-Arg-Gly-Pro-Leu-Arg-Pro-Leu-Cys-Gln-Pro-Ile-Asn-Ala-Thr-Leu-Ala-Ala-Glu-Lys-Glu-Ala-Cys-Pro-
pLH-β                    Arg                                                    Asp
hLH-β     — Glx —  — Trp —  — Gly —  — Val —  Gly —
hCG-β     Lys-Gln —  — Arg —  — Asx-Ala-Ile —  — Val —  Gly —
hFSH-β    ——(Asx-Ser) —  Glu-Leu-Thr —  Ile —  Ile —  Glu —— Arg-

                        30                                              40
hTSH-β    Tyr —  Leu —  Ile-Asn —  Thr —— |  Met, Thr)Arg-Asx-Ile-Asx-Gly-Lys-Leu-Phe-
pTSH-β    Tyr —  Leu —  Val-Asn-Ser ——  Met-Thr-Arg-Asx-Phe-Asx-Gly-Lys-Leu-Phe-
bTSH-β    Tyr —  Leu —  Ile-Asn-Thr-Val ——  Met-Thr-Arg-Asx-Val-Asx-Gly-Lys-Leu-Phe-
b,oLH-β   Val-Cys-Ile-Thr-Phe-Thr-Thr-Ser-Ile-Cys-Ala-Gly-Tyr-Cys-Pro-Ser-Met-Lys-Arg-Val-Leu-Pro-Val-Ile-
pLH-β                                                          Arg ——   — Ala-Ala-
hLH-β     — |  — |  Val-Asx — |  Thr — |  — Thr ——  Arg(Met)Leu —  Glx-Ala-Val-
hCG-β     — |  — |  Val-Asn — |  Thr — |  — Thr ——  Thr —  Gln-Gly-Val-
hFSH-β    Phe —  — Ser-Ile-Asn —  Thr( †) — |  Tyr-Lys-Arg-Asp-Leu —  Tyr-Lys-Asp-Pro-

                        50                              60                              70
hTSH-β    Lys-Tyr-Ala-Leu-Ser —  Asx — |  Arg-Asp-Phe-Ile-Tyr-Arg-Thr —  Glx-Ile —
pTSH-β    Lys-Tyr-Ala-Leu-Ser —  Asx — |  Arg-Asp-Phe-Met-Tyr-Lys-Thr-Val-Glx-Ile —
bTSH-β    Lys-Tyr-Ala-Leu-Ser —  Asp — |  Arg-Asp-Phe-Met-Tyr-Lys-Thr-Ala-Glu-Ile —
b,oLH-β   Leu-Pro-Pro   Met-Pro —  Gln-Arg-Val-Cys-Thr-Tyr-His-Glu-Leu-Arg-Phe-Ala-Ser-Val-Arg-Leu-Pro-
pLH-β     — |  Val — |  Pro —  — Arg-Glu —  Ile —  Ser —
hLH-β     — |  Val — |  Pro —  — Arg-Asx-Val —  Glx —  Ile —
hCG-β     — |  Ala —  Leu —  — Arg-Asp-Val —  Glu —  Ile —
hFSH-β    Ala-Lys-Pro-Arg-Ile —  Lys-Thr —  Phe-Lys-Glu —  Val-Tyr-Glu-Thr —  Val —
```

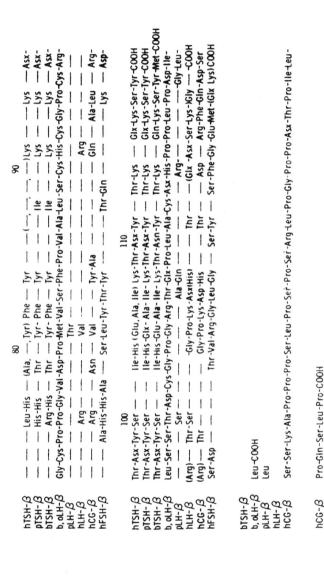

Fig. 2. Amino acid sequences of β-subunits of glycoprotein hormones. Some sequences are incomplete in ordering of peptides, amide assignments and incomplete sequences. Bovine–ovine LH-β is used as the reference sequence. A ─── indicates identical residues and a blank space a deletion to obtain maximum homology. Parentheses indicate areas of uncertainty or alignment based on composition only; · indicates residues to which carbohydrate is attached. Because of limitations of space, sequences of procine TSH and LH which are similar but not identical to bovine TSH and LH are omitted. From Pierce (1976).

(3) *Dissociation and recombination.* As mentioned earlier many efforts were made to show that TSH like LH is comprised of two different subunits.

Success was achieved finally when Liao and Pierce (1970) showed that after treatment of bTSH with 1 M propionic acid the reaction mixture could be separated into three components by gel filtration (Fig. 3). The three components seen in Fig. 3 were found to be undissociated TSH followed by two components termed α and β which we now know to be the bTSHα and bTSHβ subunits. Since this demonstration of the disaggregation of TSH in 1 M propionic acid others have shown that the dissociation is pH dependent. Using a fluorescent probe 1,8 anilino-napthylsulphonic acid,

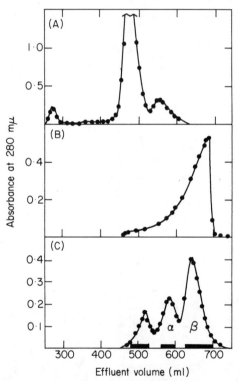

Fig. 3. The separation of the subunits of bovine TSH by gel filtration on Sephadex G-100 after treatment with propionic acid. (A) gel filtration in the presence of 0·126 M ammonium bicarbonate; TSH activity is in the large peak. (B) gel filtration through the same column in the presence of 1 M propionic acid. No separation into two components is obvious (C) the pattern given by the same material, after removal of the propionic acid by freeze-drying, when again subjected to gel filtration in the presence of ammonium bicarbonate. (Bars) fractions taken for analysis. From Liao and Pierce (1970).

Ingham, Aloj and Edelhoch (1974) found that the rate of dissociation followed first order reaction kinetics and was pH and temperature dependent. The dissociation into subunits was accompanied by changes in configuration of both subunits. Unlike hCG and hLH, bTSH is relatively insensitive to the effect of urea or guanidine hydrochloride.

Fractionation of the subunits was originally carried out by Pierce and collaborators by gel filtration on long columns two or more metres in length. Sairam and Li (1973) showed subsequently that the subunits can be separated by a simple counter-current distribution system (see Section A.2.c).

The separated, purified subunits of TSH will recombine to regenerate biological and immunological activity (Liao and Pierce (1970). These authors demonstrated not only that the α-chains from bTSH and bLH could combine with bTSHβ to form TSH but that the bTSHα could recombine with bLHβ or oLHβ to yield LH activity.

5. TSH in Other Species

Pituitary TSH has been studied in several other species beside the human and bovine. oTSH resembles bTSH in its behaviour on DEAEC columns and in gel electrophoresis. Several active components were detected (Wynston et al., 1960). During chromatography on the cation exchange IRC-50, Ellis (1958) found that sheep TSH contained two active components, one of which appeared to be derived from the other during chromatography.

Whale TSH was prepared by Pierce and his colleagues (Wynston et al., 1960) and shown to be a glycoprotein with similar properties to b and oTSH. Ui and collaborators used electrofocusing to separate and purify four components of Sei-whale TSH with isoelectric points of 8·13, 8·30, 8·57 and 8·73. The separated components showed a single band when examined by disc electrophoresis (Tamura and Ui, 1970; Tamura and Ui, 1972; Tamura-Takahashi and Ui, 1976). They were also able to show that these components exist in a single pituitary gland. Rat TSH was isolated by Fontaine and Burzawa-Gerard (1968).

Hennen, Winand and Nizet (1965) prepared hog TSH (sTSH) by a method similar to that of Condliffe et al. (1959). Their preparation of sTSH was found to cross-react immunochemically with hTSH by Goetinck and Pierce (1966).

Furth (1955) has described several types of transplantable hormone-producing tumour in mice. Two strains of mTSH-producing tumour have been studied extensively by Bates, Anderson and Furth (1957), who found that they still retained their hormonal potency after five generations of transfer and contained as much thyroid-stimulating activity/mg as did the original tumour and the same as normal mouse pituitary tissue. Tumours have been harvested from several generations of transplants of these original tumour lines as well as from new tumour lines. The mTSH has been extracted and purified (Bates and Condliffe, 1960; Condliffe *et al.*, 1969). During chromatography on CMC at pH 6, a substantial part of the mTSH in either Ciereszko type extracts, or in percolates, was unadsorbed. These acidic components were considerably less active than the main fraction when further purified (Condliffe *et al.*, 1969). The main fraction, obtained by gel filtration on Sephadex G-100 chromatography on CMC, had a potency of 68 bu/mg. Its amino acid composition differed from that of hTSH and bTSH. Its carbohydrate composition was particularly interesting since it contained galactose instead of mannose and there was little or no galactosamine.

TSH has also been studied in lower vertebrates. From studies of Fontaine and Fontaine (1962) fish pituitary extracts are known to exert little or no effect on mammalian thyroids. When eel TSH was isolated it was not surprising that it differed considerably in its composition and appeared to have considerably less secondary and tertiary structure than the mammalian thyrotrophins (Fontaine and Condliffe, 1963b).

Apart from these studies on fish TSH, a number of studies have been conducted on fish gonadotrophins from salmon (*Oncorynchus tshawytscha*) (Donaldson, 1973), carp (*Cyprinus carpiol* L) (Burzawa-Gerard and Fontaine, 1972), and the snapping turtle (*Chelydia serpenterria*) (Licht and Papkoff, 1974). Idler, Bazar and Hwang (1975) used affinity chromatography to isolate gonadotrophins from chum salmon. The fish and reptilian gonadotrophins exhibit polymorphism of the sort observed in glycoprotein hormones from higher vertebrates. Burzawa-Gerard (1974) showed that carp gonadotrophin dissociates and reassociates in the same manner as do other vertebrate glycoprotein hormones. After unfolding of the tertiary structure Pierce, Faith and Donaldson (1976a), using antibodies to reduced carboxymethylated hTSHα and to reduced carboxymethylated bTSHα, were able to show cross-reactivity with unfolded salmon LH suggesting considerable homology between the α-subunit of these widely separated species.

6. Chemical and Physical Properties of LATS* and other Thyroid-stimulating Immunoglobulins

(a) *Definition and assay*

In a series of papers Adams and Purves (1953, 1955, 1957) described a method for the assay of TSH by following the rise in protein-bound iodine in the blood after intravenous injection of the hormone into guinea-pigs. This

---

* Although it is appreciated that the use of the terms long-acting thyroid-stimulator (LATS) and thyroid-stimulating immunoglobulin (TSI) are not ideal, and may be controversial, there is as yet no international agreement on nomenclature, and they have been retained and used in this chapter for this reason.

assay is described in detail later (see Section C.2.c). McKenzie (1958) modified this procedure by using the mouse. Today this assay procedure, especially in its modified version, is widely used, not only because of its sensitivity but particularly because through its use the abnormal long-acting thyroid stimulator (LATS) can be detected.

Adams and Purves (1956) applied their assay procedure to the problem of detecting TSH in human sera. They had established that in the "normal" response to bovine pituitary TSH, the ^{131}I level in the guinea-pig's blood, whose thyroid was prelabelled with the isotope, reached a maximum 3–5 hr after injection of the hormone. When human sera were assayed two types of response were observed. Sera from hypothyroid patients gave a "normal" time response. When hyperthyroid sera were injected intravenously into the guinea-pigs a maximum level of ^{131}I in the blood was not reached for 16–24 hr.

McKenzie (1958) was able to confirm this finding, using the mouse as the test animal instead of the guinea-pig. Thus the existence of LATS could be demonstrated in two species of animal after injection of hyperthyroid serum. These findings are illustrated in Fig. 4.

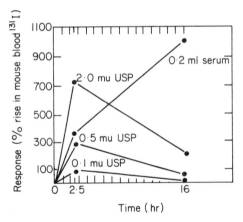

Fig. 4. The response in the McKenzie mouse assay method of the USP Thyrotrophin Reference Standard at three dosage levels and at two time intervals after intravenous injection is contrasted with that of LATS in serum from a thyrotoxic patient. From Adams (1958).

(b) Fractionation of hyperthyroid serum

LATS has been found in the serum of thyrotoxic patients. Attempts to demonstrate it in pituitary tissue taken from either euthyroid or hyperthyroid patients have not been successful, as has been summarised by Dorrington and Munro (1966) and McKenzie (1967). Considerable circumstantial evidence (Becker, Furth, Nunez, Horwith, Stokes, Berman and Ray, 1961; Becker and Furth, 1965) suggests that LATS persists in the blood of hypophysectomised patients suffering from hyperthyroidism. Hypophysectomy does not appear to relieve the disease. Two reports have appeared that LATS can be found in urine (Burger, Studer and Wyss, 1965; Pinchera, Pinchera and Stanbury, 1965).

The failure to demonstrate a pituitary origin for LATS began a search for the real site of origin. The development of ideas concerning the probable site of origin has been greatly influenced by the study of the chemical properties of LATS. All of these studies show that LATS activity can be recovered from the 7S γ-globulin fraction of hyperthyroid serum. Thus McKenzie (1962a) showed that during chromatography on Sephadex G-200, considerable LATS activity was present in the 7S fraction. Adams and Kennedy (1962) also demonstrated the association of LATS with γ-globulin. Bovine and human pituitary TSH have sedimentation coefficients of 2·8S (Fontaine and Condliffe, 1963; P. G. Condliffe, unpublished data) and when filtered on Sephadex G-100 or G-200 emerge after albumin (Condliffe and Porath, 1962). Percolation of hyperthyroid sera appears to destroy LATS although normal TSH can be extracted this way (Adams and Purves, 1961). Meek, Jones, Lewis and Vanderlaan (1964) have described a 10 fold purification of LATS by salt fractionation and chromatography on DEAEC during which LATS activity was recovered in the γ-globulin fraction. Kriss et al. (1964b) also reported the association of LATS activity with the 7S γ-globulin fraction by hyperthyroid serum (Kriss, Pieshakov and Koblin, 1964). Furthermore, Meek et al. (1964) showed that the thyroid-stimulating activity is associated with the A chain of the γ-globulin fraction after reduction with mercaptoethanol and separation of the chains by gel filtration on Sephadex G-75. After papain digestion, the LATS was located in fragment I of the A chain which has been found to contain antibody activity. These findings have been independently confirmed by others. Thus Dorrington, Carneiro and Munro (1965, 1966) also showed that LATS is a 7S γ-globulin; however they found that during reduction with mercaptoethanol, papain digestion and separation of the fragments, there was considerable loss of activity. What activity remained was associated with the "slow" fragment of the A chain in substantial agreement with the results of Meek et al. (1964).

Both Dorrington et al. (1965) and Meek et al. (1964) have reported that proteolytic digestion of LATS as described above alters the time course of LATS action in the McKenzie assay. Proteolysis leading to production of the A chain fragments reduces the mw of the active LATS from 150,000 to approximately 50,000. The peak of activity is then reached at about 3 hr instead of 10–20 hr after injection. The long acting time course thus appears to be related to molecular size.

Using the cytochemical assay of Bitensky *et al.* (1974), Petersen, Smith and Hall (1976) showed that serum from patients with Graves' disease had two zones of thyroid stimulating activity when examined by gel filtration on G-200. The 4S zone of activity proved to be pituitary TSH with the characteristic short time of action. The 7S fraction had a delayed response similar to LATS. Fab fragments prepared from IgG if patients with Graves' disease had a delayed response in the Bitensky assay similar to that of intact IgG in contrast to the earlier findings of Dorrington *et al.* (1964) and Meek *et al.* (1964) who found that reduction in size of the A chain fragment of LATS shortened the response time in the McKenzie assay.

Serum thyroid-stimulating immunoglobulins (TSI), including LATS, from patients with Graves' disease bind to thyroid plasma membrane receptors for TSH (Smith and Hall, 1974). Newer methods for measuring TSH will be discussed in Section D.6.

(c) Immunochemical studies

Convincing evidence that TSH and TSI differ has been obtained by immunological studies. McKenzie and Fishman (1960) showed that an anti-bovine TSH serum could not inhibit LATS although it was capable of blocking bTSH. Adams, Kennedy, Purves and Sirett (1962) showed that neither anti-TSH nor anti-TSH sera can neutralise LATS. These observations have been extended by Meek *et al.* (1964) and Kriss, Pleshakov, Rosenblum and Chien (1965) who have not only shown that anti-TSH serum will not react against TSI but that anti-γ-globulin, which is active against TSI, will not react with TSH.

Smith, Munro and Dorrington (1969) studied the TSI fractions obtained by chromatography of Graves disease serum on DEAE-Sephadex by immunoelectrophoresis and immunodiffusion. TSI activity was associated with the 7S γ-globulin and was adsorbed by thyroid homogenates in keeping with later studies by Yamashita and Field (1972) who showed that TSI could stimulate the adenyl cyclase activity of thyroid plasma membranes. No TSI activity was associated with the γM-globulin fraction of Graves' serum.

B. TSH BIOSYNTHESIS AND SECRETION

1. Biosynthesis

Early studies of TSH biosynthesis involved the incorporation of labelled alanine or glucosamine into immunoprecipable TSH by normal pituitary gland explants (Wilber and Utiger, 1969a; Wilber, 1971). However, the nature of the labelled immunoprecipitable material was not characterised by physico-chemical methods in these initial studies. Recently the mechanism of TSH biosynthesis has been greatly clarified by investigators using serially transplanted mouse thyrotrophic hormone-producing tumours (Furth, Moy, Hershman and Ueda, 1973) to provide a large number of relatively pure thyrotrophs (Blackman, Gershengorn and Weintraub, 1978). A combination of cell-free and intact cell studies have elucidated precursor–product relationships among heterogeneous forms of TSH subunits and complete TSH (Kourides and Weintraub, 1978; Weintraub and Stannard, 1978; Chin, Habener, Kieffer and Maloof, 1978).

mRNA has been extracted from the thyrotrophic tumours and initially translated in a heterologous wheat germ system that is devoid of enzymes necessary for carbohydrate attachment or for the proteolytic cleavage of polypeptide precursors. From 25–50% of the total protein synthesised by such methods is a protein of mw 14,000 that is closely related to standard TSH-α on the basis of immunoprecipitation (Kourides and Weintraub, 1978) and tryptic peptide (Chin *et al.*, 1978) analysis. This 14,000 α form has a smaller apparent mw than standard α (21,000 in SDS gels) but can be processed to a more normal α form by purified dog pancreatic membranes or by a frog oocyte translating system. Preliminary evidence suggests that the 14,000 α form contains no carbohydrate but contains a 3000 mw "pre" or "signal" peptide sequence that is necessary for attachment to membranes of the endoplasmic reticulum. Presumably, *in vivo* or *in vitro* processing involves both carbohydrate attachment and proteolytic cleavage of the "signal" peptide. Although the chemical structure of this putative α precursor has not yet been established, the structure of an analogous pre-α form in chorionic gonadotrophin (hCG) biosynthesis has been partially elucidated (Landefeld, McWilliams and Boime, 1976; Birken, Fetherston, Desmond, Canfield and Boime, 1978). The hCG-pre-α peptide contains a 24-amino acid, hydrophobic signal peptide extension at the N-terminus, but no "propeptide" piece containing trypsin-sensitive, basic amino acids.

Although the TSH pre-α peptide is smaller than the normal α form and does not react immunologically with TSH-β, free TSH-β has not yet been clearly identified in the cell free synthetic studies. Similarly, the hCG-β subunit has not yet been identified in such studies. These data suggest that there is excess α-subunit compared with TSH-β RNA in glycoprotein hormone-synthesising tissues. Such a hypothesis is consistent with a number of observations of excess unlabelled free α-subunits compared with free TSH-β-subunits in such tissues (Kourides, Weintraub, Ridgway and Maloof, 1975a; Hagen and McNeilly, 1975; Vaitukaitis, Ross, Braunstein and Rayford, 1976).

TSH biosynthesis by the thyrotrophic tumour has also been studied in whole dispersed cells (Weintraub and Stannard, 1978) and in tumour explants

(Chin *et al.*, 1978) using pulse-chase methods to determine precursor–product relationships. In dispersed cells, the earliest immunoprecipitable materials detected by a 10 min pulse of ^{35}S-methionine were intracellular small α forms of mw 14,000–17,000 probably representing core-glycosylated TSH-α cleaved of the signal peptide. When the 10 min pulse was followed by a chase of excess unlabelled methionine the TSH-α progressively shifted to slightly higher molecular weight forms (presumably reflecting progressive glycosylation) and complete TSH first appeared within 30 min. Fully glycosylated TSH and excess free TSH-α were not secreted until 1–2 hr and by 4 hr most of the labelled material was secreted. No free TSH-β was detected, implying that the β-subunit is limiting and is immediately combined with TSH-α to form TSH (Weintraub and Stannard, 1978).

There is no direct biosynthetic evidence for any large molecular weight TSH precursor containing both the α and β sequences in its structure. Although large molecular weight forms of TSH or TSH-β have been described (Vanhaelst and Golstein-Golaire, 1976; Klug and Adelman, 1977; Erhardt and Scriba, 1977; Kourides, Weintraub and Maloof, 1978), these forms are likely to represent disulphide-linked aggregates. It is the authors' experience that such glycoprotein hormone or subunit aggregates may be very resistant to dissociation unless complete reduction is performed in the presence of denaturants (Weintraub, Krauth, Rosen and Rabson, 1975), conditions that invariably destroy TSH biological and immunological activity (Kourides *et al.*, 1978).

In view of the likelihood of separate α- and β-subunit synthesis, it will be important to elucidate any factors coordinating the synthesis of the two subunits. Similarly, the mechanisms of intracellular glycosylation, subunit combination, and secretion will be important to define.

2. Control of TSH Secretion

Many of the factors controlling TSH secretion have been elucidated in man and will be discussed further in the section on human TSH radioimmunoassay (see below). In general, TSH secretion is derived exclusively from amphophilic or chromophobic thyrotrophs of the anterior pituitary (Russfield, 1955; Purves and Griesbach, 1957) and is regulated by a complex feedback system involving positive and negative factors from hypophyseal portal blood as well as from the systemic circulation. The principal stimulatory factor from the hypothalamus appears to be the tripeptide, thyrotrophin-releasing hormone and the principal hypothalamic inhibitory factor appears to be the tetradecapeptide, somatostatin. These hypothalamic hormones probably regulate TSH secretion by rapid (within minutes) intracellular effects not involving *de novo* protein synthesis (Wilber and Utiger, 1968). Although the detailed mechanisms of these rapid effects are still to be elucidated, it is likely that they involve hormone binding to specific membrane receptors followed by changes in intracellular ion and cyclic nucleotide concentrations, at least in certain important subcellular compartments (Wilber, Peake and Utiger, 1969; Bowers, 1971; Labrie, Barden, Poirier and DeLean, 1972; Grant, Vale and Guillemin, 1972; Curry and Bennett, 1974). The principal inhibitory factors in the systemic circulation appear to be the thyroid hormones, thyroxine (T_4) and triiodothyronine (T_3), although glucocorticoids are inhibitory under certain conditions (see Sections D.3–6). Thyroid hormones exert their inhibitory action more slowly (over hours) than somatostatin and their action may involve the *de novo* biosynthesis of an inhibitory protein (Bowers, Lee and Schally, 1968). However, no such protein has as yet been identified. There do not appear to be major stimulatory factors in the systemic circulation, although oestrogens may stimulate TSH secretion under certain circumstances (Ramey, Burrow, Polack-Wich and Donabedian, 1975; DeLean, Ferland, Drouin, Kelly and Labrie, 1977). There also does not appear to be any "short loop" feedback of TSH upon its own secretion (Nelson, Johnson and Odell, 1972).

Thyrotrophin-releasing hormone (TRH) was the first hypothalamic hormone purified, chemically characterised and synthesised. These achievements resulted from a laborious purification of the material from hundreds of thousand of porcine hypothalami by Schally and co-workers (Boler, Enzmann, Folers, Bowers and Schally, 1969) and from ovine hypothalami by Guillemin and co-workers (Burgus, Dunn, Desiderio, Vale and Guillemin, 1969). Both groups determined the correct structure, L-pyroglutamyl-L-histidyl-L-proline amide, and this knowledge led to the synthesis of large amounts of the hormone (Baugh, Krumdieck, Hershman and Pittman, 1970). Although this tripeptide is clearly a potent stimulus of TSH secretion when given exogenously to animals or man (see below), the exact physiological role of TRH is not yet clear. The same tripeptide also causes the secretion of prolactin (Tashjian, Barowsky and Jensen, 1971; Bowers, Friesen, Hwang, Guyda and Folkers, 1971; Jacobs, Snyder, Utiger and Daughaday 1973) and, under certain circumstances, growth hormone (Irie and Tsushima, 1972; Gonzalez-Barcena, Kastin, Schalch, Torres-Zomora, Perez-Paslen, Kato and Schally, 1973). Moreover, TRH has been found to be widely distributed throughout the brain (Bassiri and Utiger, 1974; Oliver, Eskay, Ben-Jonathan and Porter, 1974b) and even in the gastro-intestinal tract (Morley, Garvin, Pekary and Hershman, 1977). Thus the tripeptide is unlikely to be a specific trophic hormone for TSH secretion.

Efforts to measure endogenous TRH and the factors controlling its biosynthesis and secretion have been hampered by major technical problems. TRH is rapidly degraded both in the hypothalamus (Bauer and Lipmann,

1973; Bassiri and Utiger, 1974; Bauer and Lipmann, 1976) and in serum (Redding and Schally, 1969; Bassiri and Utiger, 1972; Jeffcoate and White, 1974) causing very low or undetectable concentrations in peripheral serum or urine (Bassiri and Utiger, 1972; Bassiri and Utiger, 1973; Eskay, Oliver, Warberg and Porter, 1976). The groups that have apparently measured TRH in peripheral blood, urine, or cerebro-spinal fluid (Ishikawa, 1973; Oliver, Charvet, Codaccioni and Vague, 1974a; Jackson and Reichlin, 1974; Montoya, Seibel and Wilber, 1975; Mitsuma, Hirooka and Nihei, 1976) might be measuring hormone derived from an extra-hypothalamic source. Moreover, urinary assays are particularly subject to technical problems or non-TRH competing substances (Vagenakis, Roti, Mannix and Braverman, 1975b; Emerson, Frohman, Szabo and Thakkar, 1977). Assays of TRH in rat blood have shown an increase during cold stress but, except for one report (Mitsuma *et al.*, 1976); there is no TRH change in hyperthyroidism or hypothyroidism, conditions associated with major decrements or increments of TSH, respectively (Montoya *et al.*, 1975; Eskay *et al.*, 1976).

Somatostatin was isolated from ovine (Brazeau, Vale, Burgus, Ling, Butcher, Rivier and Guillemin, 1973) and porcine (Schally, Dupont, Arimura, Redding and Linthicom, 1975) hypothalami. This tetradecapeptide is widely distributed both inside and outside the central nervous system and has multiple endocrine actions including the inhibition of secretion of growth hormone, TSH, insulin and glucagon (Vale, Brazeau, Rivier, Brown, Boss, Rivier, Burgus, Ling and Guillemin, 1975; Dubois, 1975). Like TRH the factors regulating somatostatin biosynthesis and secretion from the hypothalamus have not been elucidated.

In spite of the difficulties in measuring endogenous TRH and somatostatin and their lack of specificity for TSH, they probably are major factors controlling TSH secretion. One powerful line of evidence supporting such physiological role stems from experiments in which either endogeneous TRH or somatostatin were neutralised by the *in vivo* administration of specific antibodies. Under certain conditions it could be demonstrated that anti-TRH antibodies resulted in decreased TSH secretion (Koch, Goldhaber, Fireman, Zor, Shani and Tal, 1977; Szabo, Kovathana, Gordon and Frohman, 1978; Harris, Christianson, Smith, Fang, Braverman and Vagenakis, 1978) while anti-somatostatin resulted in increased TSH secretion (Arimura and Schally, 1976; Florsheim and Kozbur, 1976; Ferland, Labrie, Jobin, Arimura and Schally, 1976). Hypothalamic hormone effects on TSH secretion have not yet been clearly differentiated from effects on TSH biosynthesis. TRH appears to stimulate both TSH secretion and biosynthesis, the latter process occurring more slowly than the former (Wilber, 1971). However, it is not yet clear whether synthesis results from a separate action of TRH or is secondary to any secretory event.

Free thyroid hormone concentrations are undoubtedly major physiological factors inhibiting TSH secretion and biosynthesis. The principal inhibitory action of T_4 and T_3 is at the level of the pituitary, since increased thyroid hormone concentrations block the TSH response to exogenous TRH (see Sections D.4–6). However, because of the problems discussed above, it is not clear whether thyroid hormones also affect hypothalamic TRH or somatostatin secretion. Although T_3 is more potent than T_4 in inhibiting TSH secretion, T_4 circulates at much higher concentrations. It is probable that T_3 is usually the major circulating thyroid hormone controlling TSH secretion; nevertheless, T_4 clearly has an important independent inhibiting action (see Section D.11). However, it is still not clear whether the inhibition of TSH by T_4 is a direct action or results from intrapituitary conversion of T_4 to T_3 (Silva and Larsen, 1978).

3. Sources of Thyroid-stimulating Activity

(a) Pituitary

As discussed in the section on the chemistry of TSH, it can be purified from pituitary glands of many animal species (Section A). TSH activity has been demonstrated in the pituitary glands of representative species of all vertebrate classes (Bates and Condliffe, 1966). Human pituitaries have been reported to have widely differing TSH concentrations. These differences are undoubtedly due to differences in species specificity of the assays used, the lack until recently of a human reference standard and probably most importantly, variations in the way glands are collected and processed (Elrick, Yearwood-Drayton, Arai, Leaver and Morris, 1963; Bakke, 1965b). The recent adoption of a research standard for human TSH should help in resolving these discrepancies.

(b) Non-pituitary sources of thyroid-stimulating activity

The best known thyroid-stimulating factor of non-pituitary origin is LATS, the TSI discovered by Adams and Purves (1956) (see Section A.6). Since LATS appeared to be a 7S γ-globulin the question arose as to whether it is an immunoglobulin and if so against what antigen is its activity directed. Logically, since it is also a thyroid-stimulator, the presumed antigen would be of thyroidal origin. Beall and Solomon (1966) reported that LATS can bind some microsomal components of the human thyroid. The demonstration by Kriss et al. (1964a) that LATS has many of the properties of an IgG γ-globulin immediately suggested that a possible site of its origin might be the lymphocyte. McKenzie (1967) has shown that LATS may be a product of antibody-forming lymphoid tissue. When leucocytes from patients with Graves' disease were cultured in the presence of phytohaemagglutinin the protein fraction of the culture medium contained LATS. Attempts to stimulate *in vitro* LATS production with thyroidal fractions were not successful.

Another source of thyroid-stimulating activity in man are the chorion carcinomas described by Odell *et al.* (1963). A bacterial thyroid-stimulating factor has been described by Macchia, Bates and Pastan (1967). This factor was purified from culture media of *Clostridium perfringens* by fractionation with ammonium sulphate, gel filtration on Sephadex G-100 and chromatography on DEAEC. The factor appears to be a protein of mw *ca* 30,000. The purified factor stimulates (^{32}P)-phosphate incorporation into phospholipid and $^{14}CO_2$ production from (I-^{14}C)-glucose in beef or dog thyroid slices, as well as the formation of intracellular colloid droplets in dog thyroid slices. It also stimulates depletion of ^{131}I from the thyroids of newly hatched chicks in the assay system of Bates and Cornfield (1957). Thus it appears to have many actions in common with TSH.

C. ACTION OF TSH AND METHODS OF ASSAY

In the first phases of research on a hormone, it is of necessity recognised only by its biological action. As knowledge about the chemistry of the substance associated with hormonal activity is accumulated, it becomes possible to use this chemical information both to detect and to determine quantitatively the amount of the hormone present in blood or in other tissues and fluids. At the time the first and second editions of this book were prepared, measurements of TSH could only be carried out by biological assay procedures. The development of radioimmunochemical assays of protein and peptide hormones (Berson and Yallow, 1958, 1959) has since revolutionised research in this field. In this section we shall present in detail only those proven methods of bioassay which have produced significant estimates of TSH concentration in blood. For a detailed discussion of the assay of TSH the reader is referred to reviews by Brown (1959), McKenzie (1960) and Kirkham (1966).

Bioassay methods for TSH may be classified as gravimetric, histological or biochemical depending upon the end point employed. We shall only be concerned here with primary bioassays which measure the effect of TSH on the thyroid. This excludes such responses as tadpole metamorphosis, or increase in metabolic rate, since these are secondary manifestations of TSH activity mediated through the release of thyroid hormone from the thyroid. Of the primary assays that have been employed for the determination of TSH, only certain histometric or biochemical procedures are of sufficient sensitivity and precision to be used for estimation of the hormone in blood.

In the case of biochemical procedures they are divided into *in vivo* and *in vitro* techniques.

The development of successful radioimmunoassays for TSH by Utiger (1965a, b) and Odell, Wilber and Paul (1965a, b) introduced a purely chemical assay of TSH for the first time. While the purified antigen and the various antisera employed are of biological origin they are nonetheless employed as chemical reagents. The estimate of TSH concentration in the unknown sample of plasma is a function of the interaction of the various reagents. For purposes of standardisation, biological assays are of great importance but the development of a chemical assay has drastically altered the study of TSH and other protein hormones in blood.

Table 2 lists certain characteristics of representative assays for TSH. The estimates of the sensitivity have been taken from published information. The estimate of the lowest level of TSH that can be detected in plasma is a function of the volume of sample that can be injected into an animal in the case of *in vivo* assays and the minimum amount of TSH required to produce a significant response. When these two factors are taken into account there is much less difference between various bioassays than appears to be the case from a consideration of their absolute sensitivities alone. All of them can detect plasma TSH concentrations of at least 10^{-4} bu/ml or *ca* 10 bmu/100 ml. At given times, with particular strains of animal and under particular laboratory conditions, these bioassays can all detect the elevated levels of hTSH found in hypothyroid sera. Except in particular instances, they cannot usually detect hTSH in euthyroid plasma unless the activity is concentrated. They may or may not respond to hyperthyroid plasma depending upon their responsiveness to TSI. The chick thyroid does not respond to TSI whereas the mouse and the other mammalian thyroids do (Bates, 1963; Lepp and Oliner, 1967).

Attempts to improve the sensitivity of *in vivo* bioassays have not been successful. The limit of their usefulness may be said to lie between 10^{-4} and 10^{-5} bu/ml. Assuming hTSH to have a specific activity of 20 bu/mg and a mw of 30,000, this corresponds to a concentration of *ca* $1 \cdot 7 \times 10^{-10}$ mol/l. While *in vivo* assays may be not quite as sensitive as the *in vitro* group they have an advantage in that they respond readily to small changes in the amount of TSH present, i.e. their dose response curves tend to be steeper. The *in vitro* assays are more sensitive by an order of magnitude but their ability to discriminate between concentration levels that are not very different is less than is the case of the *in vivo* assays. Since the resting level of TSH appears to be about 10^{-10} mol/l, *in vivo* bioassays cannot detect it in euthyroid plasma (Odell *et al.* 1967). The stimulated levels are about 10^{-9}–10^{-8} mol/l in hypothyroid plasma, which is within the range of many *in vivo* bioassays.

Table 2

Characteristics of assay methods for hTSH.

Method	Animal	Injection volume ml Usual	Max.	Smallest detectable amount (u)[a]	Lowest detectable level in plasma u/ml	Index of precision λ
In Vivo:						
Colloid droplet (de Robertis, 1948)	Guinea-pig	1·0	—	2×10^{-5}	2×10^{-5}	—
Stasis (d'Angelo and Traum, 1958)	Tadpole *Rana pipiens*	0·1	0·4	2×10^{-4}	5×10^{-4}	0·14
Iodine uptake (Querido *et al.*, 1955)	Mouse	2·0	4·0	2×10^{-3}	5×10^{-4}	0·15
Iodine depletion (Bates and Cornfield, 1957)	Chick	0·2	6·0	5×10^{-4}	8×10^{-5}	0·2
Increase in plasma I (Adams and Purves, 1953, 1955; McKenzie, 1958, 1966)	Guinea-pig	0·1	2·0	1×10^{-4}	5×10^{-5}	0·2
	Mouse	0·1	0·5	$2 \cdot 5 \times 10^{-5}$	5×10^{-5}	0·24
In Vitro		Vol. of medium plus sample				
Weight response in slices (Bakke *et al.*, 1957)	Bovine	1·0	3·0	8×10^{-6}	8×10^{-6}	0·28
^{131}I depletion from slices (Kirkham, 1962)	Guinea-pig	0·2	—	7×10^{-6}	$1 \cdot 4 \times 10^{-6}$	0·2
^{131}I discharge from slices (Bottari and Donovan, 1958; El Kabir, 1962)	Guinea-pig	0·2	0·5	5×10^{-5}	1×10^{-5}	0·2
Cytochemical (Bitensky *et al.*, 1974)	Human	—	—	?	4×10^{-9}	
Radioreceptor (Smith and Hall, 1974)	Human	—	—	1×10^{-5}	?	—
Immunochemical:		Vol. of sample (ml)				
Inhibition of binding (Utiger, 1965;	—	0·005	0·05	$7 \cdot 5 \times 10^{-6}$	$1 \cdot 5 \times 10^{-5}$	—
Odell *et al.*, 1965c)	—	0·01	0·4	1×10^{-5}	$2 \cdot 5 \times 10^{-5}$	—

[a] Activities are expressed as international units to the bovine reference standard. See Section A.1.*a*.

1. Biochemical Effects of TSH and its Mechanism of Action

As pointed out in the introduction to this section many effects of TSH have been used as the basis for bioassays. The mechanism of action of TSH however remains unsolved although recently several hypotheses have been put forward in an attempt to explain the plethora of observed biochemical and morphological effects of the hormone.

(a) Initial reaction of TSH with the thyroid cell

(1) *Binding of TSH to a receptor site.* Since the first observations that bTSH is bound to the surface of dog thyroid cells (Pastan, 1966; Pastan, Roth and Macchia, 1966) evidence has accumulated that there is a specific receptor site for TSH which can be solubilized and whose properties have been described.

After these original observations Yamashita and Field (1970, 1972) isolated thyroid plasma cell membranes which could bind TSH. Adenyl cyclase was activated after binding of TSH. Amir *et al.* (1973) described the binding of purified bTSH labelled with tritium (Winand and Kohn, 1970) to purified bovine thyroid membranes. The membrane preparations had less than 1 % contamination by mitochondrial and other subcellular components. The activity of adenosine triphosphatase, adenyl cyclase and other membrane-bound enzymes was increased 10–40 fold and there was a comparable decrease in activity of non-membraneous enzymes. Binding studies showed a high degree of specificity for bTSH. Labelled bTSH could be displaced by cold hormone. hTSH is less potent than bTSH even on human thyroid membranes. Purified hTSH is not as potent as bTSH in many assay systems. The β-subunit of bTSH inhibited the binding of the undissociated hormone whereas the α-subunit was less effectively bound. These authors observed no effect of human serum LATS on the binding of bTSH in the assay. Smith and Hall (1974) developed a receptor assay for hTSH using normal human thyroid membranes. In their studies both hTSH and bTSH could be detected in doses as low as 10 μu.* Unlike the experiments of Amir *et al.* (1973) the binding of hTSH or bTSH to human thyroid receptors was inhibited by immunoglobulins from patients with Graves' disease. An interesting observation by Smith and Hall (1974) showed that binding curves for TSH were non-linear whereas those for TSI were linear for individual patients. This suggested that for TSH there are populations of receptor sites with different affinities but only a single population type for TSI. However it is not clear from the data whether the human thyroid membranes used in each assay were from a single

* It is not clear from the information given by Smith and Hall (1974) whether these are human or bovine units.

human thyroid or from a pool so this suggestion should be viewed with reserve.

Solubilisation and partial purification of the bovine thyroid plasma membrane receptor or receptors have been described by Tate, Holmes, Kohn and Winand (1975a). Bovine thyroids were homogenised and the plasma membranes purified as described by Amir *et al.* (1973). Solubilisation of the receptor sites was accomplished by homogenising them with lithium diiodosalicylate and then centrifuging the homogenate to remove the inactive membrane residues. The TSH binding activity was present in the supernatant. Examination of the supernatant by sucrose density centrifugation showed that the TSH binding activity was associated with a heterogeneous group of proteins having molecular weights estimated to be 280,000, 75,000 and 15,000–30,000. Trypsinisation of the solubilised receptors converted the higher molecular weight fractions into a still heterogeneous fraction in the 15,000–30,000 range. The membrane adenylate cyclase activity was associated with the TSH receptor fractions and was also converted to the 15,000–30,000 molecular weight fraction by trypsinisation (Tate, Schwartz, Holmes, Kohn and Winand, 1975b).

(2) *Effect of binding on TSH and the role of auxiliary substances.* While some progress has been made in the study of the TSH receptor site protein or proteins (see Section C.3) little is known about the conformation of either TSH or its receptor site. However in a series of papers published over the past six years Kohn, Winand and their collaborators have described experiments on the role of gangliosides in the interaction of glycoprotein hormones with receptor sites from thyroid tissues, retro-orbital tissue and testis. Interest in the role of gangliosides in the binding of TSH and other protein hormones to their receptor sites arose from the finding that certain bacterial toxins such as cholera toxin, bind to cell membranes and in so doing activate the adenylate cyclase of the intestinal mucosa and other tissues. The cholera toxin appears to bind to the G_{ml} ganglioside of the cell membrane. When the amino acid sequence of the β-chains of bTSH, bLH, hCG and hFSH are aligned with the sequence of the cholera toxin chain there is a significant similarity ($p = 0.003$ that the similarity is due to chance) in a portion of the toxin sequence (residues 8–12) and in the bTSHβ (residues 27–31) bLHβ (residues 35–39), hCGβ (residues 35–39) and hFSHβ (residues 26–30). The region in question involves a half-cystine residue which in bTSHβ occurs in a sequence Val–Cys–Ala–Glu–Tyr (Mullin, Fishman, Lee, Aloj, Ledley, Winand, Kohn and Brady, 1976b; Kurosky, Markel, Peterson and Fitch, 1977). A similar homology exists in many of the serine proteases which, however, do not bind to any cells (Kurosky *et al.*, 1977). Whether or not these sequences are the result of a limited convergence from dissimilar proteins, in which case they would be analogous, or whether they are the

result of divergence from a common ancestral protein, in which case they would be homologous, remains to be determined. As pointed out by Kurosky *et al.* (1977) the disulphide structure of the β-chain of the glycoprotein hormones has not been determined and nothing is known about its three-dimensional properties or those of the cholera toxin β-chain. Conclusions as to the significance of these similarities would therefore appear to be premature. However these observations have stimulated interest in the role of gangliosides in the initial events that occur during the binding of TSH and other glycoprotein hormones to their receptor sites. Thus a number of gangliosides inhibit the binding of ^{125}I-bTSH to the plasma membrane bTSH receptor site (Mullin *et al.*, 1976b). The inhibition appears to be due to an interaction between the ganglioside and bTSH, producing complexes of high molecular weight. The interaction is dependent upon the sialic acid content of the ganglioside; thus the most effective inhibitor was G_{D1b}, containing two sialic acid residues, and the least G_{D1a}. Cholera toxin interacts with TSH receptor sites and blocks the binding of TSH (Mullin, Aloj, Fishman, Lee, Kohn and Brady, 1976a). It also stimulates adenylate cyclase in thyroid plasma membranes. Analysis of thyroid plasma membranes shows that sialic acid-containing gangliosides that strongly inhibit the binding of TSH to its receptor site, are present in the thyroid plasma membranes in higher concentration than found in other extraneural tissue (Mullin, Fishman, Lee, Aloj, Ledley, Winand, Kohn and Brady, 1976b). On the basis of these and other findings Kohn and his collaborators have developed the hypothesis that the TSH receptor site contains a gangliosidic structure to which TSH binds, that TSH then undergoes a conformational change enabling it to fit the rest of the receptor site and that this conformational change and consequent complete interaction between the hormone and the receptor site stimulates adenyl cyclase and also turns on the thyroid cell machinery to carry out such functions as thyroid hormone synthesis and secretion. These authors have also postulated that the activation of membrane bound adenylate cyclase is not the primary event required for activation of the thyroid cell to transport iodine, synthesise thyroglobulin and secrete thyroid hormone. They suggest on the basis of complex and inconclusive evidence that, after the interaction of the TSHβ-subunit with a ganglioside in the receptor site, a change in conformation of TSH occurs which translocates the TSHα-subunit into the membrane. A change of state occurs in the membrane altering its permeability, its electrochemical gradient and ion transport properties (Kohn, Aloj, Friedman, Grollman, Ledley, Lee, Meldolesi and Mullins, 1977). They also suggest that for the thyroid this change of state precedes adenyl cyclase activiation and that cAMP is not the unique second messenger but merely one of several. Marshalling evidence concerning bacterial toxin actions and those of the glycoprotein hormones they attempt to show a common mechanism of initial reaction between cells as diverse as neurones, gastro-intestinal cells, glycoprotein hormone target cells and such molecules as interferon, cholera toxin, tetanus toxin, TSH, FSH, LH and hCG. Their speculations seem bound to stimulate experimental work in this area.

(b) Secondary effects of TSH

After binding of TSH to its receptor site a number of effects are seen some of which form the basis of the assays described in Sections C.2–C.4. The thyroid cell grows, inorganic phosphate uptake and turnover increases, iodine uptake increases and there is an increase in thyroglobulin synthesis and thyroid hormone secretion.

(*1*) *Activation of adenyl cyclase.* After the discovery that cyclic 3',5'-adenosine monophosphate (cAMP) mediates the effect of many peptide hormones on their target tissues, Klainer, Chi, Freidburg, Rall and Sutherland (1962) showed that TSH increased the level of cAMP in thyroid homogenates. Attempts at that time to mimic the effects of TSH on the thyroid with cAMP were unsuccessful (Field *et al.*, 1960). Pastan (1966) showed that dibutyryl cyclic 3',5'adenosine monophosphate (DBC) (Posternak, Sutherland and Henion, 1962) stimulated both glucose oxidation and incorporation of ^{32}P into phospholipid in dog thyroid slices. DBC also stimulates formation of intracellular colloid droplets through endocytosis in dog thyroid slices (Pastan and Wollman, 1967). DBC is an analogue of cAMP which enters cells more readily.

Since these early observations on the role of cAMP and the activation of adenyl cyclase many studies have shown that activation of adenyl cyclase by TSH is required for many of the physiological activities of the thyroid. In particular iodine metabolism and the secretion of thyroid hormone seem to be related to cAMP which mediates the stimulatory effect as indicated in Fig. 5. Thus Pastan and Katzen (1967) were able to activate adenyl cyclase in dog thyroid homogenates with bTSH. Gilman and Rall (1968) and Zor, Kaneko, Lowe. Bloom and Field (1969) showed that cAMP accumulates in thyroid homogenates to which TSH is added. Later studies from many laboratories have established that after TSH is bound to receptor sites in plasma cell membranes the membrane-bound adenyl cyclase is activated and cAMP is generated (see reviews by Schell-Frederick and Dumont, 1970 and Field, 1975). LATS and other thyroid stimulating immunoglobulins bind to TSH receptor sites and also activate membrane bound adenyl cyclase (Yamashita and Field, 1972; Smith and Hall, 1974). Once cAMP is generated, protein kinase is activated in both slices and in homogenates from pig and bovine thyroids (Field, Bloom, Kerins, Chagoth and Zor, 1975). Beyond the activation of the protein kinase and relationship of adenyl cyclase activation to the stimulation of iodine metabolism and other metabolic processes in the thyroid is not clear as indicated in Fig. 5.

Besides the effect of TSH on adenyl cyclase discussed above, the hormone has a strong stimulatory effect on phosphate turnover in the thyroid. As

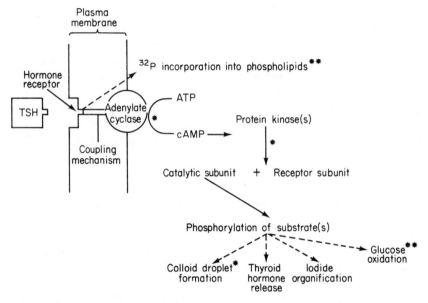

Fig. 5. Representation of mechanism of action of TSH. Phospholipids are an essential component of either the hormone receptor or the coupling mechanism. * indicates that Ca^{++} is not required for this action, while ** indicates that the effect is Ca^{++} dependent. From Field (1975).

early as 1945, Borell observed that TSH increased the turnover of ^{32}P in the gland. Later Borell and Holgren (1949) found that in guinea-pigs the uptake of ^{32}P by the thyroid was closely related to the increase in cell height of the follicular epithelium and could be used as a method of assay for TSH. Lamberg (1953a, 1955) and Crooke and Matthews (1953) described assays based upon ^{32}P uptake that detected 5×10^{-4} bu. Greenspan, Kriss and Moses (1954) and Greenspan, Kriss, Moses and Lew (1956) described a method of assay in which 2.5×10^{-4} bu could be detected. After an intra-cardiac injection of 0·1 ml test substance, the thyroids were removed and the ^{32}P uptake determined. The sensitivity of this method would be about 2.5×10^{-3} bu/ml which is not great enough to detect TSH in euthyroid plasma. These methods based upon ^{32}P uptake by the thyroid have been used for the routine assay of pituitary extracts (Pierce and Nyce, 1956). They are satisfactory for estimating the relative potencies of fractions obtained during purification of pituitary TSH. However, during the collaborative assay of the international standard of bTSH the results obtained by laboratories using the ^{32}P method were significantly different from those of others (Mussett and Perry, 1955).

The effect of TSH on ^{32}P metabolism in the thyroid gland seems to be related to fundamental stimulatory effects on thyroid metabolism (Rall, Robbins and Lewallen, 1964). Thus the incorporation of phosphate is increased into phospholipids (Lamberg, 1953; Lamberg, Wahlberg and Olin-Lamberg, 1955; Morton and Schwartz, 1953; Freinkel, 1957, 1958, 1960). TSH also increases the RNA content of the thyroid (Matovinovic and Vickery, 1959) and stimulates the rate of purine and nucleotide bio-synthesis (Hall, 1963; Hall and Tubman, 1965).

2. Histometric Assay Methods

(a) The colloid droplet method

In this method (de Robertis and del Conte, 1941 and de Robertis, 1948) guinea-pigs were starved for 24 hr before use. The animals were then divided into groups of 4–6. Each animal was injected with 1 ml of the test substance. After 30 min the animals were killed, the thyroids were dissected out, frozen, dried and then sectioned and stained with anilin-blue organe. Sections of the thyroids were examined and the droplets inside the acinar cells were counted. The concentration of droplets was expressed as the cytological coefficient C_c:

$$C_c = \frac{\text{number of droplets} \times 10}{\text{mean follicular diameter of 6 follicles}}$$

By plotting the cytological coefficient against a standard preparation it was possible to construct a dose-response curve from which unknown values could be assigned a potency in terms of Junkman–Schoeller units. Converting JSU to international units, as explained in Section A.1.a de Robertis could detect a little as 0·02 mu TSH (2×10^{-5} bu). An inspection of their data shows that the range of the method was rather wide, from 0·02–100 mu. The slope of the dose-response curve was low since a many fold change in dose was required to achieve a doubling of the response. Nonetheless, despite this lack of precision, which is a common characteristic of histological and of some biochemical methods of bioassay, de Robertis (1948) was able to obtain values for TSH in blood which agree well with those published later by other workers who employed alternative methods.

(b) The "stasis" tadpole method

In their original paper d'Angelo, Gordon and Charipper (1942) used a secondary effect of TSH by measuring the growth of the hind limb in a tadpole whose metamorphosis had been arrested by starvation. In a later version of this assay (d'Angelo and Traum, 1958), starved tadpoles of the species *Rana clamitans* are divided into groups and injected with 0·2 ml of the test solution. A plot of the mean thyroid cell height against the log of the dose in mu gives a straight line which can be fitted by the equation:

$$x = 7·22 + 1·68 \log y$$

where x is the response in microns and y is the dose expressed in mu.

From the slope of the regression line and the standard error of estimate, an index of precision of less than 0·2 has been calculated. The authors claim to be able to distinguish, at the 95% confidence level, two unknowns differing in potency by only 1·35 fold. The sensitivity of the method seems to be somewhat less than that originally claimed. An inspection of the dose-response curve (d'Angelo and Traum, 1958) shows that the stasis value of the mean cell height lies at about 5·5 μ. A dose of 2×10^{-4} bu TSH gives a height of 6 μ. If 2×10^{-4} bu is the smallest dose that can be detected and this is injected in 0·4 ml, then the method can only detect TSH at a level of 5×10^{-4} bu/ml of serum. In view of later estimates of the level of TSH in euthyroid plasma, it seems unlikely that the method can detect the hormone in the normal state.

It should be pointed out that de Robertis (1948), whose method of assay appears to have been more sensitive by an order of magnitude, found it necessary to effect some concentration of TSH in normal blood by acetone precipitation. However, the "stasis" tadpole seems to be easily capable of detecting the elevated levels that are obtained in some pathological and experimental sera. Certainly, direct assay of euthyroid sera can only give marginal responses and in many cases one can only set an upper limit to the actual level.

Asboe-Hansen, Iversen and Wichmann (1952) employed tadpoles of *Xenopus laevis* while *Rana catesbiana* has also been used by Bowers, Segaloff and Brown (1959) who report that in this case 5×10^{-4} bu could be detected in a 0·1 ml dose. This would make their sensitivity 5×10^{-3} bu/ml plasma.

3. Physiological Methods

(a) Uptake of iodine

The introduction of radiochemical techniques into the study of thyroid physiology speedily led to the discovery that the rate at which the thyroid cleared iodide from the blood was under some circumstances dependent on TSH. Numerous assay procedures for TSH have been based upon the effect. In general they can be reliable and are useful enough, but they are not sufficiently sensitive to assay blood directly without some chemical concentration of TSH. A typical procedure is that of Querido, Kassenaar and Lameyer (1955) who employ female mice, pretreated by feeding with iodocasein to decrease the endogenous TSH output. The animals are injected with the TSH solution at a dose ranging from 2×10^{-3}–1.8×10^{-7} bu/day for four days, after which ^{131}I is injected. By the use of sufficient animals, a dose response curve is obtained which has an index of precision of from 0.15–0.25.

(b) Depletion of iodine

Two versions of the iodine-depletion test have been developed. The first may be attributed to Gilliland and Strudwick (1953) who used baby chicks whose endogenous TSH output was suppressed with thyroxine. The chicks were given a dose of ^{131}I, a certain proportion of which was taken up by the thyroid glands within 24 hr. The animals were then given TSH in graded doses and it was found that the radioactivity over the thyroid, measured with four Geiger tubes placed around the neck region, decreased in proportion to the dose of TSH. A minimum sensitivity of about 6×10^{-3} bu was found in chicks which had uptakes of about 12%. Since the injection volume was about 0.25 ml the method is obviously too insensitive to detect blood levels of 5×10^{-4} bu/ml. Gilliland and Strudwick (1953), in pointing this out, also remarked that to detect TSH in euthyroid subjects it was necessary to inject chicks with large volumes of unfractionated plasma. If the value of plasma TSH is 5×10^{-4} bu/ml, one would have to inject about 5 or 6 ml per chick, rather a large volume in an animal weighing 40–50 g with a blood volume not much over 5 ml.

This assay was developed further by Bates and Cornfield (1957) who increased the sensitivity by administering propylthiouracil 24 hr after the ^{131}I dose in order to prevent reaccumulation of iodine derived from degraded hormone. Depending upon the radio–iodine uptake, which in turn is inversely related to the stable iodine content of the gland, they obtained dose response curves in which the minimal detectable dose was as low as 5×10^{-4} bu/ml. By injecting chicks with very large volumes of unfractionated normal plasma, Bates and Condliffe (1960) were able to show a positive test for TSH in some instances. However, for the reasons cited above, it is often necessary to carry out some fractionation of the plasma in order to obtain satisfactory results. Bates (1963) used this method to determine TSH levels in the plasma of hypothyroid patients directly without fractionation. Normal plasma had to be fractionated first in order to concentrate the hormone.

(c) *Increase in protein-bound iodine in blood*

The corollary of the iodine depletion technique is the method based upon the rise in protein-bound iodine in the blood following discharge of iodine from the thyroid under the influence of TSH. Adams and Purves (1953, 1955, 1957) employed guinea-pigs whose pituitaries were blocked with thyroxine after the thyroid glands had been labelled with ^{131}I. One day later a dose of TSH was administered and the rise in protein-bound radioiodine in the plasma was determined. By proper design this assay can be carried out with great precision. By means of this technique, Adams and Purves (1955, 1957) were able to detect as little as 1×10^{-4} bu which enabled them to estimate blood concentrations as low as 5×10^{-5} bu/ml when 2 ml of plasma were injected into the guinea-pigs, by way of an ear vein. The method has the drawback that it requires considerable skill and also takes several days to prepare the animals. However, the same animals can be used several times, enabling cross-over assay designs to be carried out and eliminating the problems involved in procuring and maintaining large numbers of animals. As discussed in Section A.6, this method is of importance since, by its use, an abnormally long acting thyroid-stimulator was discovered (Adams and Purves, 1956).

McKenzie (1958) has published a modification of Adams and Purves' assay in which the mouse was used as the experimental animal. This assay is undoubtedly one of the most widely used methods for the estimation of TSH. Since its introduction it has been modified in many laboratories. McKenzie and Williamson (1966) have described the version they currently use which, while unchanged in principle, has been slightly modified in practice. Mice are fed a low-iodine Remington diet for 10 days. On the tenth day they are injected with 15 μc ^{125}I and 10 μg sodium-L-thyroxine. Four days later they are used for the assay. Samples for assay are injected intravenously; the usual injection volume is 0·2 ml but volumes as large as 0·5 ml have been employed; 0·1 ml samples of blood are obtained by retro-orbital puncture just before and 2 hr and 9 hr after injection of the test samples. The samples of retro-orbital blood are counted in a well-type scintillator. The response at 2 hr was taken as being due to pituitary TSH and the 9 hr as due to LATS.

Because of the great variability of the assay, McKenzie (1967), in a study of the origins of LATS, used for comparative purposes only those results obtained in a single batch of mice. This same variability was apparent in a collaborative assay of two samples of hTSH reported by Bakke (1965a, b) in which 21 laboratories took part. Of the 21 laboratories, 10 employed the McKenzie method. The range of absolute values reported by the individual laboratories using the McKenzie assay was as great as the range of values reported by all 21. However, the potency ratio of the two hTSH preparations was remarkably similar in all laboratories.

These results illustrate the point that comparisons between laboratories are difficult to make even when the reference standards are used, whereas comparisons made by one technique in a single laboratory are probably more meaningful. The great advantage of the McKenzie method is its relative simplicity. Inbred strains of mice are readily available to almost any laboratory in all but a few parts of the world. The pretreatment by feeding a low iodine diet is important and care must be taken to ensure that the diet is truly low in iodine. The necessary counting equipment is today available in most hospitals and laboratories that employ radioisotopes. Successful use of the chick assay often involves a search for animals with a high uptake of iodine. *In vitro* techniques involve a level of sophistication which it takes time to develop. Finally, the biggest single reason behind the use of McKenzie's procedure is that not only does it enable the investigator to assay TSH but at the same time he can detect and estimate LATS that may be present in his sample.

For all its simplicity the McKenzie assay can present difficulties. Injection of too much TSH may give elevated responses at 9 hr which can be misinterpreted as being due to LATS. The quantitation of the LATS response has not been fully worked out, partly because it cannot be expressed in terms of the reference preparation of TSH. Many of the uncertain positive results obtained during assay of hyperthyroid plasma for TSH are undoubtedly related to the different time course of action of TSH and LATS in *in vivo* assays.

Failure to detect LATS in all cases of hyperthyroidism has been attributed to insufficient sensitivity of the method (McKenzie, 1965; Adams, 1965). Use of specific concentrated plasma fractions could aid in improving both the specificity and sensitivity of LATS assays.

4. *In vitro* Methods

Surviving thyroid glands or slices retain the ability to metabolise iodine and to respond to TSH when incubated in a suitable medium. Several assay procedures have been developed in which thyroid slices are used. These methods are often more sensitive than *in vivo* procedures, but they tend to have low slopes, which make them less precise.

(a) The weight response in thyroid slices

Lawrence and Bakke (1956) observed that the osmotic regulation of surviving thyroid tissue was greatly affected by the addition of TSH to the medium.

Following this observation, Bakke, Heideman, Lawrence and Wiberg (1957) developed a method for the assay of TSH based upon its ability to prevent the loss in weight which normally occurs in beef thyroid slices when they are incubated at pH 7·4 in Krebs–Ringer phosphate buffer. After 24 hr the weight of the slices usually falls to 50 % of the initial weight. In the presence of TSH this fall in weight may be reduced to only 5 or 10 %. When suitably graded concentrations of TSH are used, a dose response curve is obtained which covers a range of 8×10^{-6}–4×10^{-5} bu/ml of incubation medium. The volume of medium employed is usually about 4 ml, however it can be reduced to as little as 1·0 ml. Thus the absolute sensitivity of the method can be as low as 8×10^{-6} bu/ml. By carefully controlling the size of the slices so as to have them uniform with respect to thickness and diameter, an index of precision (λ) of about 0·28 was obtained in a number of experiments.

(b) Iodine release from pre-labelled thyroid slices

Bottari and Donovan (1958) have published a brief description of a method based on the release of ^{131}I from guinea-pig thyroid slices, previously incubated with radioiodine and thus labelled. They reported that iodine released back into the medium could be increased by adding TSH. This is analogous to the method of Adams and Purves (1953, 1955, 1957) who measured the increase of PBI in vivo. However, it is not known from Battari and Donovan's preliminary report whether or not the iodine released is organically bound. The sensitivity appears to be of similar magnitude to the uptake method described above, although it is claimed that the precision is greatly increased. The range of the dose-response curve is 10^{-6}–10^{-2} bu. Fl Kabir (1962) modified this method by using thyroids from goitrogen-treated guinea-pigs. Goitrogen treatment increased the uptake of ^{131}I and improved the precision of the method.

Kirkham (1962a, b) has published a method which also uses thyroid tissue from goitrogen-treated guinea-pigs. He maintains guinea-pigs for 100 days on a diet containing no green food. During this time the animal's drinking water contains 0·1 % methylthiouracil and 0·1 % ascorbic acid. The animals are killed at 100 days, the thyroids removed, and cut into small pieces. Approximately 28 mg of tissue are incubated in a tube containing a culture medium of 0·15 µc ^{131}I/ml. The thyroid pieces in each tube take up approximately 50 % of the ^{131}I. TSH is added in various amounts. The tubes are incubated for 40 hr when an aliquot is removed from each for counting. This aliquot is replaced with an equal volume of KSCN. After 4 hr of further incubation a second aliquot is removed and counted. The difference in radioactivity between the first and second aliquot is inversely related to the concentration of TSH added to the medium. TSH has been shown by Taurog,

Tong and Chaikoff (1958a, b) to increase the organification of ^{131}I added to guinea-pig thyroid slices. Thus in the tissue incubated with TSH more of the ^{131}I is organified and is not discharged by addition of KSCN. This method is one of the most sensitive known and has been used to measure TSH in plasma (Kirkham, 1962a, b; Kirkham and Irvine, 1963). From El Kabir's and Kirkham's experience the pretreatment of the guinea pigs with goitrogen seems to have been the key to success.

(c) Iodine release from pre-labelled thyroid glands

Brown and Munro (1967) described an *in vitro* method using mouse thyroid glands. Mice were injected with 0·1 μc ^{131}I at zero time. Two hours later the animals were killed by stunning and the thyroids placed in 1 ml Gey's solution containing TSH or other substance. The preparation was gassed with 95% O_2/5% CO_2 and shaken for 16 hr at 120 cycles/min in a 35° water bath. At the end of 18 hr the thyroids were moved, the ^{131}I remaining in the thyroid and released into the medium were determined. The glands were not sliced but were incubated whole. As a result there was relatively little ^{131}I released into the medium unless TSH was added. Mouse thyroids respond to both bTSH and to hTSH. Using the hTSH reference standard A as little as 0·1 mu could be detected. LATS also released iodine into the medium. The time course of release was the same for bTSH, hTSH and TSI.

5. Cytochemical Techniques

In 1966 Wollman (1969) showed that TSH stimulates endocytosis of colloid in the lumen of thyroid follicles. The engulfed endocytotic vesicles then fuse with lysosomes. As a result of the fusion the stability of the lysosomal membrane is affected as shown by Bitensky (1973). Based upon the cytochemical procedures of Chayen *et al.* (1973) Bitensky *et al.* (1973) showed that the rate at which leucine 2-napthylamide penetrates the lysosomal membranes measured by microdensitometry is proportional to concentration of TSH in the medium. From the published data it is not possible to estimate the minimum amount of TSH that can be detected since the weight of thyroid tissue incubated with the medium is not given nor is the volume of medium. The authors claim that hTSH can be detected at a concentration of 4×10^{-3} μu/ml. Like the earlier colloid droplet method of de Robertis and del Conte (1941) the dose-response curve of the lysosomal membrane permeability method has a low slope. A 1000 fold increase in the concentration of hTSH barely produced a doubling of the response measured by the relative increase in leucine 2-napthylamide inside the lysosomes as compared with control sections. An index of precision cannot be calculated from the data published by Bitensky *et al.* (1973). Given the low slope of the method the method must be regarded as qualitative although it appears to be two or three orders of magnitude more sensitive than most bioassays. Used as a quantal assay it is a useful addition to the range of biological methods available for detection of TSH in tissues and body fluids.

6. Radioreceptor Assays

As discussed in Section C.1 TSH binds to hormone specific receptor sites on the plasma membrane of thyroid cells. Several groups of investigators have described procedures which can be used to estimate TSH activity in serum and in tissues. They all have the following steps:

  (i) thyroid membranes are isolated and incubated with labelled TSH;

  (ii) unlabelled TSH is added to the membrane-labelled TSH preparation;

  (iii) the displacement of label is proportional to the amount of unlabelled TSH added.

In principle a receptor binding assay is no different from any other ligand-binding assay. Through use of appropriate standards the amount of unlabelled TSH can be estimated as in radioimmunoassays.

The method is more sensitive than many bioassays. Using human thyroid membranes Smith and Hall (1974) were able to detect as little as 10 μu of bTSH. In the various versions of the techniques most investigators find that standard Scatchard plots of bound/free hormone versus bound are non-linear suggesting that there are populations of TSH receptor sites with differing affinities for the hormone.

7. Immunochemical Assay

(a) *Production of anti-TSH antisera*

Repeated injection of rats with crude TSH produces a refractory state to further administration of the hormone (Anderson and Collip, 1934). This "anti-hormone" effect was shown by Werner (1936a, b) to be due to the formation of antibodies to TSH. Werner, Otero-Ruiz, Seegal and Bates (1960) showed that anti-bTSH antisera could be produced in rabbits by injection of crude commercial bovine TSH (Thytropar) which had a potency of about 1 u/mg. They administered the TSH by repeated multiple injections with Freund's adjuvant. Similar results were obtained by Cline, Selenkow and Brooke (1960). These antisera to bTSH were capable of neutralising its biological effectiveness in the McKenzie (1958) mouse assay and in the chick assay of Bates and Cornfield (1957).

After these first demonstrations of the antigenicity of bTSH, other investigators also prepared anti-bTSH antisera with the aim of developing immunological techniques for the estimation of TSH in human blood.

Potent antisera to highly purified hTSH and bTSH were produced in rabbits by the injection of a total of 0·6 mg of each hormone in three doses (Utiger et al., 1963). Each dose was administered in complete Freund's adjuvant. These antisera were subsequently used for the development of a radioimmunoassay for hTSH (see below).

(b) Species specificity

McKenzie and Fishman (1960) showed that while anti-bTSH antisera would neutralise bTSH and also showed some degree of cross-reaction with hTSH, they could not inhibit long acting thyroid stimulating (LATS, thyroid-stimulating immunoglobulin) activity. Levy, McGuire and Heideman (1962) noted that antisera to crude bTSH could be produced in rabbits which neutralised the homologous hormone in high dilutions but which had only 1/20 the neutralising ability against hTSH. Levy et al. (1962) also showed that inhibition of haemagglutination by these anti-bTSH antisera was not proportional to the TSH content of several preparations of both bTSH and hTSH. Pascasio and Selenkow (1962) also observed non-specific effects when anti-bTSH antisera were tested against other pituitary hormone preparations by haemagglutination-inhibition techniques.

The extent of immunological cross-reaction between the bovine and human forms of TSH is debatable. Firstly, all the anti-TSH antisera prepared against bTSH display a limited cross-reactivity with hTSH as shown by their ability to neutralise hTSH in several bioassay procedures when used in excess (McKenzie and Fishman, 1960; Werner et al., 1960; Levy et al., 1962; Utiger et al., 1963). Secondly, because of the low degree of this cross-reactivity, anti-bTSH antisera have not been used successfully for radioimmunoassay of hTSH in plasma with the exception of the procedure described by Lemarchand-Béraud and Vanotti (1965). When examined in Ouchterlony gels and by a radioimmunological precipitation technique, the species specificity (Utiger et al., 1963) of antisera to highly purified hTSH and bTSH was complete. This was also true of antisera prepared against partly purified hTSH (Odell, Wilber, and Utiger, 1967b). Similar findings were earlier obtained by Adams et al. (1962) who showed only weak cross-reactions between anti-bTSH antisera and hTSH in the sera of myxoedematous patients. Antisera to hTSH reacted weakly with the bovine hormone. Quantitatively 25 times as much anti-hTSH was required to neutralise bTSH as hTSH ,which is in accord with findings of Levy et al. (1962) and Utiger et al. (1963).

(c) Radioimmunoassay of hTSH

The development of radioimmunoassay by Berson and Yalow (1966) provided the first method capable of measuring TSH precisely and specifically in unextracted plasma or serum. hTSH radioimmunoassays were first reported by Utiger (1965) and Odell, Wilber and Paul (1965b). Both groups used similar methods including chloramine T iodination (Greenwood, Hunter and Glover, 1963) of highly purified human TSH (*ca* 10 u/mg) prepared by Condliffe (1963). The antibody was also prepared from purified Condliffe material and was relatively specific for human TSH. However, it was soon discovered that virtually all anti-TSH antisera cross-reacted with other human glycoprotein hormones, particularly hCG and luteinising hormone (hLH). Such cross-reactivity might have been related to a small amount of hLH contaminating the hTSH preparation; more likely, it resulted from the common α-subunit determinant shared by the glycoprotein

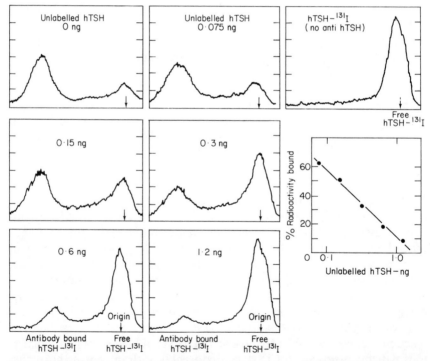

Fig. 6. Standard curve and radioactivity scans of paper strips following separation of free and antibody-bound TSH ^{131}I by chromatoelectrophoresis. The standard curve data represents a plot of the percentage of total radioactivity bound to antibody at each dose of unlabelled hTSH. From Utiger (1965a).

hormones (see above). The anti-hTSH antibody was rendered specific by absorption with 10–100 u of hCG, which neutralised the population of cross-reacting antibodies (Odell et al., 1965b). Antibody-bound labelled TSH was separated from free-labelled TSH by either ethanol-saline precipitation, chromatoelectrophoresis (Fig. 6) or, preferably, a double antibody technique (Odell, Wilber and Utiger, 1967b). TSH standards were initially arbitrary lots of purified Condliffe material but subsequently assay results were expressed in terms of an International Thyrotrophin Research Standard A supplied by the World Health Organisation and standardised by bioassay (Odell et al., 1967b).

Although several other radioimmunoassays for hTSH have been published subsequent to the first two reports described above, they do not differ in major respects from the original methods (Lemarchand-Béraud, 1970; Coble and Kohler, 1970; Greenberg, Gzernichow, Shelly, Winship and Blizzard, 1970; Fleischer, Burgus, Vale, Dunn and Guillemin, 1970; Hall, Tubmen and Garry, 1970; Hershman and Pittman, 1971a, b; Mayberry, Gharib, Bilstad and Sizemore, 1971; Patel, Burger and Hudson, 1971; Ridgway, Weintraub, Cevallos, Rack and Maloof, 1973; Pekary, Hershman and Parlow, 1975). However, certain methodological improvements have substantially increased the sensitivity of the assay.

The most important methodological advance was the use of antisera with higher affinity constants (ca 1–4 × 10^{11} M^{-1}) for hTSH (Ridgway et al., 1973; Pekary et al., 1975). Interestingly, these antisera were obtained with hTSH immunisation and there did not appear to be any advantage in immunising with the specific β-subunit of TSH (Binoux, Pierce and Odell, 1974). Another improvement was the use of a low tracer mass of [^{125}I] hTSH that had been highly purified from less immunoreactive labelled aggregates and subunits on a long (90 cm) gel chromatography column (Ridgway et al., 1973). Further sensitivity was obtained by optimising the non-equilibrium conditions used in the earliest assays (Moser and Hollingsworth, 1975). These improvements in sensitivity allowed a reduction in the maximum concentration of serum used in the assay to 10–20% (v/v) instead of the 40–50% used in the early assays. Moreover, unlike the early methods, later assays employed TSH-deficient serum in the diluent for the TSH standards, thus equalising the non-specific serum effects between samples and standards (Patel et al., 1971; Ridgway et al., 1973; Golstein and Vanhaelst, 1973). The reduction of artifactual serum effects led to a reduction in normal values and a clearer separation from the suppressed (and usually undetectable) basal values in hyperthyroidism (Patel et al., 1971; Ridgway et al., 1973).

Currently, hTSH radioimmunoassay reagents are available from several commercial sources as well as from the Hormone Distribution Programme of the National Institute of Arthritis, Metabolism and Digestive Diseases,

Bethesda, Maryland. The latter programme provides high quality, standardised reagents to qualified investigators throughout the world, thus assuring some degree of uniformity in TSH methods among various laboratories. The generally accepted international hTSH standard is Human Thyrotrophin Standard A or B, available from the Medical Research Council, Mill Hill, London.

D. THE CONCENTRATION OF hTSH IN PLASMA

In previous editions of this book, there was great uncertainty over the meaning of the different results obtained for hTSH in plasma by various biological assays. It now is clear that most bioassays do not have the requisite sensitivity or specificity for this measurement. Although a new ultrasensitive cytochemical bioassay holds great promise of providing information about the biological activity of normal and even low plasma TSH concentrations (see Section C.5), only a few reports describing its use have appeared. Furthermore, the chemical nature of the substances measured by this and other bioassays have not as yet been adequately characterised and could reflect additional glycoprotein hormones, immunoglobulins and other plasma thyrotrophic substances different from pituitary TSH.

In contrast, many reports have now appeared from a large number of laboratories confirming the specificity of these currently available hTSH radioimmunoassays. Such assays do not measure any of the other known thyrotrophic substances. The substances measured by radioimmunoassay usually have been found to behave similarly to monomeric pituitary TSH in gel chromatography (Dimond and Rosen, 1974; Kourides, Weintraub, Ridgway and Maloof, 1975) and different from biologically inactive TSH subunits, fragments and aggregates. However, plasma TSH is heterogenous by electrophoretic and other sensitive physicochemical techniques and it is theoretically possible that such heterogenous forms could have different ratios of immunological to biological activity. All serum TSH concentrations described in this section are based on the best available radioimmunoassay data.

1. The Normal Level

Investigators using the early TSH radioimmunoassays reported the range of plasma concentrations in normal subjects as $<1·5–15\,\mu u/ml$ (Utiger, 1965; Odell et al., 1967). Subsequently, others using more sensitive radioimmunoassays and including TSH-free serum in the diluent for standards (see above) have reported a normal range of $<0·5–3·5\,\mu u/ml$ with a mean of

1–2 µu/ml (Fig. 7) (Patel et al., 1971; Ridgway et al., 1973; Pekary et al., 1975). Similar values have been noted by Nisula and Louvet (1978) who concentrated TSH from serum by affinity adsorption with concanavalin A linked to agarose. There are similar TSH concentrations in male and female adults of all ages and in children, except for the neonatal period (Odell et al., 1967b; Mayberry et al., 1971).

TSH concentrations are normal in maternal serum throughout pregnancy, although Braunstein and Hershman (1976) found a slight TSH decrement in the first trimester. Foetal serum TSH is undetectable until 12 weeks of gestation and then rises to concentrations of 5–15 µu/ml in the 3rd trimester (Fisher, Hobel, Garza and Pierce, 1970). Similar concentrations of TSH are found in newborn cord blood (mean 9·5 µu/ml), but 10 min after delivery TSH rises to a mean value of 60 µu/ml and by 30 min peaks at 86 µu/ml (Fisher and Odell, 1969). Between 30 min and 4 hr TSH falls rapidly and then gradually to a mean value of 13 µu/ml at 48 hr. Warming infants to 37·2–41·4° (99–103°F) during the first 3 hr of life does not prevent the initial release of TSH, suggesting that a stimulus other than cooling is involved. In an anencephalic newborn with an absent hypothalamous studied by Allen, Greet, McGilyra, Castro and Fisher (1974), there was no spontaneous rise in TSH, although the infant possessed a pituitary that could secrete TSH in response to exogenous thyrotrophin-releasing hormone. Therefore it is likely that the newborn stimulus is mediated through a central mechanism involving hypothalamic hormones.

Investigators using the early, relatively insensitive radioimmunoassays were unable to demonstrate a diurnal variation in serum TSH concentrations (Utiger, 1965a; Odell et al., 1967b; Hershman and Pittman, 1971a, b; Webster, Guansing and Paine, 1972). Subsequently, others using more sensitive assays were able to define an evening peak, approximately double the values at other times, occurring between 21.00 and 01.00 hours (Vanhaelst, Van Cauter, DeGaute and Golstein, 1972; Alford, Baker, Pate, Rennie, Youatt, Burger and Hudson, 1973; Parker, Pekary and Hershman, 1976). This evening peak of TSH preceded the onset of sleep in most subjects and appears to differ from the sleep-related peaks of growth hormone, prolactin and luteinising hormone. In addition to this circadian rhythm there also appear to be episodic brief bursts of TSH secretion throughout the day and night. However, in contrast to those of several other pituitary hormones, the episodic peaks of TSH are of low amplitude.

2. Metabolic Clearance and Production Rates of TSH

The metabolic clearance rate of $[^{131}I]$ hTSH has been studied by single injection techniques (Odell, Utiger, Wilber and Condliffe, 1967a; Beckers,

Machiels, Soyez and Cornette, 1971) or by constant infusion to equilibrium methods (Ridgway, Weintraub and Maloof, 1974b). The $t_{\frac{1}{2}}$ of the disappearance curve in normal subjects is between 50 and 60 min, and the metabolic clearance rate averages 50 ml/min with a range of 30–86 ml/min. Apparent sex differences in clearance rate disappear when the data are normalised for body surface area. There is a direct correlation between serum thyroid hormone concentrations and the clearance rate of TSH (Ridgway et al., 1974b). TSH is cleared primarily by the kidney and there is no significant degradation by the thyroid gland (Ridgway, Singer, Weintraub, Lorenz and Maloof, 1974a).

The secretion rate of TSH (derived from the product of the clearance rate and the basal serum TSH concentration) in control subjects averages 104 mu/day with a range of 30–172 mu/day. In hyperthyroidism the secretion rate is less than 44 mu/day and in primary hypothyroidism averages 4440 mu/day with a wide range (Ridgway et al., 1974a). The increased serum TSH levels in hypothyroid patients result primarily from the increased pituitary secretion rate, but also, in part, from the decreased clearance rate described above.

3. Factors Affecting TSH Secretion

A variety of endocrine, metabolic and chemical factors have been examined for their ability to affect TSH secretion. There is no significant response of basal TSH to arginine, vasopressin, glucagon, oestrogen, oestrogen–progesterone combinations, changes in blood glucose, or electroconvulsive therapy (Odell et al., 1967b; Hershman and Pittman, 1971a, b). The administration of bacterial endotoxin (Odell et al., 1967b) or L-dopa (Refetoff, Fang, Rapoport and Friesen, 1974) produces no change in serum TSH in normal subjects but suppresses TSH in hypothyroid individuals. In one report the anticipation of muscular excercise by young men caused a small but significant increase in serum TSH from 3·1 to 4·0 μu/ml (Mason, Hartley, Kotchen, Wherry, Pennington and Jones, 1973). However, neither surgical stress (Charters, Odell and Thompson, 1969) nor severe illness (Utiger, 1965a, b) affects basal TSH secretion.

Although exposure to cold is a potent stimulus to TSH secretion in laboratory animals (Hershman, Read, Baily, Norman and Gibson, 1970b; Hershman and Pittman, 1971a; Jobin, Ferland, Cote and Labrie, 1975), it is a relatively ineffective stimulus in man. Adult subjects exposed to 2–4° for up to 2 hr showed no increase in serum TSH (Odell et al., 1967b; Hershman and Pittman; 1971a; Fisher and Odell, 1971). Even severe hypothermia during cardiac surgery associated with a decrease in body temperature to 30·6° did not increase serum TSH in adults (Hershman et al., 1970b). Only a seven day exposure to Arctic temperatures of −29° to −40° (−20° to −40°F) produced a 50% serum TSH increment in 12 normal men (Raud and Odell, 1969). In contrast, infants under 13 months of age undergoing hypothermia during cardiac surgery displayed a marked increase in serum TSH (Wilber and Baum, 1970). Moreover, in newborn infants kept at 37·2°–41·4° (99–103°F) for the first 3 hr of life, exposure to room temperature 22·2°–25·6° (72–78°F) between 3 and 4 hr resulted in a decrease in mean rectal temperature of 1·8° (3·3°F) and caused a marked increase in serum TSH (Fisher and Odell, 1969).

Excess endogenous or exogenous glucocorticoids can suppress basal TSH in normal and hypothyroid subjects although the effect is variable, depending on the dose and duration of therapy (Wilber and Utiger, 1969b; Otsuki, Dakoda and Baba, 1973; Re, Kourides, Ridgway, Weintraub and Maloof, 1976). A deficiency of cortisol induced by the administration of metyrapone to normal subjects results in a significant increase in TSH (Re et al., 1976). The physiological significance of such glucocorticoid effects is unclear. It is possible that the evening fall in plasma cortisol is related to the subsequent TSH rise in normal subjects and that the increase in plasma cortisol after pyrogen causes the TSH decrement in hypothyroid subjects. Somatostatin also causes a rapid inhibition of basal TSH in normal subjects (Weeke, Hansen and Lundaek, 1975), and this hypothalamic hormone is probably of physiological significance in the regulation of TSH secretion (see Section B above).

4. TSH Response to TRH

The purification, characterisation and synthesis of TRH, described in Section B, has provided a safe and potent agent to test pituitary TSH reserve in man. In normal individuals, TRH administered intravenously causes a rapid increase in serum TSH which peaks between 20–30 min and returns to baseline by 180 min (Fig. 5) (Anderson, Bowers, Kastin, Schalch, Schally, Snyder, Utiger, Wilber and Wise, 1971; Haigler, Pittman, Hershman and Baugh, 1971; Ormston, Garry, Cryer, Besser and Hall, 1971; Fleischer, Lorente, Kirkland, Kirkland, Clayton and Calderon, 1972; Snyder and Utiger, 1972a). The mean maximum increment in serum TSH after TRH is about 16 μu/ml with a range of 5–32 μu/ml. Similar responses are found in children (Foley, Jacobs, Hoffman, Doughaday and Blizzard, 1972), women of all ages and young men (Snyder and Utiger, 1972a, b). However, men over the age of 40 years often have severely blunted TSH responses, for reasons that are still unknown. Although significant TSH responses have been obtained with a few μg of TRH, doses producing maximal responses (200–500 μg in adults, 5–7 μg/Kg in children) are usually administered. TRH can also be given intramuscularly in doses up to 2 mg (Azizi, Vagenakis, Portnay,

Table 3

TSH response to TRH in four patients with primary hypothyroidism given increasing doses of L-thyroxine and sequential TRH stimulation tests (modified from Ridgway et al., 1973).

Patient	Date of TRH stimulation (200 μg i.v.)	L-Thyroxine dosage (μg)	Basal TSH (μu/ml)	Maximal TSH after TRH (μu/ml)	T_4 (μg/100 ml)	Free T_4 (ng/100 ml)	T_3 (ng/100 ml)
1	2.12.72	0	84	203	2·5	0·4	95
	3.16.72	50	46	180	4·5	1·0	140
	4.14.72	100	9	72	6·5	1·1	110
	5.12.72	150	7	45	7·0	1·2	150
	6. 9.72	200	<0·5	3	7·5	1·4	170
	7. 7.72	300	<0·5	0·5	10·5	2·4	290
2	8. 7.71	0	35	102	2·5	0·4	80
	8.25.71	100	8	36	6·5	1·2	110
	9.16.71	150	<0·5	5	8·5	1·9	190
	10.22.71	200	<0·5	<0·5	9·5	2·4	160
	12. 3.71	300	<0·5	<0·5	11·5	2·3	240
3	5.31.71	0	18	115	3·0	0·5	150
	6.26.71	0	10	88	4·5	0·7	115
	8.21.71	100	4	31	7·0	1·3	125
	9.18.71	150	4	48	6·5	1·2	175
	10. 9.71	200	<0·5	4	9·5	2·5	200
	11. 6.71	300	<0·5	<0·5	11·0	2·3	255
	12/ 4/71[a]	300	<0·5	<0·5	9·0	1·7	190
4	7.24.71	0	6	85	3·0	0·7	155
	8.10.71	100	<0·5	11	7·0	1·5	150
	8.31.71	150	<0·5	<0·5	9·0	1·7	245
	9.21.71	200	<0·5	<0·5	9·0	2·2	180
	10.19.71	300	<0·5	<0·5	12·5	2·5	360
Euthyroid controls		none	<0·5–4	6–18	4–11	0·8–2·4	150–250

[a] 1·0 mg TRH used for this study.

Rapoport, Ingbar and Braverman, 1975) or orally in doses up to 100 mg (Rabello, Snyder and Utiger, 1974) to produce more sustained increases in TSH.

The immunoactive TSH released by a TRH test is clearly biologically active in man. There is a modest increase in serum T_3 but only a minimal change in T_4 after i.v. TRH (Hollander, Mitsuma, Shenkman, Woolf and Gershengorn, 1972); changes in T_3 and T_4 are larger after intramuscular or oral TRH.

The TSH response to TRH is increased by oestrogen and/or progesterone in normal pregnancy (Hershman, Kojima and Friesen, 1973; Burrow, Polack-Wich and Donabedian, 1975) or during oral contraceptive therapy (Ramey, Burrow, Polack-Wich and Donabedian, 1975). The TSH response to TRH is suppressed by glucocorticoids (Otsuki et al., 1973; Re et al., 1976), L-dopa (Rapoport, Refetoff, Fang and Friesen, 1973; Refetoff et al., 1974), somatostatin (Siler, Yen, Vale and Guillemin, 1974; Carr, Gomez-Parr, Weightman, Roy, Hall, Besser, Thomas, McNeilly, Schally, Kastin and Coy, 1975), growth hormone (Root, Snyder, Rezvani, DiGeorge and Utiger, 1973; Lippe, Van Herle, LaFranchi, Uller, Levin and Kaplan, 1975), and aspirin (Yamamoto, Woeber and Ingbar, 1972). The most important factor affecting the TSH response to TRH is the serum concentration of free T_4 and T_3, which will be considered in detail in the next sections.

5. Hypothyroidism

Serum TSH concentrations are virtually always elevated in untreated patients with primary or thyroidal hypothyroidism (Utiger, 1965; Odell et al., 1967b). Patients with mild hypothyroidism may have only a slightly increased serum TSH while those with severe hypothyroidism usually have values greater than 25 µu/ml. In the latter group TSH concentrations vary widely, occasionally reaching values greater than 1000 µu/ml. There is no clear correlation between serum thyroid hormone levels or duration of hypothyroidism, and serum TSH.

The demonstration of a serum TSH value of greater than 10 µu/ml in a hypothyroid patient virtually establishes the diagnosis of primary hypothyroidism. There is no need to perform a TRH test in such patients since they will all show responsiveness which is of no further diagnostic value (Table 3). The TSH response to TRH in hypothyroid patients, expressed in absolute terms, is greater than in normal subjects, but the percent increment above basal values is usually less. TRH tests are of value in patients with equivocal hypothyroidism and a slight elevation of basal TSH, since an exaggerated response to TRH will help confirm the diagnosis of primary hypothyroidism (Table 3, patient 4).

Most cases of cretinism and childhood hypothyroidism are thyroidal in origin and also associated with elevated serum TSH concentrations. In recently established newborn screening programmes for congenital hypothyroidism TSH tests have been of importance in confirming the diagnosis, since many instances of low serum T_4 in newborns are secondary to decreased thyroxine binding globulin rather than hypothyroidism (Dussault, Morissette, Letarte, Guyda and Laberge, 1978; Mitchell, Larsen, Levy, Bennett and Madoff, 1978).

Hypothyroidism caused by pituitary or hypothalamic disease can be diagnosed by the presence of low or normal serum TSH (Utiger, 1965; Odell et al., 1967b; Anderson et al., 1971). The distinction between pituitary (secondary) and hypothalamic (tertiary) disease has often been based on the response to exogenous TRH. Patients with documented pituitary disease often show no responsiveness to TRH while those with presumed hypothalamic disease (usually based on the absence of demonstrable pituitary disease) often show normal or increased peak responses that may be delayed at 60 min or later (Costom, Grumbach and Kaplan, 1971; Hall, Ormston, Besser, Cryer and McKendrick, 1972; Faglia, Beck-Peccoz, Ferrari, Ambrosi, Spada, Travaglini and Paracchi, 1973). However, there are many documented exceptions to these classic patterns, particularly patients with pituitary disorders who show definite TRH responsiveness (Faglia et al., 1973; Berthezene, Mornex and Chavrier, 1974). Such responsiveness could result from larger concentrations of TRH achieved exogenously than endogenously or from abnormal hypothalamic–pituitary portal vasculature. It is also conceivable that certain patients with longstanding hypothalamic disease and atrophy of pituitary thyrotrophs could fail to respond to a single TRH test. Until assays are available for endogenous hypothalamic TRH and somatostatin it will not be possible to clarify this problem.

The presence of normal or even slightly elevated serum TSH in patients with hypothalamic and/or pituitary disorders had been noted in early studies and attributed to assay insensitivity and non-specific serum effects (Utiger, 1965; Odell et al., 1967b; Anderson et al., 1971; Faglia et al., 1973). Subsequently investigators using more sensitive assays were able to document slightly elevated TSH concentrations of 4–11 µu/ml in certain patients with such disorders (Patel and Burger, 1973; Illig, Krawczynska, Torresani and Prader, 1975). These patients had no evidence of thyroid disease, responded to exogenous bovine TSH, and usually had evidence of other anterior pituitary hormone deficiency. Serum TSH response to TRH was normal or increased (often with a delayed peak) and basal TSH could be suppressed by administration of exogenous thyroid hormone. Although the reason for central hypothyroidism and elevated immunoreactive TSH in these patients is not known, possible explanations are a gradually acquired resistance of the thyroid to TSH or to the secretion of TSH with diminished biological activity. In any case, it is clear that patients with hypothyroidism and slight elevations of serum TSH can no longer be assumed to have primary hypothyroidism without further study.

Patients with primary hypothyroidism treated with thyroid hormone show a fall in serum TSH, the rate and magnitude of which is dependent on the dose, route of administration, and type of thyroid hormone. Both the basal serum TSH and the response to TRH will be normalised in most patients by T_4 doses of 0·1–0·2 mg (Table 3) or by T_3 doses of 0·05 to 0·1 mg (Cotton, Gorman and Mayberry, 1971; Ridgway et al., 1973; Saberi and Utiger, 1974). In two large studies, the average dose of T_4 necessary for restoration of normal TSH was 169 µg/day or 2·25 µg/day/Kg and for suppression of TSH was 172 µg/day or 2·6 µg/day/Kg (Stock, Surks and Oppenheimer, 1974; Hoffman, Surks, Oppenheimer and Weitzman, 1977). In an individual patient such a change from normal to suppressed TSH is achieved by 25–50 µg changes in T_4 dosage associated with only small changes in serum thyroid hormone levels within the "normal range" for groups of control subjects (Table 3). Thus serum TSH before and after TRH can serve as a guide for appropriate replacement or suppressive therapy in an individual patient. In the former case, however, it is still not established whether peripheral tissues have the same sensitivity as the pituitary to thyroid hormone levels and whether there is a real clinical benefit from such fine titration of thyroid hormone therapy.

6. Hyperthyroidism

Serum TSH is virtually always low or undetectable in patients with hyperthyroidism, since pituitary hypersecretion of TSH is only rarely the cause of hyperthyroidism. The common forms of hyperthyroidism either are not related to the production of any thyrotrophic substance or are caused by thyrotrophic substances other than TSH. Hyperthyroidism not caused by thyrotrophic substances include hyperfunctioning solitary thyroid nodules or multinodular goitres, subacute thyroiditis, exogenous administration of thyroid hormone, ectopic thyroid tissue, or thyroid carcinoma. Hyperthyroidism caused by non-TSH thyrotrophic substances include Graves' disease and hyperthyroidism associated with trophoblastic neoplasms. In all of these forms of hyperthyroidism, elevated concentrations of free T_4 and/or T_3 suppress basal pituitary TSH secretion as well as the pituitary response to TRH, as described above in Figs 7–8. Reduction of serum thyroid hormone levels invariably leads to recovery of normal serum TSH levels although there is usually a transient period when TSH remains low and unresponsive to TRH despite normal or low serum T_4 and T_3 (see below).

Graves' disease is a term often applied to any chronic form of hyperthyroidism associated with a diffuse goitre. More precisely, it should be reserved for patients with characteristic ophthalmopathy, pretibial myxedema, or those in whom serum LATS or other thyroid-stimulating immunoglobulins (TSI) have been demonstrated. It is likely that such stimulating antibodies are pathogenic in the disease, but there have been considerable difficulties in developing assays of sufficient specificity, sensitivity and precision to measure them adequately. The original LATS assay (Adams and Purves, 1956) and several later modifications (McKenzie, 1958; Kriss, Pleshakov and Chien, 1964a) are relatively insensitive, imprecise and subject to artifacts (Florsheim, Williams and Schönbaum, 1970). Moreover, such assays only measure those human antibodies capable of also stimulating animal thyroid tissue. Subsequently a "LATS-protector" assay was developed that measures human antibodies capable of competing with ("protecting") those in a known LATS-positive serum for binding sites on human thyroid tissue (Adams and Kennedy, 1967; Adams and Kennedy, 1971). This assay is able to measure abnormal immunoglobulins in many Graves' sera negative for LATS but is relatively cumbersome and imprecise. Later a TSH receptor assay was developed that directly measured antibodies capable of competing with labelled bovine TSH for binding to the TSH receptor on human thyroid membranes (Smith and Hall, 1974; Hall, Smith and Mukhtar, 1975). This assay is very convenient and precise, and the initial reports showed almost all Graves' sera positive in the receptor assay. However, recent reports have shown a lower rate of positivity, in the range of 50–60% (Schleusener, Kotulla, Kruck, Kruck, Geissler and Adlkofer, 1975; Endo, Kasagi, Konishi, Ikekubo, Okuno, Takeda, Mori and Torizuka, 1978). Recently other workers have used *in vitro* bioassays to measure antibodies that directly stimulate colloid droplet formation or adenyl cyclase in human thyroid (Onaya, Kotani, Yamada and Ochi, 1973; McKenzie and Zakarija, 1976). Such assays might correlate better with thyroid function, since the LATS-protector and receptor assay could measure antibodies that bind to thyroid tissues but are not capable of stimulating the thyroid cell.

The new assays represent a major advance and have strengthened the hypothesis that autoantibodies are the cause of Graves' disease. However, none has yet been proved to be completely specific for Graves' disease (Strakosch, Joyner and Wall, 1978a, b) or has been shown to correlate well with the state of thyroid function in Graves' patients. Such correlation may be hampered by additional factors, such as intrathyroidal lymphocytes and cytotoxic antibodies that may modify the response to the stimulatory antibodies as in "euthyroid" Graves' disease.

7. Hyperthyroidism Associated with Trophoblastic Neoplasms

Hyperthyroidism has been demonstrated in patients with a variety of trophoblastic neoplasms including molar pregnancy and choriocarcinoma (Odell, Bates, Rivlin, Lipsett and Hertz, 1963; Cohen and Utiger, 1970; Hershman and Higgins, 1971). Serum and tumour extracts from such patients contain a thyrotrophic substance physicochemically and immunologically different from TSH, LATS or other thyroid-stimulating immunoglobulins. In gel chromatography the thyrotrophic substance, termed "molar thyrotrophin," appeared of higher mw than TSH but considerably less than that of immunoglobulins. Subsequently, it was found that this substance was indistinguishable, by a variety of physicochemical and immunologic criteria, from human chorionic gonadotrophin (hCG) (Nisula and Ketelslegers, 1974; Kenimer, Hershman and Higgins, 1975). Purified hCG has weak, but definite, thyrotrophic TSH activity. However, even this weak thyrotrophic activity is sufficient to cause a significant effect in these patients who invariably have very high concentrations of serum hCG (10^4–10^6 ng/ml) compared with the normal concentration of TSH (<0.5 ng/ml).

Hyperthyroidism has not yet been demonstrated in patients with nontrophoblastic cancers associated with ectopic hCG secretion, probably because the serum hCG concentrations are usually considerably lower than in patients with trophoblastic cancer. There are no documented reports of the ectopic production of TSH or thyroid-stimulating immunoglobulins.

A thyrotrophic substance, human chorionic thyrotrophin (HCT), has been extracted from the normal placenta and partially characterised (Hennen, Pierce and Freychet, 1969; Hershman and Starnes, 1969). This substance is immunologically different from TSH and hCG but cross-reacts in radioimmunoassays for porcine or bovine TSH. One group has developed a radioimmunoassay for HCT and has found third trimester peak concentrations of 10–50 µg/ml in serum from normal pregnant women and 50–100 µg/ml in serum from patients with molar pregnancy (Tojo, Kanazawa, Nakamura, Kitagaki and Mochizuki, 1973; Tojo, Kanazawa, Saida and Nakamura, 1976). However, the physiological role of this substance in normal pregnancy and in patients with trophoblastic neoplasms is unknown. The thyrotrophic substance in patients with molar pregnancy appears to be hCG (see above) and is clearly different from HCT (Hershman, Higgins and Starnes, 1970a).

8. Hyperthyroidism Caused by Pituitary Hypersecretion of TSH

Several cases of hyperthyroidism caused by excessive and inappropriate secretion of pituitary TSH have been described. The syndrome appears to encompass a heterogenous group of patients, some of whom have documented pituitary tumours; in others there is no evidence of tumours, but the histopathology of the pituitary has not yet been directly examined.

The association of hyperthyroidism and a pituitary tumour has long been recognised, and in two cases a thyrotrophic substance was demonstrated in the serum by bioassay (Jailer and Holub, 1960; Lamberg, Ripatti, Gordin, Juustila, Sivula and Bjorkesten, 1969). However, secretion of TSH as measured in a specific radioimmunoassay was first documented by Hamilton, Adams and Maloof (1970). These workers described a 50-year-old man with hyperthyroidism, elevated serum TSH (17 ng/ml) and an enlarged sella turcica who, at craniotomy, was found to have a pituitary chromophobe adenoma. After partial resection of the tumour and radiotherapy, serum TSH fell to normal and the clinical and chemical signs of hyperthyroidism remitted. Since this study at least 10 other reports have appeared describing patients with pituitary tumours, hyperthyroidism, and increased serum immunoreactive TSH as high as 35 μu/ml (Hamilton and Maloof, 1972; Faglia, Ferrari, Neri, Beck, Poccoz, Ambrosi and Valenti, 1972; Mornex, Tommasi, Cure, Farcot, Orgiazzi and Rousset, 1972; Hrubesch, Bockel, Vosberg, Wagner and Hauss, 1972; O'Donnell, Hadden, Weaver and Montgomery, 1973; Baylis, 1976; Horn, Erhardt, Fahlbrusch, Pickhardt, Werder and Scriba, 1976; Reschini, Giustina, Cantalomessa and Peracchi, 1976; Kourides, Ridgway, Weintraub, Bigos, Gershengorn and Maloof, 1977b; Tolis, Bird, Bertrand, McKenzie and Ezrin, 1978). Certain of the tumours have also been reported to secrete growth hormone or prolactin.

In other reports of TSH-induced hyperthyroidism, the patients have shown no evidence of a pituitary tumour despite careful clinical and radiographic follow-up over many years (Emerson and Utiger, 1972; Gershengorn and Weintraub, 1975; Elewaut, Mussche and Vermeulen, 1976; Hood, Vaughn-Jackson and Farid, 1976; Kourides et al., 1977b; Novogroder, Utiger, Boyar and Levine, 1977). TSH concentrations have been variable, ranging from about 9 to 160 μu/ml. Several of the patients had been first studied after previous insults to the thyroid gland including ^{131}I therapy (Emerson and Utiger, 1972), thyroidectomy (Gershengorn and Weintraub, 1975; Elewaut et al., 1976; Kourides et al., 1977b; Novogroder et al., 1976) or thyroiditis (Hood et al., 1976). However, one patient clearly had inappropriate TSH secretion before thyroidectomy (Gershengorn and Weintraub, 1975), and in another study several untreated, asymptomatic family members were noted to have a similar syndrome (Elewaut *et al.*, 1976). It is likely that these patients have a partial target organ resistance to the action of thyroid hormone that is relatively selective for the pituitary (Gershengorn and Weintraub, 1975). After thyroid insult and a period of hypothyroidism the thyrotrophs may become "reset" to secrete even more TSH for a given level of circulating thyroid hormone.

There are major differences between the neoplastic and non-neoplastic syndromes of TSH-induced hyperthyroidism (Kourides *et al.*, 1977b). The neoplasms are usually autonomous in their secretion of TSH with very little stimulation by TRH or suppression by thyroid hormone. Moreover, the tumours also secrete a large excess of the common α-subunit of the glycoprotein hormones (see below). In contrast, the patients with non-neoplastic syndromes usually show some degree of TSH suppression by thyroid hormone, hyperresponsiveness to TRH, and relatively low α-subunit levels. The differences in TSH and subunit secretion in the tumour versus the non-tumour patients with pituitary hyperthyroidism make it unlikely that the latter patients actually have an occult microadenoma.

Although the pathogenesis of these syndromes is not known, both the tumour and non-tumour cases show definite, albeit variable, degrees of resistance to the usual suppressive effects of thyroid hormone on pituitary TSH secretion. In contrast to recognised syndromes of generalised target organ resistance to the action of thyroid hormone (Refetoff, DeWind and DeGroot, 1967; Lamberg, 1973; Bode, Danon, Weintraub, Maloof and Crawford, 1973) these cases show qualitatively appropriate peripheral thyroid hormone effects, although more subtle quantitative abnormalities cannot be excluded by the currently available methodology. Also unclear is the significance of absent TRH responses in all but one (Mornex *et al.*, 1972) of the tumour patients studied and the presence of increased TRH responses in all but one (Emerson and Utiger, 1972) of the non-tumour patients. Endogenous TRH concentrations cannot be reliably measured at present but hypersecretion of TRH, alone, would not appear to explain increased TSH secretion in the face of thyroid hormone levels that normally totally inhibit the TSH response to large doses of exogenous TRH. Similarly, a deficiency in hypothalamic somatostatin secretion would not appear to explain the syndrome, since thyroid hormones inhibit TSH secretion *in vitro*, even in the absence of somatostatin. Moreover, the normal suppressive action of glucocorticoids on TSH secretion has been demonstrated in all cases examined.

A possible relationship of these syndromes to Graves' disease is also unclear. Only one patient had exophthalmos (Hamilton and Maloof, 1972), and this patient was later found to have hyperthyroidism with suppressed TSH, probably resulting from Graves' disease (Sandler, 1976). Neither LATS nor "LATS-protector" has been detected in the patients studied. The demonstration of a relationship with Graves' disease would be an extremely provocative finding and these patients clearly should be studied with more sensitive assays for thyroid-stimulating immunoglobulins. However, most of the patients have demonstrated a good correlation between changes in serum TSH and changes in thyroidal radioiodine uptake and hormone secretion.

Increased recognition of these syndromes should be facilitated by the increased availability of specific and sensitive TSH radioimmunoassays. Such recognition is not only clinically important but also should lead to fundamental advances in our knowledge of TSH and thyroid hormone physiology.

9. Exophthalmos

Malignant exophthalmos is a complication of thyrotoxicosis that has been frequently attributed to TSH. The reason for this supposition is that pituitary extracts that contain TSH often contain some factor that causes proptosis in experimental animals.

With the development of radioimmunoassay techniques for pituitary hTSH it seems clear that in clinical exophthalmos pituitary hTSH is not correlated with the presence of hTSH (Odell et al., 1967b). On the other hand, LATS is frequently present in sera of patients with malignant exophthalmos. The explanation for the persistence of exophthalmos or its occurrence when the hyperthyroidism is otherwise controlled, might be that LATS persists and can still cause hypertrophy of the retro-orbital tissues of the eye. The suggestion made by Adams (1958) that the causative factor in exophthalmos might be an abnormal thyroid-stimulating substance has received support from the work of Kriss et al. (1964d), Pinchera et al. (1965) and Kriss, Pleshakov, Rosenblum, Holderness, Sharp and Utiger (1967). However, McKenzie (1962b) and Major and Munro (1962) were unable to correlate exophthalmos with the presence of LATS.

In view of this lack of correlation the question arises as to the significance of the exophthalmos-producing substances (EPS) that are found in some pituitary fractions and which stimulate proptosis in fish and other animals (Dobyns, 1966). Similar substances have been described in hyperthyroid sera from patients with exophthalmos (Dobyns and Wilson, 1954). Dobyns (1966) has reviewed the various factors and conditions that affect the development of exophthalmos in fish. The possibility remains that proptosis can be caused in fish by a number of factors including LATS and some pituitary fractions that contain TSH activity. Despite the frequent association of TSH and EPS, situations have been reported where TSH is present without EPS or where a partial separation can be effected. Dobyns and Steelman

(1953) showed that bTSH was separable from EPS by precipitation of EPS with trichloroacetic acid, leaving TSH in the soluble fraction. Brunish (1958) found that while TSH activity in a given preparation was reduced by treatment with pepsin, EPS was unaffected. Brunish, Hayashi and Hayashi (1962) showed that bTSH and EPS could be separated on DEAEC columns. Bates, Albert and Condliffe (1959) were unable to demonstrate EPS in extracts of mouse pituitary tumours which were rich in mTSH. However, Kohn, Winand and Bates (1975) later demonstrated EPS in mTSH and showed that pepsin digestion of mTSH, bTSH, and hTSH destroyed thyrotrophic activity at a more rapid rate than EPS activity. These workers (Kohn and Winand, 1975) isolated an early pepsin digestion fragment of bTSH with selective EPS activity and showed that it contained the intact TSH-β-subunit and a fragment of the α-subunit. This material bound to guinea-pig retro-orbital tissue (Harderian gland) membranes, and the binding was enhanced in the presence of γ globulin from patients with exophthalmos (Bolonkin, Tate, Luber, Kohn and Winand, 1975).

It is, however, doubtful that the EPS activity of TSH or of its proteolytic digestion products are relevant to human exophthalmos. There is no evidence for the presence of either TSH or TSH-β immunoactivity in the serum of patients with exophthalmos (Kourides, Weintraub, Ridgway and Maloof, 1975). Nevertheless, it would be interesting to examine extracts of normal and Graves' retro-orbital tissue for high local concentrations of such materials. It seems probable that exophthalmos is another autoimmune manifestation of Graves' disease, possibly related to thyroglobulin-antithyroglobulin (Konishi, Herman and Kriss, 1974) or other immune complexes. Hopefully, the measurement of exophthalmos-producing antibodies and a description of their relationship to thyroid-stimulating antibodies will be achieved by the next edition of this book.

10. Other Thyroid Diseases

Serum TSH may be elevated in patients with various thyroid diseases despite normal serum thyroid hormone concentrations and no clinical signs or symptoms of hypothyroidism. The patients include those with certain stages of Hashimoto's thyroiditis (Gordin and Lamberg, 1975), subacute thyroiditis (Ogihara, Yamamoto, Azukizawa, Miyai and Kumahara, 1973), endemic goitre (Delange, Hershman and Ermans, 1971); patients who have been treated with [131]I (Toft, Irvine, Hunter and Seth, 1974), external neck irradiation (Glatstein, McHardy-Young, Brast, Eltringham, and Kriss, 1971) or drugs that impair thyroid hormone synthesis or secretion (Emerson, Dyson and Utiger, 1973). These patients show TSH hyperresponsiveness to TRH similar to those with mild hypothyroidism, and may progress to clinical and

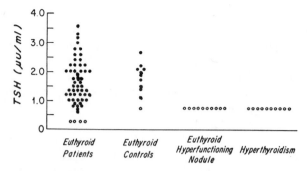

Fig. 7. Basal serum TSH concentration in euthyroid patients, euthyroid controls, euthyroid patients with hyperfunctioning thyroid nodules, and patients with hyperthyroidism. Open circles denote undetectable TSH concentrations ($< 0.5-1.0 \, \mu u/ml$). Reproduced from Ridgway *et al.* (1973).

chemical hypothyroidism with time. However, the rate of such progression is variable, and many patients may remain euthyroid indefinitely.

Serum TSH may also be suppressed and unresponsive to TRH in certain patients despite clinical and chemical euthyroidism. The patients include those receiving small doses of thyroid hormone (Snyder and Utiger, 1972b), those with hyperfunctioning solitary and multiple thyroid nodules (Figs 7–8) (Ridgway *et al.*, 1975), "euthyroid" Graves' disease (Clague, Mukhtar, Pyle, Nutt, Clark, Scott, Evered, Smith and Hall, 1976), and virtually every other condition that can also be associated with frank hyperthyroidism.

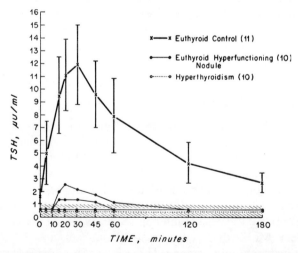

Fig. 8. Serum TSH response to TRH stimulation in euthyroid controls, euthyroid patients with hyperfunctioning thyroid nodules, and patients with hyperthyroidism. Reproduced from Ridgway *et al.* (1973).

Moreover, patients who have had chronic suppression of TSH secondary to exogenous thyroid hormone therapy (Vagenakis, Braverman. Azizi, Portnay and Ingbar, 1975a; Krugman, Hershman, Chopra, Levine, Pekary, Geffner and ChuaTeco, 1975) or various forms of hyperthyroidism (Sanchez-Franco, Garcia, Cacicedo, Martin-Zurro, Del Ray and De Escobar, 1974) may continue to show low and TRH-unresponsive serum TSH for 1–4 weeks after serum thyroid hormone concentrations become normal or low.

These instances of increased or suppressed TSH in clinically euthyroid patients with normal T_4 and T_3 are usually regarded as "subclinical" hypothyroidism or hyperthyroidism, respectively. Although the free and total thyroid hormone concentrations are "normal" with regard to a group of subjects, they must be regarded as abnormal by the sensitive pituitary feedback mechanism of each individual. Since peripheral tissues do not appear to be as sensitive as the pituitary to these minimal changes in thyroid hormone levels, such fine modulation of TSH may serve to protect these tissues from thyroid hormone deficiency or excess. There is no evidence that patients with such subclinical disease require immediate therapy, although thyroid hormones may be given to patients with elevated TSH to prevent or shrink goitres. However, these patients must be followed closely to detect disease progression requiring treatment.

Most patients with nonendemic goitre of unknown aetiology have normal serum TSH (Odell *et al.*, 1967b; Hershman and Pittman, 1971b). This could mean that excess TSH plays no role in the development of such goitres or that the thyroid is hypersensitive to normal TSH concentrations. Alternatively, some factor impairing thyroid hormone secretion could lead to a transient increase in TSH, which causes growth of thyroid tissue; the resulting increase in thyroid hormone production might then restore TSH to normal levels. Patients with non-toxic goitres treated with thyroid hormones to suppress TSH show a variable decrease in goitre size (Astwood, Cassidy and Aurbach, 1960).

11. Other Diseases

Patients with a variety of severe diseases including hepatic cirrhosis, infection, malignancy, congestive heart failure, bronchitis and malnutrition have reduced serum total and free T_3 because of reduced peripheral conversion of T_4 to T_3 (Chopra, Solomon, Chopra, Young and Chua Teco, 1974; Portnay, O'Brian, Bush, Vagenakis, Azizi, Arky, Ingbar and Braverman, 1974; Bermudaz, Surks and Oppenheimer, 1975; Moshang, Parks, Baker, Vaidya, Utiger, Bongiovanni and Snyder, 1975). However, these patients appear euthyroid and usually have normal or only slightly elevated basal TSH and responses to TRH. Patients with chronic renal failure also have reduced T_3 and normal basal TSH, but the TSH response to TRH is often diminished and delayed (Czernichow, Dauzet, Broyer and Rappaport, 1976; Lim, Fang, Katz and Refetoff, 1977). These data suggest that, despite low serum T_3, the normal or slightly elevated serum free T_4 in patients with chronic disease has a major effect in inhibiting TSH secretion. Alternatively, chronic disease may impair the pituitary or hypothalamic response to reduced T_3.

E. THE CONCENTRATION OF TSH SUBUNITS IN PLASMA

Using purified hTSH-α and hTSH-β subunits, two groups initially developed radioimmunoassays for free TSH subunits in human plasma (Kourides, Weintraub, Ridgway and Maloof, 1975; Edmonds, Molitch, Pierce and Odell, 1975). The TSH-α assay actually measures all free α-subunits of the glycoprotein hormones, since they are chemically and immunologically indistinguishable; the TSH-β assay is specific and does not measure gonadotrophin β-subunits. Certain subunit antisera show appreciable cross-reactivity with intact TSH, requiring correction of the apparent subunit values for the TSH component as measured in a separate assay (Edmonds et al., 1975). However, other antisera have been developed to free subunit determinants that are not exposed in intact TSH, yielding subunit assays with no significant TSH cross reactivity (Kourides et al., 1975). The nature of the materials measured by these specific assays has been confirmed as free α and free TSH-β by their elution in gel chromatography.

In normal subjects serum α concentrations range from <0.5–5.0 ng/ml, being slightly higher in postmenopausal women than in men or premenopausal women, and TSH-β is not detectable (<0.5 ng/ml) (Kourides et al., 1975). Both subunits increase in serum after TRH and their peak response is slightly earlier than that of TSH. In patients with primary hypothyroidism the concentrations of both α and TSH-β are increased roughly in proportion to the elevation of intact TSH and both hyperrespond to TRH. Patients with hyperthyroidism have only slightly lowered serum α-subunit since most of the basal serum α-subunit derives from gonadotrophin subunits. However, hyperthyroid subjects show no response of α or TSH-β to TRH.

Serum α and TSH-β subunits are not derived from the dissociation of TSH but are directly secreted from the pituitary both in vitro (Blackman, Gershengorn and Weintraub, 1978) and in vivo. The infusion of labelled (Kourides et al., 1975) or unlabelled (Edmonds et al., 1975) TSH into patients with primary hypothyroidism or normal subjects does not lead to any dissociation of TSH into subunits. The normal pituitary contains a large pool of free α-subunits even greater than that of TSH, but there is relatively little free TSH-β. These data support the biosynthetic data described in Section B showing that the α-subunit is present in excess and the β-subunit is limiting in TSH biosynthesis.

The metabolic clearance rates of hTSH-α and hTSH-β are both two to three times faster than that of TSH (Kourides, Re, Weintraub, Ridgway and Maloof, 1977b). The secretion rate of α in normal subjects is 91 μg/day/m², greater than that of TSH and much greater than that of TSH-β, which is usually undetectable.

Elevated serum α/TSH ratios have been described in patients (Kourides et al., 1977b) and animals (Blackman et al., 1978) with TSH-secreting pituitary tumours. The excess α production from such tumours has been of value in differentiating patients with neoplastic from non-neoplastic causes of TSH-induced hyperthyroidism (see Section D.8). Elevated serum TSH-β/TSH ratios have been described in two patients, one with an enlarged thyroid and one with an enlarged pituitary (Kourides, Weintraub and Maloof, 1978). The TSH-β in both cases had an apparently large mw (160,000–200,000), displayed immunologic properties different from standard TSH-β, and was unresponsive to TRH. Although this unusual form of TSH-β has been partially characterised, its significance remains unknown.

REFERENCES

Adams, D. D. (1958). *Proc. Univ. Otago med. Sch.* **36**, 10.
Adams, D. D. (1965). *Br. med. J.* **i**, 1015.
Adams, D. D. and Kennedy, T. H. (1962). *Proc. Univ. Otago med. Sch.* **40**, 6.
Adams, D. D. and Kennedy, T. H. (1967). *J. clin. Endocr. Metab.* **27**, 173.
Adams, D. D. and Kennedy, T. H. (1971). *J. clin. Endocr. Metab.* **33**, 47.
Adams, D. D., Kennedy, T. H., Purves, H. D. and Sirett, N. E. (1962). *Endocrinology*, **70**, 801.
Adams, D. D. and Purves, H. D. (1953). *Proc. Univ. Otago med. Sch.* **31**, 38.
Adams, D. D. and Purves, H. D. (1955). *Endocrinology*, **57**, 17.
Adams, D. D. and Purves, H. D. (1956). *Proc. Univ. Otago med. Sch.* **34**, 11.
Adams, D. D. and Purves, H. D. (1957). *Metabolism*, **6**, 26.
Adams, D. D. and Purves, H. D. (1961). "Advances in Thyroid Research", p. 184. Pergamon Press, Oxford.
Albert, A. (1949). *Ann. N.Y. Acad. Sci.* **50**, 466.
Alford, F. P., Baker, H. W. G., Patel, Y. C., Rennie, G. C., Youatt, G., Burger, H. G. and Hudson, B. (1973). *J. clin. Endocr. Metab.* **36**, 108.
Allen, J. P., Greer, M. A., McGilvra, R., Castro, A. and Fisher, D. A. (1974). *J. clin. Endocr. Metab.* **38**, 94.
Amir, S. M., Carraway, T. F. and Kohn, L. D. (1973). *J. biol. Chem.* **248**, 4092.
Anderson, E. M. and Collip, J. B. (1934). *J. Physiol.* **82**, 11.
Anderson, M. S., Bowers, C. Y., Kastin, A. J., Schalch, D. S., Schally, A. V., Snyder, P. J., Utiger, R. D., Wilber, J. F. and Wise, A. J. (1971). *New Engl. J. Med.* **285**, 1279.

Asboe-Hansen, G., Iversen, K. and Wichmann, R. (1952). *Acta endocr., Copenh.***11**, 376.

Arimura, A. and Schally, A. V. (1976). *Endocrinology*, **98**, 1069.

Astwood, E. B., Cassidy, C. E. and Aurbach, G. (1960). *J. Am. med. Assoc.* **174**, 459.

Azizi, F., Vagenakis, A. G., Portnay, G. I., Rapoport, B., Ingbar, S. H. and Braverman, L. E. (1975). *New Engl. J. Med.* **292**, 273.

Bakke, J. L. (1965a). *In* "Current Topics in Thyroid Research" (M. Andreoli and C. Cassano, eds). Academic Press, New York and London.

Bakke, J. L. (1965b). *J. clin. Endocr. Metab.* **25**, 545.

Bakke, J. L., Heideman Jr., M. L., Lawrence, N. L. and Wiberg, C. (1957). *Endocrinology*, **61**, 352.

Bakke, J. L. Kammer, M. and Lawrence, N. (1964). *J. clin. Endocr. Metab.* **24**, 281.

Bakke, J. L. and Lawrence, N. (1956). *Endocrinology*, **58**, 531.

Bakke, J. L. and Lawrence, N. (1959). *J. clin. Endocr. Metab.* **19**, 35.

Bassiri, R. M. and Utiger, R. D. (1972). *Endocrinology*, **90**, 722.

Bassiri, R. M. and Utiger, R. D. (1973). *J. clin. Invest.* **52**, 1616.

Bassiri, R. M. and Utiger, R. D. (1974). *Endocrinology*, **94**, 188.

Bates, R. W. (1963), "Evaluation of Thyroid and Parathyroid Functions", p. 44. J. B. Lippincott Co., Philadelphia.

Bates, R. W., Albert, A. and Condliffe, P. G. (1959). *Endocrinology*, **65**, 860.

Bates, R. W., Anderson, E. and Furth, J. (1957). *Endocrinology*, **61**, 549.

Bates, R. W. and Condliffe, P. G. (1960). *Rec. prog. Horm. Res.* **16**, 309.

Bates, R. W. and Condliffe, P. G. (1966). "The Pituitary Gland", Vol. 1, Chap. 9. Butterworths, London.

Bates, R. W. and Cornfield, J. (1957). *Endocrinology*, **60**, 225.

Bates, R. W., Garrison, M. M., Cooper, J. A. and Condliffe, P. G. (1968), *Endocrinology*, **83**, 721.

Bates, R. W., Garrison, M. M. and Howard, T. B. (1959). *Endocrinology*, **65**, 7.

Bauer, K. J. and Lipmann, F. (1973). *Fed. Proc.* **32**, 489.

Bauer, K. and Lipmann. F. (1976). *Endocrinology*, **99**, 230.

Baugh, C. M., Krumdieck, C. L., Hersham, J. M. and Pittman Jr., J. A. (1970). *Endocrinology*, **87**, 1015.

Baylis, P. H. (1976). *Clin. Endocr.* **5**, 145.

Beall, G. N. and Solomon, D. H. (1966). *J. clin. Invest.* **45**, 552.

Becker, D. V. and Furth, E. D. (1965). *In* "Current Topics in Thyroid Research" (M. Andreali and C. Cassano, eds), p. 596. Academic Press, New York and London.

Becker, D. V., Furth, E., Nunez, E., Horwith, M. Stokes, P. E., Berman, M. and Ray, B. (1961). "Advances in Thyroid Research", p. 87. Pergamon Press, Oxford.

Beckers, C., Machiels, J., Soyez, C. and Cornette, C. (1971). *Horm. metab. Res.* **3**, 34.

Bermudez, F., Surks, M. I. and Oppenheimer, J. H. (1975). *J. clin. Endocr. Metab.* **41**, 27.

Berson, S. A. and Yalow, R. S. (1958). *Adv. biol. med. Phys.* **6**, 350.

Berson, S. A. and Yalow, R. S. (1959). *J. clin. Invest.* **38**, 1996.

Berson, S. A. and Yalow, R. S. (1966). "The Hormones", Vol. IV, p. 577. Academic Press, New York and London.

Berthezene, F., Mornex, R. and Chavrier, B. (1974). *J. clin. Endocr. Metab.* **38**, 1068.

Binoux, M., Pierce, J. G. and Odell, W. D. (1974). *J. clin. Endocr. Metab.* **38**, 674.

Birken, S., Fetherston, J., Desmond, J., Canfield, R. and Boime, I. (1978). Prog. 60th Endocr. Soc. Meet., Miami, 434 A.

Bitensky, L., Alayhband-Zadek, J. and Chayen, J. (1974). *Clin. Endocr.* **3**, 363.

Blackman, M. R., Gershengorn, M. C. and Weintraub, B. D. (1978). *Endocrinology*, **102**, 499.

Bloomfield, G. A., Faith, M. R. and Pierce, J. G. (1978). *Biochim. biophys. Acta*, **533**, 371.

Bode, H. H., Danon, M., Weintraub, B. D., Maloof, F. and Crawford, J. D. (1973). *J. clin. Invest.* **52**, 776.

Boler, J., Enzmann, F., Folkers, K., Bowers, C. Y. and Schally, A. V. (1969). *Biochem. biophys. Res. Commun.* **37**, 705.

Bolonkin, D., Tate, R. L., Luber, J. H., Kohn, L. D. and Winand, R. J. (1975). *J. biol. Chem.* **250**, 6516.

Borell, U. (1945). *Acta med. scand.* Suppl. **161**.

Borell, U. and Holmgren, H. (1949). *Acta endocr., Copenh.* **3**, 331.

Bottari, P. M. and Donovan, B. T. (1958). *J. Physiol.* **140**, 36P.

Bowers, C. Y. (1971). *Ann. N.Y. Acad. Sci.* **185**, 263.

Bowers, C. Y., Friesen, H. G., Hwang, P., Guyda, H. J. and Folkers, K. (1971). *Biochem. biophys. Res. Commun.* **45**, 1033.

Bowers, C. Y., Lee, K. I. and Schally, A. V. (1968). *Endocrinology*, **82**, 75.

Bowers, C. Y., Segaloff, A. and Brown, B. (1959). *Endocrinology*, **65**, 882.

Braunstein, G. D. and Hershman, J. M. (1976). *J. clin. Endocr. Metab.* **42**, 1123.

Brazeau, P., Vale, W., Burgus, R., Ling, M., Butcher, M., Rivier, J. and Guillemin, R. (1973). *Science*, **189**, 77.

Brown, J. R. (1959). *Acta endocr., Copenh.* **32**, 289.

Brown, J. and Munro, D. S. (1967). *J. Endocr.* **38**, 139.

Brunish, R. (1958). *Endocrinology*, **62**, 437.

Brunish, R., Hayashi, K. and Hayashi, J. (1962). *Archs biochem. Biophys.* **98**, 135.

Burger, A., Studer, H. and Wyss, F. (1965). In "Current Topics in Thyroid Research" (M. Andreoli and C. Cassano, eds), p. 624. Academic Press, New York and London.

Burgus, R., Dunn, T. F., Desiderio, D., Vale, W., Guillemin, R. (1969) *C. r. Acad. Sci (D) (Paris)*, **269**, 226.

Burrow, G. N., Polackwich, R. and Donabedlan, R. (1965). "Perinatal Thyroid Physiology and Disease", p. 1. Raven Press, New York.

Burzawa-Gerard, E. (1971). *Biochimie*, **53**, 545.

Burzawa-Gerard, E. (1974). *C. r. Acad. Sci. (Paris)*, Ser. D. **279**, 1681.

Burzawa-Gerard, E. and Fontaine, Y. A. (1972). *Gen. comp. Endocr.* Suppl. **3**, 715.

Carr, D., Gomez-Pan, A., Weightman, D. R., Roy, V. C. M., Idall, R., Bessen, G. M., Thorner, M. O., McNeilly, A. S., Schally, A. V., Kastin, A. J. and Coy, D. H. (1975). *Br. med. J.* **3**, 67.

Carsten, M. E. and Pierce, J. G. (1960). *J. biol. Chem.* **235**, 78.

Charters, A. C., Odell, W. D. and Thompson, J. C. (1969). *J. clin. Endocr. Metab.* **29**, 63.

Chayen, J., Bitensky, L. and B., and Cher, R. G. (1973). "Practical Histochemistry." Wiley, London.

Chin, W. W., Habener, J. F., Kieffer, J. D. and Maloof, F. (1978). Prog. 60th Endocr. Soc. Meet., Miami, 427A.

Chopra, I. J., Solomon, D. H., Chopra, U., Young, R. T. and Chuateco, G. N. (1974). *J. clin. Endocr. Metab.* **39**, 501.

Ciereszko, L. S. (1945). *J. biol. Chem.* **160**, 585.

Clague, R., Mukhtar, E. D., Pyle, G. A., Nutt, J., Clark, F., Scott, M., Evered, D., Smith, B. R. and Hall, R. (1976). *J. clin. Endocr. Metab.* **43**, 550.

Cline, M. J., Selenkow, H. A. and Brooke, M. S. (1960). *Endocrinology*, **67**, 273.

Coble, Y. D. and Kohler, P. O. (1970). *J. clin. Endocr. Metab.* **31**, 220.

Cohen, J. D. and Utiger, R. D. (1970). *J. clin. Endocr. Metab.* **30**, 423.

Condliffe, P. G. (1963). *Endocrinology*, **72**, 893.

Condliffe, P. G. (1969). Biochemical specificity of thyrotropins. In "La Specificite

Zoologique des Hormones Hypophysaires et de Leurs Activities". Colloques Internationaux du CNRSN. 177.

Condliffe, P. G. and Bates, R. W. (1956). *J. biol Chem.* **223**, 843.

Condliffe, P. G. and Bates, R. W. (1957). *Archs biochem. Biophys.* **68**, 229.

Condliffe, P. G., Bates, R. W. and Fraps, R. M. (1959). *Biochim. biophys. Acta*, **34**, 430.

Condliffe, P. G. and Mochizuki, M. (1965). *In* "Current Topics in Thyroid Research" (M. Andreoli and C. Cassano, eds), p. 415. Academic Press, New York and London.

Condliffe, P. G., Mochizuki, M., Fontaine, Y. A. and Bates, R. W. (1969). *Endocrinology*, **85**, 453.

Condliffe, P. G. and Porath, J. (1962). *Fed. Proc. Abst.* **21**, 2, A-199.

Cornell, J. S. and Pierce, J. G. (1973). *J. biol. Chem.* **248**, 4327.

Costom, B. H., Grumbach, M. M. and Kaplan, S. L. (1971). *J. clin. Invest.* **50**, 2219.

Cotton, G. E., Gorman, C. A. and Mayberry, W. E. (1971). *New Engl. J. Med.* **285**, 529.

Crigler Jr., J. F. and Waugh, D. F. (1955). *J. Am. chem. Soc.* **77**, 4407.

Crooke, A. C. and Matthews, J. D. (1953). *Ciba Fdn Colloq. Endocr.* **5**, 25.

Curry, D. L. and Bennett, L. L. (1974). *Biochem. biophys. Res. Commun.* **60**, 1015.

Czernichow, P., Dauzet, M. C., Broyer, M. and Rappaport, R. (1976). *J. clin. Endocr. Metab.* **43**, 630.

d'Angelo, S. A., Gordon, A. S. and Charipper, M. A. (1942). *Endocrinology*, **31**, 217.

d'Angelo, S. A. and Traum, R. E. (1958). *Ann. N.Y. Acad. Sci.* **72**, 239.

Delange, F., Hershman, J. M. and Ermans, A. M. (1971). *J. clin. Endocr. Metab.* **33**, 261.

De Lean, A., Ferland, L., Drouin, J., Kelly, P. A. and Labrie, F. (1977). *Endocrinology*, **100**, 1496.

De la Llosa, P., Courte, C. and Jutisz, M. (1967). *Biochem. biophys. Res. Comm.* **26**, 411.

de Robertis, E. (1948). *J. clin. Endocr. Metab.* **8**, 956.

de Robertis, E. and del Conte, E. (1941). *Rev. Soc. argent. Biol.* **20**, 88.

Dimond, R. C. and Rosen, S. W. (1974). *J. clin. Endocr. Metab.* **39**, 316.

Dobyns, B. M. (1966). "The Pituitary Gland", Vol. 1, p. 411. Butterworths, London.

Dobyns, B. M. and Steelman, S. L. (1953). *Endocrinology*, **52**, 705.

Dobyns, B. M. and Wilson, L. A. (1954). *J. clin. Endocr.* **14**, 1393.

Donaldson, E. M., Yamazaki, F., Dye, H. M. and Philleo, W. W. (1972). *Gen. comp. Endocr.* **18**, 469.

Dorrington, K. J., Carneiro, L. and Munro, D. S. (1965). *In* "Current Topics in Thyroid Research" (M. Andreoli and C. Cassano, eds), p. 455. Academic Press, New York and London.

Dorrington, K. J. and Munro, D. S. (1966). *Clin. Pharmac. Ther.* **7**, 788.

Dubois, M. (1975). *Proc. natn. Acad. Sci. USA*, **72**, 1340.

Dussault, J. H., Morissette, J., Letarte, J., Guyda, H. and Laberge, C. (1978). *J. Pediatr.* **92**, 274.

Edmonds, M., Molitch, M., Pierce, J. and Odell, W. D. (1975). *Clin. Endocr.* **4**, 525.

Elewaut, A., Mussche, M. and Vermeulen, A. (1976). *J. clin. Endocr. Metab.* **43**, 575.

El Kabir, D. J. (1962). *Nature, Lond.* **194**, 688.

Ellis, S. (1958). *J. biol. Chem.* **233**, 63.

Elrick, H., Yearwood-Drayton, V., Arai, Y., Leaver, F. and Morris, H. G. (1963). *J. clin. Endocr. Metab.* **23**, 694.

Emerson, C. H., Dyson, W. L. and Utiger, R. D. (1973). *J. clin. Endocr. Metab.* **36**, 338.

Emerson, C. H., Frohman, L. A., Szabo, M. and Thakkar, I. (1977). *J. clin. Endocr. Metab.* **45**, 392.

Emerson, C. H. and Utiger, R. D. (1972). *New Engl. J. Med.* **287**, 328.

Endo, K., Kasagi, K., Konishi, J., Ikekubo, K., Okuno, T., Takeda, Y., Mori, T. and Torizuka, K. (1978). *J. clin. Endocr. Metab.* **46**, 734.

Erhardt, F. W. and Scriba, P. C. (1977). *Acta endocr., Copenh.* **85**, 698

Eskay, R. L., Oliver, C., Warberg, J. and Porter, J. C. (1976). *Endocrinology*, **98**, 269.

Faglia, G., Beck-Peccoz, P., Ferrari, C., Ambrosi, B., Spada, A., Travaglini, P. and Paracchi, S. (1973). *J. clin. Endocr. Metab.* **37**, 595.

Faglia, G., Ferrari, C., Neri, V., Beck-Peccoz, P., Ambrosi, B. and Valentini, F. (1972). *Acta endocr., Copenh.* **69**, 649.

Fawcett, J. S., Dedman, M. L. and Morris, C. J. O. R. (1969). *FEBS Lett.* **3**, 250.

Ferland, L., Labrie, F., Jobin, M., Arimura, A. and Schally, A. V. (1976). *Biochem. biophys. Res. Commun.* **68**, 149.

Field, J. B. (1975). *Metabolism*, **24**, 381.

Field, J. B., Bloom, G., Kerins, M. E. Chagoth, R. and Zor, U. (1975). *J. biol. Chem.* **250**, 4903.

Field, J. B., Pastan, I., Johnson, P. and Herring, B. (1960). *J. biol. Chem.* **235**, 1863.

Fisher, D. A., Hobel, C. J., Garza, R. and Pierce, C. A. (1970). *Pediatrics*, **46**, 208.

Fisher, D. A. and Odell, W. D. (1969). *J. clin. Invest.* **48**, 1670.

Fisher, D. A. and Odell, W. D. (1971). *J. clin. Endocr.* **33**, 859.

Fleischer, N., Burgus, R., Vale, W., Dunn, T. and Guillemin, R. (1970). *J. clin. Endocr. Metab.* **31**, 109.

Fleischer, N., Lorente, M., Kirkland, J., Kirkland, R., Clayton, G. and Calderon, M. (1972). *J. clin. Endocr. Metab.* **34**, 617.

Florsheim, W. H. and Kozbur, X. (1976). *Biochem. biophys. Res. Commun.* **72**, 603.

Florsheim, W. H., Williams, A. D. and Schönbaum, E. (1970). *Endocrinology*, **87**, 881.

Foley Jr. T. P., Jacobs, L. S., Hoffman, W., Daughaday, W. H. and Blizzard, R. M. (1972). *J. clin. Invest.* **51**, 2143.

Fontaine, Y. A. (1967). Thesis, Paris.

Fontaine, Y. A. and Burzawa-Gerard, E. (1968). *Gen. comp. Endocr.* **11**, 160.

Fontaine, Y. A. and Condliffe, P. G. (1963a). *Biochemistry*, **2**, 290.

Fontaine, Y. A. and Condliffe, P. G. (1963b). *Bull. soc. Chim. Biol. (Paris)*, **45**, 681.

Fontaine, M. and Fontaine, Y. A. (1962). *J. comp. Endocr. Suppl.* **1**, 63.

Freinkel, N. (1957). *Endocrinology*, **61**, 448.

Freinkel, N. (1958). *Biochem. J.* **68**, 327.

Freinkel, N. (1960). *Endocrinology*, **66**, 851.

Furth, J. (1955). *Rec. Prog. Hormone Res.* **11**, 221.

Furth, J., Moy, P., Hershman, J. and Ueda, G. (1973). *Arch. Path.* **96**, 217.

Gershengorn, M. C. and Weintraub, B. D. (1975). *J. clin. Invest.* **56**, 633.

Giudice, L. C. and Pierce, J. G. (1977). *Endocrinology*, **101**, 776–781.

Gilliland, I. C. and Strudwick, J. I. (1953). *Clin. Sci.* **12**, 265.

Gilman, A. G. and Rall, T. W. (1968). *J. biol. Chem.* **243**, 5867.

Glatstein, E., McHardy-Young, S., Brast, N., Eltringham, J. R. and Kriss, J. P. (1971). *J. clin. Endocr. Metab.* **32**, 833.

Goetinck, P. F. and Pierce, J. G. (1966). *Archs biochem. Biophys.* **115**, 277.

Golstein, J. and Vanhaelst, L. (1973). *Clin. chim. Acta*, **49**, 141.

Gonzalez-Barcena, D., Kastin, A. J., Schalch, D. S., Torres-Zamora, M., Perez-Pasten, E., Kato, A. and Schally, A. V. (1973). *J. clin. Endocr. Metab.* **36**, 117.

Gordin, A. and Lamberg, B. A. (1975). *Lancet*, **i**, 1234.

Grant, G., Vale, W. and Guillemin, R. (1972). *Biochem. biophys. Res. Commun.* **46**, 28.

Greenberg, A. H., Czernichow, P., Shelley, W., Winship, T. and Blizzard, R. M. (1970). *J. clin. Endocr. Metab.* **30**, 293.

Greenspan, F. S., Kriss, J. P. and Moses, L. E. (1954). *Am. J. Med.* **17**, 106.

Greenspan, F. S., Kriss, J. P., Moses, L. E. and Lew, W. (1956). *Endocrinology*, **58**, 767.

Greenwood, F. C., Hunter, W. M. and Glover, J. J. (1963). *Biochem. J.* **89**, 114.
Hagen, C. and McNeilly, A. S. (1975). *J. Endocr.* **67**, 49.
Haigler, E. D., Pitman, J. A., Hershman, J. M. and Baugh, C. M. (1971). *J. clin. Endocr. Metab.* **33**, 573.
Hall, R. (1963). *J. biol. Chem.* **238**, 306.
Hall, R., Ormston, B. J., Besser, G. M., Cryer, R. J. and McKendrick, M. (1972). *Lancet*, **i**, 759.
Hall, R., Smith, B. R. and Mukhtar, E. D. (1975). *Clin. Endocr.* **4**, 213.
Hall, R. and Tubman, J. (1965). *J. biol. Chem.* **240**, 3132.
Hall, R., Tubman, J. and Gatry, R. (1970). *Clin. Sci.* **38**, 18.
Hamilton Jr., C. R. and Maloof, F. (1972). *J. clin. Endocr. Metab.* **35**, 659.
Hamilton Jr., C. R., Adams, L. C. and Maloof, F. (1970). *New Engl. J. Med.* **283**, 1077.
Hara, K., Rathnam, P. and Saxend, B. B. (1978). *J. biol. Chem.* **253**, 1582.
Harris, A. R. C., Christianson, D., Smith, M. S., Fang, S.-L., Braverman, L. E. and Vagenakis, A. G. (1978). *J. clin. Invest.* **61**, 441.
Hays, E. E. and Steelman, S. L. (1955). "The Hormones", Vol. III. Academic Press, New York and London.
Hays, M. T., Solomon, D. H., Pierce, J. G. and Carsten, M. E. (1961). *J. clin. Endocr.* **21**, 1469.
Heideman, M. L. (1953). *Endocrinology*, **53**, 640.
Heideman, M. L., Bakke, J. L. and Lawrence, N. (1959). *Archs biochem. Biophys.* **82**, 62.
Hennen, G., Pierce, J. and Freychet, P. (1969). *J. clin. Endocr. Metab.* **29**, 581.
Hennen, G., Winand, R. and Nizet, A. (1965). *In* "Current Topics in Thyroid Research" (M. Andreali and C. Cassano, eds), p. 464, Academic Press, New York and London.
Hershman, J. M. and Higgins, H. P. (1971). *New Engl. J. Med.* **284**, 573.
Hershman, J. M., Higgins, H. P. and Starnes, W. R. (1970a). *Metabolism*, **19**, 735.
Hershman, J. M., Kojima, A. and Friesen, H. G. (1973). *J. clin. Endocr. Metab.* **36**, 497.
Hershman, J. M. and Pittman Jr., J. A. (1971a). *Ann. int. Med.* **74**, 481.
Hersham, J. M. and Pittman Jr., J. A. (1971b). *New Engl. J. Med.* **258**, 997.
Hershman, J. M., Read, D. G., Bailey, A. L., Norman, V. D. and Gibson, T. B. (1970b). *J. clin. Endocr. Metab.* **30**, 430.
Hershman, J. M. and Starnes, W. (1969). *J. clin. Invest.* **48**, 923.
Hoffman, D. P., Surks, M. I., Oppenheimer, J. H. and Weitzman, E. D. (1977). *J. clin. Endocr. Metab.* **44**, 892.
Hollander, C. S., Mitsuma, T., Shenkman, L., Wolf, P. and Gershengorn, M. C. (1972). *Science*, **175**, 209.
Hood, S., Vaughan-Jackson, J. D. and Farid, N. R. (1976). *J. clin. Endocr. Metab.* **43**, 1360.
Horn, K., Erhardt, F., Fahlbusch, R., Pickhardt, C. R., v. Werder, K. and Scriba, P. C. (1976). *J. clin. Endocr. Metab.* **43**, 137.
Hrubesch, M., Böckel, K., Vosberg, H., Wagner, H. and Hauss, W. H. (1972). *Verh. Deutsch. Ges. Inn. Med.* **78**, 1529.
Idler, D. R., Bazar, L. S. and Hwang, S. J. (1975). *Endocr. Res. Comm.* **2**, 237.
Illig, R., Krawczynska, H., Torresani, T. and Prader, A. (1975). *J. clin. Endocr. Metab.* **41**, 722.
Ingham, K. C., Aloj, S. M. and Edelhoch, M. (1974). *Archs biochem. Biophys.* **163**, 589.
Irie, M. and Tsushima, T. (1972). *J. clin. Endocr. Metab.* **35**, 97.
Ishikawa, H. (1973). *Biochem. biophys. Res. Commun.* **54**, 1203.
Jackson, I. M. D. and Reichlin, S. (1974). *Life Sci.* **14**, 2259.

Jacobs, L. S., Snyder, P. J., Utiger, R. D. and Daughaday, W. H. (1973). *J. clin. Endocr. Metab.* **36**, 1069.

Jailer, J. W. and Holub, D. A. (1960). *Am. J. Med.* **28**, 497.

Janssen, S. and Loeser, A. (1931). *Arch. exp. Path. Pharmak.* **163**, 517.

Jeffcoate, S. L. and White, N. (1974). *J. clin. Endocr. Metab.* **38**, 155.

Jobin, M., Ferland, L., Côté, J. and Labrie, F. (1975). *Neuroendocrinology,* **18**, 204.

Junkmann, K. and Schoeller, W. (1932). *Klin. Wschr.* **11**, 1176.

Kenimer, J. G., Hershman, J. M. and Higgins, H. P. (1975). *J. clin. Endocr. Metab.* **40**, 482.

Kirkham, K. E. (1962a). *J. Endocr.* **25**, 259.

Kirkham, K. E. (1962b). *Acta endocr., Copenh.* **67**, 62.

Kirkham, K. E. (1966). "Vitamins and Hormones", p. 173. Academic Press, New York and London.

Kirkham, K. E. and Irvine, W. J. (1963). *J. Endocr.* **26**, xxviii.

Klainer, L. M., Chi, Y. M., Freidberg, S. L., Rall, T. W. and Sutherland, E. W. (1962). *J. biol. Chem.* **237**, 1239.

Klug, T. L. and Adelman, R. C. (1977). *Biochem. biophys. Res. Commun.* **77**, 1431.

Kohn, L. D., Aloj, S. M., Friedman, R. M., Grollman, E. F., Ledley, F. D., Lee, G., Meldolesi, M. F. and Mullin, B. R. (1978). *In* "Advances in Carbohydrate Chemistry", Symposium on Cell Surface Carbohydrate Chemistry, pp. 103–133. Academic Press, New York and London.

Koch, Y., Goldhaber, G., Fireman, I., Zor, U., Shani, J. and Tal, E. (1977). *Endocrinology,* **100**, 1476.

Kohn, L. D. and Winand, R. J. (1975). *J. biol. Chem.* **250**, 6503.

Kohn, L. D., Winand, R. J. and Bates, R. W. (1975). *Endocrinology,* **96**, 1329.

Konishi, J., Herman, M. M. and Kriss, J. P. (1974). *Endocrinology,* **95**, 434.

Kourides, I. A., Re, R. N., Weintraub, B. D., Ridgway, E. C. and Maloof, F. (1977a). *J. clin. Invest.* **59**, 508.

Kourides, I. A., Ridgway, E. C., Weintraub, B. D., Bigos, S. T., Gershengorn, M. C. and Maloof, F. (1977b). *J. clin. Endocr. Metab.* **45**, 534.

Kourides, I. A. and Weintraub, B. D. (1978). Prog. 60th Endocr. Soc. Meet., Miami, 150A.

Kourides, I. A., Weintraub, B. D. and Maloof, F. (1978). *J. clin. Endocr. Metab.* **47**, 24.

Kourides, I. A., Weintraub, B. D., Ridgway, E. C. and Maloof, F. (1975). *J. clin. Endocr. Metab.* **40**, 872.

Kriss, J. P., Pleshakov, V. and Chien, J. R. (1964a). *J. clin. Endocr.* **24**, 1005.

Kriss, J. P., Pleshakov, V. and Koblin, R. (1964b). *Clin. Res.* **12**, 116.

Kriss, J. P., Pleshakov, V., Rosenblum, A. L., Holderness, M., Sharp, G. and Utiger, R. D. (1967). *J. clin. Endocr. Metab.* **27**, 582.

Krugman, L. G., Hershman, J. M., Chopra, I. J., Levine, G. A., Pekary, A. E., Geffner, D. L. and Chua Teco, G. N. (1975). *J. clin. Endocr. Metab.* **41**, 70.

Kurosky, A., Markel, D. E., Peterson, J. W. and Fitch, W. M. (1977). *Science,* **195**, 299.

Labrie, F., Barden, N., Poirier, G. and DeLean, A. (1972). *Proc. natn. Acad. Sci., USA,* **69**, 283.

Lamberg, B. A. (1953a). *Acta endocr., Copenh.* **13**, 145.

Lamberg, B. A. (1953b). *Acta med. scand.* (Suppl.), 279.

Lamberg, B. A. (1955). *Acta endocr., Copenh.* **18**, 405.

Lamberg, B. A. (1973). *Lancet,* i, 854.

Lamberg, B. A., Ripatti, J., Gordin, A., Juustila, H., Sivula, A. and af Björkesten, G. (1969). *Acta endocr., Copenh.* **60**, 157.

Lamberg, B. A., Wahlberg, P. and Olin-Lamberg, C. (1955). *Acta endocr., Copenh.* **19**, 263.

Lamkin, W. M., Fujino, M., Mayfield, J. D., Holcomb, G. N. and Ward, D. N. (1970). *Biochim. biophys. Acta*, **214**, 290.

Landefeld, T., McWilliams, D. R. and Boime, I. (1976). *Biochem. biophys. Res. Commun.* **72**, 381.

Lawrence, N. L. and Bakke, J. L. (1956). *Biochim. biophys. Acta*, **19**, 196.

Lemarchand-Béraud, T. L. (1970). *Acta endocr., Copenh.* **64**, 610.

Lemarchand-Béraud, Th. and Vanotti, A. (1965). *Experientia*, **21**, 353.

Lepp, A. and Oliner, L. (1967). *Endocrinology*, **80**, 369.

Levy, R. P., McGuire, W. L. and Heideman, M. L. (1962). *Proc. Soc. exp. Biol. Med.* **110**, 598.

Li, C. H. and Starman, B. (1964). *Nature, Lond.* **202**, 291.

Liao, T. H. and Pierce, J. G. (1970). *J. biol. Chem.* **245**, 3275.

Licht, P. and Papkoff, H. (1974). *Gen. comp. Endocr.* **22**, 218.

Lim, V. S., Fang, V. S., Katz, A. I. and Refetoff, S. (1977). *J. clin. Invest.* **60**, 522.

Limanova, E. E. (1962a). *Problemý Endokr. Gormonoter*, **8**, 41.

Limanova, E. E. (1962b). *Problemý Endokr. Gormonoter*, **8**, 69.

Lippe, B. M., Van Herle, A. J., Lafranchi, S. H., Uller, R. P., Lavin, N. and Kaplan, S. A. (1975). *J. clin. Endocr. Metab.* **40**, 612.

Macchia, V., Bates, R. W. and Pastan, I. (1967). *J. biol. Chem.* **242**, 3726.

Major, P. W. and Munro, D. S. (1962). *Clin. Sci.* **23**, 463.

Mason, J. W., Hartley, L. H., Kotchen, T. A., Wherry, F. E., Pennington, L. L. and Jones, L. G. (1973). *J. clin. Endocr. Metab.* **37**, 403.

Matovinovic, J. and Vickery, A. L. (1959). *Endocrinology*, **64**, 149.

Mayberry, W. E., Gharib, H., Bilstad, J. M. and Sizemore, G. W. (1971). *Ann. int. med.* **74**, 471.

McKenzie, J. M. (1958). *Endocrinology*, **63**, 372.

McKenzie, J. M. (1960). *Physiol. Rev.* **40**, 398.

McKenzie, J. M. (1962a). *J. biol. Chem.* **237**, PC3571.

McKenzie, J. M. (1962b). *Proc. R. Soc. Med.* **55**, 539.

McKenzie, J. M. (1965). *J. clin. Endocr. Metab.* **25**, 424.

McKenzie, J. M. (1967). *Rec. prog. Horm. Res.* **23**, 1.

McKenzie, J. M. and Fishman, J. (1960). *Proc. Soc. exp. Biol. Med.* **105**, 126.

McKenzie, J. M. and Williamson, A. (1966). *J. clin. Endocr. Metab.* **26**, 518.

McKenzie, J. M. and Zakarija, M. (1976). *J. clin. Endocr. Metab.* **42**, 778.

Meek, J. C., Jones, A. E., Lewis, U. J. and Vanderlaan, W. P. (1964). *Proc. natn. Acad. Sci. USA*, **52**, 342.

Mitchell, M. L., Larsen, P. R., Levy, H. L., Bennett, A. J. E. and Madoff, M. A. (1978). *J. Am. med. Assoc.* **239**, 2348.

Mitsuma, T., Hirooka, Y. and Nihei, N. (1976). *Acta endocr., Copenh.* **83**, 225.

Montoya, E., Seibel, M. J. and Wilber, J. F. (1975). *Endocrinology*, **96**, 1413.

Morley, J. E., Garven, T. J., Pekary, A. E. and Hershman, J. M. (1977). *Biochem. biophys. Res. Commun.* **79**, 314.

Morley, J. E., Jacobson, R. J., Melamed, J. and Hershman, J. M. (1976). *Am. J. Med.* **60**, 1035.

Mornex, R., Tommasi, M., Cure, M., Farcot, J., Orgiazzi, J. and Rousset, B. (1972). *Ann. Endocr. (Paris)*, **33**, 390.

Morton, M. E. and Schwartz, J. R. (1953). *Science, N.Y.*, **117**, 103.

Moser, R. J. and Hollingsworth, D. R. (1975). *Clin. Chem.* **21**, 237.

Moshang Jr., T., Parks, J. S., Baker, L., Vaidya, V., Utiger, R. D., Bongiovanni, A. M. and Snyder, P. J. (1975). *J. clin. Endocr. Metab.* **40**, 470.

Mullin, B. R., Aloj, S. M., Fishman, P. H., Lee, G., Kohn, L. D. and Brady, R. O. (1976a). *Proc. natn. Acad. Sci. USA, 73, 842.*

Mullin, B. R., Fishman, P. H., Lee, G., Aloj, S. M., Ledley, F. D., Winand, R. J., Kohn, L. D. and Brady, R. O. (1976b). *Proc. natn. Acad. Sci. USA*, **73**, 842.

Musset, M. V. and Perry, W. L. M. (1955). *Bull. Wld Hlth Org.* **13**, 917.

Nelson, J. C., Johnson, D. E. and Odell, W. D. (1972). *Ann. int. Med.* **76**, 47.

Nisula, B. C. and Ketelslegers (1974). *J. clin. Invest.* **54**, 494.

Nisula, B. C. and Louvet, J. P. (1978). *J. clin. Endocr. Metab.* **46**, 729.

Novogroder, M., Utiger, R., Boyar, R. and Levine, L. S. (1977). *J. clin. Endocr. Metab.* **45**, 1053.

Odell, W. D., Bates, R. W., Rivlin, R. S., Lipsett, M. B. and Hertz, R. (1963). *J. clin. Endocr. Metab.* **23**, 658.

Odell, W. D., Utiger, R. D., Wilber, J. F. and Condliffe, P. G. (1967a). *J. clin. Invest.* **46**, 953.

Odell, W. D., Wilber, J. F. and Paul, W. E. (1965a). *Metabolism*, **14**, 465.

Odell, W. D., Wilber, J. F. and Paul, W. E. (1965b). *J. clin. Endocr.* **25**, 1179.

Odell, W. D., Wilber, J. F. and Utiger, R. D. (1967b). *Rec. Prog. horm. Res.* **23**, 47.

O'Donnell, J., Hadden, D. R., Weaver, J. A. and Montgomery, D. A. D. (1973). *Proc. R. Soc. Med.* **66**, 441.

Ogihara, T., Yamamoto, T., Azukizawa, M., Miyai, K. and Kumahara, Y. (1973). *J. clin. Endocr. Metab.* **37**, 602.

Oliver, C., Charvet, J. P., Codaccioni, J. L. and Vague, J. (1974a). *J. clin. Endocr. Metab.* **39**, 406.

Oliver, C., Eskay, R. L., Ben-Jonathan, N. and Porter, J. C. (1974b). *Endocrinology*, **95**, 540.

Onaya, T., Kotani, M., Yanada, T. and Ochi, Y. (1973). *J. clin. Endocr. Metab.* **36**, 859.

Orgiazzi, J., Williams, D. E., Chopra, I. J., Solomon, D. H. (1976). *J. clin. Endocr. Metab.* **42**, 341.

Ormston, B. J., Cryer, R. J., Garry, R., Besser, G. M. and Hall, R. (1971). *Lancet*, **ii**, 10.

Otsuki, M., Dakoda, M. and Baba, S. (1973). *J. clin. Endocr. Metab.* **36**, 95.

Papkoff, H. and Samy, T. S. A. (1967). *Biochim. biophys. Acta*, **147**, 175.

Parker, D. C., Pekary, A. E. and Hershman, J. M. (1976). *J. clin. Endocr. Metab.* **43**, 318.

Parlow, A. F., Condliffe, P. G., Reichert, L. E. and Wilhelmi, A. E. (1965). *Endocrinology*, **76**, 27.

Pascasio, F. M. and Selenkow, H. A. (1962). *Endocrinology*, **71**, 254.

Pastan, I. (1966). *Biochem. biophys. Res. Comm.* **25**, 14.

Pastan, I. and Katzen, R. (1967). *Biochem. biophys. Res. Comm.* **29**, 792.

Pastan, I., Roth, J. and Macchia, V. (1966). *Proc. natn. Acad. Sci. USA*, **56**, 1802.

Pastan, I. and Wollman, S. H. (1967). *J. cell Biol.* **35**, 262.

Patel, Y. C. and Burger, H. G. (1973). *J. clin. Endocr. Metab.* **37**, 190.

Patel, Y. C., Burger, H. G. and Hudson, B. (1971). *J. clin. Endocr.* **33**, 768.

Pekary, A. E., Hershman, J. M. and Parlow, A. F. (1975). *J. clin. Endocr. Metab.* **41**, 676.

Petersen, V. B., Smith, B. R. and Hall, R. (1975). "Thyroid Research", p. 610. Excerpta Medica, Amsterdam.

Pierce, J. G. (1974). Chemistry of thyroid-stimulating hormones. *In* Handbook of Physiology and Endocrinology, Vol. IV, Part 2, pp. 79–101. Am. Physiol. Soc., Washington, DC.

Pierce, J. G. (1976). Excerpta Medica International Congress Series No. 403 Endocrinology. Proc. 5th Int. Cong. Endocr., Hamburg, Vol. 2, p. 99.

Pierce, J. G. and Carsten, M. E. (1957). *J. Biol. Chem.* **229**, 61.

Pierce, J. G., Carsten, M. E. and Wynston, L. K. (1970). *Ann. N.Y. Acad. Sci.* **86**, 612.

Pierce, J. G., Faith, M. R. and Donaldson, E. M. (1976a). *Gen. comp. Endocr.* **30**, 47

Pierce, J. G., Faith, M. R., Giudice, L. C. and Reeve, J. R. (1976b). "Structure and Structure–Function Relationships in Glycoprotein Hormones; in Polypeptide Hormones: Molecular and Cellular Aspects". Ciba Foundation Symposium 41 (new series), pp. 225–249. Elsevier/Excerpta Medica, North Holland.

Pierce, J. G., Liao, T. H., Howard, S. M., Shome, B. and Cornell, J. S. (1971). *Rec. prog. Hormone Res.* **27**, 165.

Pierce, J. G. and Nye, J. F. (1956). *J. biol. Chem.* **222**, 777.

Pinchera, A., Pinchera, M. and Stanbury, J. B. (1965). *J. clin. Endocr. Metab.* **25**, 189.

Porath, J. O. and Flodin, P. (1959). *Nature, Lond.* **183**, 1657.

Portnay, G. I., O'Brian, J. T., Bush, J., Vagenakis, A. G., Azizi, F., Arky, R. A., Ingbar, S. H. and Braverman, L. E. (1974). *J. clin. Endocr. Metab.* **39**, 199.

Posternak, T., Sutherland, E. W. and Henion, W. F. (1962). *Biochim. biophys. Acta,* **65**, 558.

Purves, H. D. and Griesbach, W. E. (1957). *Ciba Fdn Colloq. Endocr.* **10**, 51.

Querido, A. A., Kassenaar, A. H. and Lameyer, L. D. F. (1955). *Acta endocr., Copenh.* **12**, 335.

Querido, A. and Lameyer, L. D. F. (1956). *Proc. R. Soc. Med.* **49**, 209.

Rabello, M. M., Snyder, P. J. and Utiger, R. D. (1974). *J. clin. Endocr. Metab.* **39**, 571.

Rall, J. E., Robbins, J. and Lewallen, C. G. (1964). "The Hormones", Vol. 5, p. 159. Academic Press, New York and London.

Ramey, J. N., Burrow, N., Polack-Wich, R. J. and Donabedian, R. K. (1975). *J. clin. Endocr. Metab.* **40**, 712.

Ramey, J. N., Burrow, G. N., Spaulding, S. W., Donabedian, R. K., Speroff, L. and Frantz, A. G. (1976). *J. clin. Endocr. Metab.* **43**, 107.

Rapoport, B., Refetoff, S., Fang, V. S. and Friesen, H. G. (1973). *J. clin. Endocr. Metab.* **36**, 256.

Raud, R. and Odell, W. D. (1969). *Br. J. Hosp. Med.* **2**, 1366.

Re, R. N., Kourides, I. A., Ridgway, E. C., Weintraub, B. D. and Maloof, F. (1976). *J. clin. Endocr. Metab.* **43**, 338.

Redding, T. W. and Schally, A. V. (1969). *Proc. Soc. exp. Biol. Med.* **131**, 420.

Refetoff, S., DeWind, L. T. and DeGroot, L. J. (1967). *J. clin. Endocr. Metab.* **27**, 279.

Refetoff, S., Fang, V. S., Rapoport, B. and Friesen, H. G. (1974). *J. clin. Endocr. Metab.* **38**, 450.

Reisfeld, R. A., Lewis, U. J., Brink, N. G. and Steelman, S. L. (1962). *Endocrinology,* **71**, 559.

Reschini, E., Giustina, G., Cantalamessa, L. and Peracchi, M. (1976). *J. clin. Endocr. Metab.* **43**, 924.

Ridgway, E. C., Singer, F. R., Weintraub, B. D., Lorenz, L. and Maloof, F. (1974a). *Endocrinology,* **95**, 1181.

Ridgway, E. C., Weintraub, B. D., Cevallos, J. L., Rack, M. C. and Maloof, F. (1973). *J. clin. Invest.* **52**, 2783.

Ridgway, E. C., Weintraub, B. D. and Maloof, F. (1974b). *J. clin. Invest.* **53**, 895.

Root, A. W., Snyder, P. J., Rezvani, I., DiGeorge, A. M. and Utiger, R. D. (1973). *J. clin. Endocr. Metab.* **36**, 103.

Russfield, A. B. (1955). *J. clin. Endocr. Metab.* **15**, 1393.

Saberi, M. and Utiger, R. D. (1974). *J. clin. Endocr. Metab.* **39**, 923.

Sairam, M. R. and Li, C. H. (1973). *Biochem. biophys. Res. Comm.* **51**, 336.

Sairam, M. R. and Li, C. H. (1977a). *Can. J. Biochem.* **55**, 747.

Sairam, M. R. and Li, C. H. (1977b). *Can. J. Biochem.* **55**, 755.

Sanchez-Franco, F., Garcia, M. D., Cacicedo, L., Martin-Zurro, A., Del Rey, F. E. and De Escobar, G. M. (1974). *J. clin. Endocr. Metab.* **38**, 1098.

Sandler, R. (1976). *J. clin. Endocr. Metab.* **42**, 163.

Schally, A. V., Dupont, A., Arimura, A., Redding, T. W. and Linthicom, G. L. (1975). *Fed. Proc.* **34**, 584.

Schell-Frederick, E. and Dumont, J. E. (1970). "Biochemical Actions of Hormones", Vol. 1, p. 415. Academic Press, New York and London.

Schleusener, H., Kotulla, P., Kruck, I., Kruck, G., Geissler, D. and Adlkofer, F. (1975). "Thyroid Research", p. 414. Excerpta Medica, Amsterdam.

Schneider, P. B., Robbins, J. and Condliffe, P. G. (1965). *J. clin. Endocr. Metab.* **25**, 514.

Shome, B. D., Brown, D. M., Howard, S. M. and Pierce, J. G. (1968a). *Arch. biochem. Biophys.* **126**, 456.

Shome, B. D., Parlow, A. F., Ramirez, V. D., Elrick, H. and Pierce, J. G. (1968b). *Arch. biochem. Biophys.* **126**, 444.

Siler, T. M., Yen, S. S. C., Vale, W. and Guillemin, R. (1974). *J. clin. Endocr. Metab.* **38**, 742.

Silva, J. E. and Larsen, P. R. (1978). *J. clin. Invest.* **61**, 1247.

Smith, B. R., Dorrington, K. J. and Munro, D. S. (1969). *Biochim. biophys. Acta*, **192**, 277.

Smith, B. R. and Hall, R. (1974). *Lancet*, **ii**, 427.

Smith, P. E. and Smith, I. P. (1922). *J. med. Res.* **43**, 267.

Snyder, P. J. and Utiger, R. D. (1972a). *J. clin. Endocr. Metab.* **34**, 380.

Snyder, P. J. and Utiger, R. D. (1972b). *J. clin. Invest.* **51**, 2077.

Sonenberg, M. (1958). "Vitamins and Hormones", Vol. 16, p. 205. Academic Press, New York and London.

Stock, J. M., Surks, M. I. and Oppenheimer, J. H. (1974). *New Engl. J. Med.* **290**, 529.

Stockell-Hartree, A. (1966). *Biochem. J.* **100**, 754.

Stockell-Hartree, A., Butt, W. R. and Kirkham, K. E. (1964). *J. Endocr.* **29**, 61.

Strakosch, C. R., Joyner, D. and Wall, J. R. (1978a). *J. clin. Endocr. Metab.* **46**, 345.

Strakosch, C. R., Joyner, D. and Wall, J. R. (1978b). *J. clin. Endocr. Metab.* **47**, 361.

Szabo, M., Kovathana, N., Gordon, K. and Frohman, L. A. (1978). *Endocrinology*, **102**, 799.

Tamura, H. and Ui, N. (1970). *Biochim. biophys. Acta*, **214**, 566.

Tamura, H. and Ui, N. (1972a). *J. Biochem.* (*Japan*), **71**, 201.

Tamura, H. and Ui, N. (1972b). *J. Biochem.* (*Japan*), **71**, 531.

Tamura-Takahashi, H. and Ui, N. (1977). *J. Biochem.* **81**, 1155.

Tashjian, A. H., Barowsky, N. J. and Jensen, D. K. (1971). *Biochem. biophys. Res. Commun.* **43**, 516.

Tate, R. L., Holmes, J. M., Kohn, L. D. and Winand, R. J. (1975a). *J. biol. Chem.* **250**, 6527.

Tate, R. L., Schwartz, H. I., Holmes, J. M., Kohn, L. D. and Winand, R. J. (1975b). *J. biol. Chem.* **250**, 6509.

Taurog, A., Tong, W. and Chaikoff, I. L. (1958a). *Endocrinology*, **62**, 646.

Taurog, A., Tong, W. and Chaikoff, I. L. (1958b). *Endocrinology*, **62**, 664.

Toft, A. D., Irvine, W. J., Hunter, W. M. and Seth, J. (1974). *Br. med. J.* 3, 152.

Tojo, S., Kanazawa, S., Nakamura, A., Kitagaki, S. and Mochizuki, M. (1973). *Endocrinology* (*Japan*), **20**, 505.

Tojo, S., Kanazawa, S., Saida, K. and Nakamura, A. (1976). *Acta obstet. gynecol. scand.* **55**, 348.

Tolis, G., Bird, C., Bertrand, G., McKenzie, J. M. and Ezrin, C. (1978). *Am. J. Med.* **64**, 177.

Ui, N., Tamura-Takahashi, H., Yora, T. and Condliffe, P. G. (1977). *Biochim. biophys. Acta*, **497**, 812.

Utiger, R. D. (1965a). *In* "Current Topics in Thyroid Research" (M. Andreoli and C. Cassano, eds), p. 513. Academic Press, New York and London.

Utiger, R. D. (1965b). *J. clin. Invest.* **44**, 1277.

Utiger, R. D., Odell, W. D. and Condliffe, P. G. (1963). *Endocrinology*, **73**, 359.

Vagenakis, A. G., Braverman, L. E., Azizi, F., Portnay, G. I. and Ingbar, S. H. (1975a). *New Engl. J. Med.* **293**, 681.

Vagenakis, A. G., Roti, E., Mannix, J. and Braverman, L. E. (1975b). *J. clin. Endocr. Metab.* **41**, 801.

Vaitukaitis, J. L., Ross, G. T., Braunstein, G. D. and Rayford, P. L. (1976). *Rec. Prog. Horm. Res.* **32**, 289.

Vaitukaitis, J. L., Ross, G. T., Pierce, J. G., Cornell, J. S. and Reichert, L. E. (1973). *J. clin. Endocr. Metab.* **37**, 653.

Vale, W., Brazeau, P., Rivier, C., Brown, M., Boss, B., Rivier, J., Burgus, R., Ling, N. and Guillemin, R. (1975). *Rec. Prog. Horm. Res.* **31**, 367.

Vanhaelst. L. and Golstein-Golaire, J. (1976). *J. clin. Endocr. Metab.* **43**, 836.

Vanhaelst, L., Van Canter, E., De Gaute, J. P. and Golstein, J. (1972). *J. clin. Endocr. Metab.* **35**, 479.

Webster, B. R., Guansing, A. R. and Paice, J. C. (1972). *J. clin. Endocr. Metab.* **34**, 899.

Weeke, J., Hansen, A. P. and Lundaek, K. (1975). *J. clin. Endocr. Metab.* **41**, 168.

Weintraub, B. D., Krauth, G., Rosen, S. W. and Rabson, A. S. (1975). *J. clin. Invest.* **56**, 1043.

Weintraub, B. D. and Stannard, B. S. (1978). *FEBS Lett.* **92**, 303.

Werner, S. C. (1936a). *Proc. Soc. exp. Biol. Med.* **34**, 390.

Werner, S. C. (1936b). *Proc. Soc. exp. Biol. Med.* **34**, 392.

Werner, S. C., Otero-Ruiz, E., Seegal, B. C. and Bates, R. W. (1960). *Nature, Lond.* **185**, 472.

White, A. (1944). "Chemistry and Physiology of the Hormones", Am. Ass. Adv. Sciences, Washington, DC.

Wilber, J. F. (1971). *Endocrinology*, **89**, 873.

Wilber, J. F. and Baum, D. (1970). *J. clin. Endocr. Metab.* **31**, 372.

Wilber, J. F., Peake, G. T. and Utiger, R. D. (1969). *Endocrinology*, **84**, 758.

Wilber, J. F. and Utiger, R. D. (1968). *Proc. Soc. exp. Biol. Med.* **127**, 488.

Wilber, J. F. and Utiger, R. D. (1969a). *Endocrinology*, **84**, 1316.

Wilber, J. F. and Utiger, R. D. (1969b). *J. clin. Invest.* **48**, 2096.

Winand, R. J. and Kohn, L. D. (1970). *J. biol. Chem.* **245**, 967.

Wollman, S. H. (1969). "Lysosomes in Biology and Pathology" (J. T. Dingle and H. B. Fell, eds), Vol. 2, p. 483. North Holland, Amsterdam.

Wynston, L. K., Free, C. A. and Pierce, J. G. (1960). *J. biol. Chem.* **235**, 85.

Yamamoto, T., Woeber, K. A. and Ingbar, S. H. (1972). *J. clin. Endocr. Metab.* **34**, 423.

Yamashitu, K. and Field, J. B. (1970). *Biochem. biophys. Res. Comm.* **40**, 171.

Yamashitu, K. and Field, J. B. (1972). *J. clin. Invest.* **51**, 463.

Yora, T. and Ui, N. (1978). *J. Biochem. (Japan)*, **83**, 1173.

Zor, U., Kancko, T., Lowe, I. P., Bloom, G. and Field, J. B. (1969). *J. biol. Chem.* **244**, 5189.

XII. The Iodine-containing Hormones

J. ROBBINS and J. E. RALL

INTRODUCTION

The thyroid hormones are unusual in several respects. First, they are amino acids having a unique diphenyl ether structure which contains the element iodine. Second, they exist in very different forms in the thyroid gland, where they are integral units of the peptide chain of thyroglobulin, and in the blood, where they are attached to specialised plasma proteins by non-covalent linkage. Third, the major secretory product, thyroxine, has an unusually high affinity for its transport protein, leading to an extraordinarily slow and steady hormone action. Fourth, the major active form, triiodothyronine, is mainly a product of the extraglandular metabolism of thyroxine. Because of these unusual features, this chapter will deal with several diverse subjects: the broad aspect of iodine-containing compounds and their metabolic transformations in mammals, the properties of natural iodoproteins and the thyroxine-binding proteins, and the influence of the latter on thyroid hormone kinetics and measurements.

The historical landmarks in the developing knowledge about the thyroid hormones and related substances have been summarised in several places (Pitt-Rivers and Tata, 1959; Roche and Michel, 1951; Robbins and Rall, 1960, 1967; Chopra, 1978a). These include the discovery of the role of iodine in 1896, of thyroglobulin in 1899, of thyroxine in 1915 and triiodo-thyronine in 1952, and thyroxine-binding globulin in 1952. Characterisation of the circulating hormone as a small molecule was first clearly indicated by Trevorrow in 1939, thus dispelling the earlier belief that it was thyro-globulin. The major hormone in blood was subsequently shown to be thy-roxine by recrystallisation to constant specific activity (Taurog and Chaikoff, 1948) and by chromatography (Laidlaw, 1949; Taurog, Chaikoff and Tong, 1950; Gross, Leblond, Franklin and Quastel, 1950). Later work identified 3,5,3'-triiodothyronine (Gross and Pitt-Rivers, 1953a, b; Roche, Lissitzky and Michel, 1952a, b), 3,3'-diiodothyronine and 3,3',5'-triiodothyronine (Roche, Michel, Wolf and Nunez, 1956; Roche, Michel and Nunez, 1959) as minor components of the blood iodine, and in the past several years, the important role of peripheral monodeiodination of thyroxine to give the hormone triiodothyronine, as well as other metabolites, has been clarified (Chopra, 1978b). As we shall see, still other minor components have been identified.

In the years since this chapter was first published, the methods for measuring the thyroid hormones in blood have shifted from iodine analysis to displace-ment techniques, and most recently to radioimmunoassay. The reader should consult the earlier editions for detailed consideration of the older methods as well as for the chronological development of each of the subjects covered in this review.

A. CHEMICAL AND PHYSICAL PROPERTIES

1. The Iodoamino Acids

Thyroid hormones like the catecholamines are derivatives of tyrosine. In the case of thyroid hormones the two critical steps are iodination of tyrosine and coupling of two iodotyrosines to form an iodothyronine. If a second hydroxyl residue is added to tyrosine, the catecholamine pathway is begun.

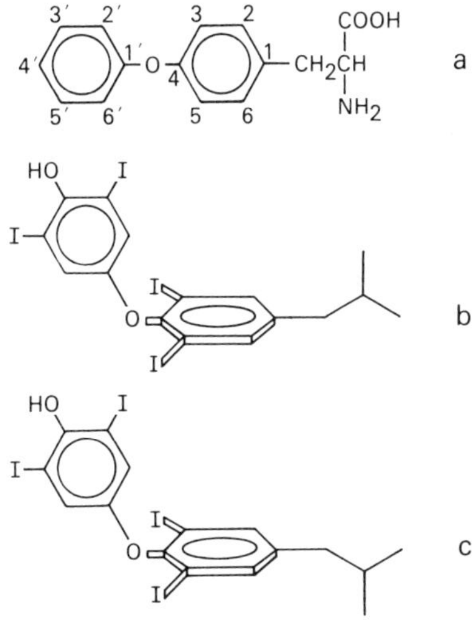

Fig. 1.

The numbering system used in describing thyroxine and its various derivatives, and the steric relationships of thyroxine, are shown in Fig. 1. The angle formed by the atoms C_4-O-C_1', is 120°. Free rotation is possible about this angle if there are no substituents on the phenyl rings. When fully iodinated as in thyroxine or in triiodothyronine, the bulky iodine atoms cause the preferred orientation of the phenyl rings to be perpendicular. In the case of T_3* both NMR studies and molecular orbital calculations

* Although the biochemical literature refers to the various thyroid hormones as thyronine derivatives, in chemical abstracts they are referred to as derivatives of alanine. Hence, thyroxine is alanine,-3-[4-(4-hydroxy-3,5-diiodophenoxyl)-3,5-diiodophenyl]. We shall use as abbreviations, T_4 for thyroxine, T_3 for 3,5,3'-triiodothyronine, rT_3 for 3,3'5'-triiodothyronine, $3,3'T_2$ for 3,3'diiodothyronine, etc. In all cases, the L isomer is implied unless specific note is made.

show no preference for the 3′-iodine atom to be in either the proximal (closest to the inner ring) or distal position (Kollman, Murray, Nuss, Jorgensen and Rothenberg, 1973). Furthermore, crystals may be prepared of T_3 in which the 3′-iodine is either proximal or distal, apparently depending on the conditions of crystallisation (Camerman and Camerman, 1972; Cody, 1974). Also, at 37° although rotation about the ether bond is somewhat restricted, there is rapid interconversion of the two forms (Emmett and Pepper, 1976). Some time ago Jorgenson and collaborators synthesized several iodothyronines with bulky groups in the 6′ position. This totally prevented rotation about the ether linkage. They were then able to compare the biological activities of methyl derivatives of 3,5-T_2 in which the 3′ position contained a CH_3 group in one case fixed proximally, and in the other case fixed distally. The compound substituted in the distal 3′ position was almost half as active as T_4. The analogue with the methyl group in the proximal position was only about 1 % as active as T_4 (Jorgensen, 1964, Jorgensen, 1976). The alanine side chain plays a role in determining the exact orientation of the two phenyl rings (Cody, Hazel, Langs and Duax, 1977) (see Fig. 1). Furthermore, the outer ring may be either cis or trans with respect to the side chain. Detailed crystallographic studies have related exact structures of thyronine derivatives with their binding affinities for plasma and nuclear binding proteins (Cody et al., 1977).

Thyroxine forms chelates with a variety of divalent metals (Cu^{++}, Fe^{++}, Mn^{++}, Mg^{++}) and the chelate with magnesium is so extremely insoluble it may be employed in an analytical method (Kuby, Noda and Lardy, 1954; Sterling and Brenner, 1966). Most iodothyronines are relatively insoluble in water at neutral pH. In phosphate buffer $\Gamma/2 = 0.04$, at 25°, pH 7·4 the solubility of T_4 is 4×10^{-5} mol/l (Evert, 1960). Increase in pH to 9 or 10 greatly increases the solubility of both T_3 and T_4. Reasonably good solvents are alkaline methanol, propylene glycol and butanol. The pK of the phenolic hydroxyl varies with the iodine substituents (Table 1) as does their extinction coefficient. These differences, as noted below, permit a spectrophotometric determination of T_4, MIT and DIT in protein solutions. Under certain conditions, a relatively stable free radical of T_4 may be formed (Borg, 1965). An excellent review of iodamino acid chemistry is available (Cahnmann, 1972).

The reactive groups on T_4 undergo the usual biological transformation (see Section B.5). The amino group may be removed by transamination to form the pyruvate derivative or it may undergo oxidative deamination to form the acetic acid analogue. The phenolic hydroxyl may be conjugated with either glucuronic acid or sulphate. Both of these reactions occur largely in the liver and these compounds are secreted in the bile. Apparently they are hydrolysed in the gut but not reabsorbed (Galton and Nisula, 1972). Deiodination is the major pathway for metabolism of both hormones. T_4

Table 1

Dissociation constants (pK) of phenolic hydroxyls and extinction coefficients for tyrosine and its iodinated derivatives. (From Edelhoch, 1962 and Gershengorn, et al., 1977a.)

| Compound | pK | Unionised[a] | | Ionised[b] | |
		$\varepsilon \times 10^{-3c}$	λ mμ	$\varepsilon \times 10^{-3c}$	λ mμ
Tyrosine	10·13	1·40	274·5	2·40	293
Mono-iodotyrosine	8·20	2·75	283	4·10	305
Di-iodotyrosine	6·36	2·75	287	6·25	311
Tri-iodothyronine	8·45	4·09	295	4·66	322
Thyroxine	7·0	4·20	298	6·18	325

[a] In 0·1 M HCl except tri-iodothyronine which is in 0·04 M HCl.
[b] In 0·1 M NaOH except tri-iodothyronine which is in 0·04 M NaOH.
[c] ε = molar extinction coefficient for 1 cm light path.

and T$_3$ are readily deiodinated in acid. Furthermore, ultraviolet light will deiodinate T$_4$ and cause the formation of a variety of poorly identified derivatives. Thyroxine (and T$_3$) can also be readily deiodinated under a variety of conditions with flavin mononucleotide, certain proteins, or amino acids and metals (Reinwein and Rall, 1966).

2. Iodoproteins

(a) Thyroglobulin and related proteins

In most mammals a crude aqueous extract of the thyroid gland contains about 80% of the protein as thyroglobulin (19S), about 5% as the 27S iodoprotein and 15% as proteins with sedimentation values of 4–7S. Thyroglobulin is a glycoprotein of 665,000 mw with an iodine content which varies as a function of iodine intake. In the U.S. in most common mammals (cow, pig, sheep) and man an iodine content of about 1% is common. This gives about 50 atoms of iodine per molecule of thyroglobulin which usually yields, after hydrolysis, about five molecules of T$_4$, less than half of T$_3$, 10 of DIT and 10 of MIT. Thyroglobulin crystallises in chains and rows of chains but not in large crystals (Jakoby, Labaw, Edelhoch, Pastan and Rall, 1966). Both hydrodynamic studies and electron microscopic examinations show thyroglobulin to be a flexible molecule (Labaw and Rall, 1968; Berg and Ekholm, 1975; Bloth and Bergquist, 1968; Edelhoch and Steiner, 1966). Some electron microscope pictures show a twisted molecule apparently composed of two subunits (Berg and Ekholm, 1975). Thyroglobulin is easily denatured by acid, alkali, urea or guanidine and half molecules of 12S are formed (Metzger and Edelhoch, 1961; Edelhoch and Lippoldt, 1964). Between pH 5 and 11 denaturation is reversible. The isoelectric point of thyroglobulin is about 4·4 although a careful study by isoelectric focusing shows multiple values and 4·4 is average (Ui, 1971). Thyroglobulin is irreversibly denatured below pH 5·0. Thyroglobulin shows an interesting effect of cold which confused interpretations for some years. Dissociation of thyroglobulin into 12S subunits under mild conditions is enhanced as the temperature is lowered (Schneider, Bornet and Edelhoch, 1971). Furthermore, less heavily iodinated thyroglobulin unfolds and dissociates more easily than fully iodinated thyroglobulin. This is explained, at least in part, by more S–S bonds being formed as thyroglobulin is progressively iodinated. Hence lightly iodinated thyroglobulin consists of two subunits not connected by disulphide bridges, whereas highly iodinated thyroglobulin has a certain proportion of the thyroglobulin molecules with the 12S subunits linked by disulphide bridges. Thus, lightly iodinated thyroglobulin or newly synthesised thyroglobulin examined in the centrifuge at 4° shows a considerable fraction of 12S molecules. If studied at 25° essentially only the mature 19S molecule is seen.

The subunit composition of thyroglobulin has been a subject of controversy for some years. The two subunits of 12S (330,000 daltons) were first thought to be dissociated by reduction and alkylation into four elementary chains of 165,000 (De Crombrugghe et al., 1966). This view is still held by some (Pitt-Rivers, 1976). However, in many species, analysis of thyroglobulin after reduction and alkylation showed multiple polypeptides with molecular weights as low as 80,000 (Pierce, Rawitch, Brown and Stanley, 1965; Lissitzky, Rolland, Reynaud, Savary and Lasry, 1968; Rolland and Lissitzky, 1970; Rawitch and Brown, 1973; Spiro, 1973; Roland and Lissitzky, 1976; Spiro, 1977a). Studies of guinea-pig thyroglobulin showed only three major bands with molecular weights of about 300,000, 210,000 and 110,000 (Haeberli, Bilstad, Edelhoch and Rall, 1975). Such large subunits were also found in sheep and hog thyroglobulin when care was taken to prevent proteolysis during and after extraction of the thyroids and a subunit and elementary chain mw of 330,000 was proposed (Lissitzky, Mauchamp, Reynaud and Rolland, 1975). This viewpoint was strengthened when a large mRNA from thyroid was isolated, and upon translation of Xenopus oocytes gave a protein of 330,000 (Vassart, Refetoff, Brocas, Dinsart and Dumont, 1975). However, in another study, three mRNAs were found in the thyroid which directed the synthesis of polypeptides of about 300,000, 200,000 and 100,000 (De Nayer, 1977). Yet another examination of the products of thyroid mRNA found a major mRNA giving a 300,000 polypeptide, albeit with minor fractions giving polypeptides two-thirds and one-third that value (Chebath, Chabaud, Becarevic, Cartouzou and Lissitzky, 1977).

Analysis of thyroglobulin for amino-(N) and carboxy-terminal (C) amino acids should resolve the problem. Although earlier reports identified three or four N-terminal amino acids, more recent data suggest that all N-terminal amino acids are blocked (Bilstad, Edelhoch, Lippoldt, Rall and Salvatore, 1972; Marriq, Rolland and Lissitzky, 1977). Recently the C-terminal amino acids of thyroglobulin have been studied using carboxypeptidase A. It was suggested that two leucine residues were C-terminal, thus giving two elementary chains to thyroglobulin (Marriq *et al.*, 1977). The data are not inconsistent, however, with an additional one or two serine residues also C-terminal. It is now clear that thyroglobulin is composed of two subunits, which may be of different composition (van der Walt, Kotze, van Jaarsveld and Edelhoch, 1978). Whether these may be composed of polypeptide chains of 110,000 and 220,000 is unresolved.

The amino acid composition of thyroglobulin is unremarkable except for iodoamino acids noted above. Additionally, traces of monoiodohistidine and diiodohistidine may be found in thyroglobulin. Both T_3 and T_4 are formed by coupling of iodotyrosines. In this process a derivative of the alanine side chain remains in peptide linkage. Whether this is alanine, serine, dehydroalanine, or something else is not clear. However, this reaction occurs without splitting of a peptide bond. The iodothyronines T_4 and T_3 are formed in thyroglobulin with particular ease whether chemical iodination is performed *in vitro* or whether iodination occurs *in vivo*. The native structure of thyroglobulin is required for substantial T_4 synthesis at low levels of iodine. Presumably this structure favouring T_4 synthesis with little iodine is a major biological function of thyroglobulin. Unfolding of thyroglobulin with urea decreases the efficiency of T_4 synthesis *in vitro* with I_2 as the iodinating agent (Edelhoch, 1962).

Thyroglobulin also contains several branched carbohydrate chains amounting to about 10% of the molecular weight. The A chain consists of multiple mannose residues attached to three *N*-acetylglucosamine residues attached in turn to an asparagine (Spiro, 1965; Arima, Spiro and Spiro, 1972). The B chain also has *N*-acetylglucosamine attached to asparagine but contains, in addition to mannose, galactose, *N*-acetylglucosamine and sialic acid residues (Fukuda and Egami, 1971; Toyoshima, Fukuda and Osawa, 1973). A third carbohydrate chain has been identified but not characterised chemically (Arima *et al.*, 1972). In human thyroglobulin a fourth chain has recently been described which contains galactosamine, glucuronic acid, galactose, xylose and sulphate and is attached to a serine residue (Spiro, 1977b). The function of the carbohydrates of thyroglobulin is not entirely clear except for one interesting finding in a transplantable rat thyroid tumour. This tissue synthesised thyroglobulin but apparently was unable to secrete it into the colloid. Careful biochemical studies showed that this abnormal thyroglobulin lacked sialic acid and the enzyme, sialyl transferase, was missing (Monaco and Robbins, 1973). The strong suggestion is that terminal sialic acids are required for thyroglobulin to be secreted into the colloid.

The so-called 27S iodoprotein has a mw of $1·3 \times 10^6$ in accord with a dimer of thyroglobulin, and its amino acid and sugar content are very close to or identical to that of thyroglobulin (Salvatore, Vecchio, Salvatore, Cahnmann and Robbins, 1965; Bilstad et al., 1972). The level of 27S protein is decreased by iodine deficiency or the administration of antithyroid drugs and appears to increase when thyroglobulin metabolism is slowed by large amounts of dietary iodine (Sinadinovic, Jovanovic, Kraincanic and Djardjevic, 1973; Frati, Bilstad, Edelhoch, Rall and Salvatore, 1974). In general, 27S has a higher iodine and T_4 content than thyroglobulin (Salvatore et al., 1965), although there is overlap between the two proteins. The 27S protein is easily dissociated into thyroglobulin and 12S proteins by denaturants, indicating that it is not held together by disulphide bonds. Although it has been difficult to form the 27S from 19S thyroglobulin and iodination of thyroglobulin in vitro does not produce the 27S species, protein synthesis is not required for the 19S → 27S transition (Frati et al., 1974).

Another polymer of thyroglobulin has been isolated, the 37S iodoprotein. A mw of 2×10^6 suggests that it is a trimer of thyroglobulin (van der Walt and van Jaarsveld, 1972).

(b) Other iodoproteins

In addition to thyroglobulin, its subunits, and polymers, an iodinated protein similar or identical to serum albumin has been found in the thyroid (Shulman, Mates and Bronson, 1967). Recent evidence suggests that iodination and perhaps synthesis of this protein occurs in the thyroid (Shimaoka and Thompson, 1965; Otten, Jonckheer and Dumont, 1971). An iodoprotein of unknown structure is also found in normal blood (Surks and Oppenheimer, 1969; Rall and Conard, 1966), and its concentration may be increased in carcinoma of the thyroid, in certain congenital defects in thyroxine synthesis and in a variety of other diseases of the thyroid.

An ill-defined group of insoluble iodoproteins may also be found in thyroid tissue. Some of these undoubtedly are incompletely synthesised thyroglobulin (Rall, Robbins and Edelhoch, 1960).

B. BIOSYNTHESIS, SECRETION AND METABOLISM

1. Iodide Concentration

The thyroid gland must cope with the problem that iodine is a necessary constituent of the thyroid hormone but is a trace element nutritionally.

The thyroid has evolved a special mechanism for concentration of the iodide ion from the very low levels usually found in blood, a property also exhibited by several other tissues—salivary glands, stomach, choroid plexus, mammary gland (Brown-Grant, 1961; Wolf, 1964). Anatomically, iodide appears first to be concentrated in thyroid cells (Andros and Wollman, 1967) and later in the colloid, implying that the basal cell membrane actively transports iodide. The mechanism of iodide concentration is fundamentally unknown but several pertinent facts must be considered (Wolff, 1964):

(i) concentration of iodide requires energy (dinitrophenol and CN^- are inhibitory),

(ii) concentration of iodide is non-specific in the sense that a variety of other monovalent anions of similar size (BF_4^-, TcO_4^-, ReO_4^-, ClO_4^-, $SeCN^-$, etc.) are also transported into the thyroid and compete with I^- transport,

(iii) K^+ is required for I^- transport and digitalis glycosides inhibit transport.

(iv) I^- transport can be saturated with excess I^-: the half saturation value in thyroid (and salivary gland and stomach) is $\sim 30\ \mu M$.

(v) certain phospholipids extractable from thyroid tissue will concentrate iodide *in vitro* in two phase systems (Schneider and Wolff, 1965),

(vi) the thyroid cell is electrically negative (~ 50 mV) compared to both colloid and extracellular fluid (Woodbury and Woodbury, 1963).

At present it is not possible to integrate these (and other) findings into a coherent scheme for iodide transport into the thyroid.

An important aspect of iodide concentration is the "Wolff-Chaikoff" phenomenon (Wolff, 1969). This effect is produced when large quantities of I^- are given acutely and consists of a virtual abolition of iodination and hormone synthesis. The effect is usually transitory even in the presence of high levels of I^- in serum, but is undoubtedly the cause of "iodide goitre," seen not infrequently in man. The cause of the inhibition could reside in the following equilibrium:

$$I^- + I_2 \leftrightarrows I_3^- \, ; k = \frac{I_3^-}{I_2 \times I^-} = 770\ l/mol$$

Thus, large quantities of I^- drive this equilibrium towards I_3^-. It seems reasonable on chemical grounds that the latter form of iodine is inactive in iodination reactions. Release from inhibition of iodination, as suggested by Braverman and Ingbar (1963), may be due to inhibition by large quantities of I^- on the iodide-concentrating mechanism itself. This causes a decrease in intrathyroidal iodide so that the equilibrium reverts towards normal. Excess iodide also inhibits adenyl cyclase activation (Van Sande et al., 1975) and colloid droplet formation (Yamamoto et al., 1972).

2. Iodination and Iodothyronine Synthesis

The simplest series of reactions which take iodine and tyrosine and form thyroxine are as follows:

$$2I^- \xrightarrow{-2e} I_2$$

The first reaction is generally assumed to utilise H_2O_2 as the oxidising agent. By analogy with chloroperoxidase (Hager, Morris, Brown and Eberwein, 1966) which at pH 3 and supplemented with I^-, H_2O_2 and tyrosine or thyroglobulin will effect DIT synthesis, it is possible that the intermediate is a complex as:

$$\text{Enzyme} + H_2O_2 + I^- \rightarrow \text{Enzyme–I} + OH^-$$

There are probably several peroxidases in the thyroid which are attached to various cell membranes (Hosoya *et al.*, 1971) including the apical plasma membrane (Tice and Wollman, 1972). Thyroid peroxidase is a haemoprotein which is still incompletely characterised (Taurog, 1977; Morrison and Schonbaum, 1976), and the identity of the peroxide-generating system is still obscure. In the thyroid the only tyrosine iodinated is in a peptide bond, largely in thyroglobulin. The non-polar environment of many of these tyrosyl residues probably accounts for the relatively greater formation of diiodotyrosine rather than monoiodotyrosine, compared with iodination of free tyrosine (Mayberry and Hockert, 1970; Van Zyl and Edelhoch, 1967).

Thyroxine synthesis also takes place in the intact thyroglobulin molecule. Iodination chemically with I_2 or enzymatically with H_2O_2, I^- and peroxidase will cause the formation of thyroxine in thyroglobulin as well as in other proteins such as serum albumin. The thyroglobulin structure favours the synthesis of five or six iodothyronine residues (Edelhoch, 1965; Van Zyl and Edelhoch, 1967) derived from the first iodotyrosines that are formed (Lamas *et al.*, 1974; Edelhoch and Robbins, 1978). An alternative model for the synthesis of thyroxine involves the coupling of diiodotyrosine in the peptide chain with free diiodohydroxphenylpyruvic acid (DIHPPA) (Ogawara and

Cahnmann, 1972; Blasi et al., 1969; Surks et al., 1968). It is not entirely certain which of these paths for thyroxine synthesis is the physiologically important one but the "coupling enzyme" appears to be thyroid peroxidase (Taurog, 1978; Lamas et al., 1972).

Triiodothyronine is formed by intramolecular coupling if one of the reactant molecules is monoiodotyrosine. The coupling reaction between DIT and monoiodohydroxyphenylpyruvic acid also can form triiodothyronine, but in lower yield than is the case with thyroxine formation from DIHPPA (Shiba and Cahnmann, 1964). Very little triiodothyronine in the thyroid is formed by monodeiodination of thyroxine (Haibach, 1971).

3. Thyroglobulin Synthesis

The recent understanding of some of the mechanisms involved in protein synthesis had led to a large amount of work concerned with the synthesis of thyroglobulin (Edelhoch and Robbins, 1978). It was first shown, using labelled amino acids and thyroid slices, that the sequential appearance of thyroglobulin-related polypeptides appeared to progress from a 3–8S species to 12S and finally the 19S molecule (Seed and Goldberg, 1963; Ui, 1974; Salvatore and Edelhoch, 1973). Subsequent work indicated that newly formed thyroglobulin has a slower sedimentation rate (14–17S) than normal thyroglobulin (Seed and Goldberg, 1965b; Nunez et al., 1965; Inoue and Taurog, 1968) and was readily dissociated into smaller fragments (Sellin and Goldberg, 1965). It is now clear that this molecular instability is related to the low iodine and disulphide content of "immature" thyroglobulin (Edelhoch and Robbins, 1978), and it has been demonstrated that the thyroid contains a 33s mRNA which codes for a 300,000 mw protein leading to formation of 19S thyroglobulin (Vassart et al., 1975). Synthesis of the complete protein in the thyroid cell requires about four hours (Nadler et al., 1964), most of which involves the post-transcriptional insertion of carbohydrates into the oligosaccharide units (Spiro and Spiro, 1966; Edelhoch and Robbins, 1978). Iodination is a late event, occurring after completion of the oligosaccharide chains (Monaco et al., 1975) and probably during or after secretion of the molecule into the follicle lumen (Ekholm and Wollman, 1975). Some further iodination occurs in the colloid (Inoue and Taurog, 1968) and may be the mechanism by which thyroglobulin is formed (Bilstad et al., 1972).

4. Secretion

Since the storage form of the thyroid hormone is the protein thyroglobulin and the secreted hormones are the amino acids thyroxine and triiodothyronine, it is apparent that proteolytic enzymes must be involved in the process of secretion of hormone. A series of studies by Wollman, Nadler and collaborators described the morphologic sequence of events leading to release of thyroid hormones (Wetzel, Spicer and Wollman, 1965; Nadler, Sarkor and Leblond, 1962; Wollman, 1969). The first step appears to be the enclosing of a small droplet of colloid by endocytosis. This droplet migrates towards the basal end of the cell and shows histochemical evidence of hydrolases only after fusion with dense granules, or lysosomes. Cathepsin is liberated from thyroid cell particles by agents which free typical lysosomal enzymes such as acid phosphatase and β-glucuronidase (Herveg, Beckers and DeVisscher, 1966; Reinwein, 1964; Balasubramanian and Deiss, 1965). Thyroid extracts contain proteases with an acid pH optimum (McQuillan and Trikojus, 1966; Rall et al., 1964) as well as several peptidases (Laver and Trikojus, 1956). TSH or other treatments which stimulate the thyroid do not increase protease activity (Loughlin, McQuillan and Trikojus, 1960) although, after TSH treatment in vivo, iodoprotein isolated with thyroid particles releases iodoaminoacids more readily (Deiss et al., 1966).

The final step by which the liberated iodothyronines obtain entry to the blood stream is unclear. There is some evidence that lymph draining the thyroid in several species, including baboons, has a substantial content of iodoprotein (70–90%) and also thyroxine and triiodothyronine (Daniel, Plaskett and Pratt, 1966; Wollman, 1969). Although this route probably accounts for only about 1% of thyroid iodine secretion, it may represent a way by which iodoprotein reaches the blood (see below). Immunologic evidence shows that much of this is thyroglobulin (Daniel, Pratt, Roitt and Torrigiani, 1967).

In all events, thyroid vein blood contains a higher concentration of thyroxine and triiodothyronine than does thyroid artery blood and the gradient is increased with TSH stimulation. One function of the thyroxine-binding proteins of serum may be to establish a gradient for iodothyronine from cell and extracellular fluid of thyroid to the blood. Direct studies of thyroid vein blood show mainly thyroxine (Taurog, Portes and Thio, 1964; Matsuda and Greer, 1965) and very small quantities (0–5% of the total ^{131}I) of either mono- or diiodotyrosine. The iodotyrosines liberated by hydrolysis of thyroglobulin are normally deiodinated by a microsomal, NADPH-requiring enzyme and this enzyme appears to be inactive against iodothyronines (see Stanbury, 1960). After TSH, appreciable triiodothyronine is found; and in the rabbit a substantial amount (20–25%) of iodoprotein as well (Taurog et al., 1964).

5. Extrathyroidal Metabolism of Iodoamino Acids

The peripheral metabolism of thyroxine, the major amino acid secreted by the thyroid, is now known to be the final step in synthesis of most of the T_3, the main active thyroid hormone. Furthermore, this step is affected by a variety of physiological conditions. The metabolism of all the other iodo-amino acids, T_3, rT_3, MIT, DIT, etc., corresponds more to normal degradative steps for inactivation of hormones or metabolism and excretion of by-products. The first indication of peripheral conversion of T_4 to T_3 was observed in the kidney many years ago (Albright and Larson, 1959). Since that time, *in vivo* studies in man have shown that T_4 is converted extra-thyroidally to both T_3 and rT_3 (Braverman, Ingbar and Sterling, 1970; Pittman, Chambers and Head, 1971; Chopra, 1976; Gavin, Castle, McMahon, Martin, Hammond and Cavalieri, 1977). Although some T_3 is secreted by the thyroid most of it is produced peripherally by monodeiodination of T_4. Almost all of the rT_3 is derived from peripheral deiodination of T_4. These are critical reactions since T_3 is highly active and rT_3 is either inactive or a weak thyroxine antagonist. Furthermore, as seen in Table 2, drugs and ill-nesses may affect the relative rates of conversion of T_4 to T_3 and rT_3. In

Table 2

Synthetic rates for T_3 and rT_3.

	T_3	rT_3	References
Conditions			
Starvation	↓	↑	Vagenakis *et al.* (1975)
Carbohydrate feeding	↑	↓	Harris *et al.* (1977)
Immediate neonatal period	↓	↑	Fisher *et al.* (1977a)
Severe illness (malaria)	↓	↑	Wartofsky *et al.* (1977)
Drugs			
Cortisol	↓	↑	Chopra *et al.* (1975)
Propylthiouracil	↓	↑	Hershman and Van Middlesworth (1962)
Propanolol	↓	↑	Wiersinga and Rouber (1977)

general, in most of these situations, T_3 synthesis is decreased. The neonatal period is of particular interest. The newborn has a level of rT_3 in blood of about 200 ng/100 ml (3·1 nmol/l) and a level of T_3 of 50 ng/100 ml (0·8 nmol/l) (Fisher, Dussault, Sack and Chopra, 1977a). Within a few days the T_3 level rises to a normal adult of $\sim$ 140 ng/100 ml (2·2 nmol/l) and rT_3 falls to normal. This adjustment with the results in Table 2 strongly suggest that either there are separate enzymes for $T_4 \rightarrow T_3$ and $T_4 \rightarrow rT_3$ or some allosteric effector changes the relative activities of a single enzyme. At present a deiodinase present in the microsomal fraction of liver, kidney, pituitary and probably other tissues appears to represent the T_4 deiodinase. This activity seems to be the physiologically important one since there is a close

correlation between the rate of T_4 deiodination measured *in vivo* and *in vitro*
with this system when rates are changed by inducing the microsomal drug
metabolising enzymes by administration of, for example, phenobarbital
(Schwartz, Kozyreff, Surks and Oppenheimer, 1969; Visser, van der Does-
Tobe, Docter and Hennemann, 1976). NADPH seems to stimulate deiodination, perhaps by increasing the free sulphydryl content (Sakurada, Rudolph,
Fang, Vagenakis, Braverman and Ingbar, 1978; Kaplan, 1978) of the cytosol.
Recently a kidney 5′ deiodinase has been shown to be largely localised to the
plasma membrane (Leonard and Rosenberg, 1978). Problems involved in
studying the T_4 deiodinase are 2 fold: firstly, the activity is low—of the order
of (in man) 0·003 μg (3·9 pmol) of T_4 deiodinated/g liver/h; secondly, T_4 is
sensitive to deiodination by non-enzymatic reactions usually involving
visible light (Morreale de Escobar, Escobar del Ray and Rodriguez, 1962;
Reinwein, Rall and Durrer, 1968). In addition to T_3 and T_4 a whole panoply
of variously deiodinated thyronines are produced (Flock, Bollman and
Grindley, 1960; Sorimachi and Robbins, 1977). These are listed in Fig. 2.
Cultured monkey hepatocarcinoma cells have proved a useful tool for these
studies (Sorimachi and Robbins, 1977). Also, as noted in Fig. 2, most of the

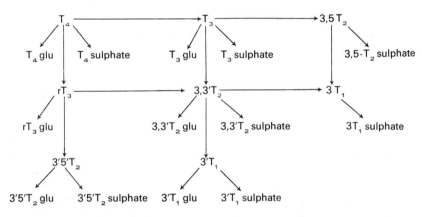

Fig. 2. Metabolism of thyroxine (glu = glucuronide).

iodothyronines can be conjugated with either sulphate or glucuronic acid.
These conjugates are excreted in the bile where they may be hydrolysed and
reabsorbed or excreted. In general, T_3 is more likely to undergo conjugation
as a sulphate and T_4 more likely to undergo glucurono-conjugation as a
glucuronoside. Additionally, any of these iodothyronines may be deaminated
to form lactic, pyruvic or acetic acid derivatives (Roche, Michel and Tata,
1954; Michel, Pitt-Rivers, Roche and Varrone, 1962). Splitting of the ether

linkage does not occur, at least in man (Pittman, Read and Chambers, 1970). There is a report, however, that DIT is formed from T_4 during incubation with human leucocytes (Burger, 1977). A little-understood pathway of T_4 and T_3 metabolism results in the formation of an iodoprotein (Surks and Oppenheimer, 1969).

The iodotyrosines are biologically inactive and in normal man almost none of them escape from the thyroid. There is, however, a deiodinase for both MIT and DIT present both in the thyroid and in liver and kidney (Foster and Gutman, 1930; Stanbury and Morris, 1958). Certain patients with absence of the iodotyrosine deiodinase have been described.

6. Quantitative Aspects of Thyroid Hormone Turnover

The entire system which describes the metabolism of iodine as it is either excreted in the urine or taken up by the thyroid, stored and then secreted as T_4 and T_3 and metabolised can be modelled on a computer but a minimum of some 15 compartments is required (Berman, 1972). The problems with this type of analysis have been discussed and values for the important parameters derived from the model are available (Berman, 1972).

In simplified form the kinetics of iodide metabolism in man show that the thyroid clears about 10–15 ml/min of blood and the kidney approximately 30 ml/min. The thyroid clearance varies as a function of the intake of stable iodine but the absolute iodine uptake (AIU) (i.e. μg iodine/hr) is reasonably constant. In Scotland where the iodine intake is low and the 24 hr uptake of radioiodine about 40% of the dose, the AIU is 2·2 μg/hr (Wayne, Koutras and Alexander, 1964). In the Eastern United States where the dietary intake of iodine is considerably higher and the average 24 hr uptake of iodine is about 20%, the AIU is about 2·9 μg/hour.

The initial step in uptake of iodine by the thyroid, the active transport of I^-, is generally rate limiting. Oxidation of I^- and iodination of tyrrosyl residues is normally so rapid that negligible amounts of free I^- are present in the thyroid. Since the normal human thyroid contains 15–20 mg of iodine and since it secretes about 70 μg iodine/day, the turnover of iodine in the thyroid is quite slow, with a half time of 50–100 days.

Table 3 lists data on production rates, pool sizes and plasma disappearance rates of the thyroid hormone. Reverse T_3 is included because, as noted above, it is a major metabolite of thyroxine and exists in the blood in significant quantity 50 ng/dl (0·8 nmol/l) (Gavin et al., 1977). It should be noted that thyroxine is metabolised slowly, less than 1% as fast as steroid or pituitary hormones. Triiodothyronine is considered to be turned over rapidly but even this rate is slower than any other hormone. As will be discussed below, binding of T_3 and T_4 to specific plasma proteins probably accounts for this

U

slow disappearance. About 15–20% of T_4 is excreted in the stool. In hyperthyroidism the rates of metabolism of both T_3 and T_4 are increased (Ingbar and Freinkel, 1958; Cavalieri, Steinberg and Searle, 1970).

Table 3

Kinetic parameters of thyroid hormone metabolism in man.

	T_4	T_3	rT_3
Production rate	87 μg/day[a]	24–34 μg/day[a,c]	33–36 μg/day[a,c]
Pool size	850 μg[b]	30 μg[c]	5 μg[c]
Half life in blood	6 day[b]	1 day[d]	0·4 day[c]

[a] Chopra (1976)
[b] Oppenheimer et al. (1967)
[c] Gavin et al. (1977)
[d] Woeber et al. (1970a)

C. THYROID HORMONE TRANSPORT IN BLOOD AND EXTRAVASCULAR FLUIDS

1. Nature of Thyroxine-binding Proteins

Several proteins participate in the transport of the thyroid hormones in human blood (Robbins and Rall, 1960; Robbins, 1976; Robbins, Cheng, Gershengorn et al., 1978a). Thyroxine-binding globulin (TBG), a trace α-globulin with very high affinity for the hormones, carries the majority of the circulating thyroxine and triiodothyronine and has no other known function. Prealbumin (PA), with a 20 fold higher concentration, binds about 15% of the circulating T_4 and 25% or less of the circulating T_3, and also participates in vitamin A transport through its interaction with the retinol-binding protein. Albumin, despite its far greater concentration, carries only about 10% of the T_4 and 25% of the T_3. In addition, several lipoproteins bind small amounts of the hormones (Hoch and Lewallen, 1974), and in abnormal states, anti-thyroid immunoglobulins may also participate in thyroid hormone transport (cf. E_5).

TBG and PA have been investigated intensively in recent years, and many of their molecular properties are now known. Adequate purification of TBG was achieved only recently through the application of affinity chromatography on columns of T_4-agarose (Pensky and Marshall, 1969; Robbins, 1976) or T_3-agarose (Cavalieri, 1975). Interestingly, PA is not retained on these columns, but has been prepared by more conventional methods

(Schultze, Schonenberger and Schwick, 1956; Purdy, Woeber, Holloway and Ingbar, 1965; Raz and Goodman, 1969; Peterson, 1971).

Some chemical and physical properties of TBG and PA are given in Tables 4 and 5. TBG is a glycoprotein containing about 23 % carbohydrate and 10 residues of sialic acid (Gershengorn, Cheng, Lippoldt et al., 1977a),

Table 4

Physical properties of human thyroxine-binding proteins. The data on TBG are from Gershengorn et al. (1977a) and Gershengorn et al., (1977b). Those on PA are from Branch, Robbins and Edelhoch (1971). For other references see Robbins (1975), Robbins (1976) and Robbins et al. (1978a). Albumin data are from Peters (1975).

	TBG	PA	ALB
mw	54,000	54,000	66,000
β-structure	28 %	45 %	15 %
α-helix	24 %	1 %	48 %
Peptide chains	1	4	1

Table 5

Chemical properties of human thyroxine-binding proteins. Data on TBG are from Gershengorn et al. (1977a), those on PA are from Raz and Goodman (1969) and Raz et al. (1970). For other data see Robbins (1975, 1976) and Robbins et al. (1978a). Albumin data are from Peters (1975).

	TBG	PA tetramer	ALB
Half-cystine residues	5	4	35
S–S bonds	2	0	17
Total carbohydrate	23 %	0	0
Sialic acid residues	10	0	0
$E_{280}^{1\%}$	6·17	14·1	5·31

whereas PA contains no sugars. Their amino acid compositions are also quite different (Robbins, Cheng et al., 1978a). The sequence of the 20 N-terminal amino acids in TBG has been determined (Cheng, 1978) and has no homology with any part of the PA molecule, the entire sequence of which is known (Kanda, Goodman, Canfield, Morgan, 1974). PA has an unusually high tyrosine and tryptophan content (8 residues/mol), accounting for its high extinction coefficient.

Both TBG and PA have molecular weights near 55,000 and are compact, globular proteins (Branch, Edelhoch, Robbins, 1971; Gershengorn, Lippoldt, Edelhoch, Robbins, 1977b). TBG, however, consists of a single polypeptide chain (Gershengorn et al., 1977a) whereas PA is a tetramer of identical

chains (Kanda, Goodman, Canfield, Morgan, 1974; Blake, Geisow et al.,
1974). The stability of the two proteins is also very different. TBG is easily
unfolded by heat, acid, or denaturing agents (Takemura, Hocman, Sterling,
1971; Gershengorn, Lippoldt et al., 1977b) whereas dissociation of the PA
tetramer or unfolding of its polypeptide backbone is extraordinarily difficult
(Branch, Robbins and Edelhoch, 1972). This may be related to the high
content of β-structure in PA, which is arranged in a "β-barrel" configuration
in each of the subunits (cf. Robbins, Cheng et al., 1978a). These β-sheets
are involved in the interface between subunits as well as in the wall of the
binding channel.

The nature of the hormone-binding site on TBG is still unknown. It
appears reasonably clear, however—despite some differences of opinion
(Korcek and Tabachnik, 1976)—that TBG possesses a single site whose
affinity is about $2 \times 10^{10} \, \text{M}^{-1}$ for T_4 and $7 \times 10^8 \, \text{M}^{-1}$ for T_3 (Table 6).

Table 6

Affinities of thyroid hormones for the transport proteins. The data are from the following studies using purified proteins at pH 7·4, 25° in phosphate or phosphate–chloride
buffer: TBG (0·06 M PO_4), Korcek and Tabachnik, 1976; PA–T_4 (0·05 M PO_4–
0·1 M Cl), Ferguson et al., 1973; PA–T_3 (0·05 M PO_4–0·1 M Cl), Cheng et al., 1977a;
ALB (0·1 M PO_4) Steiner et al., 1966. For PA, the independent sites model was used.
Other data have been listed by Prince and Ramsden, 1977. At 37°, the affinities for
TBG and PA are about 30% lower (Green Marshall, Pensky and Stanbury, 1972;
Nilsson and Peterson, 1971). In 0·1 M NaCl the affinity for albumin is about 50%
lower (Tabachnik, 1967).

	TBG (M^{-1})	PA (M^{-1})		ALB (M^{-1})	
	k	k_1	k_2	k_1	k_{2-4}
T_4	$1·5 \times 10^{10}$	$1·0 \times 10^8$	$9·5 \times 10^5$	$1·3 \times 10^6$	$6·0 \times 10^4$
T_3	$6·5 \times 10^8$	$2·0 \times 10^7$	$7·9 \times 10^5$	$2·0 \times 10^5$	—

Preliminary data with the affinity label, N-BrAc T_4, indicate that the side
chain is located near a lysyl and a tyrosyl residue, and that the site can
accommodate small thyroxyl peptides (Tabachnik, Hao and Korcek, 1971).
In contrast, the hormone-binding site of PA has been mapped out in great
detail by X-ray diffraction studies (Blake, Swan et al., 1971; Blake, Geisow
et al., 1974; Blake and Oatley, 1977), and affinity labelling (Cheng, Wilchek
et al., 1977b). The PA tetramer has 2 fold symmetry, and two identical binding
sites occupying a nearly cylindrical channel which penetrates completely
through the molecule. The phenolic hydroxyl group of the bound thyroxine
is located near the centre of the molecule and interacts with water in a hydro-

phylic patch consisting of the hydroxyls of the Ser-117 and Thr-119 pairs of residues. The alanine side chain of thyroxine is positioned near the channel entrance where the carboxyl and amino groups of the hormone are close to Lys-15 and Glu-54, respectively. Despite the obvious symmetry of the two binding sites, the first thyroxine is bound with an affinity (10^8 M^{-1}) which is two orders greater than that of the second (Cheng, Pages et al., 1977a). This strong negative cooperativity explains the earlier belief that PA possessed only a single hormone binding site (Pages et al., 1973; Raz and Goodman, 1969).

The mechanism for the negative cooperativity is still unexplained, but the dimensions of the binding channel and the location of the ligands clearly excludes a steric effect. A negative charge on the hydroxyl of the ligand enhances the negative cooperativity (Cheng, Pages et al., 1977a; Robbins, Cheng et al., 1978a) but an allosteric effects on the protein has not been ruled out.

The hormone-binding site of serum albumin has not yet been investigated in detail, despite the progress which has been made on this protein's structure (Peters, 1975). It is known that albumin possesses one rather strong binding site ($k_{T_4} = 1.3 \times 10^6$ M^{-1}) in addition to an undefined number of secondary sites (Steiner, Roth, Robbins, 1966; Sterling, 1964; Tabachnik, 1967) and that binding is weakened by acetylation (Sterling, Rosen, Tabachnik, 1962; Tabachnik, 1964), iodination (Rabinovitch, 1959) and arylation of the terminal Asp (Tritsch and Tritsch, 1963) of the protein. Fatty acids, other anions and chloride also decrease binding (cf. Robbins and Rall, 1967).

Thermodynamic studies with each of the transport proteins has implicated an hydrophobic component in the binding reactions (Green, Marshall, Pensky and Stanbury, 1972; Nilsson and Peterson, 1971).

Studies with thyroxine analogues have clarified some of the features of the hormone molecule which are responsible for binding to the serum proteins. Some of the more recent data are presented in Table 7. In the case of TBG, all aspects of thyroxine structure are important for binding since no analogue with affinity greater than that of L-T_4 has been found. Four halogen substituents, an intact L-alanine side chain, an unsubstituted phenolic group and a diphenyl ether bridge are all required for maximal affinity. It is of interest that rT_3, according to Snyder et al. (1976a) (but not Hao and Tabachnik, 1971), is bound more strongly than T_3, and that desamino analogues have very low affinity. The binding to PA and albumin are less stringent, and show enhanced binding of the desamino analogues. However, these two proteins have not been as completely studied.

The foregoing description of the transport proteins pertains to human blood. There is, however, a considerable body of data concerning species variations (Robbins and Rall, 1960; Rall et al., 1964; Refetoff, Robin and

Table 7

Relative affinities of some thyroxine analogues for thyroid hormone transport proteins. The data are from the following studies done at pH 7·4: TBG: Snyder *et al.*, 1976a, except those in parenthesis which are from Hao and Tabachnik, 1971; PA: Cheng, *et al.*, 1977a; ALB: Tabachnik and Giorgio, 1964.

Analogue	TBG	PA(k_1)	ALB
Thyroxine	100	100	100
Ring substitutions			
T_3	9	8	55
rT_3	38 ($<$0·1)		100
3,3'-T_2	1·3		
3',5'-T_2	0·07		100
3'-isopropyl-T_3	3·5		
3,5,3',5'-methyl-T_4	0		
Side chain substitutions			
D-T_4	54		
N-acetyl-T_4	(77)	12	
T_4-propionic acid	3·6	160	135
T_4-acetic acid	1·7 (38)	160	110
T_3-acetic acid	0·3		
Phenol substitutions			
4'-methyl-T_3	3·5		
4'-deoxy-T_3	1·9		
Ether bridge substitutions			
Sulphur bridge T_4	63		
Methylene bridge T_4	35		

Fang, 1970; Tanake, Ishii and Tamaki, 1969). All vertebrates exhibit some form of thyroxine binding in serum, but the affinity is generally less in the lower vertebrates. Only the higher mammals appear to have a protein analogous to human TBG. Despite some evidence to the contrary (e.g. Davis, Spaulding and Gregerman, 1970; Gordon and Coutsoftidies, 1969), recent studies have indicated that some commonly used laboratory animals such as the rat and the rabbit (Sutherland and Brandon, 1976) lack a high affinity, low capacity transport protein which could, by these criteria, be equated to TBG. On the other hand, rat serum contains a prealbumin, which has recently been isolated and characterised (Navab, Mallia, Kanda and Goodman, 1977a). It not only binds thyroxine but also interacts with the retinol transport system, as in man, and has structural and amino acid similarity to human PA. Similarly, bovine and canine prealbumin have been isolated recently (Fex and Lindgren, 1977; Fex, Laurell and Thulin, 1977). Thus, the earlier failure to find prealbumin in many species (Farer, Robbins, Blumberg and Rall, 1962) appears due to its co-migration with serum albumin in electrophoresis. Of special interest is the variation in primate prealbumins which is discussed in the section on genetic disorders. Recently, it has been shown that TBG (Glinoer, Gershengorn and Robbins, 1976) and presumably PA (Navab, Smith and Goodman, 1977b) are synthesised in the liver. As will be discussed later, alteration in the rates of synthesis are responsible for many of the abnormalities seen with the circulating thyroid hormone.

2. Physiological Role of Thyroid Hormone-Protein Interactions

Unlike other transport proteins, such as low density lipoproteins (Brown and Goldstein, 1976; Gwynn, Mahafee, Brewer and Ney, 1976) and retinol-binding protein (Heller, 1975; Rask and Peterson, 1976) which interact with the plasma membrane of specific target cells in order to transfer the ligand into the cell, there is no evidence that the thyroxine-binding proteins perform other than a passive role in the transfer of the thyroid hormones (Robbins and Rall, 1960 and 1967; Ingbar and Freinkel, 1960; Oppenheimer, 1968). Nonetheless, the thyroid hormone transport system has an important influence on the distribution of the hormones in body fluids and tissues. In general, it appears to function in such a way as to limit cellular access to the large pool of circulating hormone. This has several implications: the transport proteins modulate fluctuations in hormone availability which might result from changes in hormone secretion, they tend to minimise the need for rapid hormone synthesis, and they may protect sensitive tissues from excessive hormone effects. In the case of TBG and albumin, the proteins may be totally absent, as in the congenital anomalies described later, without altering the health of the affected individual; yet a state of complete absence of all transport proteins has never been described.

TBG and PA are found in lymph and other extravascular fluids (cf. Robbins and Rall, 1960, 1967) where the higher protein-bound iodine to total protein ratio compared with serum suggests that TBG and PA are preferentially concentrated. Even the cerebrospinal fluid contains thyroxine transport proteins, especially PA, but at very low levels (Alpers and Rall, 1955; Robbins and Rall, 1957; Siersbaek-Nielsen and Molholm Hansen, 1971; Hagen and Elliott, 1973). Kinetic evidence, however, shows clearly that a barrier to TBG diffusion exists at the capillary wall (Irvine and Simpson-Morgan, 1974). The liver is a special case, since its capillary bed does not restrict entry of plasma proteins, but neither hepatocyte cytosol nor that of other tissues contains serum transport protein in appreciable amounts

(Spaulding and Davis, 1971; Sterling *et al.*, 1974; Hamada *et al.*, 1970a; Davis *et al.*, 1974). The kidney also has a large extravascular triiodothyronine space (Cavalieri, Moser, Martin *et al.*, 1975b).

A comparison of the metabolic disposal rates of the thyroid hormones and their transport proteins (Table 8) indicates that the hormones, T_3 in particular, disappear from blood more rapidly than would be the case if the hormone–protein complex disappeared as a unit. In the liver and kidney, there is an even faster flux of T_4 and T_3 (Table 9) and it is evident that unmetabolised hormone returns from these organs to blood. Since all the

Table 8

Disappearance rate of thyroid hormones and binding proteins and theoretical disappearance rates of hormone–protein complexes.

Fraction per day[a]		nmol/day[a]			
T_4	0·10	T_4	112		
T_3	0·57			T_3	36
TBG	0·13	T_4-TBG	62	T_3-TBG	0·58
PA	0·36	T_4-PA	28	T_3-PA	1·2
ALB	0·054	T_4-ALB	7·6	T_3-ALB	0·23

[a] Disappearance rates are from the following references: T_4 and T_3: Rall, Robbins and Lewallen, 1964, p. 159; Oppenheimer and Surks, 1974, p. 197. TBG: Cavalieri, 1975; Refetoff, Fang, Marshall and Robin, 1976, PA: Oppenheimer, Surks, Bernstein and Smith, 1965. ALB: Becken, Volwiler, Goldworth *et al.*, 1962.

[b] Absolute disppearance rates for T_4 and T_3 are from the above references. For the proteins, the calculations used an assumed distribution volume of 7 l, the concentrations of TBG, PA and ALB in Table 11, and the theoretical distribution of T_4 and T_3 among the proteins as listed in Table 18. The hormone–protein complexes were assumed to disappear from the plasma at the same rate as the uncomplexed protein. For example: T_4-TBG concentration (nmol/l) × TBG clearance (l/day) = T_4-TBG disappearance rate (mol/hr).

Table 9

Acute thyroid hormone clearance. Clearance rates are from Cavalieri and Searle, 1966 (liver T_4); Cavalieri, Steinberg and Searle, 1970 (liver T_3) and Cavalieri, 1975b (kidney T_3). To calculate the fraction of free hormone cleared/min, the following values were used: hepatic blood flow, 1500 ml/min; renal blood flow, 1200 ml/min; plasma free T_4, 2 ng/dl (25·7 pmol/l); plasma free T_3, 0·4 ng/dl (6·1 pmol/l); hematocrit 45%.

	Liver T_4	Liver T_3	Kidney T_3
ml plasma/min	48	231	11
µg hormone/min	3·8	0·25	0·012
Fraction free hormone/min	230	75	5

evidence indicates that only free hormone enters the cells, one can calculate that the free thyroxine pool in the capillary circulation turns over 8 times/min in peripheral tissues in general (Robbins, 1975) and 230 times/min in the liver (Table 9). The dissociation rates of T_4 from TBG and PA (Hillier, 1971, 1975a) are much faster than required to meet this need (Table 10). If the ratio T_4-TBG to T_4-PA is 68 to 11, then the replenishment rate of the free T_4 pool

Table 10

Hormone–protein dissociation rates (37°). T_4: adapted from Hillier (1971) using TBG:PA = 68:11; T_3: adapted from Hillier (1975b) using TBG:PA = 38:27.

	T_4		T_3	
	TBG	PA	TBG	PA
$t_{\frac{1}{2}}$ (sec)	39	7·4	4·2	~ 1[a]
Hormone equivalents (ng/sec)	95	81	8·1	24
Free hormone renewal (times/sec)	35	30	15	45

[a] Too fast to measure accurately.

from either carrier is about 30 times/sec. In the case of T_3 the dissociation rate is still faster, and the entire serum T_3 pool dissociates once every 3 sec (Hillier, 1975b). Therefore, the fractional turnover of T_3 in both liver and kidney of 75 and 5 times/min, respectively, are easily accommodated. Consequently, the binding proteins appear capable of maintaining the free hormone at a relatively constant level. It is of interest that PA appears to contribute at least as much as TBG to the hormone flux. Albumin, and even minor building proteins, could also participate to a greater extent than their affinity for the hormone and their concentration in blood might suggest.

Several lines of evidence indicate that the concentration of free hormone in blood plays a central role in hormone availability and in the maintenance of a euthyroid state (Robbins and Rall, 1957, 1960, 1967). Of particular importance is the finding of a normal free hormone level and a normal hormone disposal rate (μg/day) in euthyroid subjects with altered transport protein concentrations (see below). Hepatic thyroxine clearance (Cavalieri and Searle, 1966; Oppenheimer, Bernstein and Hasen, 1967), hepatic T_3 clearance (Cavalieri, Steinberg and Searle, 1970) and renal T_3 clearance (Cavalieri, Moser, Martin et al., 1975b) have also been shown to vary directly with the free hormone level. Inasmuch as the dissociation rate of the hormone is so much faster than its disappearance rate it is likely that equilibrium between free and bound hormone exists in blood and in extravascular fluids. *In vitro* studies have shown that binding is freely reversible. The mass law equation governing such an interaction can be written as:

$$(T) = \frac{(TP_i)}{k_i(P_i)} = \frac{\sum(TP_i)}{\sum k_i(P_i)} \tag{1}$$

where $(\ ) =$ molar concentration; $k =$ intrinsic association constant; $P =$ unoccupied binding sites; $TP =$ occupied binding sites, or bound T_4 or T_3; $T =$ free hormone; subscript $i =$ any class of binding site.

If $T^t =$ total hormone:

$$\sum(TP_i) = (T^t) - (T) \tag{2}$$

and

$$(T) = \frac{(T^t)}{\sum k_i(P_i) + 1}. \tag{3}$$

It can be seen that the free hormone concentration at equilibrium is a direct function of the total hormone concentration and an inverse function of the sum of the products of the association constant and concentration of unoccupied binding sites of each type.

If the disposal rate of serum thyroxine or triiodothyronine is proportional to the concentration of free hormone, and since hormone disposal follows first order kinetics after the initial mixing period:

$$T_{dis} = KV(T) \tag{4}$$

where $T_{dis} =$ quantity of hormone disposed of per unit time (mol/time); $K =$ proportionality constant or fractional disposal rate of the hormone pool (time^{-1}); $V =$ volume of distribution of free hormone (l).

Since the experimentally determined *fractional* rate is related to the total rather than the free hormone pool:

$$\frac{T_{dis}}{V^t(T^t)} = \frac{KV(T)}{V^t(T^t)} = \frac{KV}{V^t} \cdot \frac{1}{\sum k_i(P_i) + 1} \tag{5}$$

where $V^t =$ volume of distribution of total hormone. Unlike the *absolute* disposal rate, this fractional rate can evidently vary independently of (T).

In addition to the role of the free hormone concentration, other factors clearly have an influence on hormone disposal. For example, variations in intracellular metabolic processes can be independent of the free hormone level (Oppenheimer and Surks, 1974) and would, therefore, change the value of K in equations (4) and (5). It has been shown that the metabolism of T_3 is influenced by the amount of T_4 present in the organism, since this will affect binding of T_3 to intracellular as well as extracellular hormone binding sites (Woeber, Hecker and Ingbar, 1970).

An intriguing feature of prealbumin is its interaction with the retinol transport protein (RBP). Although there appear to be four equivalent sites for RBP on PA (Robbins, Cheng, Gershengorn et al., 1978a), the concentrations in the serum are such that the circulating complex consists of one RBP molecule attached to the PA tetramer, with each protein carrying a single molecule of retinol or thyroxine, respectively. The physiological role of this hormone–vitamin complex is obscure, although it is known that the protein–protein complex retards the renal clearance of the smaller retinol-binding protein (mw 21,000) (Goodman, 1976). Whereas binding of thyroxine to PA is unaffected by the complex and does not alter the protein–protein interaction (van Jaarsveld et al., 1973a, b), retinol affinity and the protein–protein interaction are mutually enhancing (Raz et al., 1970; Horwitz and Heller, 1974; Peterson, 1971; Peterson and Rask, 1971).

Another remarkable feature of prealbumin is the finding that its surface contains two depressions which are complementary to double-helical DNA, and which has led Blake and Oatley (1977) to postulate that PA may be a model for a hormone receptor protein. Up to the present time, no direct evidence exists for such a function.

3. Theoretical Scheme for Free and Bound Hormone in Serum

In the preceding section we presented the general mass law equation for the reversible interaction of thyroid hormone with multiple hormone binding sites and related this to the role of free or unbound hormone in thyroid physiology. Here we extend these equations to a consideration of hormone distribution among each of the binding sites and develop equations which can be applied to specific questions of hormone distribution in health and disease and to certain of the methods which will be discussed later.

Theoretical treatments of this kind have been presented previously by ourselves (Robbins and Rall, 1960, 1967) and by others (Oppenheimer and Surks, 1974). In particular, several recent publications have expanded the scope and utility of these analyses by the use of computer techniques (Brown-Grant, Brennan and Yates, 1970; Di Stefano and Chang, 1971; Wosilait, 1977; Prince and Ramsden, 1977). This has permitted the evaluation of the more complicated system which actually exists in serum, i.e. multiple binding sites on individual proteins, and multiple hormone forms competing for the same binding sites with different affinities. The results have shown that almost all of the thyroxine carried by PA is bound to only one of the two sites on this protein, whereas in the case of albumin, the strong and the weaker sites bind thyroxine in the ratio of 3 or 7 to 1 (Wosilait, 1977; Prince and Ramsden, 1977). They have also shown that variations in one of the hormones can have significant effects on the distribution and unbound level of the other (Di Stefano and Chang, 1971; Prince and Ramsden, 1977).

In contrast to the treatment described by others, we have employed a general solution which can include all known elements of the hormone–protein interactions. The equations and computer analysis have been developed by Dr. Michael L. Johnson (unpublished). The free concentrations T_4 and T_3 were determined by finding a simultaneous root of two equations; i.e. values of free T_4 and free T_3 which satisfy both equations. These two equations express the total concentrations of both hormones in terms of the free concentrations and the amount of hormone bound to each class of bonding sites. Using the same notation as in equation (1) and subscripts 4 and 3 for thyroxine and triiodothyronine, respectively,

$$(T_4^t) = (T_4) + \sum(T_4 P_i) \tag{6}$$

$$(T_3^t) = (T_3) + \sum(T_3 P_i) \tag{7}$$

If k_{T_4} and k_{T_3} are the respective site affinities for T_4 and T_3 the amount of hormone bound per class of site is expressed as,

$$(T_4 P_i) = (P_i^t) \left[\frac{k_{T_4}(T_4)}{1 + k_{T_3}(T_3) + k_{T_4}(T_4)} \right] \tag{8}$$

where $k_{T_4}(T_4)/[1 + k_{T_3}(T_3) + k_{T_4}(T_4)]$ is the fraction of sites, of a given class, which are occupied by T_4; and the concentration of sites of each class is (P_i^t). The amount of T_3 bound to each class of site is similarly expressed. The mathematical procedure used to find this simultaneous root is the Marquardt-Levenberg minimisation procedure as implemented in MLAB, a modelling programme developed at NIH.

For PA, we have employed the 2-site model, which is mathematically equivalent to the interacting-site model (Ferguson et al., 1975). For albumin, we have arbitrarily used $n = 5$ for the second class of sites. Any value of n could be used, so long as nk remains constant.

We have excluded the minor binding proteins, such as the lipoproteins (Hoch and Lewallen, 1974); their very low affinity for the hormones justify the prediction that they would have an insignificant effect on hormone distribution among the major binding proteins or on free hormone levels. We have also excluded thyroid hormone metabolites, which would be expected to occupy a small proportion of the hormone binding sites. The most important of these is 3,3′,5′-triiodothyronine, which has a serum concentration of about 0·5 nmol/l (Chopra, 1976; Gavin et al., 1977; Kaplan et al., 1977), an affinity constant for TBG of about $4 \times 10^9 \text{ M}^{-1}$ (Snyder et al., 1976a), and an affinity for albumin equal to that of T_4 (Tabachnik and Giorgio, 1964). Since there are no data on its affinity for PA, and since its influence on the T_4 and T_3 interactions would be small because of its low concentration, this exclusion seems justifiable.

In further contrast to other analyses, we have used binding parameters approaching as closely as possible the physiological conditions of temperature, pH and chloride concentration. These are given in Table 11, together

Table 11

Parameters for iodothyronine-serum protein interaction at 37° in PO_4-buffered 0·1 M NaCl, pH 7·4.

Protein	Parameter	Value[a]	References
TBG	P^t	0·27 µmol/l (1·5 mg/dl)	Gershengorn, Larsen and Robbins (1976)
	$k - T_4$	$1·0 \times 10^{10} \text{ M}^{-1}$ (0·06 M PO_4)	Korcek and Tabachnik (1976)
	$k - T_3$	$4·6 \times 10^8 \text{ M}^{-1}$ (0·06 M PO_4)	Korcek and Tabachnik (1976)
PA	P^t	4·6 µmol/l (25 mg/dl)	Smith and Goodman (1971
	$k_1 - T_4$	$7·0 \times 10^7 \text{ M}^{-1}$	Ferguson et al. (1973)
	$k_2 - T_4$	$6·7 \times 10^5 \text{ M}^{-1}$	Ferguson et al. (1973)
	$k_1 - T_3$	$1·4 \times 10^7 \text{ M}^{-1}$	Cheng et al. (1977a)
	$k_2 - T_3$	$5·5 \times 10^5 \text{ M}^{-1}$	Cheng et al. (1977a)
ALB	P^t	640 µmol/l (4·2 g/dl)	Peters (1975)
	$k_1 - T_4$	$7·0 \times 10^5 \text{ M}^{-1}$	Tabachnik (1967)
	$k_{2-6} - T_4$	$4·8 \times 10^4 \text{ M}^{-1}$	Tabachnik (1967)
	$k_1 - T_3$	$1·0 \times 10^5 \text{ M}^{-1}$	50 % of value by Steiner et al. (1966)
	$k_{2-6} - T_3$	$6·9 \times 10^3 \text{ M}^{-1}$	Estimated

[a] P^t is the concentration in normal serum by direct protein measurement; k-T_4, k-T_3 for TBG and PA are calculated values at 37°, using $k^{25°}$ from Table 6 and $k^{35°}/k^{25°} = 0.7$. The latter value measured for TBG by Green et al. (1972) was 0·60, for TBG by Korcek and Tabachnik (1976) was 0·74, and for PA by Nilsson and Peterson (1971) was 0·71. In the case of albumin, Tabachnik (1967) found k_1-T_4 at 37° was very close to that obtained by Steiner et al. (1966) at 25° but was reduced 50% by 0·1 M Cl^-.

with the normal levels of the hormones and the transport proteins used as the basis of our computations. As indicated in the table, significant temperature effects on binding to TBG and PA, and an important effect of chloride on binding to albumin, have been described. It is evident, therefore, that the distribution of the hormones in vivo will be significantly different from that in various test systems that have been used. These influences will be discussed in later sections, and also come up for consideration in the effects of physiological and pathological changes on hormone levels. It is of interest that the parameters we have adopted for T_4 binding agree within a factor of two with those experimentally determined by Sutherland and Simpson-Morgan (1975) on a small number of normal human sera by an equilibrium method at physiological pH, Cl^- and temperature.

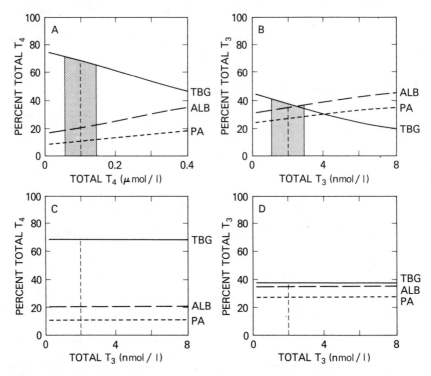

Fig. 3. Theoretical distribution of T_4 and T_3 among the transport proteins as a function of total hormone concentration. The vertical dashed line indicates the mean normal hormone concentration, and the stippled area is the normal range. A and B—total T_4 and T_3 varied with a constant mol ratio of 50; C and D—total T_4 was constant at 0·1 μmol/l while total T_3 varied.

Some results of these computations are presented in Figs 3–5. The theoretical distribution of the hormones among the transport proteins as a function of total hormone, when T_4 and T_3 vary in parallel at a fixed mole ratio of 50, is shown in Figs 3A and B. The range of hormone concentrations varies from below normal to four times the mean normal value. It is apparent that an increasing hormone level, even over the normal range, results in a decreasing fraction of both T_4 and T_3 bound to TBG, which is present in limiting amounts. As expected, both PA and albumin bind more hormone as the levels increase. The calculations in Figs 3C and D, however, show that a change in concentration of T_3, while T_4 remains constant at the mean normal level, has virtually no effect on the distribution of either hormone.

The effects of varying protein concentration on the distribution of hormones is shown in Fig. 4. As expected, variations in TBG have a considerable

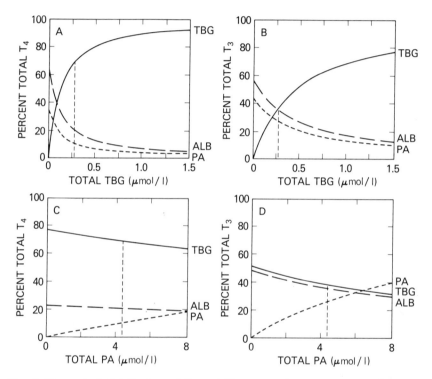

Fig. 4. Theoretical distribution of T_4 and T_3 among the transport proteins as a function of TBG or PA concentration. In all computations, free T_4 and free T_3 were maintained constant at the mean normal concentration. The vertical dashed line indicates the mean normal TBG or PA concentration.

influence on the fraction of hormone bound by PA and albumin, whereas variations in PA have a relatively small effect.

Figure 5 shows the effects of variations in total hormone concentration, over a pathophysiologically relevant range, on the free hormone levels. It can be seen that variation in total T_4 has a significant effect on free T_3 (Fig. 5B) but variation in total T_3 has almost no effect on free T_4 (Fig. 5D). Whereas the relation between free hormone and total T_4 is non-linear, that of free T_3 and total T_3 is linear. Thus, the effect of a 3 fold increase of total T_4 above normal is to increase free T_4 4·6 fold while T_3 increases 2·7 fold (Figs 5A and B). When both total T_3 and total T_4 vary at a constant ratio (Fig. 5C), the absolute increase in free T_3 is much less than the absolute increase in free T_4, but the relative increase in free T_3 is almost as great as

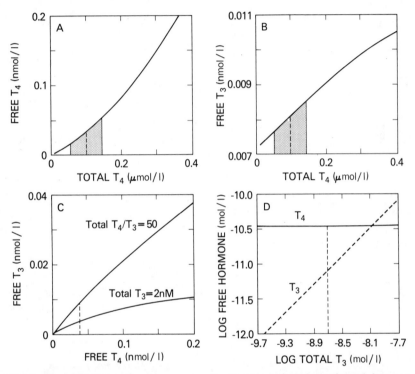

Fig. 5. Theoretical free hormone concentration as a function of total hormone concentration. In all of these computations, TBG, PA, and ALB were constant at their "normal" concentration (Table 11). The vertical dashed line indicates the mean normal hormone level, and the stippled area is the normal range. A and B—total T_3 was constant at 2 nmol/l while total T_4 varied; C—total T_3 was constant while total T_4 varied (lower curve) or both total T_4 and total T_3 varied with a constant mole ratio; D—total T_4 was constant at 0·1 μmol/l while total T_3 varied.

that of T_4. This was also seen by Prince and Ramsden (1977) and is probably more relevant to the hormone's action.

It is of interest to note that in the work of Sutherland and Simpson-Morgan (1975), the relation of the free fraction of T_4 to total T_4 was used to compute the binding constants and the concentrations of the transport proteins in serum.

D. METHODS OF DETERMINATION

This section is arranged in a somewhat arbitrary manner in order to permit a more or less systematic discussion of the various methods used to characterise and to quantitate the iodine compounds of blood. Many of the techniques are complementary, and are used in combination. Thus, the measurement of total blood thyroxine may include extraction and/or chromatography to separate the hormone from other iodocompounds and proteins, and either iodimetry or one of the "displacement" methods to quantitate it. For clinical measurement of thyroid hormones, however, many of the modern procedures have been simplified by the use of radioimmunoassay with highly specific antisera. The literature, both old and recent, contains such a wealth of methods that a thorough treatment is impractical. The discussion which follows is intended to be a guide rather than an exhaustive review and is necessarily selective.

1. Iodimetry and Activation Methods

In mammals only the thyroid hormones and their metabolites contain iodine and for many years estimation of organic iodine in blood was almost the only way to measure the level of circulating thyroid hormone. Recently more specific ways to measure the levels of T_4, T_3 and their metabolites in blood have become available which are specific, sensitive, and precise (see below). In the last six volumes of a major journal for clinical analyses not one article has appeared on iodine analysis. Nonetheless, this procedure may still be of value. The absolute iodine uptake by the thyroid, for example, requires an analysis of the iodine content of urine; urine iodine analyses are required to estimate the dietary level of iodine; occasionally iodine analyses of food, iodoproteins, thyroid tissue, etc., may be required. Hence, several methods will be briefly described and the reader is referred to the previous edition of this volume, to Foss, Hankes and Van Slyke, (1960) and to Smith (1964) for details.

There are, in general, two aspects to iodine analysis. The first involves the method whereby organic material in the sample is destroyed. The second part is the measurement of iodine itself. There are two main digestion procedures: in one, strong alkali (K_2CO_3 or KOH) and digestion at high temperature is used (Barker, Humphrey and Soley, 1951; Vilkki, 1958; Stolc, 1966). Another method is wet digestion using chloric and perchloric acids (Zak, Willard, Myers and Boyle, 1952; Schahrokh, 1954; Spitzy and Muller, 1966). Both methods are satisfactory although perchloric acid is potentially explosive and may volatilise and be deposited in the fume hood. At least one serious accident has occurred due to an explosion from this cause.

It is possible to avoid digestion althogether if thyroxine is extracted from blood by an organic solvent (n-butanol, isoamyl alcohol) because under appropriate conditions thyroxine itself catalyses the cerate–arsenite reaction (Masen, 1967; Passen and von Saleski, 1969; Kessler and Pilegi, 1970). Usually chlorine or bromine is required to destroy unidentified materials which inhibit the cerate–arsenite reaction. Bromine in strong sulphuric acid seems well suited when utilised on column eluates which contain thyroxine (Kessler and Pillegi, 1970). In that study thyroxine was more than 90 % as active as iodide in accelerating the cerate–arsenite reaction.

Chemical iodimetry is usually done utilising the catalytic effect of I^- on the reduction of ceric ion by arsenious acid (Sandell and Kolthoff, 1937; Barker, 1962). This reaction is modified by many anions and metals, and conditions must be strictly controlled to obtain reproducible results (Smith, 1964). Usually the reaction is monitored by measurement in a spectrophotometer of the rate of disappearance of the yellow $ceric^{4+}$ ion. Automated systems for analysis of iodine in blood have been described (Benotti and Benotti, 1963; Welshman, Bell and McKee, 1966).

Qualitative or semiquantitative analyses for iodine are a convenient method for locating iodoamino acids on paper or on thin layer plates. Since iodotyrosines and iodothyronines also catalyse the ceric arsenate reaction, it can be used on chromatograms to identify iodoamino acids (Bowden, Maclagan and Wilkinson, 1955; Barker, 1964). Also, the ferriferrocyanide–arsenite reaction is quite sensitive (Gmelin and Virtanen, 1959; Postmes, 1964). Both of these have been adapted for quantitative use on paper but this now seens largely unnecessary.

Iodine may also be determined with great sensitivity by activation analysis. This method consists of irradiating an unknown amount of ^{127}I with neutrons to produce a different isotope which is radioactive. Measurement of the radioactivity can be done with great sensitivity. In general, the $^{127}I(n,r) \rightarrow$ ^{128}I reaction is used which requires a high flux of thermal neutrons. Usually, it is necessary to purify the sample before irradiation to remove elements which may show induced radioactivity and post-irradiation purification may also be necessary. The energy spectrum of the radioactivity produced is analysed as is the half life of the radioactivity, for obtaining greater specificity. Although activation analysis has been used to measure the iodine content of blood it is somewhat tedious and has been superseded by other methods (Dimitriadou, Fraser and Turner, 1966). Nonetheless, for accurate measurements of small quantities of iodine it may be useful (Bowden *et al.*, 1955; Smith, Mozley and Wagner, 1964). Another but quite different method of iodine analysis employs ^{129}I. This is a very weakly radioactive isotope (half life 1.6×10^7 years) so that relatively large amounts of it may be safely administered to humans. Its utility arises from the fact that it may be assayed with a high degree of sensitivity by activation analysis. This is made possible because of its high thermal neutron cross-section area (31 barns) and a fairly distinctive product, ^{130}I, with a half life of 12.5 hr (Edwards, Rhodes and Wagner, 1966). This method of analysis has not been generally used, probably because of its tedious nature.

An important recent development in measurement of iodine uses ^{241} Americium to generate monochromatic γ-rays. These are specifically absorbed by ^{127}I which then emits a characteristic 28.5 keV X-ray. These can be readily detected. Suitably standardised, this technique permits the *in vivo* measurement of the total amount of iodine in the thyroid (Hofer and Gottschalk, 1971), and can be done with relatively little radiation exposure and with reasonable accuracy. In addition to the physiological importance of knowing the amount of iodine in the thyroid, it has also been reported that this quantity has diagnostic significance particularly for differentiating benign from malignant tumors (Patton, Hollifield, Brill, Lee and Patton, 1976).

2. Methods Employing Radioiodine and Iodine Analysis

Strictly speaking, only labelling to equilibrium with a radioactive isotope of iodine of known specific activity will permit the use of a radioisotope for measurement of the quantity of endogenously synthesised materials such as thyroid hormones or their metabolites. This method is reasonably satisfactory in experimental animals, although the time required for equilibrium may be long (Van Middlesworth, 1956; Pitt-Rivers and Rall, 1961). It cannot be used in humans because of the large amounts of radiation necessary. Furthermore, except for special analyses it is rarely used even in experimental animals nowadays since radioimmunoassay techniques of high sensitivity and specificity have been developed.

Measurement of the absolute amount of iodine taken up by the human thyroid, however, still requires the use of a radioisotope of iodine. This is because of the lack of a precise means of measuring the 5 μg/1 (0.04 μmol/l) of iodine in human blood. The test depends on the facts that in an hour or less after its ingestion iodide is evenly distributed in body fluids and that no iodinated organic compounds are returned to the blood before 6–12 hr. Furthermore, iodide is concentrated in the urine ranging from 50–150 μg/1

$(0.4–1.2\ \mu mol/l)$ in England to $300\ \mu g/l$ $(2.4\ \mu mol/l)$ or more in the USA. With less protein and very little organic iodine to complicate the analysis, measurement of urinary iodine is rapid and accurate (see above for method of iodine analysis). Between 1 and 4 hr the following relationship holds:

$$\frac{I_u^*}{I_u} = \frac{I_b^*}{I_b}$$

where u and b refer to urine and blood, and * refers to amount of radioactivity. Knowing the mean concentration of iodide in the blood during a time period when the uptake of radioiodine is measured, the absolute uptake of iodine (AIU) can be calculated. Extensive investigations of this measure of thyroid function have been reported from England, Greece and the USA (Wayne, Koutras and Alexander, 1964). This parameter of thyroid function is clearly physiologically and diagnostically important.

Another interesting technique for study of thyroid hormone secretion employs two isotopes of iodine. Usually a single injection of ^{125}I is used to label the thyroid. After a week or 10 days, when the labelled thyroid hormone levels in blood are relatively constant, a single injection of ^{131}I thyroxine is administered. A day or so later, when thyroxine is evenly distributed one can measure the ratios of $^{125}I/^{131}I$ in blood and urine. These can be utilised to calculate non-thyroxine leaks from the thyroid, variations in hormone secretion and intrathyroidal cycling of iodine (Wartofsky and Ingbar, 1971; Nicoloff, 1976). A large non-thyroxine leak of iodine from the thyroid of thyrotoxic patients has been found and a diurnal variation in the rate of thyroxine secretion noted.

The choice of isotope for these various procedures depends on whether γ-radiation is required and the length of study. Particularly in humans it is important to keep the radiation dose to a minimum. Table 12 lists several available isotopes. Although ^{131}I is convenient for many studies, it emits strong γ- and β-rays, and for some work has too long a half life. Recently, ^{123}I has become more generally available and for procedures such as the

Table 12

Radioisotopes useful in the diagnosis of thyroid disease.

Isotope	Half life	γ- or X-rays	β-rays	Availability
^{125}I	60 day	Weak	No	Readily
^{131}I	8·05 day	Yes	Yes	Readily
^{132}I	2·3 hr	Yes	Yes	Special order
^{99m}Tc	6·0 hr	Weak	No	Readily
^{123}I	13 hr	Weak	No	Special order

AIU it is particularly well-suited, giving a low radiation dose. Since ^{123}I emits only a weak X-ray, certain precautions are required for its accurate measurement in the thyroid (Martin and Rollo, 1977). ^{132}I is also satisfactory for measurement of the AIU but it is not now readily available. For long term studies, ^{125}I is particularly satisfactory. If one desires only to measure the early uptake of iodine or to image the thyroid, ^{99m}Tc is satisfactory. Pertechnetate is a monovalent anion which is concentrated by the thyroid quantitatively very much like iodide. It is not substituted on tyrosine residues, however.

3. Iodoamino Acids

(a) Extraction

Formerly, solvent extraction was the main method for characterising and isolating the iodoamino acids (cf. Radichevich and Volpert, 1966). Although supplanted by chromatographic and, more recently, displacement methods, they still have a place in the preparation of blood or tissue for chromatography, and are also used in some of the current displacement assays.

The classical method follows closely the original procedures of Leland and Foster (1932) and Blau (1933). Extraction of serum with water-saturated butanol at pH 2–4 recovers most of the iodothyronines, about 50% of iodotyrosines and about 80% of iodide (Robbins et al., 1952; Ingbar, Freinkel, Hoeprich and Athens, 1954). Back extraction of the butanol phase with 2 M sodium hydroxide (Leland and Foster, 1932) or 4 M sodium hydroxide–5% sodium carbonate (Blau, 1933) removes iodotyrosines and iodide. Iodoproteins are mainly, but not entirely, insoluble in butanol (Robbins, Rall and Rawson, 1955). A reducing substance (e.g. bisulphite) guards against the formation of I_2 with consequent iodine exchange, iodination (Acland, 1952) and oxidative degradation; however, butyl esters of the iodothyronines may form on storage (Maclagen, Bowden and Wilkinson, 1957; Bellabarba and Sterling, 1969). Extraction is often done after preliminary precipitation of the organic iodine (Tong et al., 1952; Block et al., 1958).

Other solvents, such as ethanol, methanol, or acetone (Trevorrow, 1959; Werner et al., 1957; Maclagen et al., 1957), are also effective and have the advantage of being more easily evaporated. Ethanol, as used in many of the current displacement assays for T_4 (see below), gives a recovery of 70–80% (Murphy, Pattee and Gold, 1966; Ekins, Williams and Ellis, 1969; Larsen, Atkinson, Wellman et al., 1970), but this can be increased to 95% by extraction at 60° and alkaline pH (Watson and Lees, 1973). A combination of solvents can increase the specificity of the extraction and separate thyroxine from organic iodine contaminants in blood. Thus, hexane (West, Chavre and

Wolfe, 1966) or chloroform (Robbins, 1956) decreases the solubility of thyroxine in the organic phase after initial extraction, so that it can be transferred to an aqueous phase. In preparing extracts of serum for paper or thin layer chromatography, the quantity which can be applied is sharply limited by the extracted lipids. These can be removed by similar highly non-polar solvents (Flock and Bollman, 1955; Werner et al., 1957; Block et al., 1958; Maclagen et al., 1957).

(b) Chromatography

Chromatography is the most effective tool for the separation and identi-fication of closely related iodocompounds in blood. It was first used for this purpose by Laidlaw (1949), and soon afterward by Taurog, Chaikoff and Tong (1950). Since that time a great variety of procedures have been applied. The supporting medium may be inert, providing for true partition chromato-graphy, or may act as an adsorbant or an ion exchanger. Usually its proper-ties are not purely one or the other of these. Owing to their low solubility in water the iodothyronines are strongly adsorbed to such supports as cellulose, dextran gel, and ion exchange resins and often behave in a non-ideal manner.

(1) *Preparation of the specimen.* Since the thyroid hormones can be extracted from the serum proteins by organic solvents, it is possible to carry out partition chromatography with untreated serum as the sample. Aside from convenience and the possible avoidance of artifacts introduced during extraction and concentration, this has the advantage of displaying all of the serum iodocompounds on a single chromatogram. Thus the iodoproteins, which might otherwise escape detection, can be found at the chromatogram origin (Tong et al., 1952; Robbins, 1954). Migration of the iodoamino acids is not hindered if a small sample of serum is applied.

For paper or thin layer chromatography of unlabelled or trace-labelled serum, it is usually necessary to process a relatively large volume of serum. An effective method for concentrating the extractable iodocompounds from 20 ml or more of serum, and at the same time separating them from interfering proteins, lipids and salts was described by Block et al. (1958). The use of the butanol extract of a trichloracetic acid precipitate may result in an artifact leading to a double spot for thyroxine (Acland, 1955) which may be overcome by desalting; however, electrolytic desalting causes deiodination (Jepson and Smith, 1956).

(2) *Chromatography on sheets and thin layers.* In view of the enormous literature on paper and thin layer chromatography (tlc) applied to the iodoamino acids, as well as their decreasing utilisation in the analysis of blood, no attempt will be made to catalogue these methods. Information on

techniques and lists of applicable solvent systems can be found in the following reviews: for paper chromatography, Roche, Michel and Lissitzky (1964); Michel (1966); Pitt-Rivers and Schwartz (1967); Wilkinson and Bowden (1960); Gross (1954); Pitt-Rivers and Tata (1959); Bjorksten, Grasbeck and Lamberg (1961); Plaskett (1964); Cahnmann (1972); for tlc, Pataki (1969); Schorn and Winkler (1965); Cahnmann (1972). New solvents for tlc have been described (West, Wayne and Chavre, 1965b; Sorimachi, 1979) permitting separation of many of the thyroid hormone metabolites. Ion exchange papers with organic solvents have also been used (Lowenstein, Greenspan and Spilker, 1963; Sleeman and Diggs, 1964).

Some general rules have been described and discussed by Cahnmann (1972). Acid solvents are generally better for iodotyrosine separations, and alkaline solvents for iodothyronines. In acid solvents, the R_f increases with an increasing number of iodine atoms per molecule, whereas in alkaline solvents, the R_f decreases. Descending chromatography can be used to separate slowly moving compounds. One of the more popular solvents to separate iodotyrosines on paper is n-butanol-acetic acid-water (38:5:6), and for iodothyronines, n-butanol-ethanol-0·5 M NH_4OH (5:1:2) or n-butanol-dioxane-2 M NH_4OH (4:1:saturated). With tlc, silica gel plates employing ethyl acetate-methanol-2 M NH_4OH (5:2:3), ethyl acetate-methanol-1 M acetic acid (5:2:3) or n-butanol-0·2 M NH_4OH (saturated) may be used (West et al., 1965b; Sorimachi, 1978). A combination of several solvents, or two-dimensional chromatography, is needed to separate all the iodocompounds occurring in blood.

Both thin layer and paper chromatography may be used for quantitative iodine analyses by methods described above. Since losses during the procedure may be substantial, an internal radioactive standard should be used (West et al., 1965a). A special problem, especially with thyroxine, is that iodoamino acids are subject to rapid deiodination when dried on filter paper or a similar support (Taurog, 1962). This is prevented by avoiding drying of the sample or by adding protective material such as serum protein or propylene glycol. Esterification by the solvent may also occur (cf. Cahnmann, 1972). The need to prewash silica gel to remove iron has also been pointed out (West et al., 1965b).

Carrier compounds are detected by fluorescence quenching in UV light or by colour reactions. For iodoamino acids, ninhydrin or diazotized sulphanilic acid derivatives have been used, the latter having the advantage of reacting only with phenolic amino acids and giving distinguishing colours. The ninhydrin reaction is somewhat more sensitive and can be used before measurement of iodine, whereas the coupling reaction in the diazotized reagent results in loss of iodine. Detection of iodoamino acids by their iodine content is considered in Section D.1. Iodide may be detected by

AgNO$_3$ spray and by the starch–iodine reaction, but PdCl$_2$ is probably more useful. Details on the preparation and use of the sprays have been described (Gross, 1954; Pitt-Rivers and Schwartz, 1967; Cahnmann, 1972).

(3) *Chromatography on columns.* Procedures using columns are of special value for blood because of the greater sample capacity. Early methods used partition chromatography on Kieselguhr (diatomaceous earth) (Gronkvist and Hellberg, 1951; Gross and Pitt-Rivers, 1953a; Braasch, Flock and Albert, 1954; Kennedy, 1958), cellulose powder (Mandl and Block, 1959; Rosenberg, 1951a) or starch (Rosenberg, 1951b; Dobyns and Barry, 1953) with organic solvents similar to those used for paper or thin layer chromatography. In addition, silica gel was used to separate iodohistidines in thyroid hydrolysates (Roche, Lissitzky and Michel, 1952c) and columns of AgCl as a specific adsorbent for iodine in urine (Fletcher, 1957; Cameron, 1960). At present, the common methods employ dextran gels or ion exchange resins.

Dextran gels are mainly employed as adsorbants rather than as filtration systems, and their behaviour is strongly influenced by the ratio of plasma volume to column size and by the solvent. With 3 ml of serum and a 2·5 × 20 cm column of Sephadex G-25 equilibrated with neutral buffer, most of the thyroxine is excluded with the serum proteins (Lissitzky, Bismuth and Rolland, 1962). Iodide is retarded and this separation has been used to measure protein bound iodine (Spitzy and Muller, 1961; Jacobson and Widstrom, 1962). Iodotyrosines are even more retarded than iodide (Lissitzky *et al.*, 1962) and unbound or dissociated thyroxine is retained on the column (Lissitzky *et al.*, 1962; Lee, Henry and Golub, 1964a). If, on the other hand, the serum proteins are first hydrolysed with papain (Lissitzky and Bismuth, 1963) or a preliminary extraction is done (Murphy and Pattee, 1964), the iodothyronines are retained on the dextran, and may then be eluted with an organic solvent. If the dextran gel is first equilibrated with 0·015 M NaOH and 1 ml serum is placed on a 1·5 × 22 cm or smaller column, there is complete separation of iodothyronines from the binding proteins while iodoproteins are excluded (Mougey and Mason, 1963; Makowitz, Muller and Spitzy, 1966). Partial separation of the adsorbed iodotyrosines and iodothyronines may be achieved by elution with aqueous elution systems of varying pH. Sephadex L-H20, which is more stable in organic solvents, has been used with ethyl acetate-methanol-NH$_4$OH as the eluant (Williams, Freeman and Florsheim, 1969). The tendency of dextran gels to adsorb the thyroid hormones has been utilised in competitive binding assays (see below).

Ion exchange columns have been used increasingly in iodoamino acid separations. Strong anion exchange resins, such as Dowex-1, were first employed to separate iodide from labelled protein-bound iodine (Scott and

Reilly, 1954; Dowben, 1960; Fields, Kinnory, Kaplan, Oester and Bowser, 1956). At neutral pH they retain iodide and iodotyrosines (Blanquet, Dunn and Tobias, 1955) but not the protein-bound iodine. At acid pH thyroxine is dissociated from protein and retained on the resin (Ingbar et al., 1957). This became the basis of a procedure (Galton and Pitt-Rivers, 1959) in which all serum iodocompounds other than iodoproteins were adsorbed on Dowex-1 in acetate at pH 5·6 and then eluted sequentially with increasing acidity (monoiodotyrosine at pH 3, diiodotyrosine at pH 2·2, iodothyronines at pH 1·4). Later modifications to permit a larger serum load included prior hydrolysis of the serum (Pitt-Rivers and Sacks, 1962), heating the serum to 59° (Arosenius and Parrow, 1960), or increasing the initial pH (Lewallen, 1963; Hellman, Tschudy, Robbins and Rall, 1963). Elution with a formic acid gradient was also used (Lissitzky and Lasry, 1958; Wynn, Fabrikant and Deiss, 1959). Iodide can be eluted with 3 M NaBr (Galton and Pitt-Rivers, 1959), 1M Na perchlorate (Sacks, 1964) or 0·5 M Na salicylate (Meyniel, Blanquet, Berger, Corizet and Gaillard, 1965).

It is possible to evaluate and predict the function of such columns by partitioning the individual amino acids between resin and solvents (Lewallen, 1963). From these and other data, it is clear that the iodothyronines are more strongly adsorbed than predicted from their ionic character. Although this aids in their separation from iodotyrosines, it introduces certain problems, the most troublesome being the difficulty in separating thyroxine and tri-iodothyronine. Iodothyronines can be eluted with organic solvents (Lissitzky and Lasry, 1958; Meyniel et al., 1965); and combinations of 50% dimethyl-formamide with 0·1 M ammonium acetate at pH 7·4 and pH 5·0 result in the separation of T_3 from T_4 (Cahnmann, 1972; Kologlu, Schwartz and Carter, 1966). Thyroglobulin, but not serum proteins, is retained on these columns.

Strong cation exchange resins such as Dowex 50 were also used in early procedures (Roche, Michel and Nunez, 1958; Blanquet, Meyniel and Savoie, 1960; Lerner, 1963; Reilly, Searle and Scott, 1961; Block and Mandl, 1964). Iodide and proteins are not retained by these columns, and the adsorbed iodoamino acids are eluted with ammonium salts, especially volatile ones such as ammonium acetate or carbonate, at increasing pH. Organic solvents (e.g. ethanol) are again needed for iodothyronine separation. The most recently reported methods (Ogawara, Bilstad and Cahnmann, 1972; Sorimachi and Ui, 1975; Sorimachi, 1979) using Dowex-50 at 50° permit the separation of many of the physiologically important iodothyronines in addition to T_4 and T_3.

Detailed reviews of various column chromatographic systems have been presented (Radichevich and Volpert, 1966; Cahnmann, 1972). For chromato-graphic measurement of blood thyroxine levels, the most common method has used a Dowex-1 column followed by iodimetry. This usually does not separate T_4 from T_3, is only partially successful in separating the hormones from contaminating iodinated compounds, and has largely been supplanted by the more specific displacement and RIA methods.

(4) *Gas–liquid chromatography* (glc) is a powerful method for simultaneously identifying and quantifying the iodoamino acids (Funakoshi and Cahnmann, 1969; Cahnmann, 1972). However, its technical complexity, the need for preliminary partial purification by other methods, and the advent of simpler techniques have led to its disuse in measurements on blood. Several types of volatile derivatives may be employed: N_1O-dipivalylmethyl esters (Jaakonnaki and Stouffer, 1967), tri-methylsilyl derivatives (Alexander and Scheig, 1968; Funakoshi and Cahnmann, 1969), or N_1O-diheptafluoro-butyl methyl ester (Petersen *et al.*, 1976). The more stable methyl esters can be purified after they are formed, whereas the tri-methylsilyl derivatives must be made with purified amino acids. An electron capture detector is required to achieve the sensitivity necessary for analysis of blood. Successful glc analysis of blood iodothyronines has been reported (Stouffer, 1969; Nihei, *et al.*, 1971), and a recent procedure has been applied to the measurement of free thyroxine and triiodothyronine in the dialysate from 1 ml of blood (Petersen *et al.*, 1976, 1977). The latter method can detect 0·2 pg of hormone. This procedure can be useful as a reference method, but is not suitable for routine analysis.

(c) *Electrophoresis*

Electrophoresis has been little used in the separation of iodoamino acids, as opposed to the serum transport proteins and iodoproteins. It has been used, however, to separate iodide with minimal decomposition of iodothyronines, and also to separate desamino analogs of thyroxine (cf. Roche, Michel and Lissitzky, 1964; Michel, 1966; Cahnmann, 1972). Adsorption of iodothyronines to paper in aqueous buffers causes these compounds to be markedly retarded; still, they may move as compact zones due to a process akin to adsorption chromatography (Farer, Robbins and Blumberg, 1962). Their migration can be altered by various substances which compete for binding to the paper (Myant and Osorio, 1960; Bird, 1963). High voltage electrophoresis is particularly useful and separation at acid pH (e.g. 4 N acetic acid) (Arosenius and Parrow, 1964) appears to be better than at alkaline pH (Miyamoto and Kobayoshi, 1961). The common iodoamino acids could be separated in a single dimension. Others have employed two-dimensional procedures, combining electrophoresis and chromatography (cf. Roche *et al.*, 1964; Bjorksten *et al.*, 1961; Lissitzky, Benevent, Roques and Roche, 1959; Alpers and Rall, 1955).

(d) *Displacement assay*

Also known as competitive binding assay, this method was introduced to circumvent the need for iodimetry and its attendant problems (Murphy, 1964). The method is analogous to radioimmunoassay. Its essential features are:

(i) extraction of serum iodothyronine from the proteins in the test serum,

(ii) measurement of the effect of the extract on a system which contains labelled iodothyronine, normal serum and an extrinsic adsorbent for the hormone,

(iii) comparison of the effect of the serum extract with the effect of pure reference compounds.

(Alternatively, the extrinsic adsorbant could be replaced by any method which measures the distribution of the hormone between the bound and the free state.) The specific hormone-binding protein in the normal serum is the analogue of the specific antibody in radioimmunoassay, and the distribution ratio of labelled hormone between specific protein and non-specific adsorbant depends on the total amount of hormone in the system.

The first approach used serum alone, and measured hormone distribution between TBG and albumin (separated by electrophoresis), the latter acting as the non-specific adsorbant (Ekins, 1960). In later modifications, dextran gel (Murphy and Pattee, 1964) or anion exchange resin (Murphy, 1965; Murphy, Pattee and Gold, 1966; Nakajima, Kuramochi, Horiguchi and Kuba, 1966) was the adsorbant. Many variants are commercially available as simple assay kits (Clark, 1975; Horn, 1975). The completeness of extraction of hormone from plasma (see Section (a)) should be determined, and correction applied if required. A simplified method which utilises a Sephadex column for both extraction and competitive binding has been described (Braverman, Vagenakis, Foster and Ingbar, 1971; Seligson and Seligson, 1972). Displacement methods are not foolproof since any material in blood which is extracted with the hormone in high enough quantity and which has an affinity for the thyroxine-binding sites could give a falsely high value. Dilantin is one such substance which is of practical importance but results indicate that it does not interfere (Murphy et al., 1966; Larsen et al., 1970).

When displacement assay is used for thyroxine measurement, triiodothyronine does not interfere since it is present in blood in much smaller amount and has a lower affinity for thyroxine-binding sites. The opposite is true when triiodothyronine is measured (Nauman, Nauman and Werner, 1967; Sterling, Bellabarba, Newman and Brenner, 1969). In that case, the extracted T_3 must be scrupulously separated from T_4 before it is added to the test system. These assays gave higher values for serum T_3 than later found with radioimmunoassay, and are at present little used.

(e) Radioimmunoassay

Sensitive and precise radioimmunoassay procedures for measuring both thyroxine and triiodothyronine are now widely available. They were first introduced for triiodothyronine because of the complexity of previous assays for this hormone (cf. Larsen, 1972b). The requirement for high-affinity, specific antibodies was met by utilising T_3-serum albumin conjugates as antigen (Brown, Ekins, Ellis and Reith, 1970). The need to reduce the interference by the natural transport proteins has been achieved by prior extraction of hormone (Patel and Burger, 1973) or more simply by the use of agents which inhibit protein binding. Agents that have been successfully used are 8-anilino-1-naphthalene sulphonic acid (ANS) (Chopra, Ho and Lam, 1972a), tetrachlorothyronine (Mitsuma, Gershengorn, Colucci and Hollander, 1971), diphenyl-hydantoin (Lieblich and Utiger, 1972), salicylate (Larsen, 1971) and merthiolate (Huffner and Hesch, 1973). Each of these methods requires careful validation because they can also interfere with T_3 binding to the antibody.

Antisera with adequate sensitivity and specificity for thyroxine assay can be obtained by immunisation with thyroglobulin as well as with thyroxine–protein conjugates. Inhibitors of transport protein binding used in some of these thyroxine assays are ANS (Chopra, 1972; Mitsuma, Colucci, Shenkman and Hollander, 1972) and salicylate (Larsen et al., 1973).

Detailed description of the methods for some of these assays for T_3 and T_4 have been reported (Larsen, 1976; Rall, Sterling, Gharib and Mayberry, 1972), and commercial assay kits are also widely available. A recent development has been the adaptation of T_4-RIA to blood samples collected on filter paper discs for use in neonatal screening for hypothyroidism (Larsen and Broskin, 1975; Walfish, 1975; Mitchell, 1976). This attests to the extreme sensitivity of the assays, which can measure T_3 or T_4 in a few µl of serum.

Radioimmunoassays have also been perfected for several of the thyroid hormone metabolites, which now can readily be measured in blood by these techniques. They include 3,3′,5′-triiodothyronine (reverse T_3) (Chopra, 1976), 3,3′-diiodothyronine (Burger and Sakoloff, 1977; Wu et al., 1976; Burman et al., 1977), and others (Burger, 1976; Nakamura et al., 1978).

(f) Miscellaneous

The technique of double isotope dilution is a powerful tool applicable to the quantitative analysis of substances present in blood in trace amounts. It has been applied to thyroid hormones on only a few occasions (Whitehead and Beale, 1959; Beale and Whitehead, 1960; Sterling, Bellabarba, Newman and Brenner, 1969). One method for thyroxine consisted of acetylation of whole serum by ^{3}H-acetic anhydride. Following this, ^{14}C-N-acetyl thyroxine was added, the mixture extracted several times and finally chromatographed on paper in two dimensions (Whitehead and Beale, 1959). With a known specific activity of the ^{3}H-acetic anhydride and with ^{14}C-N-acetyl thyroxine to correct for losses, the level of stable thyroxine can be calculated. An alternative method is to add ^{131}I-thyroxine to serum before acetylation. The method is reported to be accurate and precise but the numerous compounds which may be acetylated and incompletely separated from thyroxine by chromatography would appear to be a problem.

Counter current distribution is another method which has had very limited use in studying thyroid hormones. The related techniques of solvent extraction and partition chromatography have been used extensively, whereas countercurrent distribution was employed once to separate iodine contaminants from thyroid hormones (Strickler et al., 1964).

Spectral titration has been used to quantitate the iodoaminoacids in purified thyroglobulin (Edelhoch, 1962). Approximately 1 mg of protein is required. It probably has no practical use for blood hormone assay since large quantities of serum would have to be concentrated, nor has its application to crude mixtures been sufficiently evaluated.

For bioassay procedures, the reader is referred to reviews (Turner and Premachandra, 1962; Money, 1966) in which several types of procedures were summarised. Since the iodocompounds can be characterised chemically, there is little need to apply the bioassay methods to blood, and no recent studies of this kind have been reported.

4. Thyroxine-binding Proteins

(a) Identification and separation

The earliest work on the identification of thyroxine-transport proteins (cf. Robbins and Rall, 1960) used precipitation methods, and subfractions of Cohn Fraction IV were shown to be their richest source (Freinkel, Dowling and Ingbar, 1955). At present these methods are little used except for preparative purposes, and even in this case they have been largely supplanted by chromatographic procedures (Robbins, 1975). Most recently, the technique of affinity chromatography has been employed (Robbins, 1976). Thyroxine-agarose or triiodothyronine-agarose is an essential step in purification of thyroxine-binding globulin (Pensky and Marshall, 1969; Marshall, Pensky and Green, 1972; Gershengorn et al., 1977a; Cavalieri, 1975; Korcek and Tabachnick, 1974), but prealbumin is not retained by these columns. For PA, conventional chromatographic methods have been successful (Robbins, 1976), and an affinity column using human retinol-binding protein attached to Sepharose has been effective in the purification of rat PA (Navab et al., 1977b).

The identification of a specific thyroxine-binding protein was first achieved by Gordon *et al.* (1952) by zone electrophoresis in filter paper and this work was extended in a number of laboratories (Robbins and Rall, 1960). In barbital buffer, pH 8·6, with serum trace-labelled with radiothyroxine, about 85–90% of the hormone migrates in a zone intermediate between α_1 and α_2-globulin (TBG). With the reverse-flow technique (Robbins, 1956) the remaining thyroxine is entirely in the albumin region. At the same pH but with Tris (Ingbar, 1958) or other alkaline buffers (Blumberg and Robbins, 1960) more than one-third of the thyroxine moves to the prealbumin position (TBPA or PA).

In analytical electrophoresis procedures, the smallest possible amount of labelled hormone is added to the serum, bearing in mind that the endogenous level of thyroxine is about 8 µg/dl (100 nmol/l) and that of T_3 about 100 ng/dl (1·5 nmol/l). Surprisingly, however, calculation of the effects of increasing hormone level (see above) indicates that an increase of T_4 level is more likely to perturb the distribution than an increase of T_3. This is because TBG sites are about one-third saturated with T_4 at the normal level whereas very few sites are occupied by T_3 owing to its much lower concentration.

As already noted, the choice of electrophoresis buffer is important. Barbital inhibits binding of thyroxine to PA. Other buffers at about pH 9 (e.g. Tris-maleate or glycine-acetate) minimise adsorption to the support medium, which is more of a problem with PA than with TBG (Ingbar, 1958; Oppenheimer, Martinez and Bernstein, 1966; Sterling and Tabachnik, 1961a). It must be recognised, however, that at this pH the distribution of hormone is altered from the physiological state (Lutz and Gregerman, 1969; Gordon and Coutsoftides, 1969a, b; Davis and Gregerman, 1971). Filter paper is a satisfactory support medium for many purposes, but agarose (Lutz and Gregerman, 1969) or cellulose acetate (Tata, 1961) are less adsorptive and more rapid. Polyacrylamide gels can also be used (Davis and Gregerman, 1970; Roberts and Nikolai, 1969a, b), but artifacts are caused by the oxidative effects of the polymerising agent. This can be reduced by preelectrophoresis with a reducing agent (Bernstein *et al.*, 1970) or by cooling (Davis and Gregerman, 1970, 1971; Nikolai and Seal, 1966).

In abnormal serum or in studying animal species, it is useful to employ specific competitive inhibitors to assist in identifying the binding proteins; e.g. diphenylhydantoin to identify a TBG-like protein and barbital to identify a PA-like protein (Davis *et al.*, 1970). Special techniques have also been used to identify minor binding proteins (Hoch and Lewallen, 1974). One of these is a novel method which measures the altered migration of the binding protein in a gel containing T_4.

Immunoelectrophoresis is also useful for detecting minor protein components, or those which are not adequately separated by ordinary electrophoresis. Both conventional immunoelectrophoresis (Myai *et al.*, 1968) and crossed immunoelectrophoresis (Nielsen *et al.*, 1972; Freeman and Pearson, 1969) have been successfully employed. An immunoadsorption technique with anti-PA serum has also been used to assess the contribution of pre-albumin to thyroxine-binding in serum (Woeber and Ingbar, 1968).

Although the electrophoresis techniques are extremely useful for identifying the various transport proteins, they have been less than ideal for evaluating the true distribution of hormones among these proteins. Problems of pH, ionic composition and adsorption to the support medium have already been mentioned. Even with attention to these factors, it must be realised that a non-equilibrium method presents an intrinsic difficulty in attaining this goal. Therefore, even under the best conditions, the results must be considered tentative.

One other technique (Sutherland and Simpson-Morgan, 1975) deserves special mention since it is an equilibrium method which can be used with physiological conditions of temperature, pH and ion composition. It is a variant of the competitive binding techniques described later, and it employs Sephadex G-25 as the adsorbant. By computer analysis of the data over a range of hormone concentration, the complex binding curve obtained with diluted serum is fitted to a minimum number of binding components. This has enabled the authors to identify the number of different types of binding components in animal and human sera, to obtain their affinity constants and binding capacities, and to calculate the distribution of hormone among these sites.

(b) Quantification

A number of methods are available for the measurement of thyroxine-binding proteins. Direct protein measurement is applicable to prealbumin and, of course, to albumin, but not to TBG. Assay of the maximum binding capacity gives a measure of the total TBG concentration, and can also be used to measure PA. Immunoassay techniques, first applied to PA, are now being used for TBG and are likely to become the standard methods for the assay of both proteins. In addition, a variety of indirect methods have been widely used because of their ready availability in most laboratories. These have their basis in the measurement of some property related to the concentration of unoccupied binding sites, and thus are also related to the concentration of unbound hormone. They all employ labelled hormone and they measure either the distribution of hormone among the binding proteins, their rate of dialysis, or, most frequently, their competitive binding to an extrinsic substance. The latter have been especially widely used; they have been used mainly to derive clinically diagnostic indices, but can also give an absolute value for TBG—the so-called "competitive-binding" assay. In this section, we shall concern ourselves exclusively with measurement of TBG, PA and overall protein binding. Methods for albumin are well-established in clinical chemistry but have little intrinsic importance for the thyroid hormones.

(1) *Direct measurement of prealbumin.* A straightforward method for PA assay has been described (Surks and Oppenheimer, 1964; Oppenheimer, Surks, Smith and Squef, 1965; Sakurada, Saito, Inagaki, Tayama and Torikai, 1967). Thyroxine-binding prealbumin (PA-1) is separated from the slower prealbumin and all other serum proteins by starch gel or polyacrylamide gel electrophoresis, and is quantitated by densitometry after staining.

(2) *Immunoassay.* The availability of highly purified TBG and PA has permitted the development of specific radioimmunoassays (RIA) using standard techniques. TBG-RIA was first reported by Levy, Marshall and Velayo (1971) and subsequently by several other laboratories (Gershengorn, Larsen and Robbins, 1976; Cavalieri, McMahon and Castle, 1975a; Hesch et al., 1976). Although each assay gives consistent results in defining a normal range and deviations from the normal, the absolute values have been unacceptably variable. High values appear to result from instability of the TBG used as the standard. Our own experience has shown that frozen TBG, whether in reasonably high concentration or in the presence of serum albumin, and subjected only once to thawing, has a limited storage life. On the other hand, TBG in serum is stable for long periods, enabling its use in this form as a reference standard. Furthermore, the validity of an assay can be evaluated by comparing the RIA result with an independent assay based on maximum binding capacity (Gershengorn, Larsen and Robbins, 1976). Since TBG has a single binding site and its molecular weight is known, the concentration of TBG can be derived from the binding capacity.

PA-RIA has apparently not been used with human serum, but an assay for rat PA has been reported (Navab, Smith and Goodman, 1977b). Since PA is much more stable than TBG, its measurement presents fewer problems.

Simpler immunoassays have also been used with both PA and TBG. Although their precision is usually not as great as with RIA, reasonably accurate measurements can be obtained. The radial immunodiffusion method of Mancini et al. (1965) was applied to PA by a number of authors (e.g. Ingenbleek et al., 1972); a detailed description of one method has been presented (Smith and Goodman, 1971). The concentration of PA in serum is high enough to give a visible precipitation ring when a monospecific antiserum is placed in the gel. In the case of TBG, because of its low concentration, it may be necessary to incorporate radioactive thyroxine in order to identify the precipitin zone, although one report observed stainable precipitin rings (Kagedall and Kallberg, 1977). Labelled T_4 has been employed in the electrophoretic method of Laurell (1966), the so-called "Laurell rocket" (Nielsen, Burr and Weeke, 1972; Bradwell et al., 1976). With the use of a monospecific antiserum, electrophoretic separation of the serum proteins is not required, but the electric field is used to rapidly move the serum into the gel which contains the antiserum. The combination of electrophoretic separation with immunodiffusion (so-called "crossed immunoelectrophoresis") would allow the simultaneous measurement of both TBG and PA (Freeman and Pearson, 1969).

Another application of crossed immunoelectrophoresis was employed by Alper, Robin and Refetoff (1969) to quantitate the multiple polymorphic forms of PA in genetic hybrid monkeys.

A method analogous to radioimmunoassay, but employing T_4 chemically attached to glass beads to bind TBG instead of antibody, was briefly described (Castro and Ugarto, 1974). The assay was not fully validated in this preliminary report. Another assay (Corning Medical) employs anti-TBG antibody attached to glass beads and the partitioning of T_4 between TBG bound to antibody and albumin in solution.

(3) *Maximal binding capacity.* As increasing quantities of thyroxine are added to serum, the thyroxine binding capacity of TBG and, later, of PA are approached asymptotically. By the use of labelled thyroxine and zone electrophoretic separation, the proportion of the total thyroxine associated with each protein can be assessed at each thyroxine level. Saturation is assumed when a virtual plateau is reached (Albright, Larsen and Deiss, 1955; Robbins and Rall, 1955; Robbins, 1956). In order to obtain the true plateau, contamination of the TBG area by albumin-bound or PA-bound thyroxine, and loss of thyroxine form the PA area, must be prevented by using a system in which artifacts due to adsorption are minimised. Some of these are mentioned in the preceding section. Any of a number of techniques can be used, and several typical ones have been presented in some detail (Elzinga et al., 1961; Robbins, 1963; Cavalieri and Ingbar, 1975). The reverse flow method (Robbins, 1956) is suitable for TBG measurement, but not for PA. In this procedure, a fluid flow counterbalances the electrophoretic migration so that TBG moves toward the cathode while PA and albumin move toward the anode. Conventional electrophoresis in glycine-acetate buffer at pH 9 (Oppenheimer et al., 1966) appears to be the most suitable for PA, and also is adequate for TBG, although pH has an apparent effect on the measurement (Davis and Gregerman, 1971). A micro-method using agar-coated microscopic slides has been described (DiGuilio et al., 1964), and poly-acrylamide gels have also been used (Roberts and Nikolai, 1969a, b). With normal serum. TBG saturation occurs at about $1\,\mu g/ml$ ($1\cdot3\,\mu mol/l$) of thyroxine, and PA is saturated at about $6\,\mu g/ml$ ($7\cdot7\,\mu mol/l$). Levels up to

2 μg/ml (2·6 μmol/l) may be needed when TBG is elevated. The use of barbital buffer for sera with low TBG permits saturation at a lower thyroxine level, and thus greater accuracy in the measurement.

Substances in blood which block binding of thyroxine usually do not affect the thyroxine-binding capacity determination since they are diluted out in the measurement procedure, and are also displaced by the added thyroxine. Their importance may be overlooked if only maximal capacity is measured.

The maximum binding capacity is usually reported as μg thyroxine bound per unit volume of serum. Since the number of thyroxine sites per molecule and the molecular weights are known, one may also calculate the actual protein concentration. For TBG, which has a single binding site, this is straightforward, but a problem exists with PA, which has two sites of very different apparent affinity. When the concentration of PA derived from maximal binding capacity is compared with that obtained by direct measurement (see Section E.1), it is either the same or lower (Oppenheimer, Martinez and Bernstein, 1966). It appears, therefore, that only one site is occupied when the apparent plateau of thyroxine-binding to PA is reached.

(4) *Methods based on the concentration of unoccupied binding sites.* To understand the principles on which these methods are based, it is useful to consider the problem from a theoretical standpoint. In the previous editions, we presented equations for this purpose which were evaluated manually. In Section C.3 we have proposed a theoretical scheme for thyroxine and triiodothyronine binding which can be evaluated with the aid of a computer. In Figs 3 and 4, the distribution of T_4 between TBG, PA and albumin is plotted as a function of thyroid hormone or binding protein concentration. Conditions were chosen to cover the range seen in hypothyroidism and hyperthyroidism (Figs 3A and B), T_3-toxicosis (Figs 3C and D), and genetic or induced abnormalities in TBG and PA (Fig. 4) that are encountered clinically. It can be seen that T_4 and T_3 distribution is strongly influenced by the T_4 level and the TBG level, less affected by the PA level, and very little by the T_3 level. The distributions are affected most when the concentration of available binding sites becomes limiting; i.e. at high T_4 levels and at low TBG or PA levels.

Much of the early work on the thyroxine-binding proteins utilised measurement of thyroxine distribution among the electrophoretically separated proteins as a method for detecting changes in the binding proteins (Robbins and Rall, 1960). Despite the theoretical and practical problems mentioned above, it is obvious that a rise in the relative amount of thyroxine transported by one protein may be due to a rise in the concentration of that protein, a fall in the actual or effective concentration of one of the other binding proteins, or an alteration of thyroxine level. If electrophoresis is done with barbital buffer, variations in PA do not affect the distribution. Variants of this method have been applied to the diagnosis of hyper- and hypothyroidism (Burke, Metzger and Goldstein, 1964; Lamberg, Bjorksten, Jakobson, Karlsson and Axelson, 1964). The tendency to low TBG in hyperthyroidism (Guerin and Tubiana, 1964; Inada and Sterling, 1967c) and high TGB in hypothyroidism (Robbins and Rall, 1957) amplifies the changes due to variations in thyroxine level. When used to study agents which block thyroxine binding, it must be appreciated that the agent should be present in the electrophoresis buffer at the same concentration as it exists in the plasma. Although electrophoretic methods suitable for triiodothyronine are available (Braverman and Ingbar, 1965), these features of its distribution have received little attention (Mitchell, Bradford and Collins, 1964).

In the second type of method, the binding proteins in serum are generally treated as a group, although the use of separated protein fractions (Tata, 1959) or blocking agents (Ingbar, 1963) can increase the specificity of the procedure. Measurements based on solubility (Barac, 1958), thyroxine instability (Tata, 1959) or dialysis (Christensen, 1959; Gimlett, 1964) have been used. Equilibrium dialysis, to measure the absolute concentration of free thyroxine, is discussed in the next section; here we consider non-equilibrium methods giving values which are proportional to free thyroxine.

It can be shown (Robbins and Rall, 1960) that the fraction of thyroxine transferred across a membrane is:

$$\frac{K'}{\Sigma k_i(P_i) + 1}$$

where K' is the proportionality constant for transfer with dimension t^{-1}. An analogous expression can be derived for the fractional transfer of triiodothyronine in which the variable, (P_i), is the same but the constants K^1 and k_i are different. Owing especially to the lower value for k_i, the fractional transfer of triiodothyronine is greater than that of thyroxine under similar conditions of dilution and temperature. An automated method based on the rate of triiodothyronine dialysis has been presented (Pollard, Garnett and Webber, 1965). Simplified variants of equilibrium methods can also be used as diagnostic tests (Cavalieri and Searle, 1965).

Lastly, we can consider the methods which are the most widely used of all those in this category. They are also the most complex and are subject to a number of new variables depending on the adsorbing agent employed. By introducing an insoluble material capable of adsorbing thyroxine into a system which contains serum and a trace quantity of labelled thyroxine (or T_3) the distribution of hormone between serum proteins and adsorber can be measured. In such a mixture at equilibrium

$$(T) = \frac{\Sigma(TP_i)}{\Sigma k_i(P_i)} = \frac{\Sigma TR_i}{\Sigma k_{Ri}R_i} \tag{10}$$

where RT = occupied binding sites on the adsorber, R = unoccupied adsorber binding sites, and k_R = their effective association constant. If V = volume of the liquid phase and if (T) is small relative to bound thyroxine we can solve for the fraction of total thyroxine in the system which is bound to any adsorbant (Robbins, 1963)

$$\frac{\Sigma TR_i}{V\Sigma(TP_i) + \Sigma TR_i} = \frac{\Sigma k_{Ri}R_i}{V\Sigma k_i(P_i) + \Sigma k_{Ri}R_i}. \tag{11}$$

If $\Sigma k_{Ri}R_i$ is large relative to ΣR_iT, it may be treated as a constant, C, and equation (11) reduces to

$$\frac{\Sigma TR_i}{V\Sigma(TP_i) + \Sigma TR_i} = \frac{C}{V\Sigma k_i(P_i) + C} \text{ or } \frac{1}{a\Sigma k_i(P_i) + 1} \tag{12}$$

where a is a constant equal to C/V.

It is apparent that equations (3) and (12) are analogous expressions. Furthermore, these are both related to the expression $T/T^t = 1/(\Sigma k_i(P_i) + 1)$, derived from equation (3), and therefore to the free thyroxine fraction. It is also of interest to note that in the distribution of thyroxine between serum proteins, albumin plays the role of a non-specific adsorber of thyroxine and can be treated accordingly.

In all of the above, the assumption is made that the distribution of hormone is studied at equilibrium, but this is often not so in the published methods (Goolden, Gartside and Osorio, 1965). In that case, it is possible to use a kinetic analysis like that employed for non-equilibrium dialysis (see above), provided only that the reaction of free hormone with adsorber is directly proportional to free hormone concentration. It is apparent, therefore, that the non-equilibrium methods also gives results which are proportional to the free thyroxine fraction.

Variants of these procedures are so numerous that we can only refer to some representative ones and emphasise some which have contributed to the theoretical basis of the tests. Those in which labelled thyroxine is added to serum have utilised a strong anion exchange resin, such as Amberlite IRA400 (Mitchell and O'Rourke, 1958; Sterling and Tabachnik, 1961b; Harris and Oliner, 1966). Such resins have also been used with labelled triiodothyronine (Woldring, Bakker and Doorenbos, 1961; Mitchell, Harden and O'Rourke, 1960; Sterling and Tabachnik, 1961b; Nava and DeGroot, 1962). The result is dependent on temperature, time and other variables (Goolden *et al.*, 1965; Godden and Garnett, 1964; Lee, Pillegi and Segalove, 1964b; Maclagan and Howorth, 1969). When weak adsorbers are used, it is necessary either to dilute the serum or to use triiodothyronine, which is less firmly bound to serum proteins. These latter adsorbants have included Sephadex (Shapiro and Rabinowitz, 1962; Cuaron, 1966; Hansen, 1966) and coated charcoal (Herbert, Gottlieb, Lau, Gilbert and Silver, 1965).

A now little used system measures triiodothyronine distribution between plasma and erythrocytes. This was the first method of this group to be devised (Hamolsky, Stein and Freedberg, 1957; Hamolsky, 1966). The erythrocytes introduce new variables into the procedure, which then becomes sensitive to CO_2 (Hamolsky, Golodetz and Freedberg, 1959; Hamolsky, Stein, Fischer and Freedberg, 1961; Friis and Kristensen, 1961), hematocrit (Adams, Specht and Woodward, 1960; Garby, 1962), the method of washing the cells (Meade, 1960; Tauxe and Yamaguchi, 1961), the presence of immature erythrocytes (Schwartz, Carter, Kydd and Gordon, 1967; Carter, Schwartz, Kydd and Kologlu, 1964) or other erythrocyte abnormalities (Barrett, Berman and Maier, 1960), and specific effects of extraneous substances (Morreale de Escobar and Escobar del Rey, 1961).

The following references may be consulted for experimental evaluation of the theoretical basis of the "adsorber uptake" type of procedure (Lee *et al.*, 1964b; Clark and Horn, 1966; Christensen, 1960; Osorio, Jackson, Gartside and Goolden, 1961; Silverstein, Schwartz, Feldman, Kydd and Carter, 1962; Walfish, Britton, Volpe and Ezrin, 1962; Cuaron, 1966; Crispell and Coleman, 1956; Myant and Osorio, 1961; Hamada *et al.*, 1970; Goolden, Gartside and Sanderson, 1967).

Interest in these tests has continued, and many commercial kits are available (Horn, 1975). As discussed in the next section, they are used with a measurement of serum T_4 level to calculate a "free thyroxine index." In addition they have also been adapted to give a quantitative measure of TBG (the so-called competitive-binding assay). Barbital buffer is used to eliminate PA as a variable. In one approach (Nusynowitz and Benedetto, 1975) a relationship between the T_3 resin uptake, T_4 level and TBG capacity are established empirically. In others, a reference serum stripped of its thyroxine by an ion-exchange resin and standardised by a radioimmunoassay for TBG is used to obtain absolute TBG levels. The values obtained are, of course, dependent on the accuracy of the immunoassay. The adsorbants have been dextran-coated charcoal (Roberts and Nikolai, 1969a, b), ion exchange resins (Refetoff, Hagen and Selenkow, 1972a; Keane, Pegg and Johnson, 1970), Sephadex (Bastomsky, Kaloo and Frenkel-Leith, 1977) and anti-T_3 antiserum (Chopra, Solomon and Ho, 1972b; Mulaisho and Utiger, 1977). An interesting application of the competitive binding assay has been reported by Sutherland and Simpson-Morgan (1975). Using Sephadex as the adsorbant, and a computer-derived solution of the relationship of Sephadex-bound to total T_4, they could estimate the number of different binding proteins in human and animal sera, as well as their individual binding constants and capacities.

5. Free Hormone

Although closely related to the methods in the preceding section, the measurement of the free or unbound iodothyronines is discussed separately because of its special interest. It at first seemed unlikely that such measurement would be feasible because of the exceedingly low concentration of free hormone in blood. As a substitute, the calculation of so-called "free thyroxine-index" (F T_4 Index) values was employed since these are proportional to free thyroxine (F T_4). Their theoretical basis can be deduced from equations (3) and (12). They are obtained by multiplying a measurement of the total thyroxine concentration by a second measurement which is inversely proportional to the concentration of unoccupied binding sites. For the latter, early workers employed the thyroxine dialysis rate, the resin-triiodothyronine or thyroxine uptake, or the erythrocyte-triiodothyronine uptake. These indices are useful calculations which can be made from data available in routine clinical laboratories, but their intrinsic value is now diminished by the ability to measure the actual free thyroxine concentration. Nevertheless, they remain extremely popular, and a large number of variations are described in the literature and available commercially (Horn, 1975). New methods using ion exchange resins have been reported (Hamada *et al.*, 1970b, Sawin *et al.*, 1978; Mincey *et al.*, 1971; Wellby, O'Halloran and Marshall, 1974). Most of the more recent developments, however, have employed dextran gels (Levinson and Reider, 1974; Irvine, 1974; Sutherland and Simpson-Morgan, 1975; Finucane and Griffiths, 1976; Snyder, Cavalieri and Ingbar, 1976b) or polyacrylamide gels (McDonald, Robin and Segal, 1978). Some methods also combine the total T_4 assay by competitive binding, and the adsorber-T_4 uptake, into one procedure giving a single result analogous to F T_4 Index (e.g. Liewendahl and Helenius, 1975).

Although the filtration properties of the gel may be used to separate free from bound hormone, by and large, these materials are used as weak adsorbants in competitive-binding type assays. This appears to be the case even in methods which employ rapid filtration techniques (Lee, Henry and Golub, 1964a; Cavalieri, Castle and Searle, 1969; McDonald *et al.*, 1978; Finucane and Griffiths, 1976) or steady state gel filtration methods (Burke and Shakespear, 1976). As emphasised recently by several authors (Pedersen, 1974; Sutherland, Spaulding and Gregerman, 1972; Irvine, 1974; Brandon and

Simpson-Morgan, 1975), the results are dependent on a number of factors such as ionic composition (e.g. chloride content), pH and temperature. On the other hand, a valuable feature is the ability to devise conditions closely approximating the physiological ones. Ions which specifically interfere with one or another binding reaction (e.g. barbital) may be useful when the aim is to quantify a specific binding protein (e.g. TBG, see preceding section), but should be avoided when the aim is to evaluate the physiologically relevant free hormone level.

We have shown earlier (Robbins and Rall, 1957, 1967) that it is possible to calculate the level of free hormone from theoretical expressions for the protein interactions. It is obvious that accurate knowledge of the proportion of serum thyroxine bound to any one of the proteins for which the association constant, the number of sites per molecule, and the total concentration are known, would enable precise calculation of the free thyroxine concentration. Several recent publications (Brown-Grant et al., 1970; Wosilait, 1977; Prince and Ramsden, 1977; Di Stefano and Chang, 1971) have described the computation of free thyroxine and triiodothyronine and their relation to variations in hormone and binding protein levels. With the procedures and parameters presented in Section C.3 we reevaluated some of these relationships (see Fig. 5).

The theoretical relationship between free thyroxine and the expression defined in the preceding section for the so-called free thyroxine index, is presented in Fig. 6. Over a wide range of values for the constant a, the

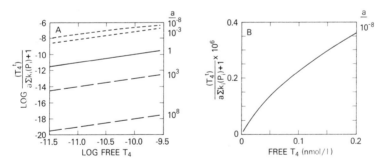

Fig. 6. Theoretical free T_4 concentration as a function of the "free T_4 index" (see text) at various values of a.

relationship is essentially linear (Fig. 6A). At very low values, however, the relation is curvilinear (Fig. 6B). Therefore, the proportionality of free T_4 and the free thyroxine index depends on the conditions of the particular assay system. To use this method properly, it should be shown empirically that the T_4 uptake or the T_3 uptake method employed does in fact give a result which is proportional to the free T_4 fraction over the clinically relevant range. Although this has been demonstrated under some conditions (Robin et al., 1971; Snyder, Cavalieri and Ingbar, 1976b; Stein and Price, 1972) it is not always the case, especially when the alterations in binding protein are large (Burr et al., 1975; Robin et al., 1971). Furthermore, the theoretical relationship may be inexact under non-equilibrium conditions, which often exist in these assays.

The fact that most of these methods give results which are not numerically related to the actual free T_4 level has led many investigators to report relative rather than absolute values and, further, to relate their results to those obtained under identical conditions with a representative or a pooled normal serum. A confusing plethora of calculation methods and terms, such as "corrected thyroxine," "effective thyroxine ratio", etc., have been used. In addition, some methods measure the nonadsorbed T_3 or T_4, rather than the adsorbed, in the competitive binding assay. Therefore, the calculation requires division rather than multiplication. A committee of the American Thyroid Association (Solomon et al., 1976) has strongly advocated the use of the terms Free Thyroxine Index or Free Triiodothyronine Index (FT$_4$ Index or FT$_3$ Index) for all these tests, the uniform use of the ratio to a standard normal serum, and multiplication of the serum thyroxine concentration by this ratio (e.g. T_4 (RIA) $\times$ T_3U (ratio) $=$ FT$_4$ Index. They also recommend that absolute units not be used in order to avoid confusion with actual T_4 or T_3 measurement.

The first actual measurement of free thyroxine was achieved by Sterling and Hegedus (1962), and several improved variants of this method have been published. They are based on the determination of the dialysable fraction of serum thyroxine after labelling with a tracer quantity of radioactive hormone. The concentration of free thyroxine is the product of this fraction times the total serum thyroxine level. The major obstacle in the procedure has been the fact that the dialysable fraction is so small that dialysable contaminants (chiefly iodide) in the radioactive thyroxine lead to a large error unless removed from the dialysate. Sterling and Hegedus used Dowex-50 chromatography for this, but Sterling and Brenner (1966) precipitate the thyroxine with magnesium. Sephadex has also been used (Liewendahl and Lamberg, 1965). In a third method (Ingbar et al., 1965) indifferent serum is added to the dialysate and the iodide then removed by dialysis against Amberlite IRA400. In a fourth method (Oppenheimer et al., 1963; Oppenheimer and Surks, 1964), the dialysable fraction of thyroxine is increased by diluting the serum 25 fold, thus permitting iodide removal by trichloracetic acid precipitation of the thyroxine. Over a limited dilution range, the dialysable fraction appears to be approximately proportional to the dilution and can be appropriately corrected.

Although all of these methods gave internally consistent results, there were a number of problems which required further evaluation. The effect of dilution in the method of Oppenheimer *et al.*, 1963 was in question since it was found that even slight dilution lowered the measured free thyroxine (Ingbar *et al.*, 1965). There is evidence, however, that a second dialysable contaminant in the radioactive thyroxine preparations leads to an overestimate of the dialysable fraction (Schussler and Plager, 1967) and so the values obtained with diluted serum were more nearly correct. The achievement of equilibrium can be a problem since thyroxine placed outside the dialysis bag behaves differently from that placed inside (Sterling and Brenner, 1966). The specific activity of available radiothyroxine is such that the amount added significantly raises the serum thyroxine level. Although this has a small effect (Sterling and Hegedus, 1962; Ingbar *et al.*, 1965; Pedersen, 1974a, b), it may not be negligible in all sera. Control of temperature is important, and most procedures are done at 37°. As discussed previously, it is important to approximate physiological ionic and pH conditions if a physiologically relevant result is desired. These matters have been discussed by Sterling (1971), who has also cited some later references, and the technique has been adapted for use in a clinical laboratory (Lee and Pileggi, 1971; Wilson *et al.*, 1974; Strickler, Link and Grauer, 1974).

A further point concerns the values used for total serum thyroxine. In the early methods, thyroxine was calculated from the PBI without regard for the fact that not all of the PBI is thyroxine. Current methods employ the more definitive estimates of serum thyroxine. The accuracy of the final result, of course, is directly related to the precision of thyroxine analysis.

Two other methods were used in early work to measure free thyroxine but were considered of insufficient reliability for general use although the values obtained were similar to those from the above methods. Ultrafiltration was employed during evaluation of the dialysis methods (Oppenheimer and Surks, 1964). A rapid gel filtration method on small columns of Sephadex showed some initial promise (Lee *et al.*, 1964a). Recently, other ultrafiltration methods have been proposed (Schussler and Plager, 1967; Chin and Schussler, 1968; Pedersen, 1974a, b; Thorson *et al.*, 1972) as well as gel filtration methods (see above). In the latter, however, it appears that adsorption to the gel is a factor even with very rapid column flow.

A recently introduced method utilises the rate of T_4 uptake from serum by an adsorber (immobilised anti-T_4 antibody—Corning Medical). As discussed in the preceding section, this parameter is proportional to the free hormone level.

The concentration of free triiodothyronine may also be measured by similar techniques. Although the dialysable fraction is greater than that for thyroxine (Ingbar *et al.*, 1965; Nauman *et al.*, 1967; Sawin *et al.*, 1978) it is

x

still very small and also requires attention to radioactive contaminants. The major obstacle in the early work was the accurate determination of total serum triiodothyronine. Even though this problem has now been solved, there has been little use of free triiodothyronine measurements, especially in the clinical laboratory (Snyder *et al.*, 1976b; Izumi, 1972; Robin, Hagen *et al.*, 1971; and Section E.1, Table 15).

Of interest are several recent reports showing that, with currently available methods of radioimmunoassay, both T_4 and T_3 can be measured in dialysates of serum (Weeke and Orskov, 1975; Ellis and Ekins, 1976; Yeo, Lewis and Evered, 1977; Jiang and Tue, 1977). This now permits direct measurement of the free hormone levels. Another direct method employs dialysis and gas–liquid chromatography of both T_4 and T_3 (Petersen, Hanson *et al.*, 1976; Petersen, Geise *et al.*, 1977), and the authors propose its use as a reference method. A direct method based on T_4 and T_3 adsorption to Sephadex LH-20 has also been described (Pennisi, Romelli and Vancheri, 1979).

Of further interest has been the attempt to use urine T_4 and T_3 excretion to evaluate free hormone levels (Robbins and Rall, 1957; Burke and Shakespear, 1976a, b). Although these have been shown to have some validity, their practical utility is severely affected by proteinuria, which alters the renal clearance of the hormones.

6. Iodoproteins

Iodoproteins in blood consist of thyroglobulin, present normally but in small amount, and poorly identified iodoproteins, a portion of which is iodinated albumin. The methods for iodoprotein separation and identification noted below, except for radioimmunoassay of thyroglobulin, are not generally specific for any one protein and they usually require larger amounts of materials than those encountered in blood. In subjects given relatively large amounts of radioiodine, radioactivity can serve to identify iodoproteins. Also, these methods are useful for analysis of iodoproteins in the thyroid where quantities involved are much greater.

(a) Salting out

Thyroglobulin has a sharp range of insolubility in ammonium sulphate or potassium phosphate and this characteristic has been used to identify labelled thyroglobulin in serum and to purify it (Derrien, Michel and Roche, 1948; Robbins, 1954). It is little used today except as a preliminary step in purification.

(b) Electrophoresis

Electrophoresis may be performed on paper or in gels. More recently, disc gel electrophoresis in polyacrylamide has found general use. If electrophoresis is performed on native proteins, separation is on the basis of the isoelectric point of the protein. Thyroglobulin has an isoelectric point of 4·5 so it is easily separated from neutral and basic proteins but poorly from acidic proteins. On paper, for example, TBG and thyroglobulin have almost identical mobilities when electrophoresis is performed at pH 7 or 8 (Robbins and Rall, 1952). PA, because of its rapid mobility is completely separated on paper electrophoresis (or disc gel) at an alkaline or neutral pH. On polyacrylamide disc gels thyroglobulin is easily separated from most proteins. Isoelectric focusing can also be used for analysis of iodoprotein and thyroglobulin has been examined with this technique (Ui, 1971). Electrophoresis can also be performed under denaturing conditions on reduced alkylated proteins in the presence of sodium dodecyl sulphate. Under these conditions, using multiple gel pore sizes and with markers, the molecular weight of proteins can be approximated (Shapiro, Vinuela and Maizel, 1967; Segrest, Jackson, Andrews and Marchesi, 1971).

(c) Ultracentrification

Centrifugation in linear density gradients of sucrose separates thyroglobulin from most other proteins, including other iodoproteins and thyroxine binding proteins (Robbins and Weathers, 1966). A refinement has recently been introduced wherein thyroglobulin is centrifuged in a density gradient of rubidium chloride (Schneider and Edelhoch, 1971). The iodine content of thyroglobulin can vary from 0·1–1·5%. The iodine changes the density of the molecule and in concentrated rubidium chloride solutions it will equilibrate at different densities. This provides a sensitive method for separating thyroglobulin molecules (or those of any iodoprotein) on the basis of their iodine content.

(d) Gel filtration

Thyroglobulin, by virtue of its size, can be separated in large quantity and fairly cleanly from most other proteins in gels. Sephadex G200 may be used but agarose is more convenient. Other iodoproteins can be separated from larger and smaller proteins on less highly linked gels. Gel filtrations in thin layers can be used for studies of small amounts of material (De Nayer, Weathers and Robbins, 1966).

(e) Immunochemical methods

Antibodies to thyroglobulin, to microsomal thyroid elements and complement fixing antibodies are found in the blood of patients with several diseases, most notably chronic lymphocytic thyroiditis. These antibodies have been studied extensively and can be measured by tanned red cell agglutination, complement fixation and immunofluorescence. More recently, a radio-immunoassay for antibodies to thyroglobulin has been developed and appears to be in some respects superior to the tanned red cell agglutination test (Salabe, Fontana and Andreoli, 1972).

Iodoproteins can also be measured by radioimmunoassay and several such techniques have been described for the quantitative measurement of thyro-globulin in blood (Van Herle, Uller, Matthews and Brown, 1973; Schneider, Favus, Stachura, Arnold, Yun Ryo, Pinsky, Colman, Arnold and Frohman, 1977). About 75% of normal individuals show detectable thyroglobulin in their blood with an average value of about 5 ng/ml. These are satisfactory assays but require considerable attention to detail to achieve the sensitivity required. Additionally, the presence of autoantibodies to thyroglobulin causes serious problems in an RIA for thyroglobulin (Schneider and Pervos, 1978). Autoantibodies to thyroglobulin are found in many types of thyroid disease and may even be noted in apparently normal individuals. These problems have recently been examined in some detail (Schneider and Pervos, 1978).

(f) Chromatography

Thyroglobulin may be chromatographed in DEAE Sephadex but little work has been done on chromatography of iodoproteins in serum (Robbins and Rall, 1966).

E. DISTRIBUTION AND CONCENTRATION

1. Normal Concentration

(a) Thyroxine and triiodothyronine

When the second edition of this volume was compiled, iodine analysis was the standard method for thyroid hormone determination in serum. Some of the previously summarised data will be briefly mentioned here since it forms the basis for much of our present knowledge. Although most of the values now reported from clinical laboratories are based on radio-immunoassay or displacement assay, we will also present results from other types of measurements. We have selected and tabulated some rep-resentative data (Tables 13–15). Those readers wishing to consult the results obtained in various laboratories can find them in many of the references given in the section on methods.

Since thyroxine comprises about 90% of the serum protein-bound iodine (PBI), the latter measurement can be used to evaluate the serum thyroxine

Table 13

Thyroid hormone levels in normal plasma based on iodine analysis.[a]

Method	No. of cases	As iodine[b]	As iodo-thyronine[b]	References
		Thyroxine (μg/dl)[d]		
Protein bound iodine PBI	609	5·48 (3·4–7·6)		Lepp et al. (1965)
Butanol extractable iodine BEI	64	4·7 (3·3–6·1)	7·2 (5·0–9·4)	Man et al. (1954)
Column chromatography T₄(C)	234	4·4 [3·1–5·9]	6·7 [4·7–9·0]	Weiss (1967)[c]
Thin layer chromatography T₄(C)	117	5·24 (3·1–7·4)	7·98 (4·7–11·2)	West et al. (1965b)
		Triiodothyronine (ng/dl)[e]		
Paper chromatography T₃(C)	18	140 (60–220)	240 (100–380)	Pind (1957)

[a] Both sexes. See text for sex difference.
[b] M. and (± 2 s.d.) or [95% confidence limits].
[c] Personal communication, performed by method of Hellman et al. (1963).
[d] 1 μg/dl = 12·87 nmol/l.
[e] 1 ng/dl = 15·36 pmol/l.

level. The values obtained in normal individuals are surprisingly uniform when measured by a variety of techniques (see Robbins and Rall, 1967, Table 8). Several factors must be considered in evaluating these data. A large number of drugs and situations affect artifactually the PBI: ovulatory suppressant drugs, pregnancy, and iodine-containing medications are a few of these. In addition, it is also affected by the method of venipuncture (Lewitus and Steinitz, 1963). A 5 min period of venous occlusion raises the PBI an average of 22% over the initial level. There is some disagreement as to whether storage of blood affects the PBI. Pileggi and Farber (1964) could find no difference in either PBI, butanol extractable iodine (BEI), or thyroxine assayed by column when measured immediately upon collection or 11 days later after the serum had been kept at 30° unsterilised. Man (1962) on the other hand found that prolonged storage of frozen serum resulted in an increase in the BEI. Addition of small amounts of thiouracil to serum prevented this increase.

The distribution of the serum PBI in normal individuals was found to be skewed toward higher values (Lowrey and Starr, 1959; Blackburn and Power, 1955; Oddie, Melby and Scroggs, 1962). In one study (Blackburn and Power, 1955), the 95% confidence limits were from 3·1–7·7 μg/dl whereas the mean value (5·2 μg/dl) plus two standard deviations on either side gave 2·8–

Table 14

Thyroid hormone levels in normal plasma based on displacement analysis or gas–liquid chromatography[a].

Method	No. of cases	Concentration[b]		References
		Thyroxine		
		µg/dl	nmol/l	
Competitive-binding		6·36	82	Murphy et al.
T$_4$(D)	M 1146[c]	[4·2–9·8]	[54–126]	(1966)
	F	6·60	85	Murphy et al.
		[3·8–9·4]	[49–121]	(1966)
	316[c]	7·26	93	Arango et al.
		[4·0–11·1]	[51–143]	(1968)
	M 1074	7·93	102	Evered et al.
		(4·5–11·3)	(58–146)	(1978)
	F 611	8·55	110	Evered et al.
		(5·0–12·1)	(64–156)	(1978)
Radioimmunoassay	40	8·33	107	Chopra (1972)
T$_4$ (RIA)		(3·5–13·2)	(45–170)	
	76[d]	7·6	98	Larsen (1976)
		(5·0–10·2)	(64–131)	
		Triiodothyronine		
		ng/dl	nmol/l	
Competitive-binding	31	220	3·38	Sterling et al.
T$_3$(D)		(166–274)	(2·7–4·2)	(1969)
Radioimmunoassay	82	138	2·12	Mitsuma et al.
T$_3$(RIA)		(92–184)	(1·4–2·8)	(1971)
	85	96	1·47	Alexander and
		(44–148)	(0·7–2·3)	Jennings (1974)
	76	111	1.70	Larsen (1976)
		(65–157)	(1·0–2·4)	
	M 176	115	1·76	Evered et al.
		(39–189)	(0·6–2·9)	(1978)
	F 211	108	1·66	Evered et al.
		(26–189)	(0·4–2·9)	(1978)
Gas–liquid chromato-	24	137	2·10	Nihei et al. (1971)
graphy T$_3$(glc)		(91–183)	(1·4–2·8)	

[a] Males and females combined except where indicated. Murphy et al. (1966) found a significant difference in the mean T$_4$ for males and females, but Arango et al. (1968) state that results in males and females were not significantly different. Data listed for Evered et al. (1978) include only women not pregnant or receiving oral contraceptives, but the number of males and females was not given.

[b] M. and (± 2 S.D.) or [95% confidence limits].

[c] Not corrected for incomplete recovery, which was $\sim 77\%$.

[d] Only subjects with normal TBG level are included.

7·6 µg/dl. There are many possible explanations for this skewness. Lowrey and Starr (1959) found in a large series of industrial workers that the average PBI in males was 5·33 µg/dl, while that in females was 5·67 µg/dl, and the difference was highly significant. On the other hand, if the series of women included 15% or so who were pregnant, this would explain their data. In later studies, Oddie and Fisher (1967) found a similar sex difference (0·21 µg/dl) in persons under the age of 20, and Murphy et al. (1966) found that serum thyroxine by displacement analysis (Table 14) was significantly higher in women. On the other hand, a large population survey by Evered et al. (1978) found that the serum T_4 and T_3 were normally distributed although there were differences related to age, sex, the use of oral contraceptives and other factors (see Section E.3). It seems likely that many of these differences involve the thyroxine-binding proteins (see below).

The rather large range of normal level of PBI or total T_4 or T_3 can have several explanations. As noted earlier, it may only reflect the fact that the parameter controlled by homeostatic mechanisms is not the total hormone level in blood, but the level of free hormone. Two methods of analysing for constancy of PBI in any one individual are twin studies and longitudinal studies in the same individual. In one investigation of monozygotic twins in humans and cattle (Long-Gilmore and Rife, 1956) it was found that three-quarters of the variation among individuals was hereditary whereas environmental factors accounted for only one-quarter. Stabenau and Pollin (1968), however, in a study of 21 pairs of monozygotic twins found that the intra-pair difference in PBI was greater than the inter-pair difference: the variances being 0·81 µg/dl and 0·66 µg/dl, respectively. This would suggest that genetic differences played a minor role. The fact that 17 of the twin pairs had at least one individual with schizophrenia may affect these data. In a later, somewhat larger sample, Stabenau and Mirsky (1970) concluded that there was, indeed, a moderately potent genetic component affecting PBI, T_4 and free T_4, but not TBG. In repeated determinations of PBI in the same individual over a period of up to seven months (Gaffney et al., 1960), the variability due to "biological sources" was stated to be 0·6–1·2 µg/dl—considerably greater than the variation due to technical factors (0·3–0·4 µg/dl). Volpe et al. (1960), however, showed smaller individual variation than group variation over periods up to four years. The average standard deviation from the mean PBI for an individual over the course of time was 0·47 µg/dl, whereas the standard deviation about the mean of 479 different normal subjects was 0·72 µg/dl. Seasonal variation in the PBI as noted below may play a role in individual variations throughout the year. Altogether, it seems likely that there is a substantial variation in thyroid hormone in the same individual and that genetic factors do not accurately determine a normal subject's precise hormone level.

Table 15

Free hormone levels in normal plasma[a].

Method	No. of cases	% of total	Concentration[b]		References
			ng/dl	pmol/l	
			Thyroxine		
Dialysis × PBI × 1·5	22	0·028	2·34	30·2	Oppenheimer et al. (1963)
		(0·022–0·034)	(1·8–2·9)	(23–38)	
	105	0·05	4·03	52·0	Ingbar et al. (1965)
		(0·03–0·07)	(1·8–6·2)	(38–66)	
Dialysis × T$_4$(D)	316	0·035	2·49	32·0	Arango et al. (1968)
		[0·016–0·064]	[0·9–5·2]	[12–67]	
Dialysis × T$_4$(RIA)	M 111	0·017	1·6	21	Sawin et al. (1978)
			(0·9–2·3)	(12–30)	
	F 110	0·015	1·4	18	Sawin et al. (1978)
			(0·8–2·1)	(10–27)	
	M 47	0·030	2·35	30·2	Parslow et al. (1977)
			(1·6–3·2)	(21–41)	
Ultrafiltration × PBI × 1·5	18	0·028	2·2	28	Chin and Schussler (1968)
		(0·018–0·038)	(1·4–3·0)	(18–39)	
Ultrafiltration × T$_4$(D)	25	0·026	2·8	36	Larsen et al. (1970)
		(0·020–0·032)	(2·2–3·4)	(28–44)	
Dialysate glc	29	0·024	1·89	24·3	Petersen et al. (1977)
			(1·0–2·8)	(13–36)	
Dialysate RIA	39	0·011	0·76	9·8	Jiang and Tue (1977)
			(0·4–1·1)	(5–14)	
	52	0·01	0·80	10	Yeo et al. (1977)
			(0·3–1·3)	(4–17)	
Dialysis curve fitting	3	0·038	2·3	30	Sutherland and Simpson-Morgan (1975)
			(0·9–2·7)	(12–35)	
Theoretical	—	0·036	3·0	38·7	Prince and Ramsden (1977)
	—	0·034	2·65	34·1	Section C.3

	n[a]		Triiodothyronine		[b]
Dialysis × T_3(D)	—	0·26 (0·18–0·34)	0·60 (0·34–0·86)	9·2 (5–13)	Sterling (1971)
Dialysis × T_3(RIA)	M 111	0·16	0·23 (0·14–0·31)	3·5 (2–5)	Sawin et al. (1978)
	F 110	0·17	0·25 (0·15–0·35)	3·8 (2–5)	Sawin et al. (1978)
	M 93	0·32	0·42 (0·28–0·57)	6·5 (4–9)	Parslow et al. (1977)
Dialysate glc	29	0·28	0·42 (0·36–0·48)	6·5 (6–7)	Petersen et al. (1977)
Dialysate RIA	F 20	0·48 (0·29–0·67)	0·51 (0·31–0·71)	7·8 (5–11)	Weeke and Orskov (1975)
	M 20	0·42 (0·28–0·56)	0·53 (0·33–0·73)	8·1 (5–11)	Weeke and Orskov (1975)
	52	0·6	0·66	10·1 (5–16)	Yeo et al. (1977)
Theoretical	—	0·30	0·36	5·6	Prince and Ramsden (1977)
	—	0·41	0·53	8·1	Section C.3

[a] Males and females combined except where indicated.

[b] M. and (±2 s.d.) or [95% confidence limits].

Although measurement of the blood iodine and thyroid hormones has been widespread throughout the world, there has been little in the way of systematic comparative study of population groups. A few studies, however, have revealed what appear to be meaningful differences. Two groups of Canadian Eskimos were found to have a higher PBI (M. = 6·5 µg/100 ml) than individuals living in the northeastern United States (M. = 5·1 µg/100 ml) (Gottschalk and Riggs, 1952; Davis and Hanson, 1965). Native inhabitants of the Marshall Islands also had a higher PBI (M. = 6·98 compared to 5·09) (Rall and Conard, 1966). The serum thyroxine levels were similar in the two groups, as was the TBG capacity, but the Marshallese had a higher iodoprotein concentration. In Congolese with or without endemic goitre, the TBG capacity was higher than in Belgians (Van den Schrieck, DeNayer, Beckers and DeVisscher, 1965). The PBI, however, was not elevated, suggesting that free thyroxine might be low.

Early measurements of thyroxine concentration in plasma (Table 13) were by butanol extractable iodine (Kydd and Peters, 1951; Man, Bondy, Weeks and Peters, 1954), or chromatography combined with iodine analysis (Pilleggi, Lee, Golub and Henry, 1961). Confusion may arise from the fact that thyroxine levels were reported either as the concentration of substance or as iodine concentration. The fractional iodine content (on the basis of molecular weight) is 0·655 for thyroxine and 0·585 for T_3. A less obvious factor is the necessity to consider the formula weight when weighed quantities of hormone are used. The commonly available preparation of thyroxine (i.e. sodium thyroxine pentahydrate) has a formula weight of 889, or 12% greater than the molecular weight of 777.

Table 14 gives values for serum hormone levels determined by displacement or radioimmunoassay. Mean thyroxine levels obtained in various laboratories are rather similar when a recovery correction is applied. A mean of about 100 nmol/l (7·8 µg/dl) with a range of ±40% (2 s.d.) is generally found. Early reports on triiodothyronine levels frequently gave mean values above 200 ng/dl (3·1 nmol/l) (Rall et al., 1972), but the lower values from radioimmunoassays in Table 14 are representative of those found in most laboratories at the present time. A mean of about 1·7 nmol/l (110 ng/dl) with a range of ±50% (2 s.d.) is representative. The weight ratio T_4/T_3 in blood is about 70 and the mole ratio is about 60. T_4 contains about 90% of the serum protein-bound iodine and T_3, about 1%.

The values for free thyroxine and free T_3 concentration (Table 15) show a greater variation among laboratories, differing by as much as a factor of three. A generally applicable value for FT_4 is 25 pmol/l (2 ng/dl) with a range of ±40% (2 s.d.) and a FT_4 fraction of 0·025%. For FT_3, representative mean values are 7 pmol/l (0·45 ng/dl), range ±35% (2 s.d.), and FT_3 fraction 0·4%. These values are comparable to the theoretical values derived from the constants for thyroxine-serum protein interactions. It should be noted that a rise in temperature from 26–37° approximately doubles the free thyroxine concentration (Bernstein and Oppenheimer, 1966; Schussler and Plager, 1967) and the important influence of pH and buffer composition has been discussed under Methods. Technical factors may explain the wide range of normal found in most laboratories. In one study (Ingbar *et al.*, 1965) the s.d. in percent free thyroxine (0·18 of the mean) was only about twice that attributable to reproducibility (0·06–0·1 of the mean) (Ingbar *et al.*, 1965) indicating that the actual range of free thyroxine concentration might be very narrow.

We have not attempted to tabulate literature values on free T_4 index or free T_3 index, or on the T_4 or T_3 uptake measurements on which these values are based. The "uptake" is dependent on the specific method employed. The "uptake ratio" (related to normal serum) is centred on 1·0, but the range of normal is variable depending on the method, and the calculated "free hormone index" is similarly variable. Although the definition of a valid "normal" range for any measurement in clinical chemistry requires that each laboratory establish its own values, this is especially pertinent in the case of the "free hormone index." Furthermore, the measurement has no meaning as a true concentration.

With respect to free hormone levels, two other findings are of interest. Refetoff, Robin and Fang (1970) reported that in a wide variety of animal species, all but a few had free thyroxine concentrations that were surprisingly similar and not very different from the human. Secondly, it was shown by Hagen and Elliot (1973) that FT_4 and FT_3 concentrations in cerebrospinal fluid were 2–6 times that found in serum, and were related to the low levels of TBG (1/75 of the serum level) and PA (1/12 of serum level). In another study (Hanson and Siersbaek-Nielsen, 1973) FT_4 and FT_3 in CSF were almost identical with serum.

(b) Non-hormonal iodine

(1) *Iodoamino acids.* There has been increasing interest in measuring non-hormonal iodoamino acids following the recent evidence that these metabolites of the hormones are found in normal human serum (Table 16). One compound in this group, 3,3′,5′-triiodothyronine (rT_3), is perhaps the most important from a clinical standpoint because of the many data showing a generally reciprocal relationship between the levels of T_3 and rT_3 in serum (see below). All of the non-hormonal iodothyronines are present at concentrations considerably below that of thyroxine. Compared to triiodothyronine, their approximate molar ratios are $T_3:T_4Ac:rT_3:3,3′-T_2:T_3Ac$ equal 100:94:37:8:8. Together they comprise about 2·5% of the

Table 16

Non-hormonal iodine components—levels in normal plasma by radioimmunoassay[a].

Component	No. of cases	Concentration[b] ng/dl	Concentration[b] nmol/l	% of PBI	References
Diiodotyrosine	92	101 |<40–432|	2·3 |<0·9–9·7|	1·1	Nelson et al. (1976)
3,3'-Diiodothyronine	44	7·6 (2·8–12·4)	0·14 (0·05–0·24)	0·07	Wu et al. (1976)
	31	4·3 (2·3–6·3)	0·082 (0·04–0·12)		Burger and Sakaloff (1977)
	18	17 (15–19)	0·32 (0·29–0·36)		Burman et al. (1977)
3,3',5'-Triiodothyronine (rT₃)	27	41 (21–61)	0·63 (0·32–0·94)	0·4	Chopra (1974)
	106	23 (7–39)	0·35 (0·11–0·60)		Kaplan et al. (1977)
T₄-acetic acid T₄Ac	—	121 (0–245)	1·6 (0–3·3)	1·5	Burger (1976)
T₃-acetic acid T₃Ac	11	8·7 |<5·5–15·2|	0·14 |<0·08–0·24|	0·1	Nakamura et al. (1978)
T₃-propionic acid	11	<8·8	<0·14		Nakamura et al. (1978)
Thyroglobulin	95[c]	510 (460–560)	0·0077 (0·0070–0·0085)	0·05	Van Herle et al. (1973)
	55	1500 (200–2800)	0·023 (0·003–0·042)		Schneider et al. (1977)

[a] Males and females combined.
[b] M. and (±2 s.d.) or \|range\|).
[c] Values are for the 75% antithyroglobulin-negative sera which has detectable thyroglobulin levels. Females had a mean level twice that of males.

serum protein-bound iodine. As these studies continue, it is likely that additional compounds will be found, as was the case in earlier studies with laboratory animals (see Section B.5).

The occurrence in normal blood of products of ether-bridge splitting— i.e. the iodotyrosines—was a matter of controversy that was reviewed in some detail in the previous edition. The original claim that the majority of the blood iodine was comprised of iodotyrosines (Werner and Block, 1959) was clearly an overestimate, as shown by later work in the same and other laboratories, as well as by comparison of total iodine in serum with the content of thyroxine measured by radioimmunoassay. It is possible, as discussed previously (Robbins and Rall, 1967), that the "iodotyrosine" fraction was derived from iodinated proteins (Weinert, Masui, Radichevich and Werner, 1967) which are known to comprise about 10 to 15% of the iodine in normal serum. More recently it was shown by radioimmunoassay (Nelson, Weiss, Lewis et al., 1974; Nelson, Weiss, Palmer et al., 1976) that the DIT level in serum extracts may be about 100 ng/dl (2·3 nmol/l) or 1% of the serum protein-bound iodine. It was also suggested that a portion of this might have an extrathyroidal origin.

(2) *Iodoproteins.* As determined by ion exchange chromatography iodine covalently bound to protein comprises about 10–15% of the total iodine in normal plasma (Pilleggi et al., 1964; Rall and Conard, 1966; Peyrin and Berger, 1965). Although available data are meager (Brown, Lowenstein, Greenspan and Mangum, 1966), it seems likely that this is iodinated serum protein which, as we shall see, may be quantitatively quite important in some thyroid diseases and is known to exist in normal thyroid glands.

Recent studies using radioimmunoassay have shown that thyroglobulin is also a constituent of normal blood (Roitt and Torrigiani, 1967; Torrigiani, Doniach and Roitt, 1969; Van Herle, Uller, Matthews and Brown, 1973) probably arising from lymphatic drainage of the thyroid gland (Daniel, Plaskett and Pratt, 1966; Daniel et al., 1967). Some recent measurements (Schneider, Favus, Stachura et al., 1977) Table 16) show that thyroglobulin accounts for only about 0·1% of the serum iodine.

Several other minor iodinated compounds described in blood were discussed in the previous edition. There has been no further work to corroborate these findings.

(3) *Iodide.* Since iodide is derived in large part from dietary intake, its concentration in blood varies with the iodine content in the food and with the time of day in relation to meals. It is possible to calculate an "average" plasma iodide level for a urinary iodine excretion of 150 µg/day and a renal clearance of 35 ml plasma/min (Rall et al., 1964). This value, 0·3 µg/dl (23·6 nmol/l), is in the range of measured values on a "usual" iodine intake

Table 17

Concentration of thyroxine-binding proteins in normal plasma[a].

Method	No. of cases	Sex	µg T$_4$/dl	TBG mg/dl	µmol/l[c]	References
Binding capacity	9	M + F	20 (14–26)		0·26 (0·18–0·33)	Robbins and Rall (1957)
	21	M + F	24·5 (19–30)		0·32 (0·24–0·39)	Oppenheimer et al. (1963)
	82	M + F	17·3 (12–23)		0·22 (0·15–0·30)	Lee et al. (1971)
Radial immunodiffusion	127	M		1·38[b] (1·0–1·8)	0·25 (0·19–0·33)	Kagedal and Kallberg (1977)
	95	F		1·54[b] [1·1–2·1]	0·29 [0·29–0·39]	Kagedal and Kallberg (1977)
Radioimmunoassay	98	M + F		1·48 (0·6–2·4)	0·27 (0·11–0·44)	Gershengorn et al. (1976).
		M		1·37 (0·6–2·1)	0·25 (0·11–0·39)	Gershengorn et al. (1976)
		F		1·66 (0·5–2·8)	0·31 (0·09–0·52)	Gershengorn et al. (1976)
	6	M + F		2·15 (1·1–3·2)	0·40 (0·20–0·59)	
Dialysis curve fitting	3	M + F	21·3 (15–28)		0·27 (0·19–0·36)	Sutherland and Simpson-Morgan (1975)

			PA		
Binding capacity	21	M + F	256 (180–332)	3·3 (2·3–4·3)	Oppenheimer et al. (1963)
Protein electrophoresis	15	M + F	27·7 (22–34)	5·1 (4·1–6·3)	Oppenheimer et al. (1966)
Radial immunodiffusion	109	M + F	25·0 (20–30)	4·6 (3·7–5·6)	Smith and Goodman (1971)
	61	M	26·3 (21–30)	4·9 (3·9–5·6)	Smith and Goodman (1971)
	57	F	23·8 (19–28)	4·4 (3·5–5·2)	Smith and Goodman (1971)
	39	M	28 (16–40)	5·2 (3·0–7·4)	Rossi et al. (1970)
	40	F	22 (12–32)	4·1 (2·2–5·9)	Rossi et al. (1970)
Dialysis curve fitting	3	M + F	258 (156–360)	3·3 (2·0–4·6)	Sutherland and Simpson-Morgan (1975)

[a] M. and (± 2 s.D.) or [95% confidence limits].
[b] Independent radioimmunoassay on the same sample gave identical results.
[c] Calculated on the basis of one T_4 site/mol, and mw 54,000.

in regions where goitre is not endemic (e.g. Fisher, Oddie and Epperson, 1965; Vought and London, 1965; Wayne, Koutras and Alexander, 1964). Plasma iodide levels derived from a number of sources have been collated (Rall *et al.*, 1964, pp. 278–281). After an overnight fast, the weighted mean was 0·25 µg/dl (19·7 nmol/l), whereas in the non-fasting state the weighted mean was 0·52 µg/dl (41·0 nmol/l).

Comparatively little attention has been paid to the iodine in blood which is associated with the blood cells. The ratio of iodide in erythrocytes to that in plasma is 0·6 (Owen and Power, 1953; Rall, Power and Albert, 1950) but the iodothyronines are virtually excluded (Riggs *et al.*, 1942; Silver, 1942) owing to their binding to the plasma proteins. This relationship was utilised as a means to evaluate the changing ratio of iodide and hormonal iodine in testing thyroid function (Scott, Reavis, Saunders and White, 1951; White, 1953). In some fish, however, iodide and iodothyronine distribution between cells and plasma is very different (Leloup and Fontaine, 1960).

(c) Thyroxine-binding proteins

Values for the concentration of the transport proteins in normal human serum are presented in Table 17. As pointed out in Section D.5, results obtained by the various competitive binding assays and some types of immunoassay do not give absolute values but are standardised by analysis of a reference serum by a reliable independent method such as RIA. Therefore, these are not listed in the Table although they have obvious clinical utility. The early data on TBG based on maximal binding capacity by electrophoretic methods gave quite uniform data in various laboratories, and are consistent with the immunoassay results in several reports. As discussed in the methods section, the rather large discrepancies between different laboratories using RIA are probably due to instability of the reference protein, and only results which we believe to be the most reliable are reported in the table. These are consistent with independent evidence that TBG contains a single hormone-binding site. Electrophoretic analysis of PA binding capacity, on the other hand, gave variable results due to experimental artifacts (see Methods) whereas more recent values based on protein measurement or immunoassay appear to be more reliable. It is also evident that binding capacity measurements do not evaluate the second PA binding site for T_4.

In several recent studies employing immunoassays, the results showed small but significant sex differences, with females having higher TBG and lower PA levels. Furthermore, the TBG values in females, and in males in some studies, showed a log-normal distribution. In two of the larger studies (TBG: Kagedall and Kalberg, 1977; PA: Smith and Goodman, 1971) it was specifically stated that the females were not receiving oral contraceptives.

The distribution of hormones among the binding proteins is reported in Table 18. Results on T_4 distribution by electrophoretic methods gave lower TBG binding and higher PA binding than obtained by immunoprecipitation and, more recently, by curve-fitting of equilibrium dialysis data and by theoretical calculations. The latter analyses give data which differ mainly

Table 18

Distribution of thyroid hormones among the transport proteins at normal hormone levels.

Method	TBG (%)	PA (%)		ALB (%)		References
		Thyroxine				
Electrophoresis[a]	43	42		15		Ingbar and
	(36–50)	(36–48)		(10–20)		Freinkel (1960)
	57	32		11		Oppenheimer et al.
	(44–71)	(21–43)		(8–13)		(1963)
Immunoprecipitation	~75	~15		~10		Woeber and Ingbar (1968)
Dialysis curve fitting	73	19		8		Sutherland and Simpson-Morgan (1975)
		PA_1 PA_2		ALB_1 $ALB_{n>1}$		
Theoretical	68	17 <0.001		10 4		Prince and Ramsden (1977)
	68	11 0.1		15 5		Section C.3
		Triiodothyronine				
Electrophoresis	72	0		15		Braverman and Ingbar (1965)
Theoretical	80	9		11		Prince and Ramsden (1977)
		PA_1 PA_2		ALB_1 $ALB_{n>1}$		
	38	26 1		26 9		Section C.3

[a] M. and (± 2 S.D.). Electrophoresis was at alkaline pH and with non-physiological buffer.

in the relative amount of binding by PA and albumin. It is noteworthy that only one site on PA accounts for most of the PA binding whereas the weak sites on serum albumin appear to account for a considerable amount of binding to this protein. Furthermore, the recent data were obtained under conditions that more closely approximate the physiological. Based on these data, it can be calculated that unoccupied sites represent about 75% of total TBG sites, 98% of total PA sites and virtually all of the albumin sites.

Y

Results on T_3 distribution are less certain. The early electrophoretic experiments are probably incorrect because the low affinity of T_3 for PA leads to dissociation during the procedure. The same may be the case in the immunoprecipitation experiments of Prince and Ramsden (1977) from which they estimated the affinity constants used in their theoretical calculation. Our own calculations, based on direct estimates of T_3-binding constants, give a surprisingly low fraction bound to TBG and a high fraction to PA as well as albumin. The method of Sutherland and Simpson-Morgan has not been applied to T_3 binding, but should be useful. As expected, T_3 occupies very few of the total sites on any of the transport proteins.

It is of interest to note from Fig. 3 in Section C.3 that there is a significant variation in the distribution of both T_4 and T_3 over the normal range of hormone concentration.

2. Artifacts Affecting Hormone Measurement

(a) Agents affecting iodine analyses

As noted above, thyroid hormones and their metabolites are nowadays almost exclusively measured by displacement techniques and radioimmunoassay is by all odds the most generally used. Iodine containing drugs, iodide itself, and those few compounds which interfere with the cerate–arsenite reaction (i.e. gold and mercury) are therefore less important than formerly. If the PBI or BEI are used iodine-containing materials cause serious problems. Iodide or any drug which liberates iodide will, of course, affect radioiodine uptake studies and may affect thyroid function. Compilations of drugs containing iodine have been published (Pileggi, Lee, Golub and Henry, 1961; Davis, 1966). It should be noted that these same drugs also alter urinary iodine and this measurement is required to determine the absolute uptake of iodine by the thyroid.

(b) Agents affecting thyroxine–protein interactions

Many drugs compete with T_4 and T_3 for binding to one or more of the binding proteins TBG, PA and albumin. In general, if the drug binds tightly to TBG or PA and is present in blood in adequate amounts, both physical and physiological adjustments ensue. Immediately upon introduction of the drug into the blood stream its binding to, say, TBG causes by displacement an increase in free T_4 in blood. This will cause a temporary decrease in TSH secretion and a slowing of T_4 secretion. Usually within a day the level of T_4 (and T_3) decreases enough so the free T_4 and T_3 are normal. Hence precise analyses of serum for total T_4 and T_3 will show levels lower than normal but the free T_4 and T_3 will be in the normal range. Some of the drugs which cause this phenomenon are shown in Table 19. In addition to these effects, however, some of these drugs may affect the actual analysis for T_4 or T_3 in serum. In general, these drugs do not interfere with radioimmunoassay of blood for T_4 or T_3 since the antibodies used are highly specific. This is true whether the method uses extraction of serum or whether it uses unextracted serum with anilinonaphthalene sulphonic acid (ANS) to prevent TBG binding.

Table 19

Drugs interacting with thyroxine binding proteins of blood.

Drug	Binds to TBG	Binds to PA	References
Salicylate		+	Larsen (1972a)
Diphenylhydantoin	+		Wolff et al. (1961)
Halofenate	+		Karch et al. (1976)
Chlorpropamide	+		Hershman et al. (1968)
Tolbutamide	+		Hershman et al. (1968)
o,p'-DDD	+		Marshall and Tompkins (1968)
Penicillin		+	Surks and Oppenheimer (1963)
Diazepam	+		Schussler (1971)

If competitive binding assay is employed, however, the offending drug, if it binds to TBG, will act like T_4 and result in a spuriously elevated value for T_4. This is likely to be the case with either the TBG competitive binding method of Murphy and Pattee (1964) or the Sephadex method of Braverman et al. (1971). Free fatty acids appear to involve thyroid hormone analyses in two ways: they somehow increase the free T_4 level in blood, perhaps by competing with T_4 for the protein binding sites, and they may interfere with the measurement of total T_4 if done by the competitive protein-binding method (Liewendahl and Helenius, 1976). Unsaturated fatty acids are more active than saturated fatty acids and these effects may be seen with mM concentrations. Total T_4 in blood measured by RIA is unaffected. Most of these perturbations caused by elevated levels of free fatty acids in serum are relatively small. There are other drugs which act physiologically to alter the concentrations of TBG or PA. These effects will be considered below.

(c) Effects of thyroid hormone replacement

Normally, thyroid hormones in human blood are comprised of about 97% thyroxine, 2% triiodothyronine and less than 1% rT_3. In a hypothyroid subject on thyroid hormone replacement therapy, or a euthyroid individual receiving enough thyroid to suppress endogenous hormone secretion, the amounts of T_4, T_3 and rT_3 in blood will depend on the nature of the material used for treatment. If T_4 is given in physiological amounts to an athyreotic subject, the T_4 in serum is generally within the normal range (Stock, Surks and Oppenheimer, 1974). Serum T_3 may be slightly below normal since as much as 30% of serum T_3 is of direct thyroidal origin. Serum rT_3 will be normal because essentially all of it is derived from peripheral deiodination of T_4. It used to be thought that with T_4 treatment the serum PBI was somewhat elevated but this may have been due to the use of larger amounts of T_4. Although the minimal amount of T_4 given to cause suppression of the thyroid should cause a slight elevation of serum T_4, this apparently does not raise its level above the normal range. If T_3 is used for therapy, the serum T_3 level may be considerably above the normal level of about 150 ng/ml (2·3 nmol/l) but this will depend on when the blood was drawn relative to the last dose of T_3. Serum T_4 levels in an individual on adequate doses of T_3 will be usually 2 μg/dl (25·7 nmol/l) or less. Recently a 4:1 mixture of $T_4:T_3$ has been formulated for therapy. This should give approximately normal blood levels for both T_4 and T_3. Desiccated thyroid glands or partially purified thyroglobulin may also be used for therapy. These preparations usually result in normal levels of T_4 and T_3 in blood when the replacement dose is accurate.

3. Physiological and Environmental Influences

(a) Age

The most dramatic changes in normal thyroid function in man occur at birth. Some years ago it was shown that normal infants showed a rise in PBI shortly after birth. This was later found to be due to a decrease in body temperature which, if prevented by a heated crib, abolished the PBI elevation (Fisher and Oddi, 1964). More recently the biochemical changes at birth have been elucidated. The normal full term infant shows a level of T_4 about the same as in the mother, which is somewhat above the adult value. The rT_3 level, however, is markedly elevated at birth (about 200 ng/dl (3·1 nmol/l)), whereas the T_3 level in serum is about 50 ng/dl (0·8 nmol/l) (one-third normal adult) (Fisher, Dussault, Sack and Chopra, 1977a). Within 24–28 hr after birth, serum T_4 in the neonate increases to about 16 μg/100 ml (206 nmol/l), free T_4 more than doubles, T_3 and free T_3 increase almost 3 fold (Erenberg, Phelps, Lam and Fisher, 1974). The level of rT_3 falls during this period to normal adult values (Fisher et al., 1977). A careful study of levels of T_3, rT_3, T_4 and TSH at very frequent intervals in the newborn shows that these levels oscillate as they approach a new steady state (Oddie, Bernard, Presley, Klein and Fisher, 1978). The oscillations dampen out as the new levels are reached. The concentration of TBG in serum, according to one report, remains more or less constant during this time at the elevated value of *ca.* 5 mg/100 ml (Erenberg *et al.*, 1974). Another study, however, suggests that the level of TBG in cord blood is about 1·1 mg/dl, rising by one month to a mean of about 1·3 mg/dl (Hesch, Gatz, Juppner and Stubbe, 1977). The reason for this discrepancy is unclear. TSH levels are elevated in cord blood and in the three-day old infant, falling to relatively low levels by six weeks of age (Abuid, Klein, Foley and Larsen, 1974).

There are changes in the levels of the thyroxine-binding serum proteins during puberty. In males in early adolescence, there appears to be a fall in PA which returns to normal by early adulthood (Malvaux, De Nayer, Beckers, van den Schrieck and de Visscher, 1966). TBG may show a slight elevation in preadolescence. In some reports the free T_4 does not change (Malvaux *et al.*, 1966; Braverman, Dawber and Ingbar, 1966) but in others a progressive fall is found (Fisher, Sack, Oddie, Pekary, Hershman, Lam and Parslow, 1977b).

Old age has been reported to involve a decrease in PBI but the most recent study of a total population showed a small progressive rise in T_4 (*ca.* 10%) with age in males and no change in females (Evered, Tunbridge, Hall, Appleton, Brewis, Clark, Manuel and Young, 1978). Serum triiodothyronine showed little change except in both males and females over 65 where it decreased slightly. Both T_3 and T_4 levels in serum were normally distributed. It is of interest that this study, in which thyroid disease and contraceptive histories were ascertained, the thyroid gland was palpated and antibodies to thyroglobulin were obtained, resulted in the exclusion of 15% of the males and 58% of the females (Evered *et al.*, 1978). This suggests that:

(i) there exists a substantial amount of thyroid disease in an unselected population,

(ii) a large number of women are either pregnant or taking oestrogens which alter thyroid hormone levels. Another study, however, has found a progressive fall in serum T_3 with age amounting to about 5 ng/dl (77 pmol/l)/decade (Rubenstein, Butler and Werner, 1973).

(b) Gonadal influences and pregnancy

Pregnancy was known for many years to increase the PBI and when TBG was studied it was found that the elevated level of thyroid hormone was due to an elevation of TBG in blood occurring early in the first trimester (Dowling, Freinkel and Ingbar, 1956a; Robbins and Nelson, 1958). It was subsequently found that administration of oestrogens also causes an increase in the level of TBG and a concentration two to three times normal may be achieved (Dowling, Freinkel and Ingbar, 1956b). The amount of oestrogens in most contraceptive medications is adequate to cause a rise in TBG. Recent studies in monkeys and in isolated monkey hepatocytes have shown that the increase in TBG levels caused by oestradiol is due to an increase in its rate of synthesis (Glinoer, Gershengorn, Dubois and Robbins, 1977a; Glinoer, McGuire, Gershengorn, Robbins and Berman, 1977b). Oestrogens also cause a decrease in the level of PA in blood (Sakurada, Saito, Inagaki, Tayama and Torikai, 1967). Since PA is of minor importance in binding of T_4, the effect of oestrogens on TBG predominates and causes the rise in serum T_4. The mechanism for this effect has been described above. Oestriol has essentially no effect on TBG, oestradiol being the major active steroid in this respect (Katz and Kappas, 1967). Antioestrogens such as clomiphene block an oestrogenic response but by themselves have little or no effect on PA or TBG (Barbosa, Seal and Doe, 1973). The reverse situation also occurs;

Table 20

Factors affecting levels of thyroxine binding proteins in blood.

Drug or condition	TBG	PA	References
Pregnancy	↑	→	Robbins and Nelson (1958)
			Dowling et al. (1956a)
Oestrogens	↑	↓	Dowling et al. (1956b)
			Sakurada et al. (1967)
Androgens	↓	↑	Federman et al. (1958)
Anabolic steroids[a]	↓	↑	Braverman and Ingbar (1967)
			Rosenberg et al. (1962)
Antiestrogens[b]	→	→	Barbosa et al. (1973)

[a] Including norethandrolone, dianabol and nilevar.
[b] Clomiphene, diphenylindine, diphenyldihydronaphthalene.

namely, a fall in TBG levels caused by exogenous androgens (Federman, Robbins and Rall, 1958). Anabolic steroids with relatively minor androgenic activity also cause a fall in TBG, usually directly related to their potency as an anabolic agent (Rosenberg, Ahn and Mitchell, 1962; Braverman and Ingbar, 1967). Table 20 lists the effects of some gonadal hormones on TBG and PA. Androgens affect PA causing an increase in the level of this protein. This appears to be due to an increased rate of synthesis of PA (Braverman, Socolow, Woeber and Ingbar, 1968). Again the main effect is on TBG which causes, by mechanisms previously described, a fall in total serum T_4. Interestingly, in the testicular feminisation syndrome in which the androgenic effects of testosterone cannot be manifested, norethandrolone had no effect on TBG although oestrogens were capable of causing an increase (Vagenakis, Hamilton, Maloof, Braverman and Ingbar, 1972).

It should be noted that with both oestrogens and androgens total T_3 parallels total T_4 rising with oestrogens or pregnancy and falling with androgens. In all circumstances, the levels of free T_4 and free T_3 remain within the normal range (Dussault, Fisher, Nicoloff, Row and Volpe, 1973).

During the normal menstrual cycle in the human there appears to be only one change in thyroid activity and even this is indirect. There is a considerably greater sensitivity to exogenous TRH in a preovulatory than in a post-ovulatory woman (Sanchez-Franco, Garcia, Cacicedo, Martin-Zurrow and Escobar del Ray, 1973). This is manifested by a greater TSH response. Curiously, women receiving contraceptive steroids show a normal response to TRH (Wenzel, Meinhold, Herpich, Adlkofer and Schleusener, 1974).

(c) Diet

One of the major effects of diet upon thyroid activity and hence the level of thyroid hormones in blood is mediated by the amount of iodine in the diet. Iodine is a trace element in soil and water so that it may easily become rate limiting in thyroid hormone synthesis as the normal human thyroid secretes about 70 μg of iodine/day, largely as T_4. The thyroid iodide-concentrating mechanism and quite possibly the deiodinating enzymes, have evolved to permit the most efficient use of the iodine available. In general, a dietary intake of 0·1 mg iodine/day is adequate to prevent goitre (Kelly and Snedden, 1960). In many areas of the world even this level is not available and endemic goitre becomes prevalent. Up to a certain point, a very efficient goitre which will capture 80% or more of the ingested iodine plus 80% of the iodine released upon deiodinative metabolism of the iodothyronines is adequate to prevent hypothyroidism. Furthermore, such an active goitre also effectively retains iodide released by the intrathyroidal deiodination of iodotyrosines. There is an obligatory faecal loss of 20–30% of the iodine from secreted thyroid hormone so a dietary level of less than 20 μg (157 nmol) of iodine/day usually results in goitrous hypothyroidism. This will be manifested by the usual clinical signs and with depressed levels of T_4 in blood (Stanbury, 1969). In severe iodine deficiency, however, there is increased secretion of T_3 (and perhaps increased T_4 to T_3 conversion) so that a low level of T_4 in serum with normal or elevated serum T_3 values may be seen (Camus and Ermans, 1972; Patel, Pharoah, Hornabrook and Hetzel, 1973; Stevenson, Silva and Pineda, 1974). The level of thyroglobulin in serum may also be increased, perhaps due to the increased TSH levels found in iodine-deficient goitre (Van Herle, Chopra, Hershman and Hornabrook, 1976). The serum iodide level is markedly reduced in iodine deficiency. In a few individuals with a goitre due to iodine deficiency hyperthyroidism may follow the intake of moderate doses of iodine presumably because the thyroid and pituitary are unable to adjust rapidly enough to this change (Matovinovic and Ramalingoswami, 1960).

Somewhat surprising is that the other major cause of goitre and hypothyroidism secondary to an unusual diet is excessive iodine. This is most commonly seen in the northern islands of Japan where seaweed is consumed in large quantity (Suzuki, Higuchi, Sawa, Ohtaki and Yoshihiko, 1965; Wolff, 1969). Large amounts of iodide inhibit thyroxine synthesis in the thyroid as was shown in the rat many years ago (Wolff and Chaikoff, 1948). The precise mechanism for this effect is still unknown. Usually in humans after several days, this inhibition is relieved, probably by a compensatory decrease in thyroid iodide concentration (Braverman and Ingbar, 1963). In Japan, iodide goitre with or without hypothyroidism is seen in 6–12% of individuals consuming a diet high in iodine (50–200 mg (400–1600 nmol) I/day) (Matovinovic and Ramalingaswami, 1960). Why these individuals are unable to adapt to a high iodine intake is still unknown. If goitre and hypothyroidism develop, depressed levels of T_4 and T_3 are found in blood.

Goitrogens of several different types have been identified in foods but whether they are present in sufficient quantity to cause goitre or hypothyroidism has still not been proved unequivocally. The first positive identification of a goitrogen in food was by Greer and Etlinger who isolated L-5-vinylthio-oxazolidone from vegetables of the brassica family (Greer, 1962). Thiocyanate may also be produced from certain foods and is goitrogenic but only in relatively large dosage (Clements, 1960). The goitrogenic effects of these agents may be enhanced in the presence of mild iodine deficiency. A large amount of soy bean products in infants' diets may be a rare cause of goitre, perhaps by increased stool bulk and hence faecal loss of thyroid hormone (Pinchera, MacGillivray, Crawford and Freeman, 1965).

There is some evidence that in South America goitre is associated with the ingestion of water derived from certain geologic formations (Gaitan, Island and Liddle, 1969). Calcium, implicated at one time, now does not appear to be involved (Harrison, Harden and Alexander, 1967). The association of goitre with microbiologically-contaminated drinking water has also been noted but not proved as a cause (Vought, Brown and Sibinovic, 1974).

Recently it has been recognised that starvation or serious undernutrition affects the metabolism of thyroxine causing a depression in the $T_4 \rightarrow T_3$ conversion and an increase in the $T_4 \rightarrow rT_3$ reaction (Vagenakis, Burger, Portnay, Rudolph, O'Brian, Azizi, Arky, Nicod, Ingbar and Braverman, 1975; Vagenakis, Portnay, O'Brian, Rudolph, Arky, Ingbar and Braverman, 1977). These effects are direct and no change in clearance of T_3 is seen. The result is a decrease in the level of T_3 in blood and an increase in rT_3. Levels of T_4 in serum are generally unchanged. Furthermore, the same effects are seen in patients receiving T_4 so this is a peripheral phenomenon and does not involve the thyroid. In spite of the low level of serum T_3 the concentration of TSH is not increased. A fall in serum T_3 can also be seen during a period of low energy intake if no carbohydrate is included in the diet; however, in this case no rise in serum rT_3 is seen (Spaulding, Chopra, Sherwin and Lyall, 1976). A diet with the same energy level all supplied by carbohydrate has no effect on T_3 or rT_3 levels in blood (Spaulding *et al.*, 1976). Hence, the type as well as a sufficiency of energy in a diet appears to modulate the peripheral metabolism of T_4. Prealbumin levels fall with malnutrition and are a very sensitive early manifestation of malnutrition (Ingenbleck, van den Schriek, De Nayer and De Visscher, 1975).

(d) Activity, stress, diurnal variation

Strenuous activity such as conditioning of race horses causes a marked increase in thyroxine secretion and turnover (Irvine, 1967). There is some evidence that a similar phenomenon can be observed in man (Irvine, 1968) although the change is not so dramatic. It should be noted that this type of exercise is chronic training for days or weeks. The effects of acute exercise are complicated by plasma and extracellular fluid changes. In spite of the increase in T_4 secretion and metabolism the level of T_4 in blood is no different between the highly trained and the untrained man (Irvine, 1968). The free T_4 level, however, appears to be elevated in the trained athlete (De Nayer, Ostyn and DeVisscher, 1970). It is not known as yet how T_3 and rT_3 are affected by prolonged exercise.

The effect of stress on the thyroid is likely to be a result of increases in cortisol and epinephrine (adrenaline) secretion, alterations in TSH levels, and changes in fluid volume and distribution. Clearly different stressful situations may also have specific effects. A variety of stresses in experimental animals (electric shock, burns, hemorrhage, etc.) produces a depression of thyroid function due to decreased levels of TSH (Brown-Grant, 1960; Brown-Grant and Pethes, 1960). Occasionally, as with injections of bacterial exotoxin, an increased secretion by the thyroid is seen (Gerwing, Long and Pitt-Rivers, 1958). The major stress studied in man has been surgery. In general, thyroid activity changes little and the serum T_4 is unchanged (Bernstein, Hasen and Oppenheimer, 1967). Surgery causes a fall in T_3 and a rise in rT_3 which could be mediated by increased adrenocortical activity (Burr, Black, Griffiths and Hoffenberg, 1975). The effects of emotional stress on thyroid function and the level of thyroid hormones in blood have been disputed for some years and no clear cut conclusion is possible. Some recent data however suggest that the anticipation of physical stress can produce a modest rise in serum TSH in young men (Mason, Hartley, Kotchen, Wherry, Pennington and Jones, 1966). Many of these studies were performed before methods were available for measurement of T_3 and rT_3 and probably should be repeated.

Cortisol (or any of the glucocorticoids, such as prednisone or dexamethasone) has definite effects on the thyroid which in general are inhibitory (Bernstein and Oppenheimer, 1966). The mechanism of the thyroidal effect seems to be that cortisol inhibits TSH secretion (Nicoloff, Fisher and Appleman, 1970). Since cortisol is secreted on a diurnal basis this produces a small diurnal variation in thyroid hormone secretion (Nicoloff et al., 1970). This is best seen with a sensitive double isotope method for measuring T_4 release from the thyroid (Nicoloff et al., 1970). Cortisol also has extra-thyroidal effects which manifest themselves on the levels of thyroid hormones in blood. A decrease in TBG and an increase in PA is produced by cortisol Oppenheimer and Werner, 1966). Since TBG is more important this tends to cause a fall in serum T_4. Cortisol also affects the metabolism of T_4 so that the level of T_3 in serum falls while that of rT_3 increases (Chopra, Williams, Orgiazzi and Solomon, 1975b). This effect is seen in individuals during treatment with T_4 so it is clearly an effect on extrathyroidal T_4 metabolism.

The data on the effects of catecholamines on the thyroid are somewhat contradictory and in many instances were obtained with very large doses. In isolated cells, with thyroid slices, or with membranes small effects may be elicited. Perhaps the main reason for interest currently is that many nerve terminals have been noted in and around thyroid follicles in the human thyroid (Melander, Sundler and Westgren, 1975).

(e) Environmental temperature, altitude

Temperature adaptation has usually been thought to involve the thyroid particularly since it has been shown that the Na^+K^+ ATPase, a major source of heat production, is under thyroid control (Ismail-Beigi and Edelman, 1971). In experimental animals, acute, moderately severe cooling produces a rise in TSH and activation of the thyroid (Yamada, Kajihara, Onaya, Kobayashi, Takemura and Shichijo, 1965). There is reason to believe that this is mediated via an increase in TRH secretion (Montoya, Seibel and Wilber, 1975). In man, however, cooling adequate to cause a fall in body temperature had no effect on the level of TSH in blood (Hershman and Pittman, 1971). As noted above, the newborn human, however, responds to hypothermia with increased secretion of TSH. In the experimental animals where acute cold stress caused TSH increases, they were followed by increased levels of T_4 in blood. In man no such changes are seen. The chronic effects of cold are different and in some species an increased metabolism of T_4 is seen (Hillier, 1968; Galton and Nisula, 1969). An increased rate of T_4 metabolism has also been noted in female divers exposed to extreme cold

(Hong, 1973). No data are as yet available on the production rates of T_3 and rT_3 in these circumstances.

Exposure of experimental animals or man to an elevated temperature also produces changes in the thyroid (Yousef and Johnson, 1965; Collins and Weiner, 1968). Acclimatisation to heat seems to cause a fall in the BMR (Chaffee and Roberts, 1971). Furthermore, thyroid uptake of ^{131}I and the degradation rate of thyroxine are lowered (Dempsey and Astwood, 1943; Lewitus, Hasenfratz, Toor, Massary and Rabinowitch, 1964; Yousef and Johnson, 1965). Concomitant effects of heat on fluid compartmentalisation, on food intake and on the secretion of other hormones such as cortisol may play such major roles that a direct effect of heat on the thyroid is not assured. It seems clear that rats are less tolerant of large doses of T_4 at elevated temperatures (Bodansky, Pilcher and Duff, 1936).

The effects of high altitude on the thyroid have also been studied. Here again known shifts in fluid causing haemoconcentration and adrenocortical stimulation are probably responsible for at least some of the change seen. Acute exposure to high altitude (usually over 3000 m) causes within a day or two considerable elevations in the serum levels of both T_3 and T_4 (Surks, 1966; Surks, Beckwitt and Chidsey, 1967; Rastoqi, Malhotra, Srivastava, Sawhney, Dua, Sridharan, Hoon and Singh, 1977). There are small discrepancies in these reports but in general the T_3 elevation is greater than that of T_4, and the level of free T_4 also increases. The level of T_3 tends to return towards normal by two weeks but the level of T_4 remains high. There is probably no change in the level of TBG or PA (Surks, 1966; Rastogi et al., 1977). Thyroxine metabolism was increased upon exposure to high altitude (Surks et al., 1967). TSH levels appear not to change (Rastogi et al., 1977). Unfortunately rT_3 levels have not been measured. It is not at all clear how these data can be put together to make sense. An elevated T_4 with an increased rate of T_4 disposal must imply an increased secretion of T_4 but TSH is not increased. The increased T_3 level could come from increased T_4 and an increased $T_4 \rightarrow T_3$ conversion. An activation of adrenal steroid secretion should cause an opposite effect, however (Mackinnon, Monk-Jones and Fotherby, 1963). Almost all of the thyroid changes have either returned to normal or are close to normal (serum T_4) in a few weeks.

4. Genetic Abnormalities in Thyroxine-binding Proteins

Congenital analbuminemia has little effect on thyroid hormone levels in blood although the levels of both TBG and PA are increased (Hollander, Bernstein and Oppenheimer, 1966). Curiously, in one case the levels of free T_4 were elevated (Hollander, et al., 1966). In bisalbuminemia one or both of the albumins may bind thyroxine (Andreoli and Robbins, 1962, Sarcione and Aungst, 1962). No genetic variation in PA has been reported for the human. In certain monkeys, mainly *M. mulata*, PA exists in polymorphic form. The mutation appears not to impair T_4 binding although one phenotype has twice the level of PA as the other (Bernstein, Robbins and Rall, 1970; Van Jaarsveld, Branch, Robbins, *et al.*, 1973a).

Congenital abnormalities in TBG have been described in which there is either an elevation or a depression in the level of TBG in blood. Usually neither of these abnormalities is associated with any clinical signs of disease. Congenital increase in TBG causes an increased total serum T_4 to twice normal values; T_3 is similarly elevated (Beierwaltes and Robbins, 1959; Refetoff, Fang, Marshall and Robin, 1976). The level of free T_4 (and presumably free T_3) in serum is normal. The T_3 resin uptake is low. All other measures of thyroid activity are normal. The mechansim for this condition appears to reside in an increased rate of synthesis of TBG (Refetoff *et al.*, 1976). No evidence for abnormal degradation of TBG or unusual affinity of TBG for either T_4 or T_3 is seen (Refetoff *et al.*, 1976). The genetics of this curious disorder show that it is an X-linked dominant (Jones and Seal, 1967). Hence, females who are heterozygous show less of an elevation of TBG than males who are homozygous and in whom TBG is about four times normal (Jones and Seal, 1967; Fialkow, Giblett and Musa, 1970; Shane, Seal and Jones, 1971). Although there is some disagreement in the literature, a recent study shows that in two women with congenital elevation of TBG, administration of oestrogens caused a further increase in TBG (Shane, *et al.*, 1971). In women half of the X chromosomes are randomly inactivated so presumably half of the cells of such heterozygous women carry a normal X chromosome which can respond to oestrogens. However, one male with elevated TBG has been reported who showed a further increase in TBG upon treatment with oestrogens (Jones and Seal, 1967). This one case suggests that even the chromosome with the defect can also respond to oestrogens. One unusual family has been reported in which congenital elevation of TBG was associated with goitres in a significant number of subjects. Linkage between a putative gene involved in goitre formation and the gene for TBG synthesis (or for the synthesis of a repressor for TBG) could result in this situation (Shane *et al.*, 1971).

The reverse situation of congenital decrease or absence of TBG occurs (Ingbar, 1961; Refetoff, Robin and Alper, 1972b). The condition is also inherited as an X-linked dominant (Nicoloff, Dowling and Patton, 1964). Since this is a rare condition, homozygosity in the female is almost never encountered. The homozygous male has absent TBG whereas the hemizygous female has a level of TBG about half normal. However, males with a low but measurable level of TBG have been reported (Emslander and Gorman, 1971; Refetoff *et al.*, 1972b). Different mutations could easily account for these differences. Included in this group is an infant with Beckwith's syndrome and low TBG (Kaufman and Frederickson, 1973). Careful studies of the TBG from such women show it to be normal with respect to affinity for T_4 and T_3, rate of degradation in blood, rate of heat inactivation, and immunological parameters (Refetoff et al., 1972b).

There are several reports that oestrogen administration does not increase TBG levels in such subjects (Ingbar, 1961; Nikolai and Seal, 1966a, b). As might be expected, the serum T_4 is quite low as is the T_3 in subjects with absent or low TBG. The T_3 resin uptake is high and the level of free T_4 in blood is normal. Treatment with thyroid or thyroxine does not usually bring the serum T_4 level to normal and can even produce symptoms of hyperthyroidism in the presence of a low serum T_4 (Kaufman and Frederickson, 1973). There have been a few cases of hyperthyroidism in individuals with low or absent TBG, and it has been suggested that there is a real association between these two conditions (Horwitz and Refetoff, 1977).

5. Diseases of the Thyroid Gland

(a) Hyperthyroidism

The hallmark of hyperthyroidism is overproduction of one or both thyroid hormones. Although peripheral degradation also increases, the net result is a rise in hormone concentration in plasma. Early studies established that an elevation of the PBI was one of the most accurate laboratory tests for hyperthyroidism (Kydd, Man and Peters, 1950; McConahey, Owen and Keating, 1956). This is now seen as a rise in serum T_4, which in the average case is increased 2·5 fold (Larsen, 1978). It should be evident that a continuum must exist between blood hormone levels in the euthyroid state, regardless of the technique of measurement, and those in which hormone secretion is mildly abnormal. Therefore, T_4 concentrations in the overlap region must be interpreted in the context of other clinical data. Diagnostic accuracy has been increased further by measurement of serum T_3 since a proportion of cases, when first examined, have elevated T_3 levels but normal T_4—so-called "T_3-thyrotoxicosis" (Hollander, Mitsuma, Shenkman, Nihei et al., 1972a, b; Sterling, 1970). The prevalence of this syndrome appears to vary inversely with dietary iodine supply. In the United States, it is about 5% of cases (Hollander, Mitsuma, Shenkman, Stevenson et al., 1972b) and may be as high as 30% in some parts of Great Britain (Shalet, Beardwell, Lamb and Gowland, 1975).

In the average case of hyperthyroidism, the serum T_3 is increased about 4·5 fold (Larsen, 1978). The relatively greater increase in T_3 compared to T_4 appears mainly to be the result of an increased relative secretion rate which in turn depends on a higher T_3/T_4 ratio in thyroglobulin (Izumi and Larsen, 1977). Although these findings suggest that measurement of the T_3 level might be the best single test in screening for hyperthyroidism, it probably can be reserved for the follow-up investigation of patients in whom there is a clinical suspicion of hyperthyroidism in the face of a normal T_4 level. A diminished T_4 to T_3 conversion caused by a complicating illness (see Section 6), or perhaps even severe thyrotoxicosis, can present a problem in interpreting the T_3 level, and there is a suggestion that hyperthyroidism with a high serum T_4 but a normal T_3 may occur occasionally (see Larsen, 1978).

Excess T_3 secretion is not the only reason for the poor correlation of the clinical severity of hyperthyroidism and the degree of thyroxine elevation (Schultz and Zieve, 1958). Another explanation is a decreased concentration of TBG, which occurs in many thyrotoxic patients (Chopra, Solomon and Ho, 1972b; Rudorff, Herrman, Kroll and Kruskemper, 1976; Guerin and Tubiana, 1964; Lemarchand-Beraud, Assayah and Vanotti, 1964). In some, especially when there is a genetic defect in TBG, the decrease is great enough to prevent an elevation of serum thyroxine above the normal (Cavalieri, 1961; Horwitz and Refetoff, 1977; Gerstner and Kaplan, 1976). A decrease in PA level also occurs (Smith and Goodman, 1971). In such cases, the free T_4 and free T_3 concentrations are elevated, as are also the entire gamut of tests, such as T_3 uptake or free T_4 index, which depend on the concentration of unoccupied thyroxine-binding sites. The measured FT_4 and FT_3 levels in hyperthyroidism are, on the average, 3–5 times normal, which is similar to the average increase of total T_3 but larger than that of total T_4 (Sterling, 1971; Ingbar et al., 1965; Oppenheimer et al., 1963; Yeo et al., 1977; Jiang and Tue, 1977; Peterson et al., 1977; Sawin et al., 1978). This is consistent with the expected relationship between free and total hormones even when the binding proteins remain normal (see Section C.3).

No consistent difference has been seen in the serum hormone patterns in various types of hyperthyroidism; i.e. Graves' disease, toxic multinodular goitre or toxic adenoma.

Many of the non-hormonal iodine components of blood also are elevated in hyperthyroidism. Reverse triiodothyronine (rT_3) is increased 2–4 fold (Chopra, 1974; Kaplan et al., 1977; Faber, Friis, Kirkegaard and Siersbaek-Nielsen, 1978) and 3,3'-diiodothyronine is increased 2–3 fold (Burger and Sakaloff, 1977; Wu et al., 1976; Burman et al., 1977). Diiodotyrosine also appears to be increased (Nelson et al., 1976). The acetic acid derivatives of T_4 and T_3, however, are unchanged (Burger, 1976; Nakamura et al., 1978).

A number of studies have described an increase in serum thyroglobulin (Hjort, Lauridsen and Persson, 1970; Torrigiani et al., 1969; Uller and Van Herle, 1978). Although the increase is substantial—averaging 35 times normal in one study (Uller and Van Herle, 1978)—thyroglobulin still comprises only a few per cent of the serum iodine in hyperthyroidism. The increase is a reflection of functional stimulation of the thyroid cells, since similar elevations are seen following stimulation of the normal thyroid by TSH (Uller, Van Herle and Chopra, 1973). In addition, a further, acute increase is seen immediately after thyroidectomy and as a delayed response after radioiodine therapy, reflecting thyroid cell damage (Uller and Van Herle, 1978; Torrigiani et al., 1969). Restoration of normal function is accompanied by normalisation of the serum thyroglobulin level, and this might be a useful indicator of remission during antithyroid drug therapy (Uller and Van Herle, 1978).

The blood iodide level can be expected to vary according to the balance between dietary intake, thyroid clearance and thyroxine degradation. Some of the values reported in hyperthyroidism have been low (Aboul-Khair and Crooks, 1965). The rapid iodide clearance coupled with an increased rate of hormone secretion in hyperthyroidism led to the adoption of measurement of hormonal radioiodine as a diagnostic test (Ingbar et al., 1954; Clark et al., 1949; and many others). This so-called "conversion ratio" requires a rather large dose of radioiodine and its use as a clinical test is no longer justified.

(b) Hypothyroidism

In hypothyroidism due to athyreosis the blood findings simply reflect a decrease in thyroidal iodide clearance and a decrease in secretion of thyroid hormones. Partial thyroid insufficiency is common, however, and overlap of values with the normal range is more troublesome than in hyperthyroidism. Recent measurements of T_4, T_3 and TSH have revealed further diagnostic difficulties. Thus an elevated serum TSH, usually taken as a sensitive indicator of primary hypothyroidism, may be accompanied by normal T_4 and T_3, indicating a compensated stage of thyroid failure. A frequent finding in such patients is a normal or even an elevated T_3 level with a subnormal T_4 level (Larsen, 1972). This is seen in endemic goitre (Pharoah, Lawton, Ellis et al., 1973) where iodine deficiency appears to cause a decrease in the T_4/T_3 ratio in thyroglobulin. It is also seen following treatment of hyperthyroidism (Sterling, Brenner, Newman et al., 1971) or, indeed, in any kind of functionally damaged thyroid gland. It is the result of a relative increase in the secretion of T_3 compared to T_4, and possibly of an increase in the peripheral conversion of T_4 to T_3 as well (Inada, Kasagi, Kurata et al., 1975).

A further complication is the fact that the serum T_3 level may be decreased in a variety of non-thyroid illnesses, or during nutritional or other stresses, as a result of diminished extrathyroidal conversion of T_4 to T_3 (see Section

E.6). Furthermore, the depressed T_3 level may be unaccompanied by clinical evidence of hypothyroidism. It is evident, therefore, that the serum T_4 level is a more appropriate screening test for hypothyroidism than the T_3 level.

An additional problem is the finding of decreased PA, and sometimes TBG levels, in many non-thyroid diseases (see Section E.6) which can result in a low total T_4 in some patients, but no clinical hypothyroidism. In such patients, the free T_4 level and free T_4 index are normal or even elevated (Harvey, 1971; Carter, Corcoran, Eastman and Lazarus, 1974). This indicates that the free hormone level, especially T_4, or any of the related tests of unoccupied binding sites, is a more discriminating test for hypothyroidism than the total hormone level in severely ill patients. It is of interest that in uncomplicated hypothyroidism the concentration of unoccupied thyroxine-binding sites, a determinant of the free hormone levels, is increased not only by virtue of the fall in thyroxine level but also by a slight increase in the concentration of TBG (Robbins and Rall, 1957; Tanaka and Starr, 1959; Lemarchand-Beraud et al., 1964; Oppenheimer et al., 1963; Rudorff et al., 1976; Cavalieri, 1975).

In hypothyroidism associated with goitre, the findings may be more complicated due to the occurrence of iodoproteins in blood (see below). Although not limited to hypothyroid patients, this finding may be more striking in them due to the low or absent thyroxine level. Extremely high circulating levels of this non-hormonal iodine may sometimes be observed in congenital goitre (Van Zyl, Schulz, Wilson and Pansegrouw, 1965). Since iodine analysis is seldom used now, these diagnostic complications are of little importance at present. In endemic and congenital goitres radioiodine studies often reveal changes indicative of hyperthyroidism despite a low hormone level (Stanbury, Brownell, Riggs, Perinetti, Itoiz and DelCastillo, 1954). Again, these tests of thyroid function, e.g. the "conversion ratio", are seldom used at the present time. In congenital goitre, the blood may reflect a specific alteration in iodine metabolism. Thus, congenital goitres due to deiodinase deficiency will have iodotyrosines in blood (Stanbury, Kassenaar, Meijer and Terpstra, 1955; McGirr, Hutchinson and Clement, 1956).

The serum hormone levels in hypothyroid patients under replacement therapy is discussed in Section E.2.c.

(c) Thyroiditis

Both subacute thyroiditis and chronic lymphocytic thyroiditis can pass through clinical phases of hyperthyroidism and hypothyroidism (cf. Robbins, Rall and Gorden, 1978b), and the serum levels of T_4 and T_3 are altered as would be expected from the preceding discussions. The special features of these diseases with respect to the blood are that they both lead to elevated levels of iodoproteins, and that sometimes autoantibodies are produced that react strongly with T_4 and T_3.

In subacute thyroiditis, the PBI is frequently elevated (Keating, Haines, Power and Williams, 1950; Robbins, Rall, Trunnell and Rawson, 1951; Volpe, McAllister and Huber, 1958) in spite of a reduced rate of iodine metabolism by the thyroid gland. A significant portion is insoluble in butanol (Ingbar and Freinkel, 1958a) and thus may be due in part to thyroglobulin liberated from disrupted thyroid follicles. Consistent elevation of Tg has indeed been found by radioimmunoassay (Van Herle, Uller, Matthews and Brown, 1973; Glinoer, Puttemans, Van Herle et al., 1974). This is not unlike the finding in the thyroiditis caused by acute irradiation with ^{131}I, where thyroglobulin liberated into the blood has been clearly identified (Robbins, 1954; Robbins, Petermann and Rall, 1954; Toro-Goyco and Matos, 1965; Uller and Van Herle, 1978).

In chronic lymphocytic thyroiditis, circulating butanol-insoluble iodine has also been found in considerable quantity (Gribetz, Talbot and Crawford, 1954; LeBouef and Bongiovanni, 1964). In this case, however, it appears to be the albumin-like iodoprotein characteristic of many types of thyroid disorder (Owen and McConahey, 1956; Torizuka, Flax and Stanbury, 1964; DeGroot, Hall, McDermott and Davis, 1962). It is quite likely that thyroglobulin exists in the blood in lymphocytic as well as in subacute thyroiditis, but, as pointed out by Torrigiani et al. (1969), the presence of anti-Tg antibodies would interfere with its detection in radioimmunoassay; with present methodology, Tg cannot be measured in the presence of these autoantibodies.

The binding of thyroxine and T_3 to circulating antithyroglobulin antibodies has been demonstrated in a significant number of cases (Premachandra and Blumenthal, 1967; Staeheli, Vallotan and Burger, 1975) but has no obvious effect on the clinical status. The high affinity of these immunoglobulins is evident from their ability to compete with TBG for the hormone. This bound form of hormone must be taken into account in evaluating thyroid status in these patients, and it may be important to measure the free hormone concentration.

(d) Non-toxic goitre and thyroid carcinoma

Sporadic goitres have been described which secrete mainly triiodothyronine (Rupp, Chevarria and Pachkis, 1959; Lissitzky, Codaccioni, Bismuth and Depieds, 1967) or other unusual compounds (Wynn, van Wyk, Deiss and Graham, 1962). In most cases, however, the abnormal finding is the non-specific one of albumin-like iodoprotein (cf. Robbins and Rall, 1960). Protein of this type, and in some cases iodoprealbumin, have been found in endemic goitre (Parker and Beierwaltes, 1962; Malamos et al., 1966), congenital goitre (Van Zyl et al., 1965; Robbins, Van Zyl and Van der Walt, 1966; Furth, Agrawal and Propp, 1970; DeGroot and Stanbury, 1959), sporadic goitre (Dowling, Ingbar and Freinkel, 1961) and autonomous thyroid nodules (Kahn, Cogan and Berger, 1962). In a few cases, immunological studies identified this material as serum albumin (Robbins et al., 1966; Lissitzky et al., 1967).

In at least two-thirds of thyroid carcinomas which contain follicular elements, a similar iodoprotein is present (Robbins et al., 1955; Tata et al., 1956; Horst and Rosler, 1953) and it may comprise most of the blood iodine. This material has the physical properties of serum albumin and may indeed be iodinated serum albumin in some cases (Robbins, 1966; Robbins and Weathers, 1966). In other instances, however, identity with serum albumin could not be established (Tata et al., 1956; Robbins, 1966; Robbins and Weathers, 1966). Functioning cancers characteristically secrete thyroxine, sometimes in sufficient quantity to cause hyperthyroidism (Robbins, 1966; Federman, 1964). Some secrete mainly T_3, and cause T_3-thyrotoxicosis (Suma and Cavalieri, 1973). There is no convincing evidence as yet for secretion of an iodinated material unique for thyroid carcinoma.

A more recent development has been the observation that differentiated thyroid cancers lead to increased levels of thyroglobulin in the blood (Van Herle and Uller, 1975). Although the levels may be extremely high, it has become increasingly clear that there is considerable overlap with the findings in non-malignant nodular goitre (Schneider et al., 1977; Torrigiani et al., 1969; Van Herle, 1977). Although the test may not be diagnostic of thyroid cancer, it remains useful in follow-up care of patients and can provide a sensitive indicator of tumour recurrence.

6. Non-thyroid Diseases

A wide variety of diseases is associated with either changes in thyroid function or with alterations in the level of thyroid hormones in blood. Some acute diseases cause increased adrenocortical activity with attendant effects on TBG and PA. Many diseases appear to influence metabolism of T_4 directly, with consequent alterations in T_3 or rT_3 levels in blood. Other diseases may affect the thyroid directly.

(a) Liver disease

Diseases of the liver can cause multiple changes in thyroid hormone levels since it is the main organ for synthesis of TBG, PA and albumin as well as the major route for metabolism of T_4. In infectious hepatitis, perhaps unexpectedly, the level of T_4 in serum is elevated due to an acute increase in

TBG (Vanotti and Beraud, 1959). Chronic liver disease can cause different changes. The serum level of T_4 is normal or low although occasionally elevated values are seen, probably depending on the severity of disease (Inada and Sterling, 1967a, b, c; Chopra, Solomon, Chopra, Young and Chua Teco, 1974). The level of serum T_4 usually reflects directly the level of TBG (Inada and Sterling, 1967a, b, c). The level of free T_4 in blood may be increased (McConnon, Row and Volpe, 1972; Chopra et al., 1974). There is frequently altered metabolism of T_4 so that serum T_3 is low and the level of rT_3 in blood is elevated (Nomura, Pittman, Chambers, Buck and Shimizu, 1975; Chopra, Chopra, Smith, Resa and Solomon, 1975a). The level of TSH in serum may be increased in chronic liver disease but its level does not appear to be related to the level of T_3 in blood (Chopra et al., 1974; Cuttelod, Lemarchand-Béraud, Magnenat, Perret, Poli and Vannotti, 1974; Nomura et al., 1975). An accumulation of partially desialated TBG in blood may be seen in severe liver disease (Marshall, Pensky and Green, 1972). The level of PA is usually low in liver disease.

Hepatocellular carcinoma of the liver is occasionally (about 10%) associated with an increase in serum TBG (Pedersen, 1974c; Gershengorn et al., 1976).

(b) Kidney disease

The wide variety of kidney diseases plus the effects of chronic haemodialysis can cause widely different effects on the thyroid. In nephrosis, the classical findings in a severely affected individual are: depressed serum T_4, TBG and PA with normal free T_4 (Robbins, Rall and Petermann, 1957; Musa, Seal and Doe, 1967). However, in the large majority of patients without large (> 20 gm/day) urinary losses of protein, both TBG and T_4 may be normal (Gavin, McMahon, Castle and Cavalieri, 1978). The free T_4 in serum may actually be increased above normal (Gavin et al., 1978). Serum T_3 is usually depressed and rT_3 is normal (Gavin et al., 1978). Levels of TSH in serum are usually in the normal range (Gavin et al., 1978). A complicating factor is treatment with corticosteroids which are given to many patients with nephrosis since these drugs act to depress TBG (Sherer and Siefring, 1956; Oppenheimer and Werner, 1966). Urinary losses of T_4 can be quite large and if the patient is in an area of low dietary iodine, can cause an iodine deficiency goitre (Gavin et al., 1978; Börner, Kammenhuber and Meissner, 1970).

Chronic renal disease with azotemia presents a different picture but one which can assume several forms. There may be sufficient retention of iodide by the impaired kidneys to depress thyroid uptake of ^{131}I. Goitre has been reported in a large fraction of patients with chronic disease but not in all reports (Baumann, Neuhaus and Thólen, 1974). Usually serum levels of T_4,

TBG and free T_4 are normal (Neuhaus, Baumann, Walser and Thólen, 1975). It has been suggested than an elevation of free T_4 occasionally noted may be due to accumulation of inhibitors of T_4 binding to TBG, such as indoles and phenols (Spaulding and Gregerman, 1972). T_3 may be depressed but rT_3 is in the normal range (Chopra, Chopra, Smith, Resa and Solomon, 1975a). In the latter study a small but significant depression of serum T_4 was seen although free T_4 was normal (Chopra et al., 1975a). TSH is probably normal (Ramírez, Jubiz, Gutch, Bloomer, Siegler and Kolff, 1973). Treatment with dialysis may cause a fall in serum T_4 (Silverberg, Ulan, Fawcett, Dossetor, Grace and Bettcher, 1973).

(c) *Endocrine diseases*

(1) *Cushing's syndrome* or hyperadrenocortical activity from any cause produces the same effects on thyroid hormones as the administration of large amounts of cortisol (see above).

(2) *Acromegaly.* The severity and duration of excessive growth hormone secretion in subjects with acromegaly and the occurrence of "burned out" cases may cause variable findings. In a significant fraction of acromegalic patients an elevated PA, a depressed TBG and depressed T_4 levels will be seen (Roth, Glick, Cuatrecasas and Hollander, 1967; Inada and Sterling, 1967a). There are old reports of a high incidence of goitre in acromegaly.

(3) *Molar pregnancy and choriocarcinoma.* It has been known for some years that subjects with hydatidiform mole or molar pregnancy frequently show laboratory evidence of hyperthyroidism (Dowling, Ingbar, and Freinkel, 1960). It would appear that most of these patients do not show evidence of clinical hyperthyroidism in spite of elevated levels of T_4 in blood (Odell, Bates, Rivlin, Lipsett and Hertz, 1963; Hershman and Higgins, 1971; Higgins, Hershman, Kenimer, Patillo, Bayley and Walfish, 1975; Nagataki, Mizuno, Sakamoto, Irie, Shizume, Nakao, Galton, Arky and Ingbar, 1977). In a recent study, over half of the patients with a molar pregnancy had elevated levels of T_4 in blood (Nagataki et al., 1977). Increased T_3 in blood was also seen in almost half the patients, occurring almost always in those with an increased serum T_4 (Nagataki et al., 1977). Free T_3 may also be increased, although it is usually normal (Osathanondh, Tulchinsky and Chopra, 1976). Estimation of the T_4 production rate in three subjects showed that it was markedly elevated, roughly in proportion to the level of T_4 (Nagataki et al., 1977). Unfortunately, measurements of rT_3 are not yet available. The reason most patients with molar pregnancy are not clinically hyperthyroid is unclear. The illness may mask mild hyperthyroidism. The rarity of frankly increased serum free T_3 with a possible shift in T_4 metabolism and some type of peripheral unresponsiveness to T_4 are all possible explanations.

The cause of the increased thyroid activity seems to reside in a circulating thyroid stimulator (Hennen, 1966; Hershman and Higgins, 1971; Kenimer, Hershman and Higgins, 1975). The present evidence seems to indicate that thyroid stimulatory activity is intrinsic to chorionic gonadotrophin and the enormous amounts of this material secreted by subjects with hydatidiform mole is sufficient to activate the thyroid (Kenimer et al., 1975). Chorio-carcinoma may produce the same results as molar pregnancy.

Toxemia of pregnancy is sometimes associated with elevated levels of T_4 and free T_4 in blood (Osathanondh et al., 1976). In some patients, T_3 and free T_3 levels were quite low. Although rT_3 was not measured, it seems likely that as in so many illnesses there is diversion of T_4 metabolism from T_3 production to rT_3 synthesis.

(d) Miscellaneous diseases

Although there are differences depending on the nature of the illness, most severe febrile infections are associated with an increase in blood of rT_3 and free rT_3 and a decrease in T_3 and free T_3 (Chopra et al., 1975a). T_4 levels are unchanged but free T_4 may be elevated. In some patients a fall in TBG may be seen (Harvey, 1971). Also it has been found that in some infections (pneumococcal pneumonia, febrile salmonella infection, perhaps malaria) there is an increased turnover of T_4 (De Rubertis and Woeber, 1973; Lutz, Gregerman, Spaulding, Hornick and Dawkins, 1973). However, some infections such as tularaemia show no such effect (Lutz et al., 1973). Fever associated with lymphoma may also cause accelerated T_4 metabolism (Gregerman and Solomon, 1967). Many febrile states also showed an increased urinary excretion of both T_3 and T_4 (Rastogi, Sawney and Talwar, 1976). It is important to note that the binding of T_4 to TBG is sensitive to temperature so that a rise from 37–40° will increase free T_4 20–30% (Bernstein and Oppenheimer, 1966; Schussler and Plager, 1967). If severe illness is associated with hypothermia, there may be a fall in free T_4 in blood (Harvey, 1971). As noted above, chronic illness tends to cause diversion of T_4 metabolism towards rT_3 rather than T_3 and to cause a fall in PA.

In anorexia nervosa, a lowered serum T_3 may also be seen, probably due to the associated malnutrition which causes reduced T_3 and increased rT_3 synthesis from T_4 (Moshang, Parks, Baker, Vaidya, Utiger, Bongiovanni and Snyder, 1975).

7. Strategy for the Choice of Thyroid Hormone Analyses

As can be seen in Table 21 it is technically feasible to measure in the blood some 19 different aspects of thyroid function or pathophysiology. Many of

Table 21

Blood tests for thyroid function or disease[a].

Thyroid hormones		Thyroid stimulating factors	Others
Bound	*Free*		
T_4	T_4	TSI	*TBG*
T_3	T_3	LATS	PA
rT_3	rT_3	*TSH*	*Unoccupied T_4 binding sites* (e.g. T_3 resin uptake)
$3,3'-T_2$			*Free T_4 index*
Thyroglobulin			Iodoproteins
			Thyroglobulin antibodies
			Thyroid microsomal antibodies
			Iodide

[a] Those in italic are now readily available in clinical laboratories.

these tests are performed by commercial or hospital laboratories. Enthusiastic house physicians and unwary practitioners can easily order an impressively complete series of tests. In most instances the cost completely overbalances any benefit to the patient. It is the authors' opinion that a rather elementary strategy in testing be employed, reserving complete testing for the rare, complicated situation or for study purposes. A diagnostic strategy includes, of course, a careful anamnesis, examination and tests related to the functional anatomy of the thyroid gland and to the action of the hormone (Robbins, Rall and Gorden, 1978b). Here we are concerned only with the levels of thyroid hormones, thyroid stimulating factors, and related substances in blood.

In suspected hyperthyroidism an elevated level of T_4 will confirm the diagnosis in the majority of cases. A normal T_4, if clinical evidence of hyperthyroidism seems solid, warrants T_3 and free T_4 determination to see if either T_3 thyrotoxicosis or depression of TBG or PA is involved. Free T_4 index can substitute for free T_4 measurement. The level of TSH is usually not diagnostically helpful in the diagnosis of hyperthyroidism.

In suspected hypothyroidism a depressed serum T_4 and an elevated TSH will confirm such a diagnosis in most instances. If the TSH is high and the T_4 is normal, investigation of TBG (free T_4 or free T_4 index) is indicated. T_3 and rT_3 determinations may finally be necessary to understand the situation. A low TSH raises the question of pituitary failure.

An alternative approach for both hyper- and hypothyroidism is to use the free T_4 level (or free T_4 index) as the initial screening test (Britton,

Quinn, Brown and Ekins, 1975). The second-line, confirmatory test is the T_3 level for hyperthyroidism and the TSH level for hypothyroidism.

Determination of antibodies to thyroid proteins is helpful in diagnosis of chronic lymphocytic thyroiditis, although the test is not uniformly positive and low levels may be present in "normal" adults. The level of thyroglobulin is of some help in diagnosing recurrent carcinoma of the thyroid. Special situations, such as suspected hyperthyroidism in an infant or possible cretinism, may require more complete testing. However, it is particularly important in these cases to understand the normal postnatal changes in thyroid physiology noted in Section E3(a) above. In large-scale neonatal screening for hypothyroidism, the accepted procedure is to measure the T_4 level in capillary blood at two or three days of age, and to use the TSH levels as a confirmatory test. Analysis of thyroid function in pregnancy or concomitant with other disease may require more extensive testing. Interactions of a variety of drugs with thyroid activity or with test procedures require exact knowledge of each situation and will modify the programs outlined above.

CONCLUSIONS

As we reviewed the development in the field of thyroid hormones since the last edition of "Hormones in Blood" we have been impressed with several important advances. Firstly, the general increase in sophistication of analysis of proteins applied to PA has permitted now a quite specific picture of the structure of thyroxine binding prealbumin and how thyroxine and triiodothyronine bind to it from both a chemical and physical viewpoint. It is clear we are within striking distance of a similar comprehension of TBG. Secondly, although barely discussed in this chapter, we are beginning to know where to look for the mechanism whereby thyroid hormones control an organism's energy expenditures. Thirdly, we now know in some detail the exact pathways of thyroxine metabolism. Radioimmunoassay has been indispensible in permitting accurate, sensitive, and specific analysis for the various metabolites of thyroxine, some active and some inactive. As emphasised throughout this chapter, this improvement in methodology allows widespread clinical use of measurements of thyroid hormones in blood both in free and bound form. Finally, we see now the regulation of thyroxine metabolism by carbohydrate and by adrenocortical hormones and, we suspect, by many factors. The mechanism whereby these conditions divert thyroxine metabolism from T_3 production to rT_3 production is almost completely obscure. Nevertheless, we now know of this totally unsuspected realm of control of thyroid activity. Another decade of work should reveal much of its mysteries.

REFERENCES

Aboul-Khair, S. A. and Crooks, J. (1965). *Acta endocr., Copenh.* **48**, 14.
Abuid, J., Klein, A. H., Foley Jr., T. P. and Larsen, P. R. (1974). *J. clin. Endocr. Metab.* **39**, 263.
Acland, J. D. (1952). *Nature, Lond.* **170**, 32.
Acland, J. D. (1955). *Nature, Lond.* **176**, 694.
Adams, R., Specht, N. and Woodward, I. (1960). *J. clin. Endocr. Metab.* **20**, 1366.
Albright, E. C. and Larson, F. C. (1959). *J. clin. Invest.* **38**, 1899.
Albright, E. C., Larson, F. C. and Deiss, W. P. (1955). *J. clin. Invest.* **34**, 44.
Alexander, N. M. and Jenning, J. F. (1974). *Clin. Chem.* **20**, 1353.
Alper, C. A., Robin, N. I. and Refetoff, S. (1969). *Proc. natn. Acad. Sci. USA*, **63**, 775.
Alpers, J. B. and Rall, J. E. (1955). *J. clin. Endocr. Metab.* **15**, 1482.
Andreoli, M. and Robbins, J. (1962). *J. clin. Invest.* **41**, 1070.
Andreoli, M., Robbins, J., Rall, J. E. and Berman, M. (1965). *In* "Current Topics in Thyroid Research" (M. Andreoli and C. Cassano, eds), p. 635. Academic Press, New York and London.
Andros, G. and Wollman, S. H. (1967). *Am. J. Physiol.* **213**, 198.
Arango, G., Mayberry, W. E., Hockert, T. J. and Elveback, L. R. (1968). *Mayo Clin. Proc.* **43**, 503.
Arima, T., Spiro, J. J. and Spiro, R. G. (1972). *J. biol. Chem.* **247**, 1825.
Arosenius, K. E. and Parrow, A. (1964). *Scand. J. clin. Lab. Invest.* **16**, 447.
Balasubramanian, K. and Deiss, W. P. (1965). *Biochim. biophys. Acta*, **110**, 564.
Barac, G. (1958). *Clin. chim. Acta*, **3**, 99.
Barbosa, J., Seal, U. S. and Doe, R. P. (1973). *J. clin. Endocr. Metab.* **36**, 666.
Barker, S. B. (1962). *In* "Methods in Hormone Research", p. 351. Academic Press, New York and London.
Barker, S. B. (1964). *Biochem. J.* **90**, 214.
Barker, S. B., Humphrey, M. J. and Soley, M. H. (1951). *J. clin. Invest.* **30**, 55.
Barrett, O., Berman, A. and Maier, J. G. (1960). *J. clin. Endocr. Metab.* **20**, 1467.
Bastomsky, C. H., Kaloo, H. and Frenkel-Leith, D. B. (1977). *Clin. chim. Acta*, **74**, 51.
Baumann, G., Neuhaus, K. and Thólen, H. (1974). *Ann. int. Med.* **81**, 706.
Beale, D. and Whitehead, J. K. (1960). *Clin. chim. Acta*, **5**, 150.
Beeken, W. K., Volwiler, W., Goldsworthy, P. D., Garby, L. E., Reynolds, W. E., Stoysdill, R. and Stemler, R. S. (1962). *J. clin. Invest.* **41**, 1312.
Beierwaltes, W. H. and Robbins, J. (1959). *J. clin. Invest.* **38**, 1683.
Bellabarba, D. and Sterling, K. (1969). *J. clin. Endocr. Metab.* **29**, 1510.
Benotti, J. and Benotti, N. (1963). *Clin. Chem.* **9**, 408.
Berg, G. and Ekholm, R. (1975). *Biochim. biophys. Acta*, **386**, 422.
Berman, M. (1972). *In* "The Thyroid and Biogenic Amines" (J. E. Rall and I. J. Kopin, eds), p. 172. North-Holland, Amsterdam. (Vol. 1 of "Methods in Investigative and Diagnostic Endocrinology", S. A. Berson, ed.)
Bernstein, G., Hasen, J. and Oppenheimer, J. H. (1967). *J. clin. Endocr. Metab.* **41**, 27.
Bernstein, G. and Oppenheimer, J. H. (1966). *J. clin. Endocr. Metab.* **26**, 195.
Bernstein, R. S., Robbins, J. and Rall, J. E. (1970). *Endocrinology*, **86**, 383.
Bilstad, J. M., Edelhoch, H., Lippoldt, R., Rall, J. E. and Salvatore, G. (1972). *Archs biochem. Biophys.* **151**, 341.
Bird, R. (1963). *Clin. chim. Acta*, **8**, 936.

Bjorksten. F.. Gräsbeck. R. and Lamberg, B. A. (1961). *Acta chem. scand*, **15**, 1165.

Blackburn, C. M. and Power, M. H. (1955). *J. clin. Endocr. Metab.* **15**, 1379.

Blake, C. C. F., Geisow, M. J., Swan, I. D. A., Rerat, C. and Rerat, B. (1974). *J. mol. Biol.* **88**, 1.

Blake, C. C. F. and Oatley, S. J. (1970). *Nature, Lond.* **268**, 115.

Blake, C. C. F., Swan, I. D. A., Rerat, C., Berthou, J., Laurent, A. and Rerat, B. (1971). *J. mol. Biol.* **61**, 217.

Blanquet, P., Dunn, R. W. and Tobias, C. A. (1955). *Archs biochem. Biophys.* **58**, 502.

Blanquet, P., Meyniel, G. and Savoie, J. C. (1960). *C.r. hebd. Séanc. Acad. Sci., Paris*, **250**, 217.

Blasi, F., Fragomele, F. and Covelli, I. (1969). *Endocrinology*, **85**, 542.

Blau, N. F. (1933). *J. biol. Chem.* **102**, 269.

Block, R. J. and Mandl, R. H. (1964). *Ann. N.Y. Acad. Sci.* **102**, 87.

Block, R. J., Mandl, R. H., Keller, S. and Werner, S. C. (1958). *Archs biochem. Biophys.* **75**, 508.

Block, R. J., Werner, S. C., Mandl, R. H., Row, V. V. and Radichevich, I. (1960). *Archs biochem. Biophys.* **88**, 98.

Bloth, B. and Bergquist, R. (1968). *J. exp. Med.* **128**, 1129.

Blumberg, B. S. and Robbins, J. (1960). *Endocrinology*, **67**, 368.

Bodansky, M., Pilcher, J. F. and Duff, V. B. (1936). *J. exp. Med.* **63**, 523.

Borg, D. C. (1965). *Proc. natn. Acad. Sci. USA* **53**, 829.

Börner, E., Kammenhuber, K. and Meissner, H. P. (1970). *Klin. Wschr.* **48**, 1320.

Bowden, C. H., Maclagan, N. F. and Wilkinson, J. H. (1955). *Biochem. J.* **59**, 93.

Braasch, J. W., Flock, E. V. and Albert, A. (1954). *Endocrinology*, **55**, 768.

Bradwell, A. R., Burnett, D., Ramsden, W. A., Burr, W. A., Prince, H. P. and Hoffenberg, R. (1976). *Clin. chim. Acta*, **71**, 501.

Branch, W. T., Robbins, J. and Edelhoch, H. (1971). *J. biol. Chem.* **246**, 6011.

Branch, W. T., Robbins, J. and Edelhoch, H. (1972). *Archs biochem. Biophys.* **152**, 144.

Braverman, L. E., Dawber, N. A. and Ingbar, S. H. (1966). *J. clin. Invest.* **45**, 1273.

Braverman, L. E. and Ingbar, S. H. (1963). *J. clin. Invest.* **42**, 1216.

Braverman, L. E. and Ingbar, S. H. (1965). *Endocrinology*, **76**, 547.

Braverman, L. E. and Ingbar, S. H. (1967). *J. clin. Endocr. Metab.* **27**, 389.

Braverman, L. E., Ingbar, S. H. and Sterling, K. (1970). *J. clin. Invest.* **49**, 855.

Braverman, L. E., Socolow, E. L., Woeber, K. A. and Ingbar, S. H. (1968). *J. clin. Endocr. Metab.* **28**, 831.

Braverman, L. E., Vagenakis, A. G., Foster, A. E. and Ingbar, S. H. (1971). *J. clin. Endocr. Metab.* **32**, 497.

Brown, B. L., Ekins, R. P., Ellis, S. M. and Reith, W. S. (1970). *Nature, Lond.* **226**, 369.

Brown, C. H., Lowenstein, J. M., Greenspan, F. S. and Mangum, J. (1966). *Metabolism*, **16**, 649.

Brown, M. S. and Goldstein, J. L. (1976). *Science*, **191**, 150.

Brown-Grant, K. (1960). *Br. med. Bull.* **16**, 165.

Brown-Grant, K. (1961). *Physiol. Rev.* **41**, 189.

Brown-Grant, K. and Pethes, G. (1960). *J. Physiol.* **151**, 40.

Brown-Grant, K., Brennan, R. D. and Yates, F. E. (1970). *J. clin. Endocr. Metab.* **30**, 733.

Burger, A. (1976). Prog. 5th Int. Conf. Endocr., p. 52, Abst. 129.

Burger, A. (1977). *Clin. Res.* **25**, 291A.

Burger, A. and Sakoloff, C. (1977). *J. clin. Endocr. Metab.* **45**, 384.

Burke, C. W. and Shakespear, R. A. (1976a). *J. clin. Endocr. Metab.* **42**, 494.

Burke, C. W. and Shakespear, R. A. (1976b). *J. clin. Endocr. Metab.* **42**, 504.

Burke, G., Metzger, B. E. and Goldstein, M. S. (1964). *J. Lab. clin. Med.* **63**, 708.

Burman, K. D., Strum, D., Dimond, R. C., Djuh, Y.-Y., Wright, F. D., Earll, J. M. and Wartofsky, L. (1977). *J. clin. Endocr. Metab.* **45**, 339.

Burr, W. A., Black, E. G., Griffiths, R. S. and Hoffenberg, R. (1975). *Lancet*, **ii**, 1277.

Cahnmann, H. J. (1972). In "The Thyroid and Biogenic Amines" (J. E. Rall and I. J. Kopin, eds), p. 27. North-Holland, Amsterdam. (Vol. 1 of "Methods in Investigative and Diagnostic Endocrinology", S. A. Berson, ed.)

Camerman, N. and Camerman, A. (1972). *Science*, **175**, 764.

Cameron, C. (1960). *Biochem. J.* **74**, 329.

Carter, A. C., Schwartz, H. L., Kydd, D. M. and Kologlu, S. (1964). *Endocrinology*, **74**, 689.

Carter, J. N., Corcoran, J. M., Eastman, C. J. and Lazarus, L. (1974). *Lancet*, **ii**, 971.

Castro, A. and Ugarto, E. (1974). *Res. Commun. Chem. Path. Pharmac.* **7**, 453.

Cavalieri, R. R. (1961). *J. clin. Endocr. Metab.* **21**, 1455.

Cavalieri, R. R. (1975). *J. clin. Invest.* **56**, 79.

Cavalieri, R. R., Castle, J. N. and Searle, G. L. (1969). *J. nucl. Med.* **10**, 565.

Cavalieri, R. R. and Ingbar, S. H. (1975). *Meth. Enzymol.* **36**, 126.

Cavalieri, R. R., McMahon, F. A. and Castle, J. N. (1975a). *J. clin. Invest.* **56**, 79.

Cavalieri, R. R., Moser, C., Martin, P., Shames and Perez-Mendez, V. (1975b). In "Thyroid Hormone Metabolism" (W. A. Harland and J. S. Orr, eds), p. 307. Academic Press, London and New York.

Cavalieri, R. R. and Searle, G. L. (1965). *J. Lab. clin. Med.* **65**, 171.

Cavalieri, R. R. and Searle, G. L. (1966). *J. clin. Invest.* **45**, 939.

Cavalieri, R. R., Steinberg, M. and Searle, G. L. (1970). *J. clin. Invest.* **49**, 1041.

Chaffee, R. R. J. and Roberts, J. C. (1971). *Ann. Rev. Physiol.* **33**, 155.

Chebath, J., Chabaud, O., Becarevic, A., Cartouzou, G. and Lissitzky, S. (1977). *Eur. J. Biochem.* **77**, 243.

Cheng, S. Y. (1977). *Biochem. biophys. Res. Commun.* **79**, 1212.

Cheng, S. Y., Pages, R. A., Saroff, H. A., Edelhoch, H. and Robbins, J. (1977a). *Biochemistry*, **16**, 3707.

Cheng, S. Y., Wilchek, M., Cahnmann, H. J. and Robbins, J. (1977b). *J. biol. Chem.* **252**, 6076.

Chin, W. and Schussler, G. C. (1968). *J. clin. Endocr. Metab.* **28**, 181.

Chopra, I. J. (1972). *J. clin. Endocr. Metab.* **34**, 938.

Chopra, I. J. (1974). *J. clin. Invest.* **54**, 583.

Chopra, I. J. (1976). *J. clin. Invest.* **58**, 32.

Chopra, I. J. (1978a). In "The Thyroid" (S. C. Werner and S. H. Ingbar, eds), p. 100. Harper and Row, Hagerstown, Md.

Chopra, I. J. (1978b). *Rec. Prog. Horm. Res.* **34**, 521.

Chopra, I. J., Chopra, U., Smith, S. R., Resa, M. and Solomon, D. H. (1975a). *J. clin. Endocr. Metab.* **41**, 1043.

Chopra, I. J., Ho, R. S. and Lam, R. (1972a). *J. Lab. clin. Med.* **80**, 729.

Chopra, I. J., Solomon, D. H., Chopra, U., Young, R. T. and Chua Teco, G. N. (1974). *J. clin. Endocr. Metab.* **39**, 501.

Chopra, I. J., Solomon, D. H. and Ho, R. J. (1972b). *J. clin. Endocr. Metab.* **35**, 565.

Chopra, I. J., Williams, D. E., Orgiazzi, J. and Solomon, D. H. (1975b). *J. clin. Endocr. Metab.* **41**, 911.

Christensen, L. K. (1959). *Scand. J. clin. Lab. Invest.* **11**, 326.

Christensen, L. K. (1960). *Endocrinology*, **66**, 138.

Clark, D. E., Moe, R. H. and Adams, S. S. (1949). *Surgery*, **26**, 331.

Clark, F. (1975). *J. clin. Path.* **28**, 211.

Clark, F. and Horn, D. B. (1965). *J. clin. Endocr. Metab.* **25**, 39.

Clark, F. and Horn, D. B. (1966). *J. clin. Endocr. Metab.* **26**, 352.

Clements, F. W. (1960). *Br. med. Bull.* **16**, 133.

Cody, V. (1974). *J. Am. chem. Soc.* **96**, 6720.

Cody, V., Hazel, J., Langs, D. A. and Duax, W. L. (1977). *J. med. Chem.* **20**, 1628.

Collins, K. J. and Weiner, J. S. (1968). *Physiol. Rev.* **48**, 785.

Crispell, K. R. and Coleman, J. (1956). *J. clin. Invest.* **35**, 475.

Cuaron, A. (1966). *J. clin. Endocr. Metab.* **26**, 53.

Cuttelod, S., Lemarchand-Béraud, T., Magnenat, P., Pettet, C., Poli, S. and Vannotti, A. (1974). *Metabolism*, **23**, 101.

Daniel, P. M., Plaskett, L. G. and Pratt, O. E. (1966). *Biochem. J.* **100**, 622.

Daniel, P. M., Pratt, O. E., Roitt, I. M. and Torrigiani, G. (1967). *Immunology*, **12**, 489.

Davies, L. E. and Hanson, S. (1965). *Can. med. Ass. J.* **92**, 205.

Davis, P. J. (1966). *Am. J. Med.* **40**, 918.

Davis, P. J. and Gregerman, R. I. (1970). *J. clin. Endocr. Metab.* **30**, 237.

Davis, P. J. and Gregerman, R. I. (1971). *J. clin. Endocr. Metab.* **33**, 699.

Davis, P. J., Spaulding, S. W. and Gregerman, R. I. (1970). *Endocrinology*, **87**, 978.

Davis, P. J., Handwerger, B. S. and Glaser, F. (1974). *J. biol. Chem.* **249**, 6208.

De Crombrugghe, B., Pitt-Rivers, R. and Edelhoch, H. (1966). *J. biol. Chem.* **241**, 2766.

De Groot, L. I. and Stanbury, J. B. (1959). *Am. J. Med.* **27**, 586.

De Groot, L. J., Hall, R., McDermott, W. V. and Davis, A. M. (1962). *New Engl. J. Med.* **267**, 267.

Deiss, W. P., Balasubramanian, K., Peake, R. L., Starrett, J. A. and Powell, R. C. (1966). *Endocrinology*, **79**, 19.

Delange, F., Camus, M. and Ermans, A. M. (1972). *J. clin. Endocr. Metab.* **34**, 891.

Dempsey, E. W. and Astwood, E. B. (1943). *Endocrinology*, **32**, 509.

De Nayer, P. (1977). *8th Ann. Meet. Eur. Thyroid Assoc.*, *Ann. Endocr.* **38**, 7A.

De Nayer, P., Weathers, B. and Robbins, J. (1966). *Prog. Am. Thyroid Assoc.*, p. 38.

De Nayer, P. H., Ostyn, M. and De Visscher, M. (1970). *Ann. Endocr. (Paris)* **31**, 721.

Derrien, Y., Michel, R. and Roche, J. (1948). *Biochim. biophys. Acta*, **2**, 454.

De Rubertis, F. R. and Woeber, K. A. (1973). *J. clin. Invest.* **52**, 78.

Di Guiulio, W. D., Michalak, Z., Weinhold, P. A., Hamilton, J. R. and Thoma, G. E. (1964). *J. Lab. Clin. Med.* **64**, 349.

Dimitriadou, A., Fraser, R. and Turner, P. C. R. (1966). *In* "Endocrinologia Experimentalis: Estimation of Iodocompounds in Biological Material" (V. Stolc, ed.), p. 87. Publishing House of the Slovak Academy of Sciences, Bratislava.

Di Stefano, J. J. and Chang, R. F. (1971). *Am. J. Physiol.* **221**, 1529.

Dobyns, B. and Barry, S. R. (1953). *J. biol. Chem.* **204**, 517.

Dowben, R. M. (1960). *J. Lab. clin. Med.* **55**, 132.

Dowling, J. T., Frienkel, N. and Ingbar, S. H. (1956a). *J. clin. Invest.* **35**, 1263.

Dowling, J. T., Freinkel, N. and Ingbar, S. H. (1956b). *J. clin. Endocr. Metab.* **16**, 1491.

Dowling, J. T., Ingbar, S. H. and Freinkel, N. (1960). *J. clin. Endocr. Metab.* **20**, 1.

Dowling, J. T., Ingbar, S. H. and Freinkel, N. (1961). *J. clin. Endocr. Metab.* **21**, 1390.

Dussault, J. H., Fisher, D. A., Nicoloff, J. T., Row, V. V. and Volpe, R. (1973). *Acta endocr., Copenh.* **72**, 265.

Edelhoch, H. (1962). *J. biol. Chem.* **237**, 2778.

Edelhoch, H. (1965). *Rec. Prog. horm. Res.* **21**, 1.

Edelhoch, H. and Lippoldt, R. E. (1964). *Biochim. biophys. Acta*, **79**, 64.

Edelhoch, H. and Robbins, J. (1978). *In* "The Thyroid" (S. C. Werner and S. H. Ingbar, eds), p. 62. Harper and Row, Hagerstown, MD.

Edelhoch, H. and Steiner, R. F. (1966). *Biopolymer*, **4**, 999.

Edwards, R. R. (1962). *Science, N.Y.* **137**, 851.

Ekholm, R. and Wollman, S. H. (1975). *Endocrinology*, **97**, 1432.

Ekins, R. P. (1960). *Clin. chim. Acta*, **5**, 453.

Ekins, R. P., Williams, E. S. and Ellis, S. (1969). *Clin. Biochem.* **2**, 253.

Ellis, S. M. and Ekins, R. P. (1976). *In* "Thyroid Research" (J. Robbins and L. Braverman, eds), p. 597, Excerpta Medica, Amsterdam.

Elzinga, K. E., Carr, E. A. and Beierwaltes, W. H. (1961). *Am. J. clin. Path.* **36**, 125.

Emmett, J. C. and Pepper, E. S. (1976). *Nature, Lond.* **257**, 334.

Erenberg, A., Phelps, D. L., Lam, R. and Fisher, D. A. (1974). *Pediatrics*, **53**, 211.

Evered, D. C., Tunbridge, W. M. G., Hall, R., Appleton, D., Brewis, M., Clark, F., Manuel, P. and Young, E. (1978). *Clin. chim. Acta*, **83**, 223.

Faber, J., Friis, T., Kirkegaard, C. and Siersbaek-Nielsen, K. (1978). *Acta endocr., Copenh.* **87**, 313.

Farer, L. S., Robbins, J., Blumberg, B. S. and Rall, J. E. (1962). *Endocrinology*, **70**, 686.

Federman, D. D. (1964). *Medicine*, **43**, 267.

Federman, D. D., Robbins, J. and Rall, J. E. (1958). *J. clin. Invest.* **37**, 1024.

Ferguson, R. N., Edelhoch, H., Saroff, H. and Robbins, J. (1975). *Biochemistry*, **14**, 282.

Fex, G., Laurell, C-B. and Thuliss, E. (1977). *Eur. J. Biochem.* **75**, 181.

Fex, G. and Lindgress, R. (1977). *Biochim. biophys. Acta*, **493**, 410.

Fialkow, P. J., Giblett, E. R. and Musa, B. (1970). *J. clin. Endocr. Metab.* **30**, 66.

Fields, T., Kinnory, D. S., Kaplan, E., Oester, Y. T. and Bowser, E. N. (1956). *J. Lab. clin. Med.* **47**, 33.

Finucane, J. F. and Griffiths, R. S. (1976). *J. clin. Path.* **29**, 949.

Fisher, D. A. and Oddie, T. (1964). *Am. J. Dis. Childh.* **107**, 574.

Fisher, D. A., Oddie, T. H. and Epperson, D. (1965). *J. clin. Endocr.* **25**, 1580.

Fisher, D. A., Dussault, J. H., Sack, J. and Chopra, I. J. (1977a). *Rec. Prog. horm. Res.* **33**, 59.

Fisher, D. A., Sack, J., Oddie, T. H., Pekary, A. E., Hershman, J. M., Lam, R. W. and Parslow, M. E. (1977b). *J. clin. Endocr. Metab.* **45**, 191.

Fletcher, K. (1957). *Biochem. J.* **67**, 136 and 140.

Flock, E. V. and Bollman, J. L. (1955). *J. biol. Chem.* **214**, 709.

Flock, E. V., Bollman, J. L. and Grindley, J. H. (1960). *Endocrinology*, **67**, 419.

Foss, O. P., Hankes, L. V. and Van Slyke, D. D. (1960). *Clin. chim. Acta*, **5**, 301.

Foster, G. L. and Gutman, A. B. (1930). *J. biol. Chem.* **87**, 289.

Frati, L., Bilstad, J., Edelhoch, H., Rall, J. E. and Salvatore, G. (1974). *Archs biochem. Biophys.* **162**, 126.

Freeman, T. and Pearson, J. D. (1969). *Clin. chim. Acta*, **26**, 365.

Freinkel, N., Dowling, J. T. and Ingbar, S. H. (1955). *J. clin. Invest.* **34**, 1698.

Friis, T. H. and Østergaard Kristensen, H. P. (1961). *Acta endocr., Copenh.* **36**, 335.

Fukuda, M. and Egami, F. (1971). *Biochem. J.* **123**, 407.

Funakoshi, K. and Cahnmann, H. J. (1969). *Ann. Biochem.* **27**, 150.

Furth, E. D., Agrawal, R. B. and Propp, R. P. (1970). *J. clin. Endocr. Metab.* **31**, 60.

Gaffney, G. W., Gregerman, R. I., Yiengst, W. J. and Shock, N. W. (1960). *J. Geront.* **15**, 234.

Gaitan, E., Island, D. P. and Liddle, G. W. (1969). *Tr. Ass. Am. Phys.* **82**, 141.

Galton, V. A. and Nisula, B. C. (1969). *Endocrinology*, **85**, 79.

Galton, V. A. and Nisula, B. C. (1972). *J. Endocr.* **54**, 187.

Galton, V. A. and Pitt-Rivers, R. (1959). *Biochem. J.* **72**, 310.

Garby, L. (1962). *Scand. J. clin. Lab. Invest.* **14**, 316.

Gavin, L., Castle, J., McMahon, F., Martin, P., Hammond, M. and Cavalieri, R. R. (1977). *J. clin. Endocr. Metab.* **44**, 733.

Gavin, L. A., McMahon, F. A., Castle, J. N. and Cavalieri, R. R. (1978). *J. clin. Endocr. Metab.* **46**, 125.

Gershengorn, M. C., Larsen, P. R. and Robbins, J. (1976). *J. clin. Endocr. Metab.* **42**, 907.

Gershengorn, M. C., Cheng, S-Y., Lippoldt, R. E., Lord, R. S. and Robbins, J. (1977a). *J. biol. Chem.* **252**, 8713.

Gershengorn, M. C., Lippoldt, R. L. Edelhoch, H. and Robbins, J. (1977b). *J. biol. Chem.* **252**, 8719.

Gerstner, J. B. and Caplan, R. H. (1976). *J. clin. Endocr.* **42**, 64.

Gerwing, J., Long, D. A. and Pitt-Rivers, R. (1958). *J. Physiol. (Lond.)* **144**, 229.

Gimlette, T. M. D. (1964). *J. clin. Path.* **17**, 58.

Gimlette, T. M. D. (1965). *J. clin. Path.* **18**, 293.

Glinoer, D., Gershengorn, M. C. and Robbins, J. (1976). *Biochim. biophys. Acta*, **418**, 232.

Glinoer, D., Gershengorn, M. C., Dubois, A. and Robbins, J. (1977a). *Endocrinology*, **100**, 807.

Glinoer, D., McGuire, R. A., Gershengorn, M. C., Robbins, J. and Berman, M. (1977b). *Endocrinology*, **100**, 9.

Glinoer, D., Puttermans, N., Van Herle, A. J., Camus, M. and Ermans, A. M. (1974). *Acta endocr., Copenh.* **77**, 26.

Gmelin, R. and Virtanen, A. I. (1959). *Acta chim. scand.* **13**, 1469.

Godden, J. D. and Garnett, E. S. (1964). *J. Endocr.* **29**, 167.

Goodman, D. S. (1976). *In* "Trace Components of Plasma Isolation and Clinical Significance" (G. A. Jamieson and T. J. Greenwalt, eds), p. 313. Alan R. Liss, New York.

Goolden, A. W. G., Gartside, J. M. and Osorio, C. (1965). *J. clin. Endocr. Metab.* **25**, 127.

Goolden, A. W. G., Gartside, J. M. and Sanderson, C. (1967). *Lancet*, **i**, 12.

Gordon, A. and Coutsoftides, T. (1969a). *Acta endocr., Copenh.* **62**, 217.

Gordon, A. and Coutsoftides, T. (1969b). *Acta endocr., Copenh.* **62**, 234.

Gordon, A. H., Gross, J., O'Connor, D. and Pitt-Rivers, R. (1952). *Nature, Lond.* **169**, 19.

Gottschalk, C. W. and Riggs, D. S. (1952). *J. clin. Endocr. Metab.* **12**, 235.

Green, A. M., Marshall, J. S., Pensky, J. and Stanbury, J. B. (1972). *Biochim. biophys. Acta*, **278**, 117.

Greer, M. A. (1962). *Rec. Prog. Horm. Res.* **18**, 187.

Gregerman, R. I. and Solomon, N. (1967). *J. clin. Endocr. Metab.* **27**, 93.

Gribetz, O., Talbot, N. B. and Crawford, J. D. (1954). *New Engl. J. Med.* **250**, 555.

Gronkvist, K. E. and Hellberg, H. (1951). *Farmac. Rev.* **50**, 189.

Gross, J. (1954). *Br. med. Bull.* **10**, 218.

Gross, J., Leblond, C. P., Franklin, A. E. and Quastel, J. H. (1950). *Science*, **111**, 605.

Gross, J. and Pitt-Rivers, R. (1953a). *Biochem. J.* **53**, 645.

Gross, J. and Pitt-Rivers, R. (1953b). *Biochem. J.* **53**, 652.

Guerin, M. T. and Tubiana, M. (1964). *Ann. Endocr., Paris*, **25**, 475.

Gwynne, J. T., Mahafee, D., Brewer, H. B. and Ney, R. L. (1976). *Proc. natn. Acad. Sci. USA*, **73**, 4329.

Haeberli, A., Bilstad, J. M., Edelhoch, H. and Rall, J. E. (1975). *J. biol. Chem.* **250**, 7294.

Hagen, G. A. and Elliot, W. J. (1973). *J. clin. Endocr. Metab.* **37**, 415.

Hager, L., Morris, D., Brown, F. S. and Eberwein, H. (1966). *J. biol. Chem.* **241**, 1769.

Haibach, H. (1971). *Endocrinology*, **88**, 918.

Hamada, S., Nakagawa, T., Mori, T. and Torizuka, K. (1970a). *J. clin. Endocr. Metab.* **31**, 166.

Hamada, S., Torizuka, K., Myake, T. and Fukase, M. (1970b). *Biochim. biophys. Acta*, **201**, 479.

Hamolsky, M. W. (1966). *In* "Endocrinologia Experimentalis: Estimation of Iodo-compounds in Biological Material" (V. Stolc, ed.), p. 259. Publishing House of the Slovak Academy of Sciences, Bratislava.

Hamolsky, M. W., Golodetz, A. and Freedberg, A. S. (1959). *J. clin. Endocr. Metab.* **19**, 103.

Hamolsky, M. W., Stein, M. and Freedberg, A. S. (1957). *J. clin. Endocr. Metab.* **17**, 33.

Hamolsky, M. W., Stein, M., Fischer, D. B. and Freedberg, A. S. (1961). *Endocrinology*, **68**, 662.

Hansen, H. H. (1966). *Scand. J. clin. Lab. Invest.* **18**, 240.

Hanson, J. M. and Siersbaek-Nielsen, K. (1969). *J. clin. Endocr. Metab.* **29**, 1023.

Hao, Y. L. and Tabachnik, M. (1971). *Endocrinology*, **88**, 81.

Harris, A., Fang, S., Ingbar, S., Braverman, L. and Vagenakis, A. (1977). *Clin. Res.* **25**, 463A.

Harris, J. C. and Oliner, L. (1966). *J. nucl. Med.* **7**, 259.

Harrison, M. T., Harden, R. M. and Alexander, W. D. (1967). *Metabolism*, **16**, 84.

Harvey, R. F. (1971). *Lancet*, **i**, 208.

Heller, J. (1975). *J. biol. Chem.* **250**, 3613.

Hellman, E. S., Tschudy, D. P., Robbins, J. and Rall, J. E. (1963). *J. clin. Endocr. Metab.* **23**, 1185.

Hennen, G. (1966). *Archs Int. Physiol. Biochem.* **74**, 303.

Herbert, V., Gottlieb, C. W., Lau, K. S., Gilbert, P. and Silver, S. (1965). *J. Lab. clin. Med.* **66**, 814.

Hershman, J. M., Craane, T. J. and Colwell, J. A. (1968). *J. clin. Endocr. Metab.* **28**, 1605.

Hershman, J. M. and Higgins, H. P. (1971). *New Engl. J. Med.* **284**, 573.

Hershman, J. M. and Pittman, J. A. (1971). *Ann. int. Med.* **74**, 481.

Hershman, J. M. and Van Middlesworth, L. (1962). *Endocrinology*, **71**, 94.

Herveg, J. P., Beckers, C. and De Visscher, M. (1966). *Biochem. J.* **100**, 540.

Hesch, R. D., Gatz, J., McIntosh, C. H. S., Janzen, J. and Hehrmann, R. (1976). *Clin. chim. Acta*, **70**, 33.

Hesch, R. D., Gatz, J., Jüppner, H. and Stubbe, P. (1977). *Horm. Metab. Res.* **9**, 141.

Higgins, H. P., Hershman, J. M., Kenimer, J. G., Patillo, R. A., Bayley, T. A. and Walfish, P. (1975). *Ann. int. Med.* **83**, 307.

Hillier, A. P. (1968). *J. Physiol. (Lond.)* **197**, 135.

Hillier, A. P. (1971). *J. Physiol.* **217**, 625.

Hillier, A. P. (1975a). *Acta endocr., Copenh.* **78**, 32.

Hillier, A. P. (1975b). *Acta endocr., Copenh.* **80**, 49.

Hjort, T., Lauridsen, V. B., Persson, I. (1970). *J. clin. Endocr. Metab.* **30**, 520.

Hoch, H. and Lewallen, C. G. (1974). *J. clin. Endocr. Metab.* **38**, 663.

Hofer, P. B. and Gottschalk, A. (1971). *Radiology*, **99**, 117.

Hollander, C. S., Bernstein, G. and Oppenheimer, J. (1966). "Program of the Endocrine Society", p. 54.

Hollander, C. S., Mitsuma, T., Nikei, N., Shenkman, L., Burday, S. Z. and Blum, M. (1972). *Lancet*, **i**, 609.

Hollander, C. S., Mitsuma, T., Shenkman, L., Stevenson, C., Pineda, G. and Silva, E. (1972b). *Lancet*, **ii**, 1276.

Hong, S. K. (1973). *Fedn. Proc.* **32**, 1614.

Horn, D. B. (1975). *J. clin. Path.* **28**, 218.

Horst, W. and Rösler, H. (1953). *Klin. Wschr.* **31**, 13.

Horwitz, D. L. and Refetoff, S. (1977). *J. clin. Endocr. Metab.* **44**, 242.

Horwitz, J. and Heller, J. (1974). *J. biol. Chem.* **249**, 4712.

Hosoya, T., Matsukawa, S. and Nagai, Y. (1971). *Biochemistry*, **10**, 3086.

Hüffner, M. and Hesch, R. D. (1973). *Clin. chim. Acta*, **44**, 101.

Inada, M. and Sterling, K. (1967a). *J. clin. Endocr. Metab.* **27**, 1019.

Inada, M. and Sterling, K. (1967b). *J. clin. Invest.* **46**, 1275.

Inada, M. and Sterling, K. (1967c). *J. clin. Invest.* **46**, 1442.

Inada, M., Kasagi, K., Kurata, S., Kazama, Y., Takayama, H., Torizuka, K., Fukase, M. and Soma, T. (1975). *J. clin. Invest.* **55**, 1337.

Ingbar, S. H. (1958). *Endocrinology*, **63**, 256.

Ingbar, S. H. (1961). *J. clin. Invest.* **40**, 2053.

Ingbar, S. H. (1963). *J. clin. Invest.* **42**, 143.

Ingbar, S. H., Braverman, L. E., Dawber, N. A. and Lee, G. Y. (1965). *J. clin. Invest.* **44**, 1679.

Ingbar, S. H., Dowling, J. T. and Freinkel, N. (1957). *Endocrinology*, **61**, 321.

Ingbar, S. H. and Freinkel, N. (1958a). *AMA Arch. Int. Med.* **105**, 339.

Ingbar, S. H. and Freinkel, N. (1958b). *J. clin. Invest.* **37**, 1603.

Ingbar, S. H. and Freinkel, N. (1960). *Rec. Prog. Horm. Res.* **16**, 353.

Ingbar, S. H., Freinkel, N., Hoeprich, P. D. and Athens, J. W. (1954). *J. clin. Invest.* **33**, 388.

Ingenbleek, Y., de Visscher, M. and De Nayer, P. (1972). *Lancet*, **ii**, 106.

Ingenbleek, Y., van den Schriek, H. G., De Nayer, P. and De Visscher, M. (1975). *Clin. chim. Acta*, **63**, 61.

Inoue, K. and Taurog, A. (1968). *Endocrinology*, **83**, 816.

Irvine, C. H. G. (1967). *J. Endocr.* **39**, 313.

Irvine, C. H. G. (1968). *J. clin. Endocr. Metab.* **28**, 942.

Irvine, C. H. G. (1974). *J. clin. Endocr. Metab.* **38**, 655.

Irvine, C. H. G. and Simpson-Morgan, M. W. (1974). *J. clin. Invest.* **54**, 156.

Ismail-Beigi, F. and Edelman, I. S. (1971). *J. gen. Physiol.* **57**, 710.

Izumi, M. (1972). *Endocr. Jap.* **19**, 259.

Izumi, M. and Larsen, P. R. (1977). *J. clin. Invest.* **59**, 1105.

Jaakonnaki, P. I. and Stouffer, J. E. (1967). *J. Gas Chromatogr.* **5**, 303.

Jacobsson, L. and Widstrom, G. (1962). *Scand. J. clin. Lab. Invest.* **14**, 285.

Jakoby, W. B., Labaw, L., Edelhoch, H., Pastan, I. and Rall, J. E. (1966). *Science*, **153**, 1671.

Jepson, J. B. and Smith, I. (1956). *Nature, Lond.* **177**, 184.

Jiang, N-S. and Tue, K. A. (1977). *Clin. Chem.* **23**, 1679.

Jones, J. E. and Seal, U. S. (1967). *J. clin. Endocr. Metab.* **27**, 1521.

Jorgensen, E. C. (1964). *Mayo Clin. Proc.* **39**, 560.

Jorgensen, E. C. (1976). *Pharm. Ther. B.* **2**, 661.

Kagedal, B. and Kallberg, M. (1977). *Clin. Chem.* **23**, 1694.

Kahn, A., Cogan, S. R. and Berger, S. (1962). *J. clin. Endocr. Metab.* **22**, 1.

Kanda, Y., Goodman, S., Canfield, R. E. and Morgan, F. J. (1974). *J. biol. Chem.* **249**, 6796.

Kaplan, M. M. (1978). "Program of the Endocrine Society", p. 119.

Kaplan, M. M., Schemmel, M. and Utiger, R. (1977). *J. clin. Endocr. Metab.* **45**, 447.

Karch, F. E., Morgan, J. P., Kubasik, N. P. and Sine, H. E. (1976). *J. clin. Endocr. Metab.* **43**, 26.

Katz, F. H. and Kappas, A. (1967). *J. clin. Invest.* **46**, 1768.

Kaufman, S. L. and Frederickson, R. (1973). *Calif. Med.* **118**, 63.

Keane, P. M., Pegg, P. J. and Johnson, E. (1970). *J. clin. Endocr. Metab.* **29**, 1126.

Keating, F. R., Haines, S. F., Power, M. H. and Williams, M. M. D. (1950). *J. clin. Endocr. Metab.* **10**, 1425.

Kelly, F. C. and Snedden, W. W. (1960). *In* "Endemic Goiter", p. 27. WHO, Geneva.

Kenimer, J. G., Hershman, J. M. and Higgins, H. P. (1975). *J. clin. Endocr. Metab.* **40**, 482.

Kennedy, T. H. (1958). *Austr. J. biol. Sci.* **11**, 106.

Kessler, G. and Pillegi, V. J. (1970). *Clin. Chem.* **16**, 382.

Kollman, P. A., Murray, W. J., Nuss, M. E., Jorgensen, E. C. and Rothenberg, S. (1973). *J. Am. chem. Soc.* **95**, 8518.

Kologlu, S., Schwartz, H. L. and Carter, A. C. (1966). *Endocrinology*, **78**, 231.

Korcek, L. and Tabachnik, M. (1974). *Biochim. biophys. Acta*, **371**, 323.

Korcek, L. and Tabachnik, M. (1976). *J. biol. Chem.* **251**, 3558.

Kuby, S. A., Noda, L. and Lardy, H. A. (1954). *J. biol. Chem.* **210**, 65.

Kydd, D. M., Man, E. B. and Peters, J. P. (1950). *J. clin. Invest.* **29**, 1033.

Labaw, L. and Rall, J. E. (1968). *J. mol. Biol.* **36**, 25.

Laidlaw, J. C. (1949). *Nature, Lond.* **164**, 927.

Lamas, L., Dorria, M. and Taurog, A. (1972). *Endocrinology*, **90**, 1417.

Lamas, L., Taurog, A., Salvatore, G. and Edelhoch, H. (1974). *J. biol. Chem.* **249**, 2732.

Lamberg, B. A., Björksten, F., Jakobson, T., Karlsson, R., and Axelson, E. (1964). *Acta med. scand.* **175**, 173.

Larsen, P. R. (1971). *Metabolism*, **20**, 976.

Larsen, P. R. (1972a). *J. clin. Invest.* **51**, 1125.

Larsen, P. R. (1972b). *Metabolism*, **21**, 1073.

Larsen, P. R. (1976). *In* "Hormones in Human Blood. Detection and Assay" (H. N. A. Antoniades *ed.*), p. 679. Harvard University Press, Cambridge, MA.

Larsen, P. R. (1978). *In* "The Thyroid" (S. C. Werner and S. H. Ingbar, eds), p. 231. Hagerstown, MD.

Larsen, P. R., Atkinson, A. J., Wellman, H. N. and Goldsmith, R. E. (1970). *J. clin. Invest.* **49**, 1266.

Larsen, P. R. and Broskin, K. (1975). *Pediatr. Res.* **9**, 604.

Larsen, P. R., Dockalova, J., Sipula, D. and Wu, F. M. (1973). *J. clin. Endocr. Metab.* **37**, 177.

Laurell, C-B, (1966). *Anal. Biochem.* **15**, 45.

Leboeuf, G. and Bongiovanni, A. M. (1964). *Adv. Pediatr.* **13**, 183.

Lee, N. D., Catz, B., Margolese, M. S. and Pileggi, V. J. (1971). *Clin. Chem.* **17**, 174.

Lee, N. D., Henry, R. J. and Golub, O. J. (1964a). *J. clin. Endocr. Metab.* **24**, 486.

Lee, N. D. and Pileggi, V. J. (1971). *Clin. Chem.* **17**, 167.

Lee, N. D., Pileggi, V. J. and Segalove, M. (1964b). *Clin. Chem.* **10**, 136.

Leland, J. P. and Foster, G. L. (1932). *J. biol. Chem.* **95**, 165.

Leloup, J. and Fontaine, M. (1960). *Ann. N.Y. Acad. Sci.* **86**, 316.

Lemarchand-Béraud, T., Assayah, M. R. and Vanotti, A. (1964). *Acta endocr., Copenh.* **45**, 99.

Leonard, J. L. and Rosenberg, I. N. (1978). *Endocrinology,* **103**, 274.
Lepp, A., Pena, H. and Hoxie, V. (1965). *Am. J. clin. Pathol.* **44**, 331.
Lerner, S. R. (1963). *Archs biochem. Biophys.* **103**, 36.
Levinson, S. S. and Rieder, S. V. (1974). *Clin. Chem.* **20**, 1568.
Levy, R. P., Marshall, J. S. and Velayo, N. L. (1971). *J. clin. Endocr. Metab.* **32**, 372.
Lewallen, C. G. (1963). *In* "Evaluation of Thyroid and Parathyroid Functions" (F. W. Sunderman and F. W. Sunderman Jr., eds), p. 19. Lippincott, Philadelphia.
Lewitus, Z. and Steinitz, K. (1963). *Clin. chim. Acta,* **8**, 629.
Lewitus, Z., Hasenfratz, J., Toor, M., Massry, S. and Rabinowitch, E. (1964). *J. clin. Endocr. Metab.* **24**, 1084.
Lieblich, J. and Utiger, R. D. (1972). *J. clin. Invest.* **51**, 157.
Liewendahl, K. and Helenius, T. (1975). *Clin. chim. Acta,* **64**, 263.
Liewendahl, K. and Helenius, T. (1976). *Clin. chim. Acta,* **72**, 301.
Liewendahl, K. and Lamberg, B.-A. (1969). *Acta endocr., Copenh.* **61**, 343.
Lissitzky, S., Benevent, M. T., Roques, M. and Roche, J. (1959). *Bull. Soc. Chim. Biol., Paris,* **41**, 1329.
Lissitzky, S. and Bismuth, J. (1963). *Clin. chim. Acta,* **8**, 269.
Lissitzky, S., Bismuth, J. and Rolland, M. (1962). *Clin. chim. Acta,* **7**, 183.
Lissitzky, S., Codaccioni, J. L., Bismuth, J. and Depieds, R. (1967). *J. clin. Endocr. Metab.* **27**, 185.
Lissitzky, S. and Lasry, S. (1958). *Bull. Soc. Chim. Biol., Paris,* **40**, 609.
Lissitzky, S., Mauchamp, J., Reynaud, J. and Rolland, M. (1975). *FEBS Lett.* **60**, 359.
Lissitzky, S., Rolland, M., Reynaud, J., Savary, J. and Lasry, S. (1968). *Eur. J. Biochem.* **4**, 464.
Long, J. F., Gilmore, L. O. and Rife, D. C. (1956). "Novant' Anni dei Leggi Mendeliane", p. 188. Rome.
Loughlin, R. E., McQuillan, M. T. and Trikojus, V. M. (1960). *Endocrinology,* **66**, 733.
Lowenstein, J. M., Greenspan, F. S. and Spilker, P. (1963). *J. Lab. clin. Med.* **62**, 831.
Lowrey, R. and Starr, P. (1959). *J. Am. med. Assoc.* **171**, 2045.
Lutz, J. H. and Gregerman, R. I. (1969). *J. clin. Endocr. Metab.* **29**, 487.
Lutz, J. H., Gregerman, R. I., Spaulding, S. W., Hornick, R. B. and Dawkins, A. T. (1973). *J. clin. Endocr. Metab.* **35**, 230.
McConahey, W. M., Owen, C. A. and Keating, F. R. (1956). *J. clin. Endocr. Metab.* **16**, 724.
McConnon, J., Row, V. V. and Volpe, R. (1972). *J. clin. Endocr. Metab.* **34**, 144.
McDonald, L. J., Robin, N. I. and Siegel, L. (1978). *Clin. Chem.* **24**, 652.
McGirr, E. M., Hutchinson, J. H. and Clement, W. E. (1956). *Lancet,* **ii**, 906.
McQuillan, M. T. and Trikojus, V. M. (1966). *In* "Glycoproteins: Their Composition, Structure and Function" (A. Gottschalk, ed.). Elsevier, Amsterdam.
Mackinnon, P. C. B., Monk-Jones, M. E. and Fotherby, D. (1963). *J. Endocr.* **25**, 55.
Maclagan, N. F., Bowden, C. H. and Wilkinson, J. H. (1957). *Biochem. J.* **67**, 5.
Maclagan, N. F. and Haworth, P. J. N. (1969). *Clin. Sci.* **37**, 45.
Malkowitz, E., Muller, K. and Spitzy, H. (1966). *Microchem. J.* **10**, 194.
Malamos, B., Miras, K., Koutras, D. A., Kostamis, P., Binopoulos, D., Mantzos, J., Levis, G., Rigopolous, G., Zerefos, N. and Tassopoulos, C. N. (1966). *J. clin. Endocr. Metab.* **26**, 696.
Malvaux, P., De Nayer, P., Beckers, C., van den Schrieck, H. G. and de Visscher, M. (1966). *J. clin. Endocr. Metab.* **26**, 457.
Man, E. B. (1962). *J. Lab. clin. Med.* **59**, 528.
Man, E. B., Bondy, P. K., Weeks, E. A. and Peters, J. P. (1954). *Yale J. biol. Med.* **27**, 90.

Man, E. B., Kydd, D. M. and Peters, J. P. (1951). *J. clin. Invest.* **30**, 531.
Mancini, G., Carbonara, A. O. and Hermans, J. F. (1965). *Immunochemistry*, **2**, 235.
Mandl, R. H. and Block, R. J. (1959). *Archs biochem. Biophys*, **81**, 25.
Marriq, C., Rolland, M. and Lissitzky, S. (1977). *Eur. J. Biochem.* **79**, 143.
Marshall, J. S., Pensky, J. and Green, A. M. (1972). *J. clin. Invest.* **51**, 3173.
Marshall, J. S. and Tompkins, L. S. (1968). *J. clin. Endocr. Metab.* **28**, 386.
Martin, D. M. and Rollo, F. D. (1977). *J. nucl. Med.* **18**, 919.
Masen, J. M. (1967). *J. clin. Pathol.* **48**, 561.
Mason, J. W., Hartley, L. H., Kotchen, T. A., Wherry, F. E., Pennington, L. L. and Jones, L. G. (1966). *J. clin. Endocr. Metab.* **37**, 403.
Matovinovic, J. and Ramalingaswami, V. (1960). *In* "Endemic Goiter", p. 385. WHO, Geneva.
Matsuda, K. and Greer, M. A. (1965). *Endocrinology*, **76**, 1013.
Mayberry, W. E. and Hockert, T. J. (1970). *J. biol. Chem.* **245**, 697.
Meade, R. C. (1960). *J. clin. Endocr. Metab.* **20**, 480.
Melander, A., Sundler, F. and Westgren, U. (1975). *Endocrinology*, **96**, 102.
Metzger, H. and Edelhoch, H. (1961). *J. Am. chem. Soc.* **83**, 1423.
Meyniel, G., Blanquet, P., Berger, J. A., Croizet, M. and Gaillard, G. (1965). *Bull. Soc. Chim. Biol., Paris*, **47**, 99.
Michel, R. (1966). *In* "Endocrinologia Experimentalis: Estimation of Iodocompounds in Biological Material" (V. Stolc, ed.), p. 139. Publishing House of the Slovak Academy of Sciences, Bratislava.
Michel, R., Pitt-Rivers, R., Roche, J. and Varrone, S. (1962). *Biochim. biophys. Acta*, **57**, 335.
Mincey, E. K., Thorson, S. C. and Brown, J. L. (1971). *Clin. Biochem.* **4**, 216.
Mitchell, A. H. (1976). *Clin. Chem.* **22**, 1912.
Mitchell, M. L., Bradford, A. H. and Collins, S. (1964). *J. clin. Endocr. Metab.* **24**, 867.
Mitchell, M. L., Harden, A. B. and O'Rourke, M. E. (1960). *J. clin. Endocr. Metab.* **20**, 1474.
Mitchell, M. L. and O'Rourke, M. E. (1958). *J. clin. Endocr. Metab.* **18**, 1437.
Mitsuma, T., Colucci, J., Shenkman, L. and Hollander, C. S. (1972). *Biochem. biophys. Res. Commun.* **46**, 2107.
Mitsuma, T., Gershengorn, M. Colucci, J. and Hollander, C. S. (1971). *J. clin. Endocr.* **33**, 364.
Miyamoto, S. and Kobayashi, T. (1961). *J. Biochem., Tokyo*, **49**, 548.
Money, W. L. (1966). *In* "Endocrinologia Experimentalis: Estimation of Iodocompounds in Biological Material" (V. Stolc, ed.), p. 265. Publishing House of the Slovak Academy of Sciences, Bratislava.
Monaco, F. and Robbins, J. (1973). *J. biol. Chem.* **248**, 2328.
Morreale de Escobar, G., Escobar del Rey, F. (1961). *J. Physiol.* **159**, 15.
Morreale de Escobar, G., Escobar del Rey, F. and Rodriguez, P. L. (1962). *J. biol. Chem.* **237**, 2041.
Morrison, M. and Schonbaum, G. R. (1976). *Ann. Rev. Biochem.* **45**, 861.
Moshang, T., Parks, J. S., Baker, L., Vaidya, V., Utiger, R. D., Bongiovanni, A. M. and Snyder, P. J. (1975). *J. clin. Endocr. Metab.* **40**, 470.
Mougey, E. H. and Mason, J. W. (1963). *Analyt. Biochem.* **6**, 223.
Montoya, E., Seibel, M. J. and Wilber, J. F. (1975). *Endocrinology*, **96**, 1413.
Mulaisho, C. and Utiger, R. D. (1977). *Acta endocr., Copenh.* **85**, 314.
Murphy, B. E. P. (1964). *Nature, Lond.* **201**, 679.
Murphy, B. E. P. (1965). *J. Lab. clin. Med.* **66**, 161.

Murphy, B. E. P. and Pattee, C. J. (1964). *J. clin. Endocr. Metab.* **24**, 187.

Murphy, B. E. P., Pattee, C. J. and Gold, A. (1966). *J. clin. Endocr. Metab.* **26**, 247.

Musa, B. U., Seal, U. S. and Doe, R. P. (1967). *J. clin. Endocr. Metab.* **27**, 768.

Myai, K., Itoh, K. F., Abe, H. and Kumahara, Y. (1968). *Clin. chim. Acta*, **22**, 341.

Myant, N. B. and Osorio, C. (1960). *J. Physiol.* **152**, 391.

Myant, N. B. and Osorio, C. (1961). *J. Physiol.* **157**, 527.

Nadler, N. J., Sarkor, S. J. and Lebland, C. P. (1962), *Endocrinology*, **71**, 120.

Nadler, N. J., Young, B. A., Leblond, C. P. and Mitmaker, B. (1964). *Endocrinology*, **74**, 333.

Nagataki, S., Mizuno, M., Sakmoto, S., Irie, M., Shizume, K., Nakao, K., Galton, V. A., Arky, R. A. and Ingbar, S. H. (1977). *J. clin. Endocr. Metab.* **44**, 254.

Nakajima, H., Kuramochi, M., Horiguchi, T. and Kubo, S. (1966). *J. clin. Endocr. Metab.* **26**, 99.

Nakamura, Y., Chopra, I. J. and Solomon, D. H. (1978). *J. clin. Endocr. Metab.* **46**, 91.

Nauman, J. A., Nauman, A. and Werner, S. C. (1967). *J. clin. Invest.* **46**, 1346.

Nava, M. and De Groot, L. J. (1962). *New Engl. J. Med.* **266**, 1307.

Navab, M., Mallia, A. K., Kanda, Y. and Goodman, D. S. (1977a). *J. biol. Chem.* **252**, 5100.

Navab, M., Smith, J. E. and Goodman, D. S. (1977b). *J. biol. Chem.* **252**, 5107.

Nelson, J. C., Weiss, R. M., Lewis, J. E., Wilcox, R. B. and Palmer, F. J. (1974). *J. clin. Invest.* **53**, 416.

Nelson, J. C., Weiss, R. M., Palmer, F. J., Lewis, J. F. and Wilcox, R. B. (1976). *J. clin. Endocr. Metab.* **41**, 1118.

Neuhaus, K., Baumann, G., Walser, A. and Tholen, H. (1975). *J. clin. Endocr. Metab.* **41**, 395.

Nicoloff, J. T. (1976). *J. clin. Invest.* **49**, 1912.

Nicoloff, J. T., Dowling, J. T. and Patton, D. D. (1964). *J. clin. Endocr. Metab.* **24**, 294.

Nicoloff, J. T., Fisher, D. A. and Appleman, M. D. (1970). *J. clin. Invest.* **49**, 1922.

Nielsen, H. A., Buus, O. and Weeke, B. (1972). *Clin. chim. Acta*, **36**, 133.

Nihei, N. N., Gershengorn, M. C., Mitsuma, T., Stringham, L. R., Cordy, A., Kushmi, B. and Hollander, C. S. (1971). *Analyt. Biochem.* **43**, 433.

Nikolai, T. F. and Seal, U. S. (1966a). *J. clin. Endocr. Metab.* **26**, 835.

Nikolai, T. K. and Seal, U. S. (1966b). *J. clin. Endocr. Metab.* **27**, 1515.

Nilsson, S. F. and Peterson, P. A. (1971). *J. biol. Chem.* **246**, 6098.

Nomura, S., Pittman, C. S., Chambers, J. B., Buck, M. W. and Shimizu, T. (1975). *J. clin. Invest.* **56**, 643.

Nusynovitz, M. L. and Benedetto, A. R. (1975). *J. nucl. Med.* **16**, 1076.

Oddie, T. H. and Fisher, D. A. (1967). *J. clin. Endocr. Metab.* **27**, 89.

Oddie, T. H., Melby, J. C. and Scroggs, J. E. (1962). *J. clin. Endocr. Metab.* **22**, 1138.

Oddie, T. H., Bernard, B., Presley, M., Klein, A. H. and Fisher, D. A. (1978). *J. clin. Endocr. Metab.* **47**, 61.

Odell, W. D., Bates, R. W., Rivlin, R. S., Lipsett, M. B. and Hertz, R. (1963). *J. clin. Endocr. Metab.* **23**, 658.

Ogawara, H. and Cahnmann, H. J. (1972). *Biochim. biophys. Acta*, **257**, 328.

Ogawara, H., Bilstad, J. M. and Cahnmann, H. J. (1972). *Biochim. biophys. Acta*, **257**, 339.

Oppenheimer, J. H., Bernstein, G. and Hasen, J. (1967). *J. clin. Invest.* **46**, 762.

Oppenheimer, J. H., Martinez, M. and Bernstein, G. (1966). *J. Lab. clin. Med.* **67**, 500.

Oppenheimer, J. H., Squef, R., Surks, M. I. and Hauer, H. (1963). *J. clin. Invest.* **42**, 1769.

Oppenheimer, J. H. and Surks, M. I. (1964). *J. clin. Endocr. Metab.* **24**, 785.

Oppenheimer, J. H. and Surks, M. I. (1965). *Science*, **149**, 748.

Oppenheimer, J. H. and Surks, M. I. (1974). *In* "Handbook of Physiology, Section 7: Endocrinology III", Vol. 3, p. 197. Am. Physiol. Soc. Washington, DC.

Oppenheimer, J. H., Surks, M. I., Smith, J. C. and Squef, R. (1965). *J. biol. Chem.* **240**, 173.

Oppenheimer, J. H. and Werner, S. C. (1966). *J. clin. Endocr. Metab.* **26**, 715.

Osathanondh, R., Tulchinsky, D. and Chopra, I. J. (1976). *J. clin. Endocr. Metab.* **42**, 98.

Osorio, C., Jackson, D. J., Gartside, J. M., and Goolden, J. M. (1961). *Clin. Sci.* **21**, 355.

Otten, J., Jonckheer, M. and Dumont, J. E. (1971). *J. clin. Endocr. Metab.* **32**, 18.

Owen, C. A. and McConahey, W. H. (1956). *J. clin. Endocr. Metab.* **16**, 1570.

Owen, C. A. and Power, M. H. (1953). *J. biol. Chem.* **200**, 111.

Pages, R. A., Robbins, J. and Edelhoch, H. (1973). *Biochemistry*, **12**, 2773.

Parker, R. H. and Beierwaltes, W. H. (1962). *J. clin. Endocr. Metab.* **22**, 19.

Parslow, M. E., Hoddie, T. and Fisher, D. A. (1977). *Clin. Chem.* **23**, 490.

Passen, S. and von Saleski, J. (1969). *J. clin. Pathol.* **51**, 166.

Pataki, G. (1969). "Techniques of Thin-Layer Chromatography", p. 94. 2nd edition. Humphrey, Ann Arbor, MI.

Patel, Y. C. and Burger, H. G. (1973). *J. clin. Endocr. Metab.* **36**, 187.

Patel, Y. C., Pharoah, P. O. D., Hornabrook, R. W. and Hetzel, B. S. (1973). *J. clin. Endocr. Metab.* **37**, 783.

Patton, J. A., Hollifield, J. W., Brill, A. B., Lee, G. S. and Patton, D. D. (1976). *J. nucl. Med.* **17**, 17.

Pedersen, K. O. (1974a). *Sc. J. clin. Lab. Invest.* **34**, 241.

Pedersen, K. O. (1974b). *Sc. J. clin. Lab. Invest.* **34**, 247.

Pedersen, O. L. (1974c). *Ugeskr. Laeg.* **136**, 1154.

Pensky, J. and Marshall, J. S. (1969). *Archs biochem. Biophys.* **135**, 304.

Pennisi, F., Romelli, P. B. and Vancheri, L. (1979). *In* "International Symposium on Free Thyroid Hormones". Exerpta Medica, Amsterdam.

Peters, T. (1975). *In* "The Plasma Proteins" (F. W. Putnam, ed.), p. 133. Academic Press, New York and London.

Petersen, B. A., Hanson, R. N., Giese, R. N. and Karger, B. L. (1976). *J. Chromatogr.* **126**, 503.

Petersen, B. A., Geise, R. W., Larsen, P. R. and Karger, B. L. (1977). *Clin. Chem.* **23**, 1389.

Peterson, P. A. (1971). *J. biol. Chem.* **246**, 34.

Peterson, P. A. and Rask, L. (1971). *J. biol. Chem.* **246**, 7544.

Peyrin, J. O. and Berger, M. (1965). *Rev. fr. Etud. clin. Biol.* **10**, 330.

Pharoah, P. O. D., Lawton, N. F., Ellis, S. M., Williams, E. S. and Ekins, R. P. (1973). *Clin. Endocr.* **2**, 193.

Pierce, J. G., Rawitch, A. B., Brown, D. M. and Stanley, P. G. (1965). *Biochim. biophys. Acta*, **111**, 247.

Pileggi, V. J. and Farber, P. (1964). *Clin. chem. Acta*, **9**, 93.

Pileggi, V. J., Lee, N. D., Golub, O. J. and Henry, R. J. (1961). *J. clin. Endocr. Metab.* **21**, 1272.

Pileggi, V. J., Segal, H. A. and Golub, O. J. (1964). *J. clin. Endocr. Metab.* **24**, 273.

Pinchera, A., MacGillivray, M. H., Crawford, J. D. and Freeman, A. G. (1965). *New. Engl. J. Med.* **273**, 83.

Pind, K. (1957). *Acta endocr., Copenh.* **26**, 263.

Pittman, C. S., Chambers, J. B. and Read, V. H. (1971). *J. clin. Invest.* **50**, 1187.

Pittman, C. S., Read, V. H. and Chambers Jr., J. B. (1970). *J. clin. Invest.* **49**, 373.

Pitt-Rivers, R. (1976). *Biochem. J.* **157**, 767.

Pitt-Rivers, R. and Rall, J. E. (1961). *Endocrinology*, **68**, 309.

Pitt-Rivers, R. and Sacks, B. I. (1962). *Biochem. J.* **82**, 111.

Pitt-Rivers, R. and Schwartz, H. L. (1969). *In* "Chromatographic and Electrophoretic Techniques" (J. Smith, ed.), p. 224. Heinemann Medical Books, London.

Pitt-Rivers, R. and Tata, J. R. (1959). "The Thyroid Hormones", p. 1378. Pergamon Press, London.

Plaskett, L. G. (1964). *Chromatogr. Rev.* **6**, 91.

Pollard, A. C., Garnett, E. S. and Webber, C. (1965). *Clin. Chem.* **11**, 959.

Postmes, T. J. L. J. (1964). *Clin. chim. Acta*, **10**, 581.

Premachandra, B. N. and Blumenthal, H. T. (1967). *J. clin. Endocr. Metab.* **27**, 931.

Prince, H. P. and Ramsden, D. B. (1977). *Clin. Endocr.* **7**, 307.

Purdy, R. H., Woeber, K. A., Holloway, M. T. and Ingbar, S. H. (1965). *Biochemistry*, **4**, 1888.

Rabinovitch, B. (1959). *J. Am. chem. Soc.* **81**, 1883.

Radichevich, I. and Volpert, E. (1966). *In* "Endocrinologia Experimentalis: Estimation of Iodocompounds in Biological Material" (V. Stolc, ed.), p. 105. Slovak Academy of Science, Bratislava.

Rall, J. E. and Conard, R. A. (1966). *Am. J. Med.* **40**, 883.

Rall, J. E., Power, M. H. and Albert, A. (1950). *Proc. Soc. exp. Biol. Med.* **74**, 460.

Rall, J. E., Robbins, J. and Edelhoch, H. (1960). *Ann. N.Y. Acad. Sci.* **86**, 373.

Rall, J. E., Robbins, J. and Lewallen, C. G. (1964). *In* "The Hormones" (G. Pincus, K. V. Thimann and E. B. Astwood, eds), p. 159. Academic Press, New York and London.

Rall, J. E., Sterling, K., Gharib, H. and Mayberry, W. E. (1972). *In* "The Thyroid and Biogenic Amines" (J. E. Rall and I. J. Kopin, eds), p. 204. North-Holland, Amsterdam. (Vol. 1 of "Methods in Investigative and Diagnostic Endocrinology", S. A. Berson, ed.)

Ramírez, G., Jubiz, W., Gutch, C. F., Bloomer, H. A., Siegler, R. and Kloff, W. J. (1973). *Ann. int. Med.* **79**, 500.

Rask, L. and Peterson, P. A. (1976). *J. biol. Chem.* **251**, 6360.

Rastogi, G. K., Malhotra, M. S., Srivastava, M. C., Sawhney, R. C., Dua, G. L., Sridharan, K., Hoon, R. S. and Singh, I. (1977). *J. clin. Endocr. Metab.* **44**, 447.

Rastogi, G. K., Sawney, R. C. and Talwar, K. K. (1976). *Horm. Metab. Res.* **8**, 409.

Rawitch, A. B. and Brown, D. M. (1973). *Biochim. biophys. Acta*, **295**, 225.

Raz, A. and Goodman, D. S. (1969). *J. biol. Chem.* **244**, 3230.

Raz, A., Shiratori, T. and Goodman, D. S. (1970). *J. biol Chem.* **245**, 1903.

Refetoff, S., Fang, V. S., Marshall, J. S. and Robin, N. I. (1976). *J. clin. Invest.* **57**, 485.

Refetoff, S., Hagen, S. R. and Selenkow, H. A. (1972a). *J. nucl. Med.* **13**, 2.

Refetoff, S., Robin, N. I. and Alper, C. A. (1972b). *J. clin. Invest.* **51**, 848.

Refetoff, S., Robin, N. I. and Fang, V. S. (1970). *Endocrinology*, **86**, 793.

Reilly, W. A., Searle, G. L. and Scott, K. C. (1961). *Metabolism*, **10**, 869.

Reinwein, D. (1964). *Acta endocr., Copenh.* **47** (Suppl.), 94.

Reinwein, D. and Rall, J. E. (1966). *J. biol. Chem.* **241**, 1636.

Reinwein, D., Rall, J. E. and Durrer, H. A. (1968). *Endocrinology*, **83**, 1023.

Rhodes, B. A. and Wagner, H. N. (1966). *Nature, Lond.* **210**, 647.

Riggs, D. S., Lavietes, P. H. and Man, E. B. (1942). *J. biol. Chem.* **143**, 363.

Robbins, J. (1954). *J. biol. Chem.* **208**, 377.

Robbins, J. (1956). *Archs biochem. Biophys.* **63**, 461.

Robbins, J. (1963). *In* "Evaluation of Thyroid and Parathyroid Functions" (F. W. Sunderman and F. W. Sunderman, Jr., eds), pp. 90 and 95. Lippincott, PA.

Robbins, J. (1966). *In* "International Colloquium Tumor Thyroid Gland, Marseilles, 1964", p. 250. Karger, Basel and New York.

Robbins, J. (1975). *In* "Thyroid Hormone Metabolism" (W. A. Harland and J. S. Orr, eds), p. 1. Academic Press, London and New York.

Robbins, J. (1976). *In* "Trace Components of Plasma: Isolation and Clinical Significance" (G. A. Jamieson and T. J. Greenwalt, eds), p. 331. Alan R. Liss, New York.

Robbins, J., Cheng, S. Y., Gershengorn, M., Glinoer, D., Cahnmann, H. J. and Edelhoch, H. (1978a). *Rec. Prog. Horm. Res.* **34**, 517.

Robbins, J. and Nelson, J. (1958). *J. clin. Invest.* **37**, 153.

Robbins, J., Petermann, M. L. and Rall, J. E. (1954). *J. biol. Chem.* **208**, 387.

Robbins, J. and Rall, J. E. (1952). *Proc. Soc. exp. Biol. Med.* **81**, 530.

Robbins, J. and Rall, J. E. (1955). *J. clin. Invest.* **34**, 1324.

Robbins, J. and Rall, J. E. (1957). *Rec. Prog. Horm. Res.* **13**, 161.

Robbins, J. and Rall, J. E. (1960). *Physiol. Rev.* **40**, 415.

Robbins, J. and Rall, J. E. (1966). *In* "Endocrinology Experimentalis: Estimation of Iodocompounds in Biological Material" (V. Stolc, ed.), p. 183. Slovak Academy of Science, Bratislava.

Robbins, J. and Rall, J. E. (1967). *In* "Hormones in Blood" (C. H. Gray and A. L. Bacharach, eds), Vol. 1, p. 383. Academic Press, London and New York.

Robbins, J., Rall, J. E., Becker, D. V. and Rawson, R. W. (1952). *J. clin. Endocr. Metab.* **12**, 856.

Robbins, J., Rall, J. E. and Gorden, P. (1978b). *In* "Diseases of Metabolism" (P. K. Bondy and L. E. Rosenberg, eds). W. B. Saunders, Philadelphia.

Robbins, J., Rall, J. E. and Petermann, M. L. (1957). *J. clin. Invest.* **36**, 1333.

Robbins, J., Rall, J. E. and Rawson (1955). *J. clin. Endocr. Metab.* **15**, 1315.

Robbins, J., Rall, J. E., Trunnell, J. B. and Rawson, R. W. (1951). *J. clin. Endocr. Metab.* **11**, 1106.

Robbins, J. and Weathers, B. (1966). *Cancer Res.* **26**, 492.

Robbins, J., Van Zyl, A. and Van der Walt (1966). *Endocrinology*, **78**, 1213.

Roberts, R. C. and Nikolai, T. F. (1969a). *Clin. Chem.* **15**, 367.

Roberts, R. C. and Nikolai, T. F. (1969b). *Clin. Chem*, **15**, 1132.

Robin, N. I., Hager, S. R., Collaco, F., Refetoff, S. and Selenkow, H. A. (1971). *Hormones*, **2**, 266.

Roche, J., Lissitzky, S. and Michel, R. (1952a). *C.r. hebd. Séanc. Acad. Sci., Paris,* **234**, 997.

Roche, J., Lissitzky, S. L. and Michel, R. (1952b). *C.r. hebd. Séanc. Acad. Sci., Paris,* **234**, 1228.

Roche, J., Lissitzky, S. and Michel, R. (1952c). *Biochim. biophys. Acta,* **8**, 339.

Roche, J. and Michel, R. (1951). *Adv. Prot. Chem.* **6**, 253.

Roche, J., Michel, R. and Lissitzky, S. (1964). *In* "Methods of Biochemical Analysis" (D. Glick, ed.), p. 143. Interscience, New York.

Roche, J., Michel, R. and Nunez, J. (1958). *Bull. Soc. Chim. Biol., Paris,* **40**, 361.

Roche, J., Michel, R. and Nunez, J. (1959). *Acta endocr., Copenh.* **32**, 142.

Roche, J., Michel, R. and Tata, J. (1954). *Biochim. biophys. Acta,* **15**, 500.

Roche, J., Michel, R., Wolf, W. and Nunez, J. (1956). *Biochim. biophys. Acta,* **19**, 308.

Roitt, I. M. and Torrigiani, G. (1967). *Endocrinology,* **81**, 421.

Rolland, M. and Lissitzky, S. (1970). *Biochim. biophys. Acta*, **214**, 282.
Rolland, M. and Lissitzky, S. (1976). *Biochim. biophys. Acta*, **427**, 696.
Rosenberg, I. N. (1951a). *J. clin. Invest.* **30**, 1.
Rosenberg, I. N. (1951b). *J. clin. Endocr. Metab.* **11**, 1063.
Rosenberg, I. N., Ahn, C. S. and Mitchell, M. L. (1962). *J. clin. Endocr. Metab.* **22**, 612.
Rossi, T., Hirvonen, T. and Toivanen, P. (1970). *Sc. J. clin. Lab. Invest.* **26**, 35.
Roth, J., Glick, S. M., Cuatrecasas, P. and Hollander, C. S. (1967). *Ann. int. Med.* **66**, 760.
Rubenstein, H. E., Butler, V. P. and Werner, S. C. (1973). *J. clin. Endocr. Metab.* **37**, 247.
Rudorff, K. H., Herrmann, J., Kroll, H. J. and Krüskemper, H. L. (1976). *J. clin. Chem. clin. Biochem.* **14**, 31.
Rupp, J. J., Chavarria, C. Paschkis, K. F. and Chablarian, G. (1959). *Ann. int. Med.* **51**, 359.
Sacks, B. I. (1964). *Nature, Lond.* **202**, 899.
Sakurada, T., Rudolph, M., Fang, S. L., Vagenakis, A. G., Braverman, L. E. and Ingbar, S. H. (1978). *J. clin. Endocr. Metab.* **46**, 916.
Sakurada, T., Saito, S., Inagaki, K., Tayama, S. and Torikai, T. (1967). *Tohoku J. exp. Med.* **93**, 339.
Salabe, G., Fontana, S. and Andreoli, M. (1972). *Hormones*, **3**, 1.
Salavatore, G. and Edelhoch, H. (1973). *In* "Hormonal Proteins and Peptides" (C. H. Li, ed.), p. 201. Academic Press, London and New York.
Salvatore, G., Vecchio, G., Salvatore, M., Cahnmann, H. J. and Robbins, J. (1965). *J. biol. Chem.* **240**, 2935.
Sanchez-Franco, F., Garcia, M. D., Cacicedo, L., Martin-Zurro, A. and Escobar Del Rey, F. (1973). *J. clin. Endocr. Metab.* **37**, 736.
Sandell, E. and Kolthoff, I. M. (1937). *Mikrochem. Acta*, **1**, 9.
Sarcione, E. J. and Aungst, C. W. (1962). *Clin. chim. Acta*, **7**, 297.
Sawin, C. T., Chopra, D., Albaro, J. and Azizi, F., (1978). *Ann. int. Med.* **88**, 474.
Schahrokh, B. K. (1954). *J. biol. Chem.* **154**, 517.
Schneider, A. B., Bornet, H. and Edelhoch, H. (1971). *J. biol. Chem.* **246**, 2835.
Schneider, A. B. and Edelhoch, H. (1971). *J. biol. Chem.* **246**, 6592.
Schneider, A. B., Favus, M. J., Stachura, M. D., Arnold, J. E., Yun Ryo, U., Pinsky, S., Colman, H., Arnold, H. J. and Frohman, L. A. (1977). *Ann. int. Med.* **86**, 29.
Schneider, A. B. and Pervos, R. (1978). *J. clin. Endocr. Metab.* **47**, 126.
Schneider, P. B. and Wolff, J. (1965). *Biochim. biophys. Acta*, **94**, 115.
Schorn, H. and Winkler, C. (1965). *J. Chromatogr.* **18**, 69.
Schultz, A. L. and Zieve, L. (1958). *J. clin. Endocr. Metab.* **18**, 629.
Schultze, H. E., Schonenberger, M. and Schwick, G. (1956). *Biochem. Z.* **328**, 267.
Schussler, G. C. (1971). *J. Pharm. exp. Ther.* **178**, 204.
Schussler, G. C. and Plager, J. E. (1967). *J. clin. Endocr. Metab.* **27**, 242.
Schwartz, H. L., Carter, A. C., Kydd, D. M. and Gordon, A. S. (1967). *Endocrinology* **80**, 65.
Schwartz, H. L., Kozyreff, V., Surks, M. I. and Oppenheimer, J. H. (1969). *Nature, Lond.* **221**, 1262.
Scott, K. G. and Reilly, W. A. (1954). *Metabolism*, **3**, 506.
Scott, K. G., Reavis, G. C., Saunders, W. W. and White, W. E. (1951). *Proc. Soc. exp. Biol. Med.* **76**, 592.
Segrest, J. P., Jackson, R. L., Andrews, E. P. and Marchesi, V. T. (1971). *Biochem. biophys. Res. Commun.* **44**, 390.

Seligson, H. and Seligson, D. (1972). *Clin. chim. Acta*, **38**, 199.

Shalet, S. M., Beardwell, C. G., Lamb, A. M. and Gowland, E. (1975). *Lancet*, **ii**, 1008.

Shane, S. R., Seal, U. S. and Jones, J. E. (1971). *J. clin. Endocr. Metab.* **32**, 587.

Shapiro, A. L., Vinuela, E. and Maizel, J. V. (1967). *Biochem. biophys. Res. Commun.* **28**, 815.

Shapiro, B. and Rubinowitz, J. L. (1962). *J. nucl. Med.* **3**, 417.

Sherer, M. G. and Siefring, B. N. (1956). *J. clin. Endocr. Metab.* **16**, 643.

Shiba, T. and Cahnmann, H. J. (1964). *J. org. Chem.* **29**, 1652.

Shimaoka, K. and Thompson, B. D. (1965). *Endocrinology*, **76**, 570.

Shulman, S., Mates, G. and Bronson, P. (1967). *Biochim. biophys. Acta*, **147**, 208.

Siersbaek-Nielsen, K. and Molholm-Hansen, J. (1971). *Acta endocr., Copenh.* **67**, 616.

Silverberg, D. S., Ulan, R. A., Fawcett, D. M., Dossetor, J. B., Grace, M. and Bettcher, K. (1973). *Can. med. Assoc. J.* **109**, 282.

Silverstein, J. N., Schwartz, H. L., Feldman, E. B., Kydd, D. M. and Carter, A. C. (1962). *J. clin. Endocr. Metab.* **22**, 1002.

Sinadinovic, J., Jovanovic, M., Kraincanic, M. and Djardjevic, D. J. (1973). *Acta endocr., Copenh.*, **73**, 43.

Sleeman, H. K. and Diggs, J. W. (1964). *Analyt. Biochem.* **8**, 532.

Smith, E. M., Mozley, J. M. and Wagner, H. W. (1964). *J. nucl. Med.* **5**, 828.

Smith, F. R. and Goodman, D. S. (1971). *J. clin. Invest.* **50**, 2426.

Smith, G. F. (1964). *In* "Cerate Oxidimetry", 2nd edition. G. Fredrick Smith Chemical Co., Columbus, Ohio.

Snyder, S. M., Cavalieri, R. R., Goldfine, I. D., Ingbar, S. H. and Jorgensen, E. C. (1976a). *J. biol. Chem.* **251**, 6489.

Snyder, S. M., Cavalieri, R. R. and Ingbar, S. H. (1976b). *J. nucl. Med.* **17**, 660.

Solomon, D. H., Benotti, J., DeGroot, L. J., Greer, M. A., Oppenheimer, J. H., Pileggi, V. J., Robbins, J., Selenkow, H. A., Sterling, K. and Volpe, R. (1976). *J. clin. Endocr. Metab.* **42**, 595.

Sorimachi, K. (1979). *Analyt. Biochem.* **93**, 31.

Sorimachi, K. and Robbins, J. (1977). *J. biol. Chem.* **252**, 4458.

Sorimachi, K. and Ui, N. (1975). *Analyt. Biochem.* **67**, 157.

Spaulding, S. W., Chopra, I. J., Sherwin, R. S. and Lyall, S. S. (1976). *J. clin. Endocr. Metab.* **42**, 197.

Spaulding, S. W. and Davis, P. J. (1971). *Biochim. biophys. Acta*, **229**, 279.

Spaulding, S. W. and Gregerman, R. I. (1972). *J. clin. Endocr. Metab.* **34**, 974.

Spiro, M. J. (1973). *J. biol. Chem.* **248**, 4446.

Spiro, M. J. (1977a). *Biochem. biophys. Res. Commun.* **77**, 874.

Spiro, M. J. (1977b). *J. biol. Chem.* **252**, 5424.

Spiro, R. G. (1965). *J. biol. Chem.* **240**, 1603.

Spitzy, H. and Muller, K. (1966). *In* "Endocrinologia Experimentalis: Estimation of Iodocompounds in Biological Materials" (V. Stolc, ed.), p. 23. Publishing House of the Slovak Academy of Sciences, Bratislava.

Stabenau, J. R. and Mirsky, H. (1970). *Acta genet. Med.* **19**, 127.

Stabenau, J. R. and Pollin, W. (1967). Personal communication.

Stabenau, J. R. and Pollin, W. (1968). *J. clin. Endocr.* **28**, 693.

Staeheli, V., Vallottan, M. B. and Burger, A. (1975). *J. clin. Endocr. Metab.* **41**, 669.

Stanbury, J. B. (1960). *Ann. N.Y. Acad. Sci.* **86**, 417.

Stanbury, J. B. (1969). "Endemic Goiter", pp. 7–10, Pan-American Health Organization, Publication No. 193.

Stanbury, J. B., Brownell, G. L., Riggs, D. S., Perinetti, H., Itoiz, J. and DelCastillo, E. B. (1954). "Endemic Goiter." Harvard University Press, Cambridge, MA.

Stanbury, J. B., Kassenaar, A. H., Meijer, J. W. A. and Terpstra, J. (1955). *J. clin. Endocr. Metab.* **15**, 1216.

Stanbury, J. B. and Morris, M. L. (1958). *J. biol. Chem.* **233**, 106.

Stein, R. B. and Price, L. (1972). *J. clin. Endocr. Metab.* **34**, 225.

Steiner, R. F., Roth, J. and Robbins, J. (1966). *J. biol. Chem.* **241**, 560.

Sterling, K. (1964). *J. clin. Invest.* **43**, 1721.

Sterling, K. (1970). *Rec. Prog. horm. Res.* **26**, 249.

Sterling, K. (1971). *Crit. Rev. clin. Lab. Sci.* **2**, 223.

Sterling, K., Bellabarba, D., Newman, E. S. and Brenner, M. A. (1969). *J. clin. Invest.* **48**, 1150.

Sterling, K. and Brenner, M. A. (1966). *J. clin. Invest.* **45**, 153.

Sterling, K., Brenner, M. A., Newman, E. S., Odell, W. D. and Bellabarba, D. (1971). *J. clin. Endocr. Metab.* **33**, 729.

Sterling, K. and Hegedus, A. (1962). *J. clin. Invest.* **41**, 1031.

Sterling, K., Rosen, P. and Tabachnik, M. (1962). *J. clin. Invest.* **41**, 1021.

Sterling, K., Saldanha, V. F., Brenner, M. A. and Milch, P. O. (1974). *Nature, Lond.* **250**, 661.

Sterling, K. and Tabachnik, M. (1961a). *Endocrinology*, **68**, 1073.

Sterling, K. and Tabachnik, M. (1961b). *J. clin. Endocr. Metab.* **21**, 456.

Stevenson, C., Silva, E. and Pineda, G. (1974). *J. clin. Endocr. Metab.* **38**, 390.

Stock, J. M., Surks, M. I. and Oppenheimer, J. H. (1974). *New Engl. J. Med.* **290**, 529.

Stolc, V. (1966). *In* "Endocrinologia Experimentalis: Estimation of Iodocompounds in Biological Materials" (V. Stolc, ed.), p. 53. Publishing House of the Slovak Academy of Sciences, Bratislava.

Stouffer, J. E. (1969). *J. Chromatogr. Sci.* **7**, 124.

Strickler, H. S., Link, S. S. and Grauer, R. C. (1974). *Clin. Chem.* **20**, 695.

Strickler, H. S., Saier, E. L., Kelvington, E., Kempic, J., Campbell, E. and Grauer, R. C. (1964). *J. clin. Endocr. Metab.* **24**, 15.

Sung, L. C. and Cavalieri, R. R. (1973). *J. clin. Endocr. Metab.* **36**, 215.

Surks, M. I. (1966). *J. appl. Physiol.* **21**, 1185.

Surks, M. I., Beckwitt, H. J. and Chidsey, C. A. (1967). *J. clin. Endocr. Metab.* **27**, 789.

Surks, M. I. and Oppenheimer, J. H. (1963). *Endocrinology*, **72**, 567.

Surks, M. I. and Oppenheimer, J. H. (1964). *J. clin. Endocr. Metab.* **24**, 794.

Surks, M. I. and Oppenheimer, J. H. (1969). *J. clin. Invest.* **48**, 685.

Surks, M. I., Weinbach, S. and Volpert, E. (1968). *Endocrinology*, **82**, 1156.

Sutherland, R. L. and Brandon, M. R. (1976). *Endocrinology*, **98**, 91.

Sutherland, R. L., Brandon, M. P. and Simpson-Morgan, M. W. (1975). *J. Endocr.* **66**, 319.

Sutherland, R. L. and Simpson-Morgan, M. W. (1975). *J. Endocr.* **65**, 319.

Suzuki, H., Higuchi, T., Sawa, K., Ohtaki, S. and Yoshihiko, H. (1965). *Acta endocr., Copenh.* **50**, 161.

Tabachnik, M. (1964). *J. biol. Chem.* **239**, 1242.

Tabachnik, M. (1967). *J. biol. Chem.* **242**, 1646.

Tabachnik, M. and Giorgio, N. A. (1964). *Archs biochem. Biophys.* **105**, 563.

Tabachnik, M., Hao, Y. L. and Korcek, L. (1971). *Endocrinology*, **89**, 606.

Takemura, Y., Herman, G. and Sterling, K. (1971). *J. clin. Endocr. Metab.* **32**, 222.

Tanabe, Y., Ishii, T. and Tamaki, Y. (1969). *Gen. Comp. Endocr.* **13**, 14.

Tanaka, S. and Starr, P. (1959). *J. clin. Endocr. Metab.* **19**, 84.

Tata, J. R. (1959). *Biochem. J.* **72**, 222.

Tata, J. R. (1961). *Clin. chim. Acta*, **6**, 819.

Tata, J. R., Rall, J. E. and Rawson, R. W. (1956). *J. clin. Endocr. Metab.* **16**, 1554.

Taurog, A. (1962). *Endocrinology*, **73**, 45.

Taurog, A. (1978). *In* "The Thyroid" (S. C. Werner and S. H. Ingbar, eds). p. 31 Harper and Row, Hagerstown, MD.

Taurog, A., Chaikoff, I. L. and Tong, W. (1950). *J. biol. Chem.* **184**, 99.

Taurog, A., Porter, J. C. and Thio, D. T. (1964). *Endocrinology*, **74**, 902.

Tauxe, W. N. and Yamaguchi, M. Y. (1961). *Am. J. clin. Path.* **36**, 1.

Thorson, S. C., Wilkins, G. E., Schaffrin, M., Morrison, R. T. and McIntosh, H. W. (1972). *J. Lab. clin. Med.* **80**, 145.

Tice, L. and Wollman, S. H. (1972). *Lab. Invest.* **26**, 63.

Tong, W., Taurog, A. and Chaikoff, I. L. (1952). *J. biol. Chem.* **195**, 407.

Torizuka, K., Flax, M. H. and Stanbury, J. B. (1964). *Endocrinology*, **74**, 746.

Torrigiani, G., Doniach, D. and Roitt, I. M. (1969). *J. clin. Endocr. Metab.* **29**, 305.

Toro-Goyco, E. and Matos, M. (1965). *J. clin. Endocr. Metab.* **25**, 916.

Toyoshima, S., Fukuda, M. and Osawa, T. (1973). *Biochem. biophys. Res. Commun.* **51**, 945.

Trevorrow, V. (1939). *J. biol. Chem.* **127**, 737.

Tritsch, G. L. and Tritsch, N. E. (1963). *J. biol. Chem.* **238**, 138.

Turner, C. W. and Premachandra, B. N. (1962). *In* "Methods in Hormone Research" (R. I. Dorfman, ed.), p. 385. Academic Press, New York and London.

Ui, N. (1971). *Biochim. biophys. Acta*, **229**, 567.

Ui, N. (1974). *In* "Handbook of Physiology, Vol. III Thyroid", p. 55. American Physiological Association, Washington, DC.

Uller, R. P. and Van Herle, A. J. (1978). *J. clin. Endocr. Metab.* **46**, 747.

Uller, R. P., Van Herle, A. J. and Chopra, I. J. (1973). *J. clin. Endocr. Metab.* **37**, 741.

Vagenakis, A. G., Burger, A., Portnay, G. I., Rudolph, M., O'Brian, J. T., Azizi, F., Arky, R. A., Nicod, P., Ingbar, S. H. and Braverman, L. E. (1975). *J. clin. Endocr. Metab.* **41**, 191.

Vagenakis, A. G., Hamilton, C., Maloof, F., Braverman, L. E. and Ingbar, S. H. (1972). *J. clin. Endocr. Metab.* **34**, 327.

Vagenakis, A. G., Portnay, G. I., O'Brian, J. T., Rudolph, M., Arky, R. A., Ingbar, S. H. and Braverman, L. E. (1977). *J. clin. Endocr. Metab.* **45**, 1305.

Vahlquist, A., Peterson, P. A. and Wibell, L. (1973). *Eur. J. clin. Invest.* **3**, 352.

Van der Walt, B. and Van Jaarsveld, P. P. (1972). *Archs biochem. Biophys.* **150**, 786.

Van der Walt, B., Kotze, B., Van Jaarsveld, P. and Edelhoch, H. (1978). *J. biol. Chem.* **253**, 1853.

Van Herle, A. J. (1977). *In* "Radiation Associated Thyroid Carcinoma" (L. J. De Groot, ed.), p. 329. Grune and Stratton, New York.

Van Herle, A. J. and Uller, R. P. (1975). *J. clin. Invest.* **56**, 272.

Van Herle, A. J., Uller, R. P., Matthews, N. L. and Brown, J. (1973). *J. clin. Invest.* **52**, 1320.

Van Herle, A. J., Chopra, I. J., Hershman, J. M. and Hornabrook, R. W. (1976). *J. clin. Endocr. Metab.* **43**, 512.

Van Jaarsveld, P. P., Branch, W. T., Robbins, J., Morgan, F. J., Kanda, Y. and Canfield, R. E. (1973a). *J. biol. Chem.* **248**, 7898.

Van Jaarsveld, P. P., Edelhoch, H., Goodman, D. S. and Robbins, J. (1973b). *J. biol. Chem.* **248**, 4698.

Van Middlesworth, L. (1956). *Endocrinology*, **58**, 235.

Vanotti, A. and Beraud, T. (1959). *J. clin. Endocr. Metab.* **19**, 466.

Van Sande, J., Grenier, G., Willema, C. and Dumont, J. E. (1975). *Endocrinology*, **96**, 781.

Van Zyl, A. and Edelhoch, H. (1967). *J. biol. Chem.* **242**, 2423.

Van Zyl, A., Schulz, K., Wilson, B. and Pansegrouw, D. (1965). *Endocrinology*, **76**, 353.

Vassart, G., Refetoff, S., Brocas, H., Dinsart, C. and Dumont, J. E. (1975). *Proc. natn. Acad. Sci. USA*, **72**, 3839.

Vilkki, P. (1958). *Scand. J. clin. Lab. Invest.* **10**, 272.

Visser, T. J., Van der Does-Tobe, I., Docter, R. and Hennemann, G. (1976). *Biochem. J.* **157**, 479.

Volpe, R., MacAllister, W. J. and Huber, N. (1958). *J. clin. Endocr. Metab.* **18**, 65.

Vought, R. L. and London, W. T. (1965). *Metabolism*, **14**, 699.

Vought, R. L., Brown, F. A. and Sibinovic, R. H. (1974). *J. clin. Endocr. Metab.* **38**, 861.

Wahner, H. W., Emslander, F. and Gorman, C. A. (1971). *Metabolism*, **33**, 93.

Walfish, P. G. (1975). *In* "Perinatal Thyroid Physiology and Disease" (D. A. Fisher and G. N. Burrows, eds), p. 239. Raven Press, New York.

Walfish, P. G., Britton, A., Volpe, R. and Ezrin, C. (1962). *J. clin. Endocr. Metab.* **22**, 178.

Wartofsky, L., Burman, K. D., Dimond, R. C., Noel, G. L., Frantz, A. G. and Earll, J. M. (1977). *J. clin. Endocr. Metab.* **44**, 85.

Wartofsky, L. and Ingbar, S. H. (1971). *J. clin. Endocr. Metab.* **33**, 488.

Watson, D. and Lees, S. (1973). *Ann. clin. Biochem.* **10**, 14.

Wayne, E. J., Koutras, D. A. and Alexander, W. D. (1964). "Clinical Aspects of Iodine Metabolism." F. A. Davis Co., Philadelphia.

Weeke, J. and Orskov, H. (1975). *Scand, J. clin. Lab. Invest.* **35**, 237.

Weinert, H., Masui, H., Radichevich, I. and Werner, S. C. (1967). *J. clin. Invest.* **46**, 1264.

Welby, M. L., O'Halloran, M. W. and Marshall, J. (1974). *Clin. Endocr.* **3**, 63.

Welshman, S. W., Bell, J. F. and McKee, G. (1966). *J. clin. Path.* **19**, 510.

Wenzel, K. W., Meinhold, H., Herpich, M., Adlkofer, F. and Schleusener, H. (1974). *Klin. Wochenschr.* **52**, 722.

Werner, S. C. and Block, R. J. (1959). *Nature, Lond.* **183**, 406.

Werner, S. C., Block, R. J., Mandl, R. H. and Kassenaar, A. A. H. (1957). *J. clin. Endocr. Metab.* **17**, 817.

West, C. D., Chavre, V. J. and Wolfe, M. (1965a). *J. clin. Endocr. Metab.* **25**, 1189.

West, C. D., Chavre, V. J. and Wolfe, M. (1966). *J. clin. Endocr. Metab.* **26**, 986.

West, C. D., Wayne, A. W. and Chavre, V. J. (1965b). *Analyt. Biochem.* **12**, 41.

Wetzel, B., Spicer, S. S. and Wollman, S. H. (1965). *J. cell Biol.* **25**, 593.

White, W. E. (1953). *J. Lab. clin. Med.* **41**, 516.

Whitehead, J. K. and Beale, D. (1959). *Clin. chim. Acta*, **4**, 710.

Wiersinga, W. M. and Touber, J. L. (1977). *J. clin. Endocr. Metab.* **45**, 293.

Wilkinson, J. H. and Bowden, C. H. (1960). *In* "Chromatography and Electrophoresis Techniques" (I. Smith, ed.), p. 166. Interscience, New York.

Williams, A. D., Freeman, D. E. and Florsheim, W. H. (1969). *J. Chromatogr.* **45**, 371.

Wilson, F., Rankel, S., Linke, E. G. and Henry, J. B. (1974). *Am. J. clin. Path.* **62**, 383.

Woeber, K. A. and Ingbar, S. H. (1968). *J. clin. Invest.* **47**, 1710.

Woeber, K. A., Sobel, R. J., Ingbar, S. H. and Sterling, K. (1970a). *J. clin. Invest.* **49**, 643.

Woeber, K. A., Hecker, E. and Ingbar, S. H. (1970b). *J. clin. Invest.* **49**, 650.

Woldring, M. G., Bakker, A. and Doorenbos, H. (1961). *Acta endocr., Copenh.* **37**, 607.

Wolff, J. (1964). *Physiol. Rev.* **44**, 45.

Wolff, J. (1969). *Am. J. Med.* **47**, 101.

Wolff, J. and Chaikoff, I. L. (1948). *Endocrinology*, **43**, 174.

Wolff, J., Standaert, M. E. and Rall, J. E. (1961). *J. clin. Invest.* **40**, 1373.

Wollman, S. H. (1969). *In* "Lysosomes in Biology and Pathology" (J. T. Dingle and H. B. Fell, eds), p. 483. North Holland, Amsterdam.

Woodbury, D. M. and Woodbury, J. W. (1963). *J. Physiol.* **169**, 553.

Wosilait, W. D. (1977). *Res. Commun. Chem. Path. Pharm.* **16**, 541.

Wu, S-Y, Chopra, I. J., Nakamura, Y., Solomon, D. H. and Bennet, L. R. (1976). *J. clin. Endocr. Metab.* **43**, 682.

Wynn, J., Fabrikant, I. and Deiss, W. P. (1959). *Archs biochem. Biophys.* **84**, 106.

Wynn, J., VanWyk, J. J., Deiss, W. P. and Graham, J. B. (1962). *J. clin. Endocr. Metab.* **22**, 415.

Yamada, T., Kajihara, A., Onaya, T., Kobayashi, I., Takamura, Y. and Schichijo, K. (1965). *Endocrinology,* **77**, 968.

Yamamoto, K., Onaya, T., Yamada, T. and Kotani, M. (1972). *Endocrinology,* **90**, 986.

Yeo, P. P. B., Lewis, M. and Evered, D. C. (1977). *Clin. Endocr.* **6**, 159.

Yousef, M. K. and Johnson, H. D. (1965). *Life Sci.* **4**, 1531.

Zak, B., Willard, H. H., Myers, G. B. and Boyle, A. J. (1952). *Analyt. Chem.* **24**, 1345.

Subject Index